Endoscopic Pituitary Surgery

Endocrine, Neuro-Ophthalmologic, and Surgical Management

Harvey Cushing

American Association of Neurological Surgeons

and the American Association of Neurosurgeons

Thieme

Endoscopic Pituitary Surgery

Endocrine, Neuro-Ophthalmologic, and Surgical Management

Theodore H. Schwartz, MD, FACS
Professor
Departments of Neurological Surgery,
Otolaryngology-Head and Neck Surgery,
and Neurology and Neuroscience
Weill Cornell Medical College
Attending Neurosurgeon
Department of Neurological Surgery
New York–Presbyterian Hospital
New York, New York

Vijay K. Anand, MD, FACS
Clinical Professor
Department of Otolaryngology-Head and Neck Surgery
Weill Cornell Medical College
New York–Presbyterian Hospital
New York, New York

Thieme
New York • Stuttgart

American Association of Neurosurgeons
Rolling Meadows, Illinois

Thieme Publishers, Inc.
333 Seventh Ave.
New York, NY 10001

American Association of Neurosurgeons (AANS)*
5550 Meadowbrook Drive
Rolling Meadows, Illinois 60008-3852

*The abbreviation AANS refers to both the American Association of Neurological Surgeons and the American Association of Neurosurgeons.

Executive Editor: Kay D. Conerly
Managing Editor: Lauren Henry
Editorial Director: Michael Wachinger
Production Editor: Print Matters, Inc.
International Production Director: Andreas Schabert
Vice President, International Marketing and Sales: Cornelia Schulze
Vice President, Finance and Accounts: Sarah Vanderbilt
President: Brian D. Scanlan
Compositor: Manila Typesetting Company
Printer: Leo Paper Group

Library of Congress Cataloging-in-Publication Data

Endoscopic pituitary surgery endocrine, neuro-ophthalmologic, and surgical management / [edited by] Theodore H. Schwartz, Vijay K. Anand.
p. ; cm.
Includes bibliographical references and index.
ISBN 978-1-60406-347-9 (alk. paper)
1. Pituitary gland–Endoscopic surgery. I. Schwartz, Theodore H. II. Anand, Vijay K., 1951-
[DNLM: 1. Pituitary Diseases–surgery. 2. Endoscopy–methods. 3. Pituitary Gland–surgery. WK 590]
RD599.5.P58E53 2010
617.4'40597--dc22
2010054493

Important note: Medical knowledge is ever-changing. As new research and clinical experience broaden our knowledge, changes in treatment and drug therapy may be required. The authors and editors of the material herein have consulted sources believed to be reliable in their efforts to provide information that is complete and in accord with the standards accepted at the time of publication. However, in view of the possibility of human error by the authors, editors, or publisher of the work herein or changes in medical knowledge, neither the authors, editors, or publisher, nor any other party who has been involved in the preparation of this work, warrants that the information contained herein is in every respect accurate or complete, and they are not responsible for any errors or omissions or for the results obtained from use of such information. Readers are encouraged to confirm the information contained herein with other sources. For example, readers are advised to check the product information sheet included in the package of each drug they plan to administer to be certain that the information contained in this publication is accurate and that changes have not been made in the recommended dose or in the contraindications for administration. This recommendation is of particular importance in connection with new or infrequently used drugs.
Some of the product names, patents, and registered designs referred to in this book are in fact registered trademarks or proprietary names even though specific reference to this fact is not always made in the text. Therefore, the appearance of a name without designation as proprietary is not to be construed as a representation by the publisher that it is in the public domain.

The material presented in this publication by the AANS is for educational purposes only. The material is not intended to represent the only, nor necessarily the best, method or procedure appropriate for the medical or socioeconomic situations discussed, but rather it is intended to present an approach, view, statement, or opinion of the faculty, which may be helpful to others who face similar situations.

Neither the content, the use of a specific product in conjunction therewith, nor the exhibition of any materials by any parties coincident with this publication, should be construed as indicating endorsement or approval of the views presented, the products used, or the materials exhibited by the AANS, or its Committees, Commissions, or Affiliates.

Printed in China
5 4 3 2 1

ISBN 978-1-60406-347-9

This book is dedicated to our patients, who have entrusted us with their health and without whom this work would not be possible. We would also like to dedicate this book to our wives, Nancy and Nanda, who have stood by our sides all along the way, providing us with unending support.

Contents

Continuing Medical Education Credit Information and Objectives

Objectives

Upon completion of this activity, participants should be able to:

Objective 1: Assess patients with a pituitary tumor to determine if they are a candidate for surgery or medical therapy.
Objective 2: Determine what the best surgical approach would be to remove pituitary tumors of varying shapes and sizes.
Objective 3: Discuss new minimally invasive endoscopic techniques for removing pituitary tumors.
Objective 4: Describe how to manage patients after pituitary surgery who may need medical care for their endocrinopathy or further adjuvant chemotherapy or radiation therapy.

Bibliographic References

Nyquist GG, Ananad VK, Singh A, Schwartz TH. Janus flap: bilateral nasoseptal flaps for anterior skull base reconstruction. Otolaryngol Head Neck Surg. 2010 Mar;142(3):327-31.

Schaberg MR, Anand VK, Schwartz TH, Cobb W. Microscopic versus endoscopic transnasal pituitary surgery. Curr Opin Otolaryngol Head Neck Surg. 2010 Feb;18(1):8-14.

Endoscopic endonasal transsphenoidal surgery for functional pituitary adenomas. Hofstetter CP, Shin BJ, Mubita L, Huang C, Anand VK, Boockvar JA, Schwartz TH. Neurosurg Focus. 2011 Apr;30(4):E10.

Endoscopic endonasal approach for pituitary adenoma: surgical complications in 301 patients. Gondim JA, Almeida JP, Albuquerque LA, Schops M, Gomes E, Ferraz T, Sobreira W, Kretzmann MT. Pituitary. 2011 Jun;14(2):174-83.

Accreditation and Designation

The American Association of Neurological Surgeons is accredited by the Accreditation Council for Continuing Medical Education to provide continuing medical education for physicians.

The AANS* designates this enduring material for a maximum of 15 *AMA PRA Category 1 credits*™.
Physicians should claim only the credits commensurate with the extent of their participation in the activity.

**The acronym AANS refers to both the American Association of Neurological Surgeons and the American Association of Neurosurgeons.*

Method of physician participation in the learning process for this text book: The Home Study Examination is online on the AANS website at: http://www.aans.org/education/books/endopitsurgery.asp

Estimated time to complete this activity varies by learner, and activity equaled up to 15 *AMA PRA Category 1 credits*™.

Release/Termination Dates

Original Release Date: October 14, 2011
CME Termination Date: October 14, 2014

Disclosure Information

The AANS controls the content and production of this CME activity and attempts to ensure the presentation of balanced, objective information. In accordance with the Standards for Commercial Support established by the Accreditation Council for Continuing Medical Education, authors, planning committee members, staff, and any others involved in planning the educational content, and the significant others of those mentioned must disclose any relationship they or their co-authors have with commercial interests which may be related to their content. The ACCME defines "relevant financial relationships" as financial relationships in any amount occurring within the past 12 months that create a conflict of interest.

Those who have disclosed a relationship* with commercial interests are listed below.

Name	Disclosure	Type of Relationship*
Paolo Cappabianca, MD	Karl Storz, Baxter BioSurgery and Covidien	Industry Grant Support
William T. Couldwell, MD, PhD	ABNS Board of Directors	Fiduciary Position
Felice Esposito, MD, PhD, FACS	Baxter BioSurgery and Covidien	Industry Grant Support
Paul A. Gardner, MD	Karl Storz, Stryker	Industry Grant Support
	KLS Martin, Covidien	Industry Grant Support
Y. Pierre Gobin, MD	Lazarus Effect, Inc.	Stock or Shareholder
Anthony Heaney, MD	Novartis Pharmaceuticals	Consultant Fee
Daniel F. Kelly, MD	Mizuho America	Royalties
David L. Kleinberg, MD	Novartis, Preclinical	Industry Grant Support
	Novartis, Clinical and Advisory Board	Industry Grant Support
	Chiasma Consulting	Consultant Fee
	Novo Nordisk Advisory Board	Speaker's Bureau
	Eli Lilly HypoCCs Board	Other financial support
Howard A. Riina, MD	New York Presbyterian	University Grant/Research Support
	Evisiom Medical Systems	Stock or Shareholder
	Neurovasx	Stock or Shareholder
Theodore H. Schwartz, MD, FACS	Medtronic, Neurologix	Stock or Shareholder
	Visionsense	Speaker's Bureau, Honorarium
Carl Snyderman, MD	Blue Belt Technology, Inc.	Consultant Fee
William Yong, MD	Stein-Oppernheimer Grant (UCLA)	University Grant

**Relationship refers to receipt of royalties, consultantship, funding by research grant, receiving honoraria for educational services elsewhere, or any other relationship to a commercial interest that provides sufficient reason for disclosure.*

Those who have reported they do not have any relationships with commercial interests:

Name:

Ammara Abbasi, BA, BS
Pietro Ameri, MD
Vijay K. Anand, MD, FACS
Beng Ti Ang, MD
John C. Ausiello, MD
Paul D. Brown, MD
Seth Brown, MD, FACS
Luigi M. Cavallo, MD, PhD
Jeroen Coppens, MD

Matteo G. De Notaris, MD
Marc J. Dinkin, MD
Joshua R. Dusick, MD
Isabella Esposito, MD
Rudolf Fahlbusch, MD
Nasrin Fatemi, MD
Juan Fernandez-Miranda, MD
Giorgio Frank, MD
Pamela U. Freda, MD
Jeffrey P. Greenfield, MD, PhD
Christoph P. Hofstetter, MD, PhD
John A. Jane Jr., MD
Jared Knopman, MD
David V. LaBorde, MD
Ilya Laufer, MD
Ehud Lavi, MD
Edward R. Laws Jr., MD, FACS
Lewis Z. Leng, MD
Richard L. Levy, MD
Mark E. Linskey, MD[†]
Christopher M. Loftus, MD, FACS[†]
Patricia Fogarty Mack, MD
Tannaz Moin, MD
Stephen J. Monteith, MD
Yaron Moshel, MD, PhD
Michael Nanaszko, MD
Manoel de Paiva Neto, MD
Andre Neubauer, MD
Gurston G. Nyquist, MD
Edward H. Oldfield, MD
Nelson M. Oyesiku, MD, PhD, FACS
Ernesto Pasquini, MD
Vincenzo Paterno, MD
Athos Patsalides, MD
C. Douglas Phillips, MD, FACR
Bruce E. Pollock, MD
Kalmon D. Post, MD
Prashant Raghavan, MD
Jonathan Roth, MD
Nathan C. Rowland, MD, PhD
Charles A. Sansur, MD, MHSc
Madeleine R. Schaberg, MD, MPH
Theresa Scognamiglio, MD
Dharambir S. Sethi, MD, FRCS
Jonathan H. Sherman, MD
Ameet Singh, MD
Brian J. Snyder, MD
Abtin Tabaee, MD
Martin H. Weiss, MD
Jacqueline M.S. Winterkorn, MD, PhD
Stefan Wolfsberger, MD
Gabriel Zada, MD

[†]Educational Content Planners.

Historical Perspective

The first resection of a pituitary adenoma was performed in 1889 by Sir Victor Horsley using the transcranial route. Techniques for chiasmal surgery were poorly developed at that time and accompanied by substantial morbidity, which led to the development of other approaches, notably the transphenoidal technique as first performed successfully by Schloffer in 1907. However, Harvey Cushing, the neurosurgical giant of the era, preferred the cranial approach, which no doubt was an important factor in slowing the adoption of transsphenoidal surgery. Cushing's preference probably was due to the lack of sophisticated radiological techniques, which made the transcranial approach attractive because it allowed the surgeon to see the pathological changes affecting the optic nerves and chiasm and to make appropriate adjustments during the course of the operation.

With the evolution of airstudies and more recently of computed tomography and magnetic resonance imaging, the diagnosis and local anatomy of a pituitary lesion can be very well pictured prior to any surgery. This made the simpler and less invasive transsphenoidal approach much more attractive, accounting for why it has been used in the surgical management of most pituitary adenomas during the last 40 years.

Now endoscopy has come on the scene and added dramatically to the surgical options. The nuances of this revolutionary technique form the basis of the present book.

Russel Patterson

Foreword

I am honored and pleased to write the foreword to this book edited by Dr. Schwartz and Dr. Anand, as I take pleasure in having initiated their collaboration nearly ten years ago. Their thoughtful team approach has led to innovative endoscopic, minimal-access techniques for surgery of the anterior skull base. In this text, they and other leaders in the field of pituitary surgery provide an excellent review of the history, diagnosis, medical management, and surgical approaches for the treatment of diseases of this gland.

This is an excellent text for the student as well as the experienced pituitary surgeon, providing a range of material from reviewing basic therapy to complex surgical approaches. The early chapters are organized to draw upon the rich history of our understanding of diseases and treatment of disorders of the pituitary gland. The later chapters build upon this knowledge base and take us into the recent endoscopic advances in the field, providing useful information for neurosurgeons and otolaryngologists of all experience levels.

Diagrams and surgical photos help the audience appreciate the nuances of endoscopic surgery. There is a steep learning curve in mastering endoscopic surgery, and this book will shorten that curve by facilitating the readers' three-dimensional understanding of this surgical corridor. Precise understanding of anatomy is the framework upon which surgeons develop their skill and judgment. The authors have helped us expand our knowledge in many critical areas.

Philip E. Stieg, PhD, MD
Professor and Chairman of Neurological Surgery
Weill Medical College of Cornell University
Neurosurgeon-in-Chief
New York–Presbyterian Hospital

Preface

For many centuries anatomists had thought the gland, formally known as the hypophysis cerebri, was somehow responsible for the excretion of brain wastes through the nasal cavities [. . .]. The gland was of no interest to surgeons because it could not be reached in living subjects. They only encountered it at autopsy.

—Michael Bliss, *Harvey Cushing: A Life in Surgery*

This book was created to form a bridge from the past to the present and future of pituitary surgery. The past ten years have witnessed a rapid growth in the use of endoscopes and minimal-access approaches in all aspects of surgical practice and, in particular, in neurosurgery and otolaryngology. Computer-guided navigation has rendered surgery more precise and less invasive. The impact of minimal-access endonasal endoscopic surgery in the treatment not only of pituitary lesions but also many other pathologies of the anterior skull base and sinuses has been profound. Yet, it is easy to fall prey to the illusion that rapid adoption of a new technology can make us better surgeons or, even less accurately, better doctors. It is imperative that we not forget the importance of experience and sound clinical judgment in the treatment of any disease entity.

Pituitary surgery has a time-honored historic tradition and it is not a coincidence that the gland fascinated Harvey Cushing, the father of modern neurosurgery. He wrote to his father in 1909, "I think of little else than the pituitary body nowadays." Indeed, the greatest contributions to pituitary surgery have come over the past 20 years by surgeons who never picked up an endoscope. The endoscope is a useful tool that allows us to see more clearly, and with a wider view, the anatomy of the gland and its pathology. However, the fundamental principles of pituitary surgery are not altered by the presence of this tool, and the wisdom of the master pituitary surgeons of the pre-endoscope era is not only extremely valuable but also essential to pass on. This book is meant as a tribute to them, and as a means of imparting their wisdom and sound clinical judgment that has developed over years of experience with pituitary disease and marrying their insights with the new technique of endoscopy.

The book is organized into two parts. The first (Chapters 1 to 8) is a comprehensive overview of the principles of pituitary surgery, which are valid regardless of the tools one uses for visualization. We hear from the masters and learn from their experience. A variety of perspectives on the subject are presented to impart a comprehensive view of the field. The second part of the book (Chapters 9 to 34) emphasizes the technical aspects of endoscopic pituitary surgery, and highlights many of the methodological nuances acquired by the new breed of endoscopic neurosurgeons and otolaryngologists. Within this section are also chapters on the technology itself that is moving this field forward into the realm of three-dimensional endoscopy and virtual reality. This section also emphasizes the team approach to surgery and the value of a close relationship between neurosurgery and otorhinolaryngology in the development and implementation of the endoscopic approaches and skull base reconstruction.

It is our hope that this textbook will serve as a guide not only for residents in training but also for practicing neurosurgeons and otolaryngologists who wish to make the transition to endoscopic pituitary surgery. Our experience with this tool has led us to the conclusion that the endoscope and the extended transsphenoidal approaches provide numerous advantages over the microscope and a speculum retractor, but only if one remains mindful of the knowledge gained by the giants on whose shoulders we stand.

Theodore H. Schwartz, MD, FACS
Vijay K. Anand, MD, FACS

Acknowledgments

We would like to acknowledge the fellows and residents in the Departments of Neurosurgery and Otolaryngology at Weill Cornell Medical College/New York–Presbyterian Hospital for their help taking care of our patients and assistance in co-authoring our manuscripts and chapters. We would also like to acknowledge the assistance of our editors at Thieme, Kay Conerly and Lauren Henry.

Contributors

Ammara Abbasi, BA, BS
Emory University
Atlanta, Georgia

Pietro Ameri, MD
Department of Medicine
Division of Endocrinology
New York University School of Medicine
New York, New York
Department of Endocrinological and Medical Sciences
University of Genova
Genova, Italy

Vijay K. Anand, MD, FACS
Clinical Professor
Department of Otolaryngology-Head and Neck Surgery
Weill Cornell Medical College
New York–Presbyterian Hospital
New York, New York

Beng Ti Ang, MBBS, FRCSEd (SN)
Associate Professor
Department of Neurosurgery
National Neuroscience Institute
Singapore, Malaysia

John C. Ausiello, MD
Department of Medicine
Columbia University
College of Physicians and Surgeons
New York, New York

Paul D. Brown, MD
Professor
Department of Radiation Oncology
MD Anderson Cancer Center
University of Texas
Houston, Texas

Seth Brown, MD, FACS
Clinical Assistant Professor
Department of Surgery
Division of Otolaryngology
University of Connecticut School of Medicine
Farmington, Connecticut

Paolo Cappabianca, MD
Professor
Department of Neurological Sciences
Division of Neurosurgery
Università degli Studi di Napoli Federico II
Naples, Italy

Luigi M. Cavallo, MD, PhD
Department of Neurological Sciences
Division of Neurosurgery
Università degli Studi di Napoli Federico II
Naples, Italy

Jeroen R. Coppens, MD
Department of Neurosurgery
University of Utah School of Medicine
Salt Lake City, Utah

William T. Couldwell, MD, PhD
Professor and Joseph J. Yager Chair
Department of Neurosurgery
University of Utah School of Medicine
Salt Lake City, Utah

Matteo G. De Notaris, MD
Associate Professor
Department of Human Anatomy and Embryology
University of Barcelona
Barcelona, Spain

Marc J. Dinkin, MD
Assistant Professor
Departments of Ophthalmology and Neurology and Neurosurgery
Weill Cornell Medical College
New York–Presbyterian Hospital
New York, New York

Joshua R. Dusick, MD
Department of Neurosurgery
David Geffen School of Medicine
University of California at Los Angeles
University of California at Los Angeles Pituitary Tumor and Neuroendocrine Program
Los Angeles, California

Felice Esposito, MD, PhD, FACS
Instructor of Neurosurgery
Department of Neurological Sciences
Division of Neurosurgery
Università degli Studi di Napoli Federico II
Naples, Italy

Isabella Esposito, MD
Department of Neurological Sciences
Division of Neurosurgery
Università degli Studi di Napoli Federico II
Napoli, Italy

Rudolf Fahlbusch, MD
Professor and Director
Center of Endocrine Neurosurgery
International Neuroscience Institute
Otto Von Gueriche University
Hannover, Germany

Nasrin Fatemi, MD
Brain Tumor Center
John Wayne Cancer Institute at Saint John's Health Center
Santa Monica, California

Juan Fernandez-Miranda, MD
Assistant Professor
Department of Neurological Surgery
University of Pittsburgh Medical Center
Pittsburgh, Pennsylvania

Patricia Fogarty Mack, MD
Associate Professor
Department of Anesthesiology
Weill Cornell Medical College
New York–Presbyterian Hospital
New York, New York

Giorgio Frank, MD
Center of Pituitary Tumor Surgery
Department of Neuroscience
Bellaria Hospital
Bologna, Italy

Pamela U. Freda, MD
Associate Professor
Department of Medicine
Columbia University
College of Physicians and Surgeons
New York, New York

Paul A. Gardner, MD
Assistant Professor
Department of Neurological Surgery
University of Pittsburgh Medical Center
Pittsburgh, Pennsylvania

Y. Pierre Gobin, MD
Professor
Director of Interventional Neuroradiology
Department of Radiology
Weill Cornell Medical College
New York–Presbyterian Hospital
New York, New York

Jeffrey P. Greenfield, MD, PhD
Assistant Professor
Department of Neurological Surgery
Weill Cornell Medical College
New York–Presbyterian Hospital
New York, New York

Anthony Heaney, MD
Associate Professor
Division of Endocrinology, Diabetes, and Hypertension
David Geffen School of Medicine
University of California at Los Angeles
Los Angeles, California

Christoph P. Hofstetter, MD, PhD
Department of Neurological Surgery
Weill Cornell Medical College
New York–Presbyterian Hospital
New York, New York

John A. Jane Jr., MD
Associate Professor
Department of Neurosurgery
University of Virginia
Charlottesville, Virginia

Daniel F. Kelly, MD
Director
Brain Tumor Center
John Wayne Cancer Institute at Saint John's Health Center
Santa Monica, California

David L. Kleinberg, MD
Professor
Neuro Endocrine Unit
Department of Medicine
New York University School of Medicine
New York, New York

Jared Knopman, MD
Department of Neurological Surgery
Weill Cornell Medical College
New York–Presbyterian Hospital
New York, New York

David V. LaBorde, MD
Department of Neurosurgery
Emory University
Atlanta, Georgia

Ilya Laufer, MD
Department of Neurological Surgery
Weill Cornell Medical College
New York–Presbyterian Hospital
New York, New York

Ehud Lavi, MD
Chief
Neuropathology Service
Professor
Department of Pathology and Laboratory Medicine
Weill Cornell Medical College
New York–Presbyterian Hospital
New York, New York

Edward R. Laws Jr., MD, FACS
Professor
Department of Neurosurgery
Brigham and Women's Hospital
Harvard University
Boston, Massachusetts

Lewis Z. Leng, MD
Department of Neurological Surgery
Weill Cornell Medical College
New York– Presbyterian Hospital
New York, New York

Richard L. Levy, MD
Assistant Professor
Director of Pediatric Ophthalmology and Strabismus
Department of Ophthalmology
Weill Cornell Medical College
New York–Presbyterian Hospital
New York, New York

Tannaz Moin, MD
Division of Endocrinology, Diabetes, and Hypertension
David Geffen School of Medicine
University of California at Los Angeles
Los Angeles, California

Stephen J. Monteith, MD
Department of Neurological Surgery
University of Virginia
Charlottesville, Virginia

Yaron Moshel, MD, PhD
Assistant Professor
Department of Neurosurgery
Division of Neuro-Oncology
Jefferson Medical College
Thomas Jefferson University
Philadelphia, Pennsylvania

Michael Nanaszko
Weill Cornell Medical College
New York, New York

André Neubauer, PhD
Industrial Materials Institute
National Research Council Canada
Boucherville, Quebec, Canada

Gurston G. Nyquist, MD
Assistant Clinical Professor
Department of Otolaryngology
Hofstra North Shore–LIJ School of Medicine
Hempstead, New York
Ear, Nose, and Throat Associates of New York
Queens, New York

Edward H. Oldfield, MD
Director
Neuro-endocrine
Professor of Neurosurgery and Internal Medicine
Department of Neurosurgery
University of Virginia School of Medicine
Charlottesville, Virginia

Nelson M. Oyesiku, MD, PhD, FACS
Vice Chair
Al Lerner Center in Neurosurgery
Professor of Endocrinology
Department of Neurosurgery
Emory University
Atlanta, Georgia

Manoel de Paiva Neto, MD
Brain Tumor Center
John Wayne Cancer Institute at Saint John's Health Center
Santa Monica, California

Ernesto Pasquini, MD
Center of Endoscopic ENT Surgery
ENT Department
Sant'Orsola-Malpighi Hospital
Bologna, Italy

Vincenzo Paternó, MD
Consulting Neurosurgeon
International Neuroscience Institute
Hannover, Germany

Athos Patsalides, MD
Assistant Professor of Radiology in Neurological Surgery
Department of Neurological Surgery
Weill Cornell Medical College
New York–Presbyterian Hospital
New York, New York

C. Douglas Phillips, MD, FACR
Professor
Director of Head and Neck Imaging
Department of Radiology
Weill Cornell Medical College
New York–Presbyterian Hospital
New York, New York

Bruce E. Pollock, MD
Professor of Neurologic Surgery and Radiation Oncology
Departments of Neurological Surgery and Radiation Oncology
Mayo Clinic College of Medicine
Rochester, Minnesota

Kalmon D. Post, MD
Chairman Emeritus
Department of Neurosurgery
Professor
Departments of Neurosurgery and Medicine
Mount Sinai School of Medicine
Mount Sinai Hospital
New York, New York

Prashant Raghavan, MD
Assistant Professor
Division of Neuroradiology
University of Virginia
Charlottesville, Virginia

Howard A. Riina, MD
Associate Professor of Neurological Surgery in Neurology
Department of Neurological Surgery
Weill Cornell Medical College
New York–Presbyterian Hospital
New York, New York

Jonathan Roth, MD
Department of Neurosurgery
Tel Aviv Sourasky Medical Center
Tel Aviv, Israel

Nathan C. Rowland, MD, PhD
Department of Neurological Surgery
University of California, San Francisco
San Francisco, California

Charles A. Sansur, MD, MHSc
Assistant Professor
Department of Neurosurgery
University of Maryland School of Medicine
Baltimore, Maryland

Madeleine R. Schaberg, MD, MPH
Assistant Professor
Department of Otolaryngology–Head and Neck Surgery
Jefferson Medical College
Thomas Jefferson University
Philadelphia, Pennsylvania

Theodore H. Schwartz, MD, FACS
Professor
Departments of Neurological Surgery, Otolaryngology-Head and Neck Surgery, and Neurology and Neuroscience
Weill Cornell Medical College
Attending Neurosurgeon
Department of Neurological Surgery
New York–Presbyterian Hospital
New York, New York

Theresa Scognamiglio, MD
Assistant Professor
Department of Anatomic Pathology and Clinical Pathology
Weill Cornell Medical College
Assistant Attending Pathologist
New York–Presbyterian Hospital
New York, New York

Dharambir S. Sethi, MD, FRCS
Department of Otolaryngology
Clinical Associate Professor
National University of Singapore
Senior Consultant
Department of Otolaryngology
Singapore General Hospital
Singapore, Malaysia

Jonathan H. Sherman, MD
Department of Neurosurgery
Memorial Sloan-Kettering Cancer Center
New York, New York

Ameet Singh, MD
Co-Director, Endoscopic Pituitary and Skull Base Surgery Program
Assistant Professor of Surgery
Division of Otolaryngology–Head and Neck Surgery
Assistant Professor of Neurosurgery
Department of Neurosurgery
George Washington University Medical Center
Washington DC

Brian J. Snyder, MD
Neurological Surgery, P.C.
Long Island, New York

Carl Snyderman, MD
Professor
Departments of Otolaryngology and Neurological Surgery
University of Pittsburgh School of Medicine
Co-Director
Center for Cranial Base Surgery
University of Pittsburgh Medical Center
Pittsburgh, Pennsylvania

Abtin Tabaee, MD
Assistant Professor
Albert Einstein College of Medicine
Director of Rhinology and Endoscopic Sinus Surgery
Department of Otolaryngology
Beth Israel Medical Center
New York, New York

Martin H. Weiss, MD
Professor and Martin H. Weiss Chair
Department of Neurosurgery
Keck School of Medicine
University of Southern California
Los Angeles, California

Jacqueline M. S. Winterkorn, MD, PhD
Clinical Professor
Departments of Ophthalmology and of Neurology and Neuroscience
Weill Cornell Medical College
New York–Presbyterian Hospital
New York, New York

Stefan Wolfsberger, MD
Department of Neurosurgery
Medical University Vienna
Vienna, Austria

William H. Yong, MD
Professor
Department of Pathology and Laboratory Medicine
Jonnsson Comprehensive Cancer Center
David Geffen School of Medicine
University of California at Los Angeles
Los Angeles, California

Gabriel Zada, MD
Clinical Instructor
Keck School of Medicine
University of Southern California Medical Center
Los Angeles, California

1 History of Pituitary Surgery

Edward R. Laws Jr.

The transsphenoidal approach is the result of an evolutionary process rather than a revolutionary one.[1] Extracranial approaches to the anterior skull base have evolved over the last hundred years. Many neurosurgical (and nonneurosurgical) pioneers have contributed to their development. The evolution of transsphenoidal surgery is a complex tale of innovative leaps in ideology coupled with periods of extensive surgical experimentation interspersed with a period of complete rejection of the technique.

Ancient Egyptians

The ancient Egyptians were one of the first groups to carefully study and document the anatomy of the human body and undoubtedly were the first to reach the brain through the transnasal route.[2] To avoid disfigurement of the face of the deceased, the brain was removed through the nose by means of special tools, which were introduced into the skull base through a sphenoethmoidal breach during the process of mummification.[3] Recently studied mummies provide clear evidence of their methods (**Fig. 1.1**).[4]

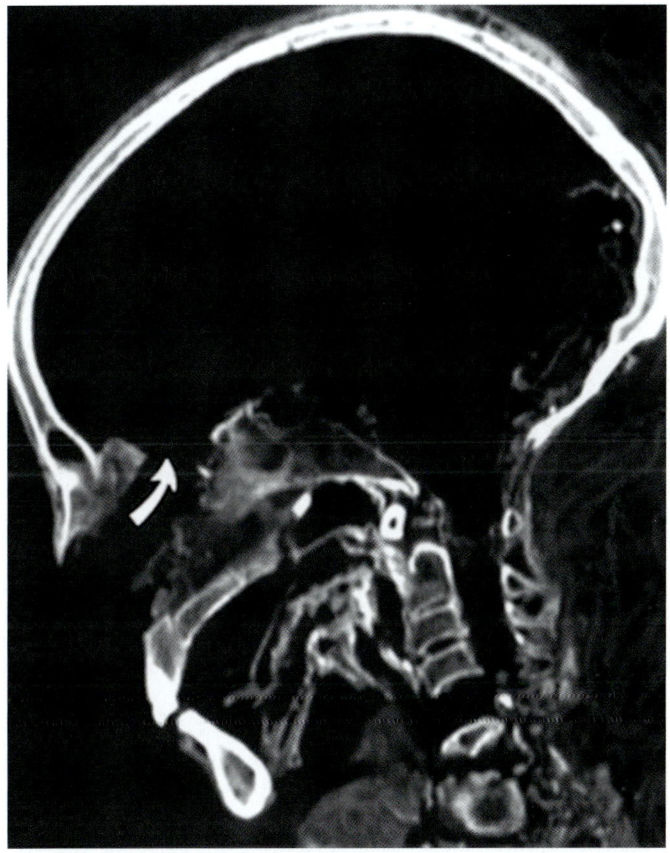

Fig. 1.1 Sagittal computed tomography (CT) scan of a mummy showing the transnasal passageway of brain removal (*arrow*). (From Hoffman H, Hudgins PA. Head and skull base features of nine Egyptian mummies: evaluation with high-resolution CT and reformation techniques. Am J Roentgenol 2002;178:1367–1376. Reprinted with permission.)

Early Neurosurgery

The transsphenoidal route remained unnoticed until 1894, when Davide Giordano, chief surgeon of the Hospital of Venice, performed an anatomical study that provided an approach to the sella turcica through an extracranial transfacial transsphenoidal exposure.[5] Based in part on these observations, the first successful transsphenoidal resection of a pituitary tumor was done by Hermann Schloffer of Vienna, Austria, in 1907 in a three-stage operation (**Fig. 1.2**).[6,7]

Before Schloffer, pituitary tumors were approached transcranially, using either the subfrontal (**Fig. 1.3**) or the subtemporal route. Sir Victor Horsley attempted the first craniotomy for a pituitary lesion. Although his first operation was unsuccessful, in 1906 he reported on 10 patients treated with craniotomy.[1,6,8] Caton and Paul had attempted to resect a pituitary tumor using the subtemporal approach of Horsley in a patient with acromegaly but were unsuccessful.[6,8] Fedor Krause of Berlin reported a successful transfrontal exposure of the optic chiasm in 1902. Kiliani developed an intradural bifrontal approach in cadavers in 1904, hoping that it would lead to improvement of the technique.[6] These approaches, however, had significant morbidity and mortality due to retraction of the frontal lobes and the lack of good antisepsis.

Theodor Kocher (Cushing's mentor) modified Schloffer's approach by submucosal removal of the septum, allowing better visualization. However, it was Oskar Hirsch, a rhinologist, who developed a completely endonasal transseptal transsphenoidal operation in 1910, based on his mentor Hajek's treatment for sphenoid sinusitis.[1,6–10] Harvey Cushing later improved the technique, using Kocher's submucosal resection of the septum and a nasal speculum (a modified pediatric vaginal speculum).

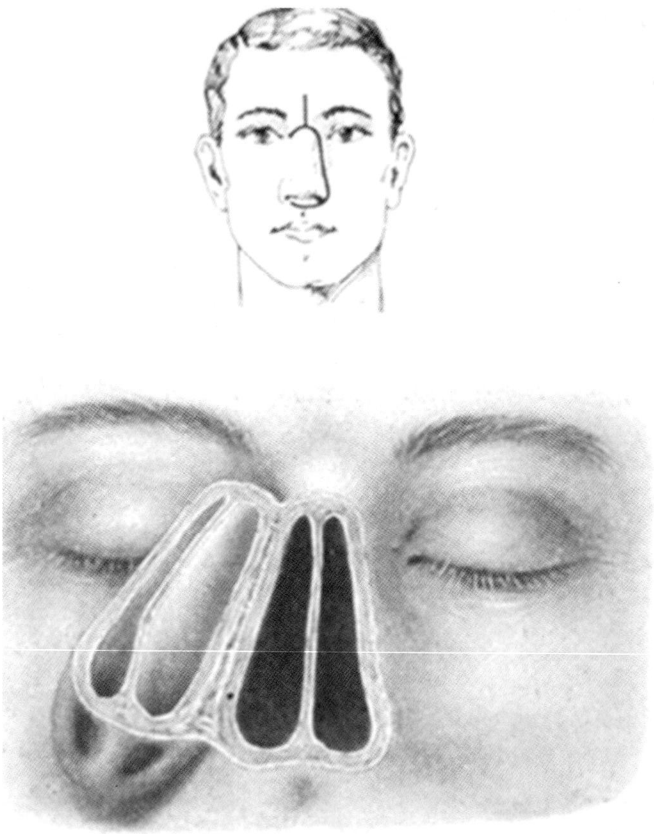

Fig. 1.2 Diagram demonstrating the lateral rhinotomy exposure of the septum and nasal turbinates of the nose just prior to exposure of the sphenoid sinus described by Schloffer.

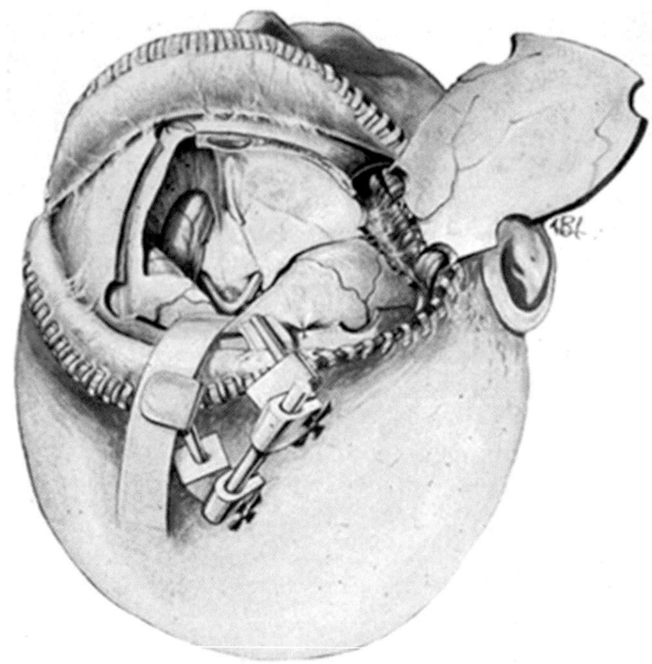

Fig. 1.3 Anatomical drawing of the subfrontal approach to the pituitary. This approach was popular both before and after the emergence of transsphenoidal operations.

At the same time, in the United States, Albert Halstead of Chicago modified the curvilinear incision through the nasolabial junction suggested by Allen Kanavel.[11–13] His sublabial gingival incision (**Fig. 1.4**) allowed more retraction of the cartilaginous septum compared with the endonasal approach, improved exposure, and provided better cosmetic results.[1,6,12,14] Other attempts at the development of sellar approaches include Ottokar Chiari's transethmoidal approach and Preysing's transpalatal approach.[6]

Driven by the discouraging results of his transcranial approaches, Harvey Cushing adopted the transsphenoidal approach,[13] initially using Schloffer's procedure. He performed his first transsphenoidal operation in 1909 for a patient with acromegaly.[6,15] By 1912, he had modified the procedure by combining Halstead's sublabial incision and Kocher's submucosal septal dissection,[6,13,16] resulting in the operation still performed by most neurosurgeons today (**Fig. 1.5**). From 1910 to 1925, Cushing operated on 231 pituitary tumors using the sublabial transsphenoidal approach, with a mortality rate of only 5.6%.[7]

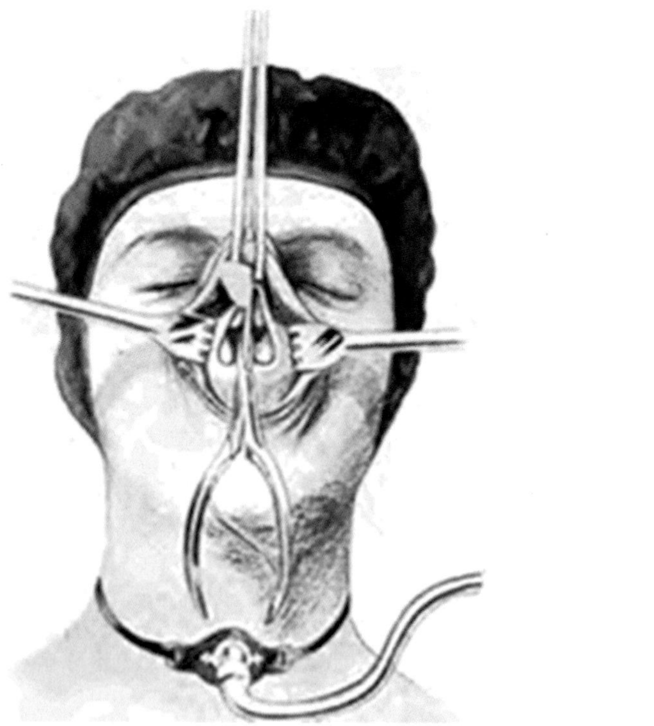

Fig. 1.4 Albert Halstead's sublabial approach. Note the use of a tracheostomy for the administration of anesthetics.

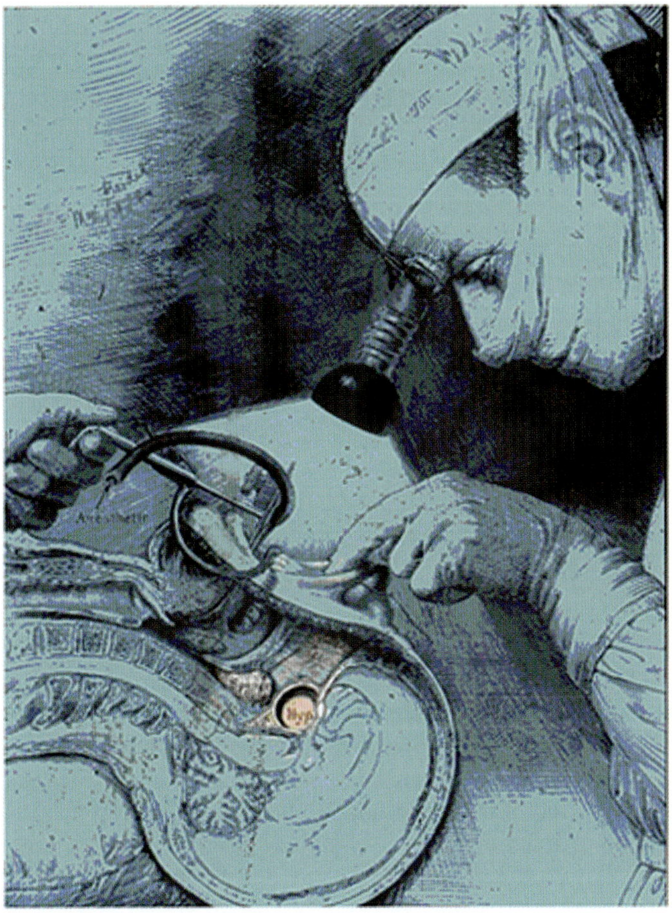

Fig. 1.5 Illustration depicting Harvey Cushing with his headlight, using a sublabial approach to the sella. Note the anesthetic tube in the special mouth gag designed by Cushing.

Abandonment of the Transsphenoidal Approach

Cushing's intense interest in intracranial surgery led him to pursue and develop transcranial approaches to the pituitary gland. As he developed expertise and confidence in these approaches, he reduced his mortality rate with the transcranial approach to 4.6%, essentially eliminating any significant difference in surgical mortality when compared with the transsphenoidal approach.[17] By the late 1920s, Cushing had treated many patients with suprasellar tumors, especially meningiomas and craniopharyngiomas, by a transfrontal approach, which enabled him to verify suprasellar tumors diagnostically and achieve a more extensive resection and decompression of the optic chiasm. The transcranial approach avoided the dreaded complications of meningitis and systemic infection, the most common causes of death associated with the transsphenoidal approach. By 1929, Cushing had virtually abandoned the transsphenoidal operation, performing pituitary surgery exclusively via the transfrontal route.[17,18] As might be expected, the majority of the neurosurgical community followed Cushing's lead.

Meanwhile, Norman Dott, who learned the transsphenoidal approach in 1923 from Cushing during a traveling fellowship at the Peter Bent Brigham Hospital in Boston, returned to Edinburgh, where he continued to advocate this procedure.[19] He designed a speculum with a lighted tip, which provided superior visualization during the operation.[1,7,10,18] This interim stage preserved the transsphenoidal approach from extinction.

Another key factor in the preservation of the transsphenoidal approach was the contribution of Hirsch and Hamlin. Oskar Hirsch immigrated to the United States after being expelled from Austria by the Nazis in 1938. He collaborated with Hannibal Hamlin, a neurosurgeon in the Boston community. Hirsch and Hamlin extolled the virtues of the transsphenoidal approach and reported excellent long-term results.[6,8] Despite their enthusiasm, transfrontal approaches remained the most popular methods throughout the 1950s and 1960s.

Revival of the Transsphenoidal Approach

Numerous innovations introduced in the 1950s played an important role in the resurgence of interest in transsphenoidal surgery. With the introduction of cortisone and antibiotic therapy, total hypophysectomy could be performed with significantly reduced mortality and better long-term success.[20]

The two persons credited for the revival of the transsphenoidal approach are Gerard Guiot and Jules Hardy. In 1956 Guiot visited Dott, observed his meticulous technique and outstanding surgical outcomes, and returned to Paris, where he reintroduced the transsphenoidal approach.[7] He further refined his technique and enhanced surgical accuracy by introducing intraoperative radiofluoroscopy to define the anatomy of the anterior skull base while maneuvering surgical instruments.[17] This allowed him to apply the transsphenoidal approach to craniopharyngiomas, clivus chordomas, and parasellar lesions, and thus he played a pivotal role in the resurrection of the transsphenoidal approach during the following two decades.[6,21,22]

The spread of the transsphenoidal approach across North America was initiated by Jules Hardy upon his return to Canada. As a trainee under Guiot in Paris, Hardy of Montreal continued the use of televised radiofluoroscopic control,[17] which gave him the opportunity to perform more extensive resections of large midline suprasellar tumors. He later adopted the routine use of preoperative angiography, polytomography of the sella, and intraoperative air encephalography.[6] In 1967, Hardy introduced the use of the operating microscope during this procedure and designed his own microsurgical instrumentation (**Fig. 1.6, 1.7, 1.8,** and **1.9**).[6,23] The microscope and microtechnique permitted safer and more effective resections of pituitary tumors and other sellar

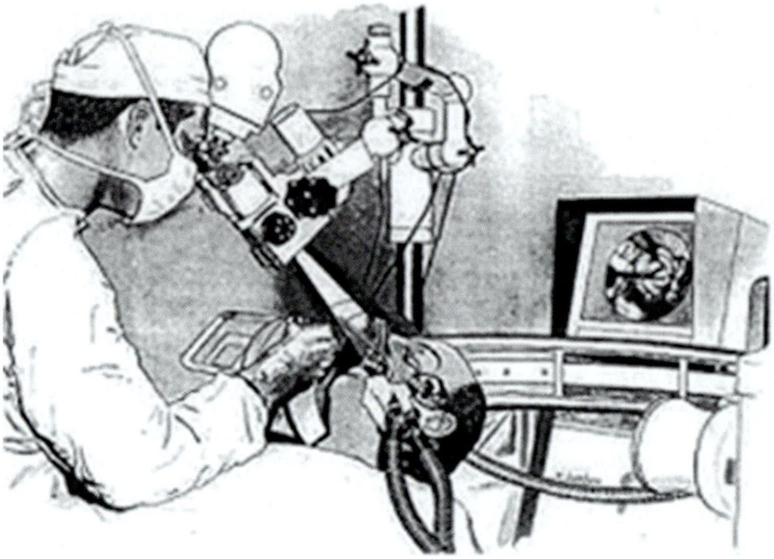

Fig. 1.6 Illustration depicting Hardy's use of the operating microscope and televised radiofluoroscopic control. (From Hardy J. Transsphenoidal hypophysectomy. J Neurosurg 1971;34:582–594. Reprinted with permission.)

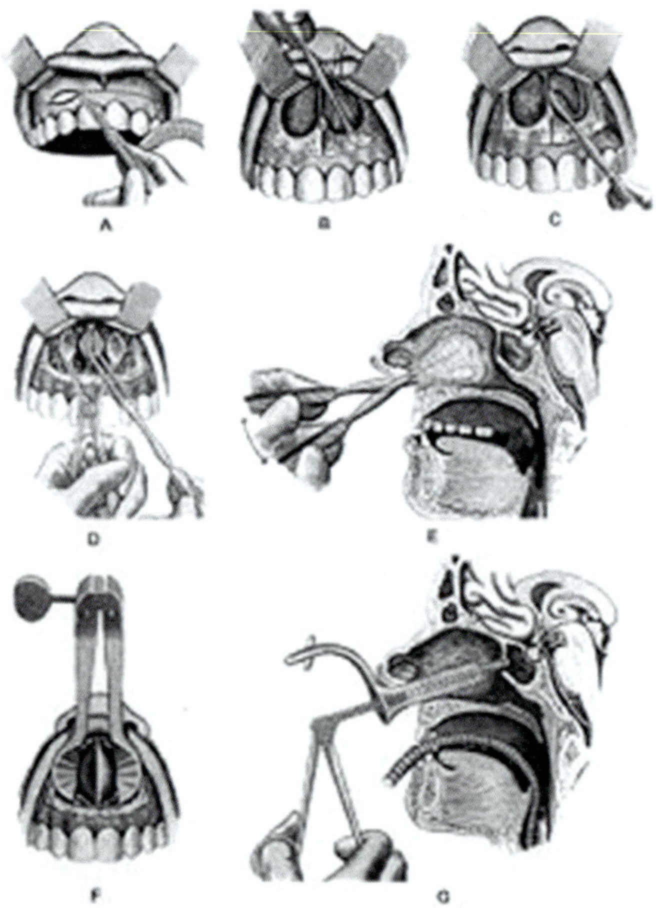

Fig. 1.7 Illustrations depicting Hardy's sublabial transseptal transsphenoidal approach. **(A)** Sublabial incision. **(B)** Elevation of nasal mucosa from the floor. **(C)** Submucosal dissection from the septum. **(D)** Resection of the cartilaginous septum with a swivel knife. **(E)** Sagittal view of the submucosal dissection. **(F)** Introduction of the self-retaining speculum that reveals the vomer, which resembles the keel of a ship. **(G)** Sagittal view of the speculum in position. (From Jho HD, et al. Endoscopic pituitary surgery: an early experience. Surg Neurol 1997;47:213–222. Reprinted with permission.)

and parasellar lesions, with no serious morbidity or mortality in the first 50 patients.[17,24] A year later, he introduced the concept of the microadenoma, a lesion that could cause endocrinologic abnormalities without producing obvious deformation of the bony sella.[25] He performed selective removal of microadenomas while preserving pituitary function. His landmark paper in 1971 described the use of the operating microscope for improved illumination and intraoperative fluoroscopy for improved localization of tumors and guidance of instruments.[1,6,7,18,26] It was at this time that the concept of pituitary surgery incorporated endocrinologic control in addition to relief of mass effect and preservation of vision.[1]

The operation as described by Hardy has undergone further refinements and has become the primary surgical procedure used by most neurosurgeons for the excision of pituitary tumors and other sellar lesions for the past 30 years.[6,27–29] Mortality rates dropped below 1% in expert hands, rendering the procedure reasonably safe and highly effective.[6,30–32]

Endoscopy and the Pituitary

Although introduced to neurosurgery almost a century ago, until recently endoscopy has been primarily limited to intraventricular procedures.[17] However, it was not commonly used in pituitary surgery until the mid-1990s, when functional endoscopic sinus surgery had virtually replaced conventional open techniques used by otorhinolaryngologists for the treatment of inflammatory sinonasal disorders.[6] The excellent visualization and better surgical results offered by the endoscope in sinus surgery prompted neurosurgeons to explore its potential use in transsphenoidal surgery.[20,33–35]

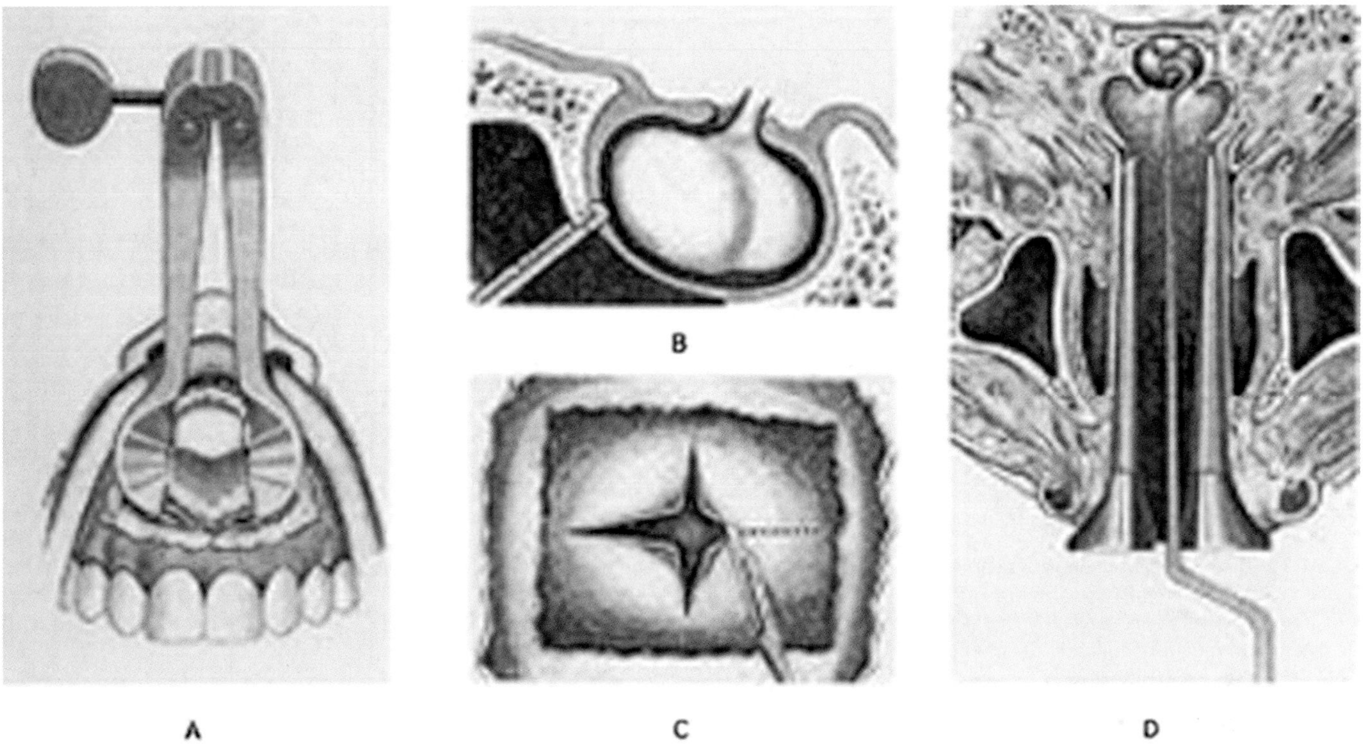

Fig. 1.8 Operative drawing depicting the sella turcica portion of the procedure. **(A)** Resection of the vomer and the floor of the sphenoid sinus, exposing the sella turcica. **(B)** Opening of the sellar floor with a rongeur. **(C)** Cruciate incision made in the dura of the sella turcica. **(D)** Horizontal view of the strict midline approach to the sella turcica. (From Kanter AS, et al. The transsphenoidal approach. Neurosurgery Focus 2005;18(4):E61–4. Modified with permission.)

The initial role of endoscopy was to augment microsurgery and allow for the viewing of structures out of the line of sight by using straight and angled endoscopes. Previously this had been achieved through the use of angled mirrors.[6,23,36,37] Guiot was the first to report the use of an endoscope during sublabial transsphenoidal surgery in 1963, but he abandoned the procedure because of lack of adequate visualization.[17,38] In the late 1970s, Apuzzo et al,[39] as well as Bushe and Halves,[6,36,40,41] reported the use of the endoscope as a technical adjunct in the microscopic resection of pituitary lesions with extrasellar extension. In 1994, Gamea and El-Guindy, otolaryngologists, and Fathi, a neurosurgeon, from Egypt reported on 10 patients with pituitary adenoma operated upon with endoscopic assistance.[42] This method has become known as endoscope-assisted transsphenoidal surgery.

Supporters of the technique went one step further, using the endoscope as the sole visualization tool for the removal of pituitary tumors—the pure endoscopic transsphenoidal approach.[20] In 1992, Jankowski et al[43] reported the first of these operations in three patients with pituitary adenomas using a middle turbinectomy approach. In 1995, Sethi and Pillay,[44] an otorhinolaryngologist and a neurologic surgeon, respectively, from the Singapore General Hospital, reported the use of an endonasal endoscopic transsphenoidal technique. Similar techniques were reported by Rodziewicz and coworkers[45] and other groups.[36,39,46]

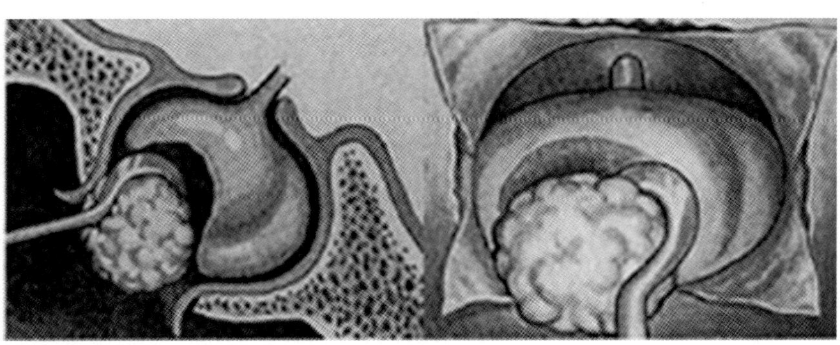

Fig. 1.9 Illustration depicting selective removal of a pituitary microadenoma while preserving pituitary function. (From Hardy J. Transsphenoidal hypophysectomy. J Neurosurg 1971;34:582–594. Reprinted with permission.)

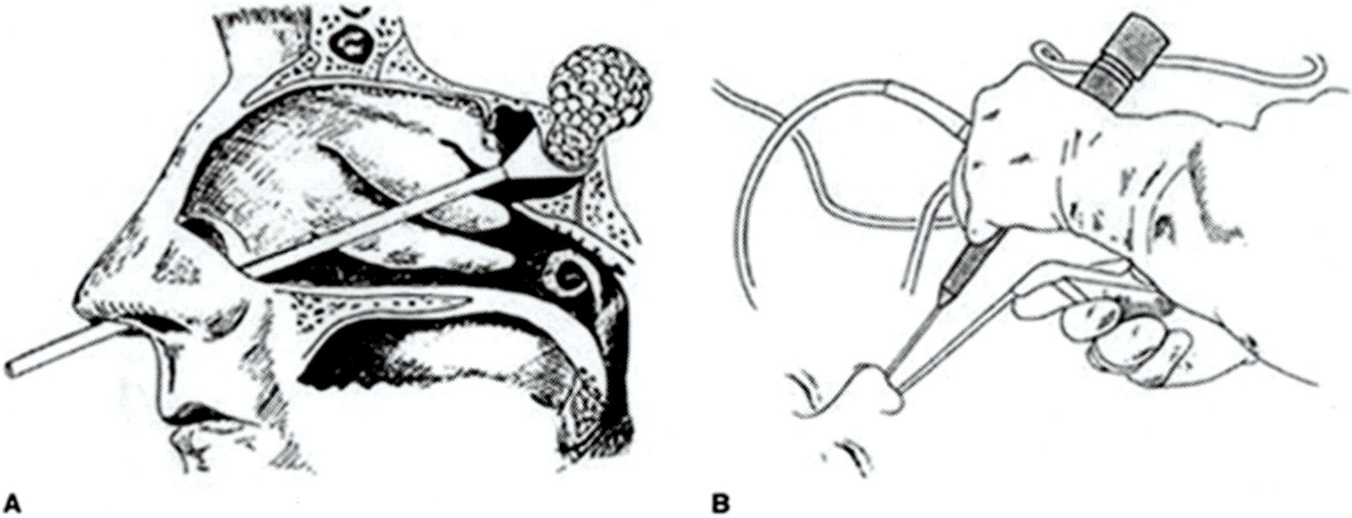

Fig. 1.10 **(A)** Illustration depicting an endonasal endoscopic approach to the sella. Note the absence of septal or alar incisions. No speculum or retractor is used. **(B)** The endoscope is held in the surgeon's nondominant hand, and instruments are held in the dominant hand until the anterior sphenoidotomy is made. (From Jho HD, Carrau RL, Ko Y, Daly MA. Endoscopic pituitary surgery: an early experience. Surg Neurol 1997;47:213–222, discussion 222–223. Reprinted with permission.)

Much credit for the development and popularization of the pure endoscopic transsphenoidal approach is given to Hae Dong Jho and Ricardo Carrau, a neurosurgeon and an otorhinolaryngologist, respectively, working at the University of Pittsburgh Medical Center. The new endoscopic transsphenoidal approach to the sellar region was strictly endonasal without the use of a transsphenoidal retractor or the operating microscope (**Fig. 1.10**).[3,47,48] They are widely recognized as the pioneers of the pure endoscopic endonasal approach for the treatment of pituitary adenomas.[7,49] They started by using the endoscope as an adjunct to the microscopic technique[37,47] and then moved to a purely endoscopic technique. In 1997, they reported on 50 patients who were treated by their purely endoscopic approach.[50]

Paolo Cappabianca and Enrico de Divitiis,[51] of Naples, epitomized the European focus of more recent progress in transsphenoidal surgery.[3] They were among the first to report their experience with the use of the purely endoscopic technique, introducing the term *functional endoscopic pituitary surgery* (FEPS).[51] They developed dedicated endoscopic instrumentation,[52] suggested technical improvements,[53,54] and significantly contributed to the scientific basis[41,54–56] and critical assessment of the technique.[41,53,57,58] These reports have been followed by many others from around the world.[41,59,60]

Conclusion

The current transsphenoidal approaches are the result of an evolutionary process. Five thousand years ago the approach was used by ancient Egyptians, and it was reintroduced in the 19th century by Giordano as an anatomical study. The operative technique was developed by a series of European and North American innovators, such as Schloffer, Kocher, Hirsch, Halstead, Cushing, Dott, Guiot, and Hardy, who validated transsphenoidal surgery, either with a sublabial or directly transnasal approach, as a surgical reality. As contemporary neurosurgical leaders (including Cappabianca, de Divitiis, Frank, Jane Jr., Jho, Kassam, Laws, Oldfield, and Schwartz) further modify the procedure and develop specialized instrumentation, the indications for this approach will continue to grow.

References

1. Kanter AS, Dumont AS, Asthagiri AR, Oskouian RJ, Jane JA Jr, Laws ER Jr. The transsphenoidal approach. A historical perspective. Neurosurg Focus 2005;18:e6
2. El Gindi S. Neurosurgery in Egypt: past, present, and future-from pyramids to radiosurgery. Neurosurgery 2002;51:789–795, discussion 795–796
3. Cappabianca P, de Divitiis E. Back to the Egyptians: neurosurgery via the nose. A five-thousand year history and the recent contribution of the endoscope. Neurosurg Rev 2007;30:1–7, discussion 7
4. Hoffman H, Hudgins PA. Head and skull base features of nine Egyptian mummies: evaluation with high-resolution CT and reformation techniques. AJR Am J Roentgenol 2002;178:1367–1376
5. Artico M, Pastore FS, Fraioli B, Giuffrè R. The contribution of Davide Giordano (1864–1954) to pituitary surgery: the transglabellar-nasal approach. Neurosurgery 1998;42:909–911, discussion 911–912
6. Liu JK, Das K, Weiss MH, Laws ER Jr, Couldwell WT. The history and evolution of transsphenoidal surgery. J Neurosurg 2001;95:1083–1096
7. Maroon JC. Skull base surgery: past, present, and future trends. Neurosurg Focus 2005;19:E1

8. Cohen-Gadol AA, Liu JK, Laws ER Jr. Cushing's first case of transsphenoidal surgery: the launch of the pituitary surgery era. J Neurosurg 2005;103:570–574
9. Liu JK, Cohen-Gadol AA, Laws ER Jr, Cole CD, Kan P, Couldwell WT. Harvey Cushing and Oskar Hirsch: early forefathers of modern transsphenoidal surgery. J Neurosurg 2005;103:1096–1104
10. Lanzino G, Laws ER Jr. Key personalities in the development and popularization of the transsphenoidal approach to pituitary tumors: an historical overview. Neurosurg Clin N Am 2003;14:1–10
11. Kanavel A. The removal of tumors of the pituitary body by an infranasal route. A proposed operation and description of the technique. JAMA 1909;53:1704–1707
12. Halstead AE. Remarks on the operative treatment of tumors of the hypophysis. With the report of two cases done by an oro-nasal method. Surg Gynecol Obstet 1910;10:494–502
13. Cushing H. The Weir Mitchell Lecture. Surgical experiences with pituitary disorders. JAMA 1914;63:1515–1525
14. Stone JL, Meglio G, Laws ER Jr. Development of pituitary surgery: the Chicago contributions. J Am Coll Surg 2005;201:784–805
15. Cushing H III. Partial Hypophysectomy for Acromegaly: With Remarks on the Function of the Hypophysis. Ann Surg 1909;50:1002–1017
16. Cushing H. The Pituitary Body and Its Disorders: Clinical States Produced by Disorders of the Hypophysis Cerebri. Philadelphia: JB Lippincott; 1912:296–305
17. Couldwell WT. Transsphenoidal and transcranial surgery for pituitary adenomas. J Neurooncol 2004;69:237–256
18. Rosegay H. Cushing's legacy to transsphenoidal surgery. J Neurosurg 1981;54:448–454
19. Dott NM, Bailey P. A consideration of the hypophyseal adenomata. Br J Surg 1925;13:314–366
20. Gandhi CD, Post KD. Historical movements in transsphenoidal surgery. Neurosurg Focus 2001;11:E7
21. Guiot G. Considerations on the surgical treatment of pituitary adenomas. In: Fahlbusch R, Werder KV, eds. Treatment of Pituitary Adenomas. 1st European Workshop. Stuttgart: Thieme; 1978: 202–218
22. Hardy J. Neurosurgeon of the year. Gerard Guiot. Surg Neurol 1979; 11:1–2
23. Hardy J. [Surgery of the pituitary gland, using the trans-sphenoidal approach. Comparative study of 2 technical methods]. Union Med Can 1967;96:702–712 (Fr)
24. Welbourn RB. The evolution of transsphenoidal pituitary microsurgery. Surgery 1986;100:1185–1190
25. Hardy J. Transsphenoidal microsurgery of the normal and pathological pituitary. Clin Neurosurg 1969;16:185–217
26. Hardy J. Transsphenoidal hypophysectomy. J Neurosurg 1971;34: 582–594
27. Laws ER Jr. Pituitary surgery. Endocrinol Metab Clin North Am 1987;16:647–665
28. Laws ER Jr. Transsphenoidal microsurgery in the management of craniopharyngioma. J Neurosurg 1980;52:661–666
29. Laws ER Jr, Piepgras DG, Randall RV, Abboud CF. Neurosurgical management of acromegaly. Results in 82 patients treated between 1972 and 1977. J Neurosurg 1979;50:454–461
30. Ciric IS, Ragin A, Baumgartner C, Pierce D. Complications of transsphenoidal surgery: results of a national survey, review of the literature, and personal experience. Neurosurgery 1997;40:225–236, discussion 236–237
31. Laws ER Jr, Kern EB. Complications of trans-sphenoidal surgery. Clin Neurosurg 1976;23:401–416
32. Wilson CB. A decade of pituitary microsurgery. The Herbert Olivecrona lecture. J Neurosurg 1984;61:814–833
33. Alfieri A. Endoscopic endonasal transsphenoidal approach to the sellar region: technical evolution of the methodology and refinement of a dedicated instrumentation. J Neurosurg Sci 1999;43:85–92
34. Carrau RL, Jho HD, Ko Y. Transnasal-transsphenoidal endoscopic surgery of the pituitary gland. Laryngoscope 1996;106:914–918
35. Jho HD, Carrau RL, Ko Y, Daly MA. Endoscopic pituitary surgery: an early experience. Surg Neurol 1997;47:213–222, discussion 222–223
36. Doglietto F, Prevedello DM, Jane JA Jr, Han J, Laws ER Jr. Brief history of endoscopic transsphenoidal surgery—from Philipp Bozzini to the First World Congress of Endoscopic Skull Base Surgery. Neurosurg Focus 2005;19:E3
37. Jane JA Jr, Han J, Prevedello DM, Jagannathan J, Dumont AS, Laws ER Jr. Perspectives on endoscopic transsphenoidal surgery. Neurosurg Focus 2005;19:E2
38. Guiot J, Rougerie J, Fourestier M, et al. [Intracranial endoscopic explorations.]. Presse Med 1963;71:1225–1228
39. Apuzzo ML, Heifetz MD, Weiss MH, Kurze T. Neurosurgical endoscopy using the side-viewing telescope. J Neurosurg 1977;46:398–400
40. Bushe KA, Halves E. [Modified technique in transsphenoidal operations of pituitary adenomas. Technical note (author's transl)]. Acta Neurochir (Wien) 1978;41:163–175
41. Prevedello DM, Doglietto F, Jane JA Jr, Jagannathan J, Han J, Laws ER Jr. History of endoscopic skull base surgery: its evolution and current reality. J Neurosurg 2007;107:206–213
42. Gamea A, Fathi M, el-Guindy A. The use of the rigid endoscope in trans-sphenoidal pituitary surgery. J Laryngol Otol 1994;108: 19–22
43. Jankowski R, Auque J, Simon C, Marchal JC, Hepner H, Wayoff M. Endoscopic pituitary tumor surgery. Laryngoscope 1992;102: 198–202
44. Sethi DS, Pillay PK. Endoscopic management of lesions of the sella turcica. J Laryngol Otol 1995;109:956–962
45. Rodziewicz GS, Kelley RT, Kellman RM, Smith MV. Transnasal endoscopic surgery of the pituitary gland: technical note. Neurosurgery 1996;39:189–192, discussion 192–193
46. Heilman CB, Shucart WA, Rebeiz EE. Endoscopic sphenoidotomy approach to the sella. Neurosurgery 1997;41:602–607
47. Carrau RL, Jho HD, Ko Y. Transnasal-transsphenoidal endoscopic surgery of the pituitary gland. Laryngoscope 1996;106:914–918
48. Jho HD, Carrau RL, Ko Y. Endoscopic pituitary surgery. In: Reganchary SS, Wilkins RH, eds. Neurosurgical Operative Atlas. Park Ridge, IL: American Association of Neurological Surgeons; 1996:1–12
49. Cappabianca P, de Divitiis E. Endoscopy and transsphenoidal surgery. Neurosurgery 2004;54:1043–1048, 1048–1050
50. Jho HD, Carrau RL. Endoscopic endonasal transsphenoidal surgery: experience with 50 patients. J Neurosurg 1997;87:44–51
51. Cappabianca P, Alfieri A, de Divitiis E. Endoscopic endonasal transsphenoidal approach to the sella: towards functional endoscopic pituitary surgery (FEPS). Minim Invasive Neurosurg 1998;41: 66–73
52. Cappabianca P, Alfieri A, Thermes S, Buonamassa S, de Divitiis E. Instruments for endoscopic endonasal transsphenoidal surgery. Neurosurgery 1999;45:392–395, discussion 395–396

53. Cappabianca P, Alfieri A, Colao A, et al. Endoscopic endonasal transsphenoidal surgery in recurrent and residual pituitary adenomas: technical note. Minim Invasive Neurosurg 2000;43:38–43
54. Cappabianca P, Cavallo LM, Valente V, et al. Sellar repair with fibrin sealant and collagen fleece after endoscopic endonasal transsphenoidal surgery. Surg Neurol 2004;62:227–233, discussion 233
55. Cappabianca P, Cavallo LM, de Divitiis E. Endoscopic endonasal transsphenoidal surgery. Neurosurgery 2004;55:933–940, discussion 940–941
56. Cappabianca P, Cavallo LM, Esposito F, de Divitiis E. Endoscopic endonasal transsphenoidal surgery: procedure, endoscopic equipment and instrumentation. Childs Nerv Syst 2004;20:796–801
57. Cavallo LM, Briganti F, Cappabianca P, et al. Hemorrhagic vascular complications of endoscopic transsphenoidal surgery. Minim Invasive Neurosurg 2004;47:145–150
58. Cappabianca P, Cavallo LM, Colao A, de Divitiis E. Surgical complications associated with the endoscopic endonasal transsphenoidal approach for pituitary adenomas. J Neurosurg 2002;97:293–298
59. Ogawa T, Matsumoto K, Nakashima T, et al. Hypophysis surgery with or without endoscopy. Auris Nasus Larynx 2001;28:143–149
60. Stamm AC, Pignatari S, Sebusiani BB, Galati M, Mitsuda S, Haetinger RG. Image-guided endoscopic sinus and skull base surgery. Rev Bras Otorrinolaringol (Engl Ed) 2002;68:502–509

2 Anatomy of the Pituitary Gland and Parasellar Region

Ameet Singh, Jonathan Roth, Vijay K. Anand, and Theodore H. Schwartz

The pituitary gland is a remarkable organ that is located at the base of the brain at the center of the skull base. The gland controls an array of endocrine functions important for human growth and metabolism. The most common pituitary-related pathologies that are surgically treated are pituitary tumors (mostly adenomas) and pituitary apoplexy. The classic indications for surgical treatment include visual loss from progressive mass effect, hormonal control in hyperfunctioning adenomas, failure of medical therapy, and necessity for a tissue diagnosis.[1] Transcranial approaches to the sella for treating pituitary pathologies have been in existence since the late 19th century. In the early 1900s, Hirsch described a transnasal approach to the sella turcica that was refined by Cushing, who standardized the translabial, transseptal, transsphenoidal approach to the pituitary gland.[2]

Recently, given the technologic enhancements in endoscopic visualization and instrumentation, the endonasal endoscopic approach has gained popularity for addressing pathology of the pituitary gland. Regardless of the surgical approach, a commanding knowledge of the anatomy of the pituitary gland and parasellar region is critical for surgeons operating in this area. This chapter addresses the anatomy of the pituitary gland and parasellar region as well as the surrounding anatomy of the cavernous sinus, suprasellar region, and third ventricle. In addition, anatomical principles emphasized by the endoscopic approach are also discussed in greater detail. Although these anatomical relationships are not new, the endoscopic approach places these anatomical concepts in a different light and therefore are important to understand and appreciate.

Pituitary Gland

The pituitary gland is composed of an anterior and a posterior lobe that are embryologically, anatomically, and functionally distinct. The anterior lobe surrounds the lower part of the pituitary stalk to form the pars tuberalis (**Fig. 2.1A**). The pituitary stalk generally attaches to the anterosuperior portion of the pituitary gland. If the anterior lobe is separated from the posterior lobe, the pars tuberalis tends to remain with posterior lobe. The anterior lobe is firmer but easily separated from the anterior and lateral sellar walls. The posterior lobe, on the other hand, is softer and gelatinous. However, it is more firmly attached to the sellar walls and thus sometimes is difficult to remove. The inferior surface of the gland conforms to the sella floor, whereas the shape of the superior and lateral surfaces of the gland is variable because they border soft tissue structures, namely, the cavernous sinus and diaphragma sellae. The superior surface is usually ovoid and may become triangular in shape if the carotid arteries compress the gland laterally and posteriorly (**Fig. 2.1B**). The width of the pituitary gland is usually equal or slightly larger than the length or depth of the gland. In addition, the superior surface of the posterior gland may be distinguished from the anterior lobe by its lighter color. This is an important anatomical point that can help to distinguish the two lobes when the pituitary is approached transcranially.[3]

Given its central location, the pituitary gland is surrounded by several critical neurovascular structures. These include the optic nerves, optic chiasm, and anterior circulation superiorly (**Fig. 2.2A**); the cavernous sinuses, internal carotid arteries, and cranial nerves laterally; and the brainstem and posterior circulation posteriorly (**Fig. 2.2B**). Anteriorly, the pituitary gland is enclosed by the sphenoid sinus and frontal lobes (**Fig. 2.2C**). These critical neurovascular structures, often separated by a few millimeters, surround the pituitary gland superiorly, laterally, and posteriorly and therefore make anterior-based approaches the preferred and safest surgical routes to the sellar region.

Sphenoid Bone

The complexity of the neurovasculature surrounding or traversing the sphenoid bone necessitates a thorough knowledge of its bony anatomy. More importantly, the sphenoid bone contributes in large measure to the anatomy of the sella and parasellar region, making its anatomy important for any pituitary surgeon. The sphenoid bone is a butterfly-shaped bone divided into the body of the sphenoid centrally, a single greater and lesser wing bilaterally, and pterygoid processes pointing inferiorly from the body of the sphenoid bone. The lesser wings originate from the superomedial part of the central bone, and the greater wings emanate from the lower part of the central bone. The lesser wing of the

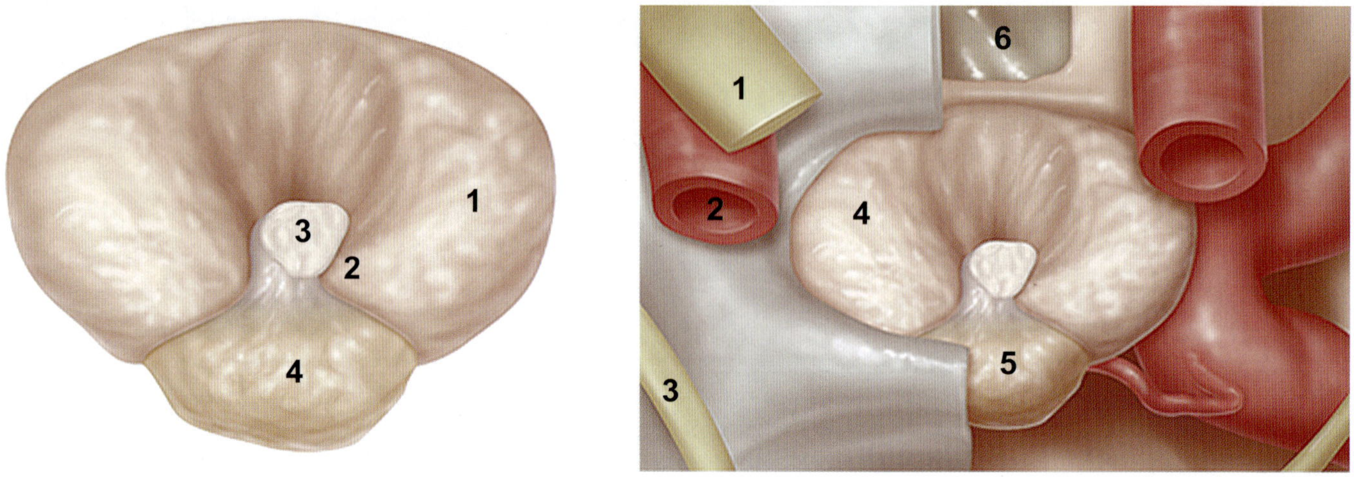

A B

Fig. 2.1 **(A)** The pituitary gland may be divided into a firmer anterior lobe and a softer, gelatinous posterior lobe. The anterior lobe surrounds the pituitary stalk to form the pars tuberalis. 1, anterior lobe; 2, pars tuberalis; 3, pituitary stalk; 4, posterior lobe. **(B)** The superior surface of the pituitary gland is usually ovoid and may become triangular if the carotid arteries compress the gland posteriorly and laterally. The posterior gland may also be distinguished from anterior lobe by its lighter color. 1, optic lobe; 2, internal carotid; 3, oculomotor nerve; 4, anterior pituitary; 5, posterior pituitary; 6, sphenoid sinus.

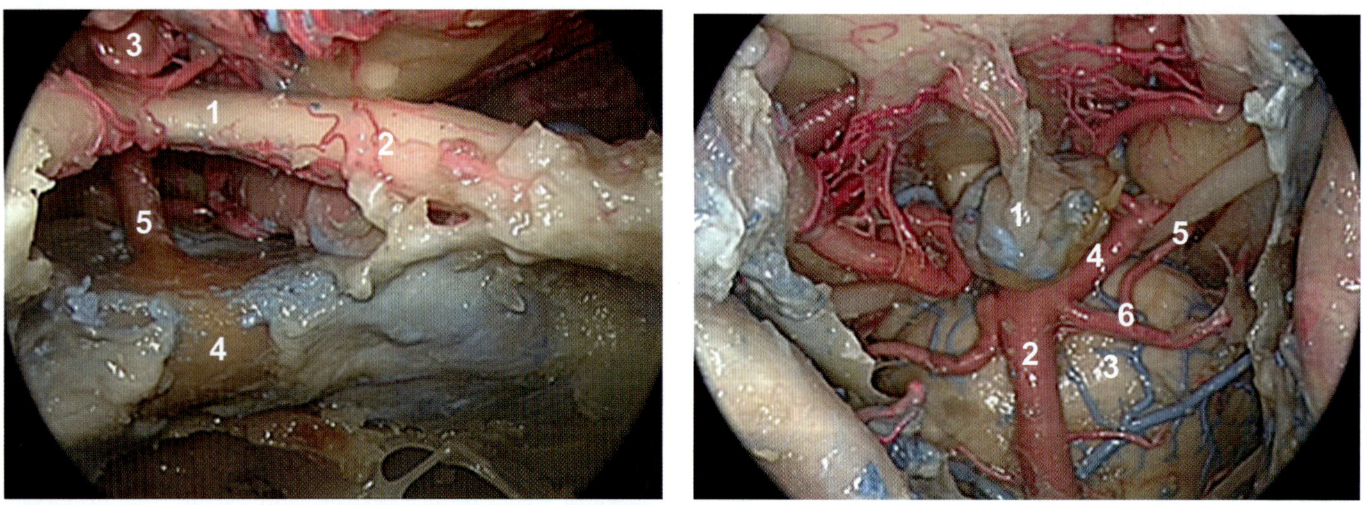

A B

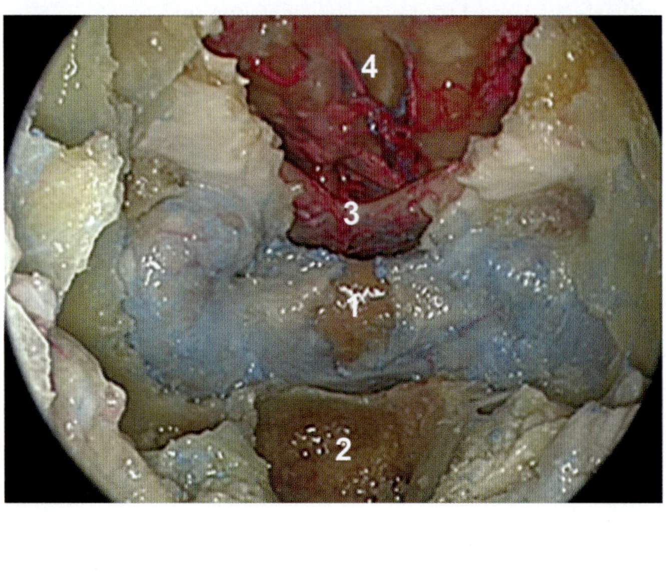

C

Fig. 2.2 **(A)** The pituitary gland is flanked by the optic chiasm and anterior cerebral circulation superiorly and the optic nerves superomedially. 1, optic chiasm; 2, optic nerve; 3, anterior cerebral circulation; 4, pituitary gland; 5, pituitary stalk. **(B)** The pituitary gland is surrounded by the brainstem and posterior circulation posteriorly. 1, pituitary gland; 2, basilar artery; 3, brainstem; 4, posterior cerebral artery; 5, oculomotor nerve; 6, superior cerebral artery. **(C)** The pituitary gland is enclosed by the sphenoid sinus anteriorly and the frontal lobes anterosuperiorly. 1, pituitary gland; 2, sphenoid sinus; 3, optic chiasm; 4, frontal lobes.

sphenoid along with the planum sphenoidale contribute to the anterior cranial base, which houses the olfactory tracts, gyrus rectus, and posterior part of the frontal lobe. The lesser wing also contributes to the posterior part of each orbit. In close association to these central bony structures lie the pituitary gland, optic chiasm, as well as several cranial nerves traversing various foramina located in the sphenoid bone. The lateral part of the middle cranial base is formed by contributions from the lesser and greater wings of the sphenoid bone, which house the temporal lobe. The greater wing also forms the lateral wall of the orbit and the roof of the infratemporal fossa[3,4] (**Fig. 2.3A**).

Several cranial nerves traverse multiple foramina formed within the sphenoid bone. The superior orbital fissure, located between the inferior margin of the lesser wing and the superior margin of the greater wing of the sphenoid bone, is negotiated by the oculomotor, trochlear, abducens, and ophthalmic branch of the trigeminal nerve. The optic canals, which transmit the optic nerves, are located above and medial to the superior orbital fissure, separated by a ridge of bone called the optic strut. Extracranially, the optic strut corresponds to the lateral opticocarotid recess, an important anatomical landmark on the lateral sphenoid wall during transsphenoidal surgery. Other important foramina embedded in the sphenoid bone, located at the junction of the body and greater wing, are the foramen rotundum, pterygoid canal, foramen ovale, and foramen spinosum. The major structures passing through these foramina are the maxillary nerve, vidian nerve, mandibular nerve, and middle meningeal artery, respectively[5] (**Fig. 2.3B**).

Important vascular structures have an intimate relationship with the sphenoid bone. The internal carotid arteries project into the sphenoid bone and form prominences in the lateral wall of the sphenoid sinus. The cavernous sinuses, discussed later in greater detail, lie on the lateral aspect of the pituitary gland and serve as a conduit for lateral extension of some pituitary adenomas. Intercavernous sinuses pass through the sellar cavity and dorsum sellae. Finally, the basilar artery lies on the posterior surface of the sphenoid bone, which contributes to the superior clivus (**Fig. 2.2B**).

A

B

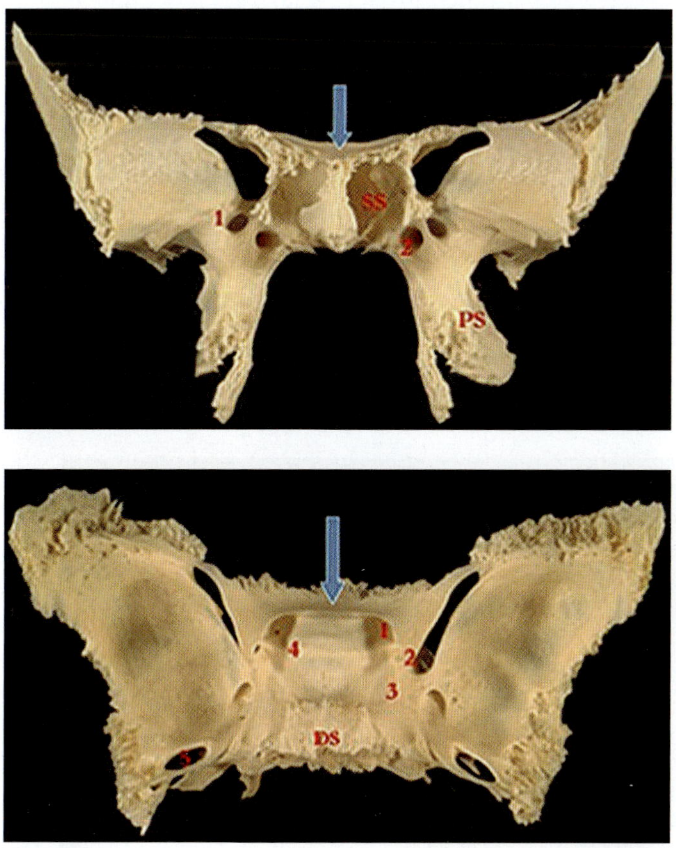

Fig. 2.3 **(A)** The lesser wing, greater wing, and pterygoid process emanating from the butterfly-shaped central sphenoid bone seen from an anterior-posterior view. 1, forcemen rotundum; 2, vidian canal; arrow, planum sphenoidale. **(B)** Anatomical landmarks and embedded foramina of the sphenoid bone as seen from a superior view. 1, optic canal; 2, anterior clinoid; 3, groove of internal carotid artery; 4, middle clinoid; 5, foramen ovale; 6, posterior clinoid; DS, dorsum sellae; arrow, planum sphenoidale.

Sellar Bone

The sella turcica is a bony region of the sphenoid bone that houses the pituitary gland. The gland is limited anteriorly by the tuberculum sellae and posteriorly by the dorsum sellae. The tuberculum is a thick ridge of bone connecting the sellar fossa to the planum sphenoidale. Between the tuberculum sellae and planum sphenoidale lies a depression bounded laterally by the optic foramina called the chiasmatic sulcus. The optic chiasm usually lies posterior to this bony landmark. The sella turcica has three bony spicules or prominences; namely, the middle, anterior, and posterior clinoid processes, the latter two of which provide attachment to the tentorium cerebelli. The anterior clinoid processes are located at the medial edge of the lesser wings, the middle clinoid processes lateral to the tuberculum sellae, and the posterior clinoid processes on the superolateral margin of the dorsum sellae (**Fig. 2.3B**). The depth or height of the sella is usually determined by the sellar floor and a perpendicular line connecting the tuberculum and dorsum. The length of the sella is the largest anterior-posterior dimension of the pituitary fossa, typically located at the level of the tuberculum. The greatest distance between the two carotid sulci is considered the sellar width.

Sphenoid Sinus

The sphenoid sinus, contained within the central part of sphenoid bone, is widely considered the gateway to the pituitary gland, parasellar region, and anterior skull base. It is a large paranasal sinus located posterior to the ethmoid

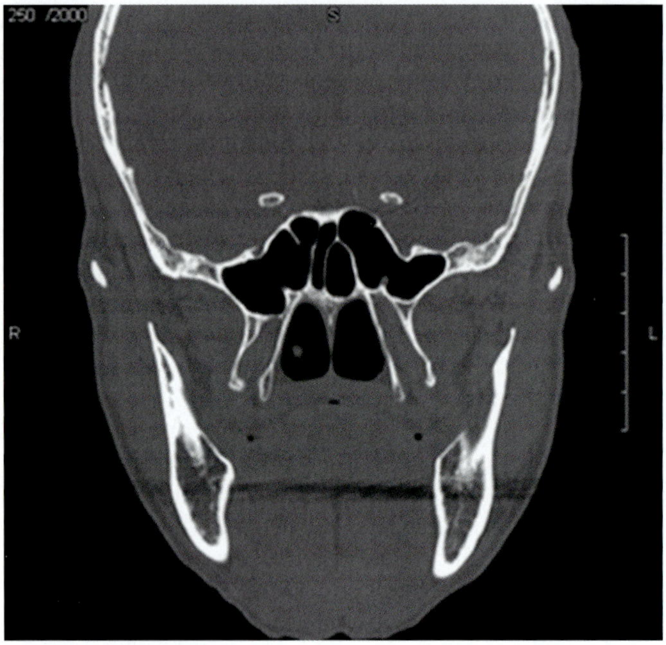

Fig. 2.4 Computed tomography image of a well-pneumatized sphenoid sinus with multiple vertical, horizontal, and oblique septations.

sinuses, typically divided into two unequal halves by a single vertical septation. However, it is not uncommon to find multiple complete and incomplete septations dividing the sinus into several cells, complicating the descriptive anatomy of this region.[3,6] The major vertical septation often continues posteriorly to the face of the sella. However, it may localize to either of the carotid siphons, emphasizing the need for atraumatic dissection while removing these septations to avoid damage to the underlying vascular structures (**Fig. 2.4**). Single septations are found 68% of the time, and these septations may be found as much as 8 mm off the midline.[7]

The natural sphenoid sinus ostium is elliptical and usually located in the anterosuperior aspect of the anterior sphenoid sinus wall approximately 1.5 cm superior to the posterior choanae in the sphenoethmoidal recess adjacent to the posterior tip of the middle turbinate and inferior edge of the superior turbinate (**Fig. 2.5**). The Onodi cell, when present, represents pneumatization of a posterior ethmoid cell into the sphenoid sinus and may distort identification of the true sphenoid sinus. It is present in 7 to 25% of patients and must be recognized radiographically and endoscopically prior to embarking on a skull base approach or endoscopic sinus surgery. This is important because of the passage of the optic nerve in the lateral wall of the cell[8] (**Fig. 2.6**).

The sphenoid sinus is variably pneumatized and is characterized by the position of the sinus in relationship to the sella turcica. Pneumatization is classified into sellar (80%), presellar (17%), and conchal (3%) types. A sellar sphenoid sinus has extensive pneumatization anteriorly and inferiorly to the sellar protuberance, making identification of intrasphenoidal anatomical landmarks easier during endoscopic transsphenoidal surgery. A presellar pneumatization pattern has pneumatization anteriorly, making the sellar protuberance and other landmarks slightly more difficult to identify. Finally, no pneumatization exists for the conchal type of sphenoid sinus, common in children younger than 12 years of age, which poses a challenging anatomical dissection for the management of any pituitary or anterior skull base lesion[8] (**Fig. 2.7**). In this pattern, the bone separating the sella from the sphenoid sinus is usually greater than 10 mm.[3]

A

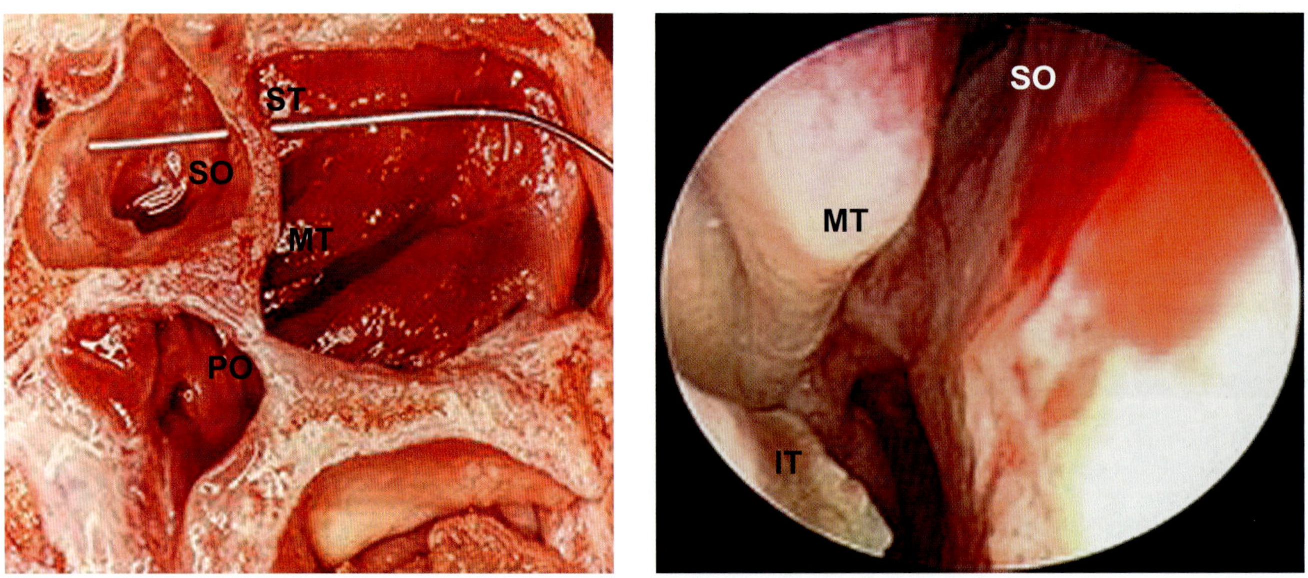

B

Fig. 2.5 **(A)** Sagittal cadaveric dissection demonstrating the location of the natural sphenoid sinus ostium. **(B)** Endoscopic image demonstrating the location of the sphenoid sinus ostium in relationship to the superior turbinate. IT, inferior turbinate; MT, middle turbinate; PC, posterior choanae; SO, sphenoid ostium.

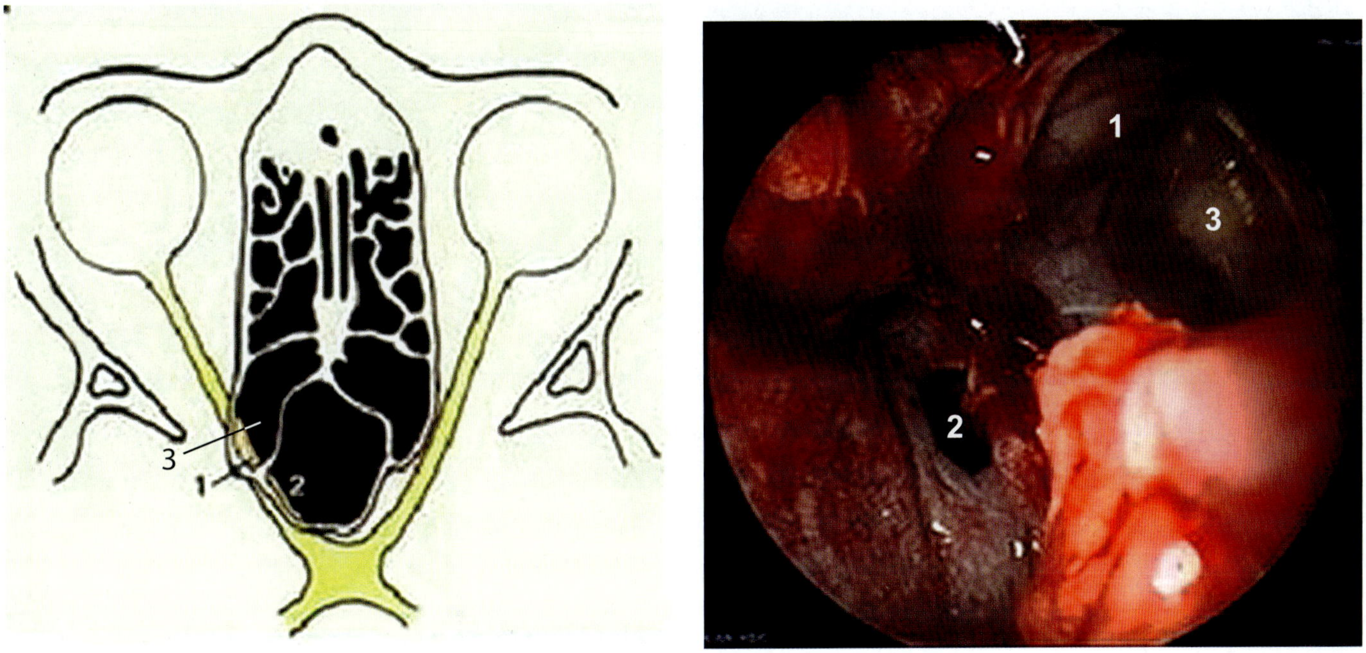

A B

Fig. 2.6 **(A)** Axial image of the posterolateral pneumatization of a posterior ethmoid cell termed an Onodi cell. **(B)** Endoscopic image of a left Onodi cell, demonstrating the optic nerve running in its superior lateral corner. 1, optic nerve; 2; sphenoid sinus; 3, onodi cell.

Image guidance is critical for a transsphenoidal approach through a conchal sphenoid sinus to avoid straying laterally while drilling.

One final additional pattern of pneumatization that has been described is called the postsellar sphenoid sinus, where, in addition to a sellar pattern, pneumatization exists posterior to the sellar prominence. Far lateral pneumatization of the sphenoid sinus occurs in a certain proportion of patients, in which the sinus extends into the roots of the pterygoid processes or the greater wing of the sphenoid. Also, as a person ages, the sphenoid sinus pneumatizes even further secondary to bony resorption, which results in direct mucosal contact with the dura. The thickness of the anterior wall of the sella ranges from 0.1 to 0.7 mm in the sellar pattern of sphenoid sinus pneumatization versus the presellar type where the thickness varies from 0.3 to 1.5 mm. The thickest bone is usually found at the tuberculum sellae and clivus, whereas the thinnest bone is found along the anterior sellar wall.[7]

A recent retrospective radiologic study of 296 patients operated on for pituitary adenomas via the transsphenoidal approach reviewed the different anatomical variations of the sphenoid sinus. There was a 77% incidence of sellar and 2% incidence of conchal sphenoid sinus pneumatization. A single intersphenoid septation was noted in 71.6%, accessory

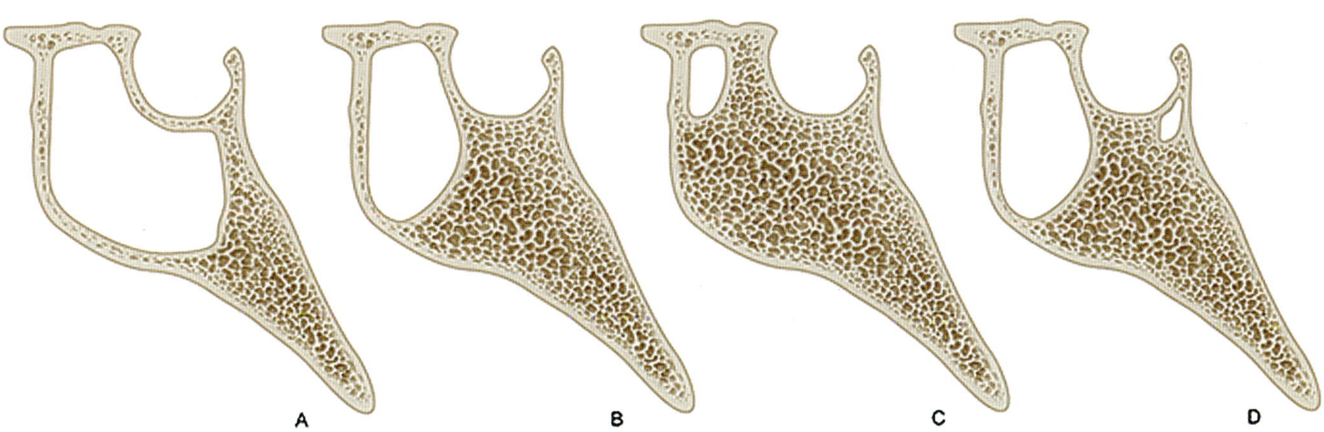

Fig. 2.7 Four types of sphenoid sinus pneumatization: **(A)** sellar, **(B)** presellar, **(C)** conchal, **(D)** postsellar.

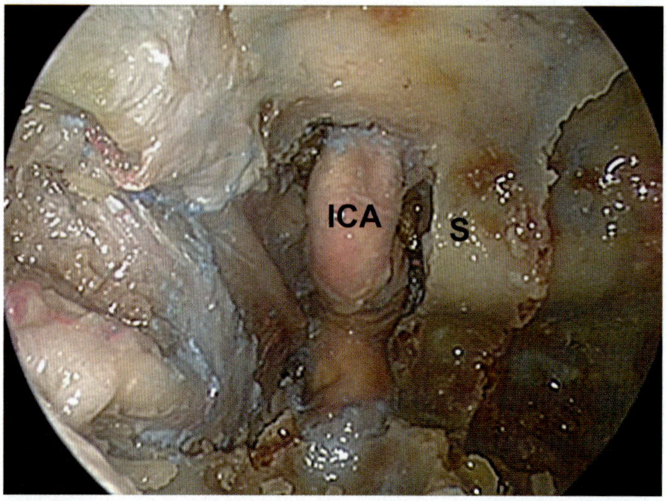

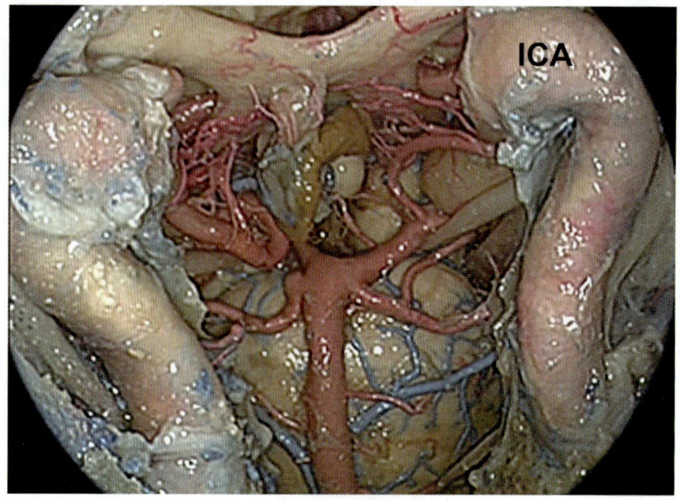

Fig. 2.8 **(A)** Location of the parasellar carotid arteries positioned in the lateral wall of the sphenoid sinus. **(B)** Complete bony removal and exposure of the presellar, infrasellar, and retrosellar segments as well as the paraclival portions of the carotid artery. ICA, internal carotid artery; S, sella.

septation in 10.8%, multiple septations in 8.7%, and no septation in 10.8% of patients. The sellar bulge was prominent in 189 patients.[9] A similar radiologic study concurred with the findings of a single sphenoid septum in 80% of cases and a double septum in 20%.[10]

The carotid artery lies directly against the lateral wall of the sphenoid sinus, making it the most important landmark to identify to avoid a catastrophic complication during pituitary surgery. The degree of sphenoid sinus pneumatization influences whether the carotid artery is seen as a small bulge or as its full course along the lateral sphenoid sinus wall (**Fig. 2.8A**). The parasellar segment of the internal carotid artery may be divided into three segments, namely the inferior horizontal portion, anterior vertical portion, and superior horizontal portion. Both the inferior and anterior segments are intracavernous, with the inferior forming the inferior limb of the parasellar region and the anterior limb forming the convexity of the C-shape located lateral and anterior to the sella wall.[4] Another classification for the carotid artery divides the carotid prominence into the retrosellar, infrasellar, and presellar segments. The retrosellar segment is located in the posterolateral aspect of the sphenoid sinus, the infrasellar segment is positioned below the sellar floor, and the presellar segment is located anterolateral to the sellar wall (**Fig. 2.8B**). In a study of 50 specimens, 98% had presellar, 80% had infrasellar, and 78% had retrosellar prominences.[7] Identifying all anatomical aspects of the carotid prominence is necessary to enhance the safety of a transsphenoidal procedure.

The distance between the lateral aspect of the pituitary gland and the medial margin of the internal carotid artery is an important anatomical consideration during transsphenoidal hypophysectomy. In one study the distance between the artery and the gland ranged from 1 to 7 mm with an average of 2.3 mm. In 25% of cases, the artery crossed the medial wall of the cavernous sinus and protruded into the pituitary gland. These cases often resulted in residual tumor and the potential for some remaining pituitary hyperfunction. In the same study, the shortest distance between the two carotid arteries was found to be in the supraclinoid region in 82% of cases, cavernous sinus in 14% of cases, and sphenoid sinus in 4% of cases.[3]

Multiple classification schemes exist regarding the organization and classification of the sphenoid sinus and pertinent neurovascular structures. Alfieri and Jho divided the sphenoid sinus into five vertical compartments: median, bilateral vertical paramedian, and bilateral lateral. The median compartment contains the sellar impression posteriorly, the planum sphenoidale superiorly and anteriorly, and the clivus inferiorly. The paramedian compartment contains the medial posterior third of the optic canal and the internal carotid artery, which is divided into paraclival and parasellar segments. The parasellar carotid protuberance is called the sellar segment and is subdivided into four segments; from superior to inferior, they are the superior horizontal segment, the vertical segment, the inferior horizontal segment, and the hidden segment. The carotid segment near the cavernous sinus is called the trigeminal segment. The paraclival segment inferiorly near the foramen lacerum is termed the foramen lacerum medium and further subdivided into the inferior lacerum segment and the superior cavernous sinus segment.[11,12]

The lateral and medial opticocarotid recesses are important landmarks. The lateral recess is bounded superomedially by the optic canal and inferomedially by the carotid protuberance. The recess corresponds to the optic strut

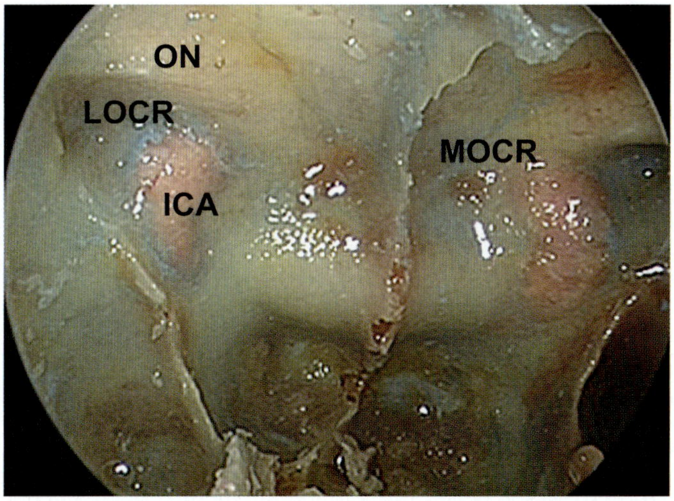

Fig. 2.9 Endoscopic view of the lateral and medial opticocarotid recesses in the lateral wall of the sphenoid sinus. ICA, internal carotid artery; LOCR, lateral opticocarotid recess; MOCR, medial opticocarotid recess; ON, optic nerve.

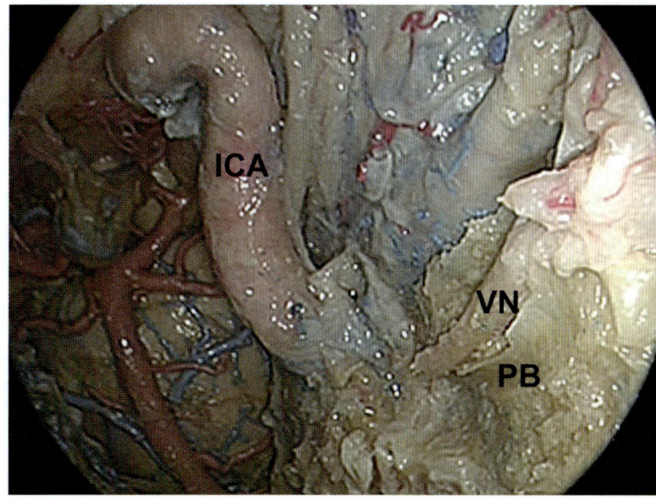

Fig. 2.10 Endoscopic anatomy of the lateral sphenoid sinus wall. ICA, internal carotid artery; PB, palatine bone; VN, vidian nerve.

and anterior clinoid process intracranially. The oculomotor nerve is also found inferiorly within the confines of this recess. The medial recess corresponds with the lateral aspect of the tuberculum sellae, is bounded superolaterally by the optic canal and inferolaterally by the carotid protuberance, and corresponds with the medial clinoid intracranially.[8] The medial opticocarotid recess is the space medial to the junction between the optic nerve and the carotid arteries and has been labeled the anatomic keyhole in endonasal skull base surgery[13] (**Fig. 2.9**).

The next recess is triangular in shape, with the base at the parasellar region of the carotid and the apex corresponding to the superior orbital fissure.[12] This region between the maxillary and mandibular divisions of the trigeminal nerve represents an embryologic fusion plane of the basi-sphenoid called Sternberg's canal. This area is an important landmark because a bony dehiscence may result in an encephalocele of the middle cranial fossa and a subsequent spontaneous cerebrospinal fluid leak.[8] The vidian nerve, which is formed by the greater superficial petrosal nerve and the deep petrosal nerve, exits the cranial cavity through the pterygoid canal that runs inferior and anterior to the internal carotid artery in its paraclival lateral segment. It courses over the mandibular branch of the trigeminal nerve into the pterygopalatine fossa anteriorly and laterally[14] (**Fig. 2.10**).

Internal carotid artery and optic nerve protrusion are commonplace among sphenoid sinus variations. The bone separating the artery from the sinus is thinnest anteriorly and thickest posteriorly, with the thinnest portion just inferior to the tuberculum sellae. Multiple studies have shown that the bone over the carotid artery is less than 0.5 mm in nearly 90% of patients. In addition, the bone might be completely missing in 10% of patients, where the sphenoid sinus mucosa rests directly on the carotid artery. The presence of anatomical variations increases the complexity of endoscopic surgery in this region. The optic canals protrude in the superolateral portion of the sphenoid sinus. Again, most studies have shown that the bone covering the optic canals is usually less than 0.5 mm in more than 80% of specimens. Thin bone or the lack of bone can easily explain the incidence of carotid artery or optic nerve injury during transsphenoidal surgery[15] (**Fig. 2.11**).

A radiologic study of 92 computed tomography scans on sphenoid sinus variations demonstrated internal carotid protrusion in 26%, optic nerve protrusion in 32%, and anterior clinoid pneumatization in 29% of patients. Protrusion was defined as the presence of 50% or more of the structure being visible in the sinus. Optic nerve dehiscence was noted in 23%, and internal carotid artery dehiscence was observed in 26% of

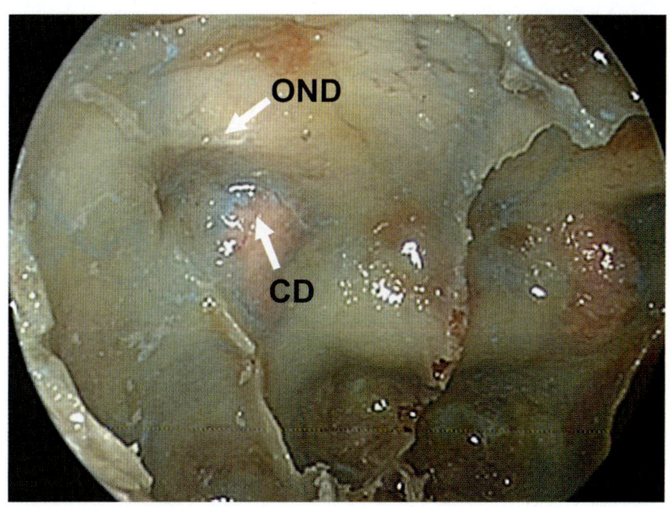

Fig. 2.11 Dehiscence of the internal carotid artery and optic nerve into the sphenoid sinus cavity. CD, carotid demiscence; OND, optic nerve demiscence.

patients. Bilateral dehiscences were noted in 16% of patients. A statistically significant relationship between pneumatization of the anterior clinoid process and optic nerve protrusion was found. The authors postulated that anterior clinoid process pneumatization may cause medial displacement of the optic nerve.[10] Occasionally, as mentioned earlier, only a mucoperiosteal covering was noted on the internal carotid artery. Optic nerve protrusion varies widely in the literature from 8 to 70%, depending on the definition of protrusion. Regardless, recognition of the types of bony prominences and depressions as well as their relative incidences is important for the endoscopic skull base surgeon.

Diaphragma Sellae

The diaphragma sellae is a dural sheath composed of two leaves of dura that form the roof of the pituitary gland. It is rectangular in shape, and it is usually convex in 54% of patients, flat in 42%, and concave in 4%. It is usually complete except centrally where the pituitary stalk descends from the third ventricle. The diaphragma sellae is thinner around the infundibulum and thicker around the periphery. The opening in the diaphragm is usually larger than the size of the pituitary stalk, and there is remarkable variability in the size and morphology of the opening. In one study the diaphragmal opening was greater than 5 mm in 56% of cases, round in 54% of cases, and elliptical in 46% of patients.[3] The size and morphology of the diaphragmal opening determine the dumbbell growth pattern of a pituitary adenoma. A large central or peripheral deficiency of the diaphragma is also thought to predispose the patient to an empty sella, where the arachnoid crosses into the sella and if opened may result in a cerebrospinal fluid leak after pituitary surgery (**Fig. 2.12**).

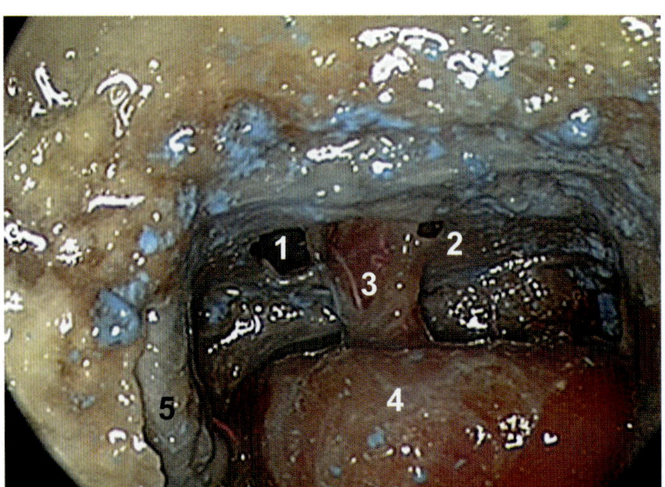

Fig. 2.12 Endoscopic view of the diaphragma sellae separated from the superior surface of the pituitary gland. 1, diaphragmal opening; 2, diaphragm; 3, pituitary stalk; 4, pituitary gland; 5, internal carotid artery.

A recent cadaveric study assessed the anatomical aspects of the diaphragma, specifically its role in guiding the superior growth of a pituitary adenoma. Twenty cadaveric heads were dissected, with various measurements taken at the level of the diaphragma sella. The authors found the diaphragma to be composed of two layers of dura with the average anteroposterior diameter 7.26 mm (range 3.4 to 10.7 mm) and average lateral distance 7.33 mm (range 2.8 to 14.1 mm). This finding demonstrated the large variability in the size and shape of the diaphragmal opening, resulting in the corresponding growth of pituitary tumors into the suprasellar cistern. The authors also proposed a classification system of the diaphragma sella with respect to the central opening to classify the growth pattern of pituitary adenomas. Group A (20% of heads studied) has an opening of less than 4 mm, group B (40% of heads studied) has an opening of between 4 and 8 mm, and group C (40% of heads studied) has an opening of greater than 8 mm.[16]

Cavernous Sinus

The cavernous sinuses are located on the lateral aspects of the sphenoid sinus, sella, and pituitary gland. They extend from the superior orbital fissure anteriorly to the petrous apex posteriorly. The medial walls of the cavernous sinuses abut the lateral walls of the pituitary gland, usually separated by a single layer of dura (**Fig. 2.13A**). Besides extending superiorly through the diaphragmal opening, large pituitary adenomas can easily spread laterally into the cavernous sinuses. Pituitary adenomas do not spread inferiorly, anteriorly, or posteriorly, given the bony confines of the sella turcica.

The cavernous sinuses contain several neurovascular structures, including portions of the internal carotid artery. The internal carotid artery enters the cavernous sinus after the lateral bend (above the foramen lacerum), lateral to the posterior clinoid processes. The artery travels anteriorly and then superiorly, medial to the anterior clinoid processes, where it penetrates the roof of the cavernous sinus. The intracavernous carotid artery is fixed at multiple points, which include the proximal and distal dural rings (**Fig. 2.13B**).

Nerves in the cavernous sinus include the oculomotor nerve superiorly, followed by the trochlear nerve, the ophthalmic division of the trigeminal nerve, and the abducens nerves, from superior to inferior. The oculomotor, trochlear, and ophthalmic nerves lie between two dural leaves of the lateral sinus wall, whereas the abducens nerve lies in the cavernous sinus abutting the lateral wall of the carotid artery and the lateral aspect of the ophthalmic nerve. The oculomotor nerve enters the cavernous sinus lateral and anterior to the dorsum sellae, whereas the ophthalmic nerve enters inferiorly and travels upward to exit the superior orbital fissure. The abducens nerve penetrates the cavernous

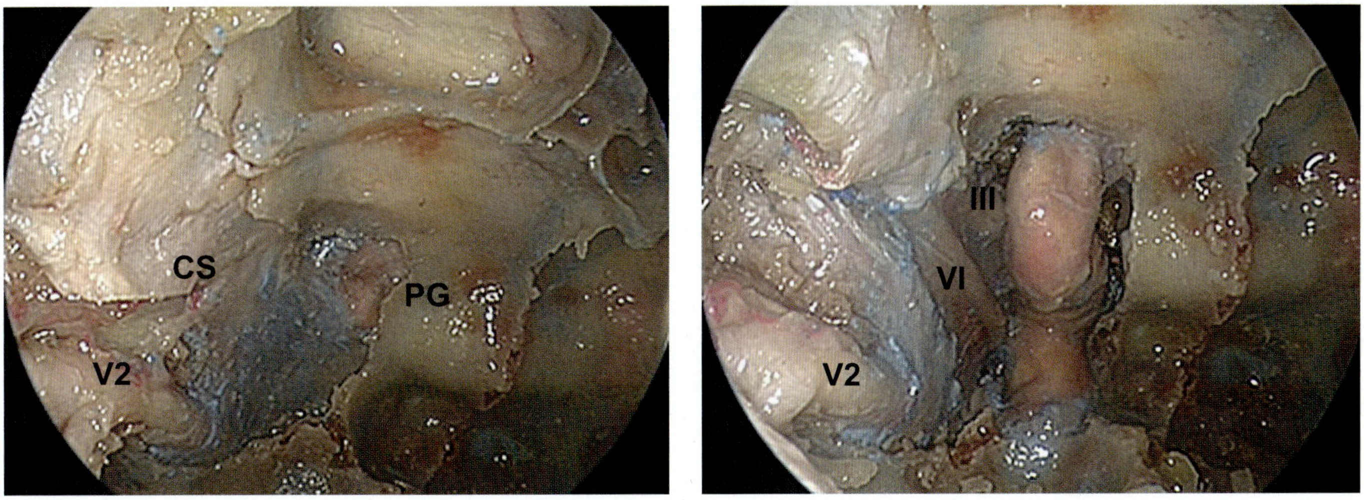

Fig. 2.13 (A) The cavernous sinus is separated by a single layer of dura from the lateral walls of the pituitary gland. **(B)** Neural and vascular structures, including the carotid artery traversing through the cavernous sinuses. CS, cavernous sinus; PG, pituitary gland; V2, maxillary nerve; III, oculomotor nerve; VI, abducens nerve.

sinus at the inferior and posterior border, bends around the intracavernous carotid, and runs parallel to the ophthalmic nerve (**Fig. 2.14**).

Several venous sinuses connect the bilateral cavernous sinuses, which are found around the diaphragma and pituitary gland. These intercavernous connections are named based on their location to the pituitary gland and may occur anterior, inferior, or posterior to the gland. The anterior intercavernous sinus passes anterior to the pituitary gland, and the posterior passes behind the hypophysis. The anterior intercavernous sinus is usually larger than its posterior counterpart and may sometimes cover the entire anterior part of the sella. This configuration can cause significant bleeding during a transsphenoidal surgery, although it is usually controlled with gentle prolonged pressure of the channel. When both the anterior and posterior intercavernous connections exist, the entire structure is called the circular sinus. The largest and most constant intercavernous sinus connection is the basilar sinus, which passes behind the dorsum sellae and upper clivus, connecting the posterior aspects of both cavernous sinuses. Multiple variations exist for intercavernous sinuses, which include combinations of anterior, posterior, and inferior connections or the complete absence of some or all of them (**Fig. 2.15**). Intercavernous

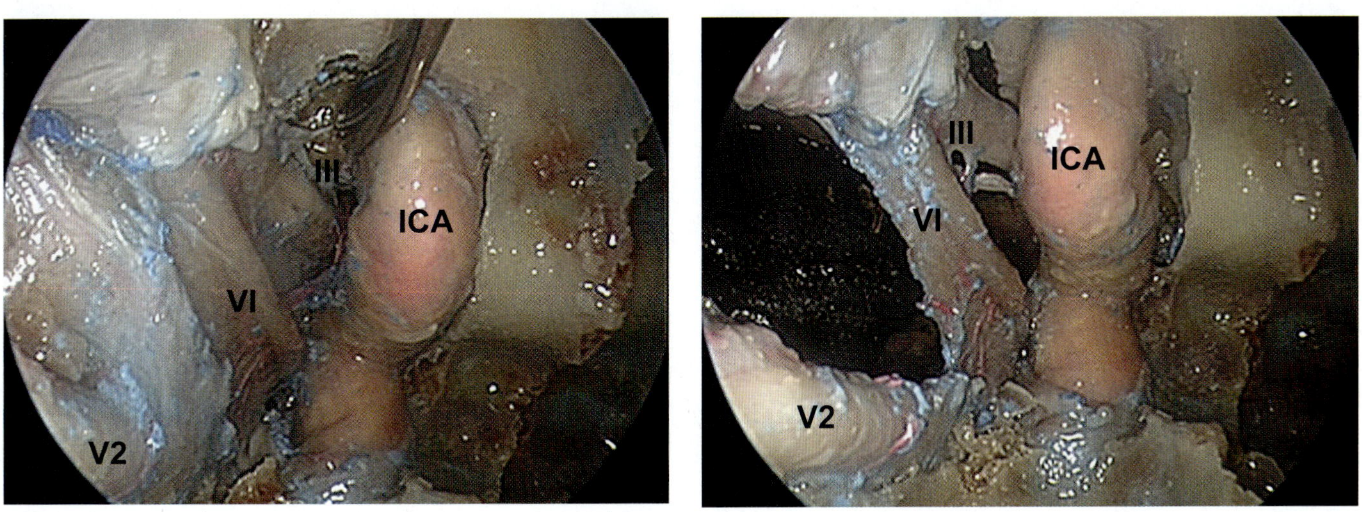

Fig. 2.14 (A,B) Neural structures traversing the cavernous sinus in the lateral wall of the sphenoid sinus. ICA, internal carotid artery; V2, maxillary nerve; III, oculomotor nerve; VI, abducens nerve.

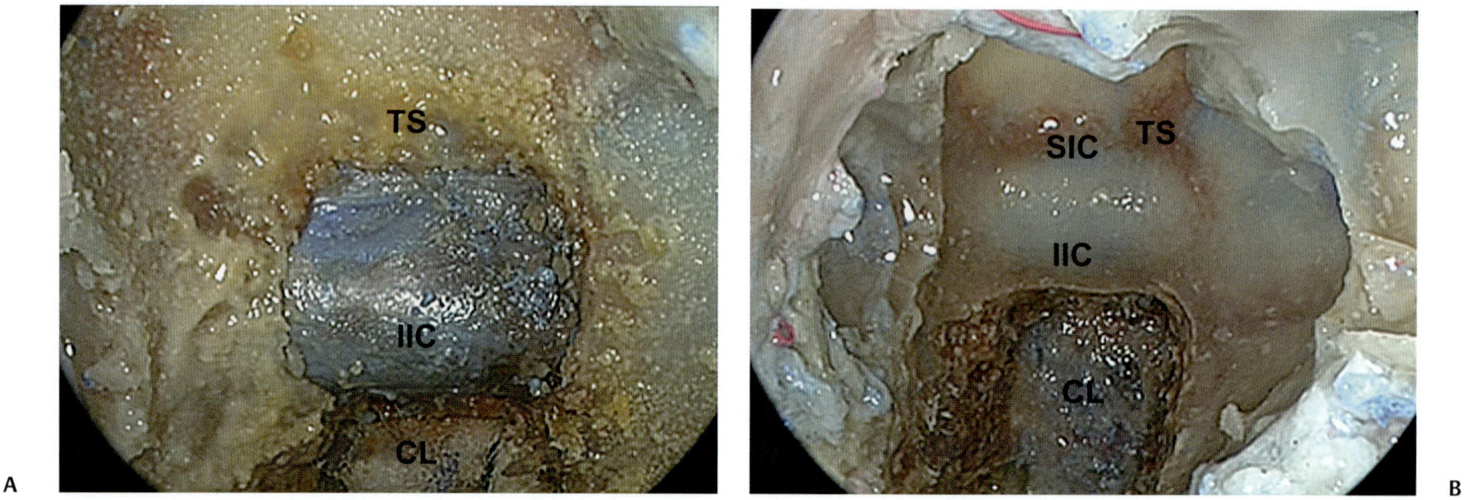

Fig. 2.15 **(A,B)** Intercavernous sinuses named based on their location to the pituitary gland. CL, clivus; IIC, inferior intercavernous sinus; SIC, superior inter cavernous sinus; TS, tuberculum sellae.

sinuses are named based on their location in relation to the pituitary gland.[7,17]

Vascular Anatomy Sella Region

The vast majority of blood supply to the sellar region is derived from the intracavernous portion of the internal carotid artery. The meningohypophyseal artery is the largest intercavernous carotid artery branch, and it exits the carotid at the level of the dorsum sellae just before the carotid turns anteriorly after leaving the carotid canal. The inferior hypophyseal artery originates from the meningohypophyseal trunk, travels medially, and supplies the posterior pituitary. This artery also anastomoses with its counterpart from the opposite side, and together they supply the dura of the sellar floor. Another artery, when present, arises from the medial side of the carotid artery and supplies the capsule of the gland and dura lining the anterior and inferior walls of the sella protuberance. The superior hypophyseal artery exits the carotid artery in the supraclinoid region, runs medially below the floor of the third ventricle, and connects with its counterpart on the contralateral side to form a vascular ring around the infundibulum. This branch also provides vascular supply to the optic nerve, chiasm, optic tract, infundibulum, and floor of the third ventricle[15] (**Fig. 2.16**).

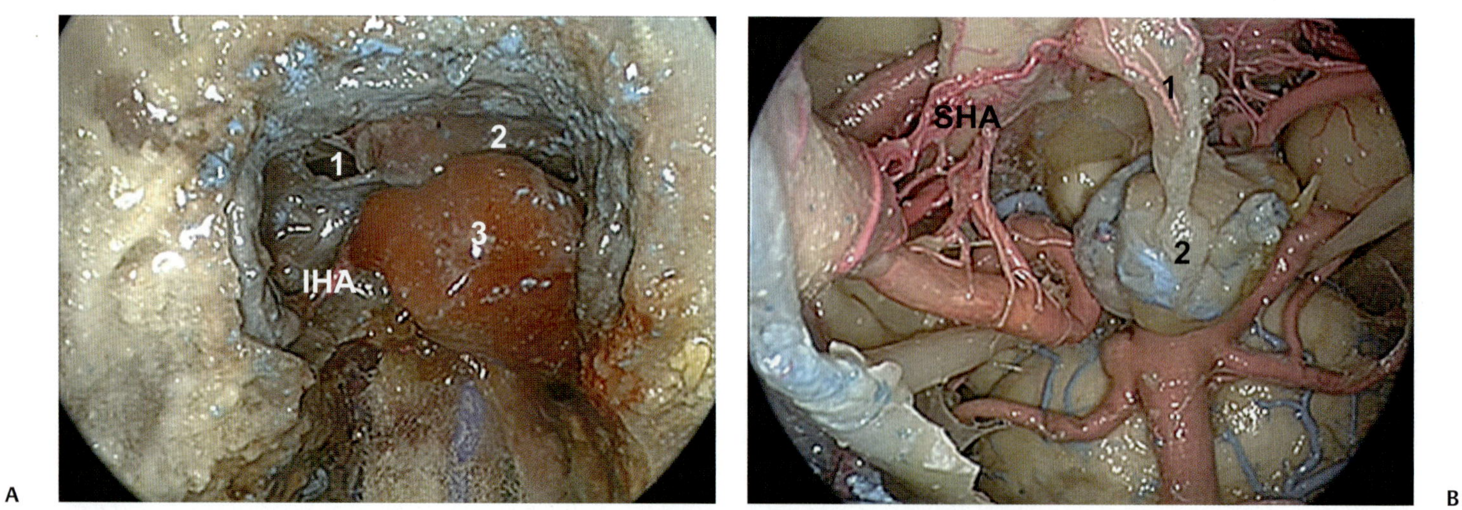

Fig. 2.16 **(A,B)** Endoscopic images demonstrating the vascular supply to the sella from branches off the intercavernous portion of the carotid artery. IHA, inferior hypophyseal artery; SHA, superior hypophyseal; 1, diaphragmal opening; 2, pituitary stalk; 3, pituitary gland.

Suprasellar Anatomy

Tumors originating from the sella such as pituitary adenomas often extend into the suprasellar cistern and the floor of the third ventricle. The suprasellar anatomy superior to the pituitary fossa has been described by Perneczky as an equilateral pyramid. The anterior wall is composed of the optic nerves, anterior optic chiasm, lamina terminalis, anterior cerebral arteries, and their communicating branches. The lateral walls are composed of the internal carotid arteries, optic tracts, anterior choroidal vessels, and posterior cerebral arteries. The posterior wall is composed of the mesencephalon, basilar artery, posterior cerebral and superior cerebellar vessels, and oculomotor nerves. The infundibulum and stalk of the pituitary form the vertical axis of the pyramid. Knowledge of this pyramid aids the endoscopic surgeon in conceptualizing the anatomical relationship of neurovascular structures during pituitary or anterior endoscopic skull base surgery.[8,18] (**Fig. 2.17**).

The optic nerves, oculomotor nerves, and olfactory tracts pass through the suprasellar region and anterior incisural space. The anterior incisural space is located between the free edges of the tentorium and the anterior part of the midbrain, roughly corresponding to the suprasellar region. The optic nerves exit the optic canals medial to the anterior clinoid processes and are directed posteriorly, medially, and superiorly toward the optic chiasm. The optic tracts leave the optic chiasm and travel posteriorly and laterally around the cerebral peduncles to enter the middle incisural space. The optic chiasm is located at the junction of the anterior wall (lamina terminalis) and the floor of the third ventricle. Major structures situated superior to the optic chiasm are the anterior cerebral and anterior communicating arteries, lamina terminalis, and third ventricle. Inferior to the optic chiasm lies the diaphragma sellae and pituitary gland, laterally lie the internal carotid arteries, and posterior-inferiorly lies the infundibulum. The infundibular recess and median eminence lie at the base of pituitary stalk behind the chiasm.

The relationship of the optic chiasm, pituitary gland, and infundibulum is important for transcranial and transsphenoidal routes to the hypophysis. Three different patterns exist: normal, pre-fixed, and post-fixed. Normally, the chiasm lies above the diaphragma and pituitary gland. The pre-fixed chiasm is situated anteriorly above the tuberculum sellae, and the post-fixed chiasm is located above the dorsum sellae. The majority of patients exhibit the normal chiasmal configuration, whereas the pre-fixed and post-fixed patterns are each noted 10 to 15% of the time. A pre-fixed configuration, a normal pattern with a small space between the tuberculum and chiasm, and prominent tuberculum sellae would restrict access to the suprasellar cistern via the transsphenoidal route. Conversely, the same chiasmal patterns would pose little difficulty in accessing the suprasellar cistern if the approach were done transcranially[5,15] (**Fig. 2.17**).[5]

Several other cranial nerves are encountered in the suprasellar region and warrant mention because they may be involved during dissection of large pituitary adenomas. The oculomotor nerve originates from the midbrain on the medial portion of the cerebral peduncle and passes through the posterior cerebral and superior cerebellar arteries. The oculomotor nerve travels through the interpeduncular cistern, pierces the roof of the cavernous sinus, and travels posteriorly in the superior and lateral corner of the cavernous sinus. The trochlear nerve also arises in the midbrain below

A

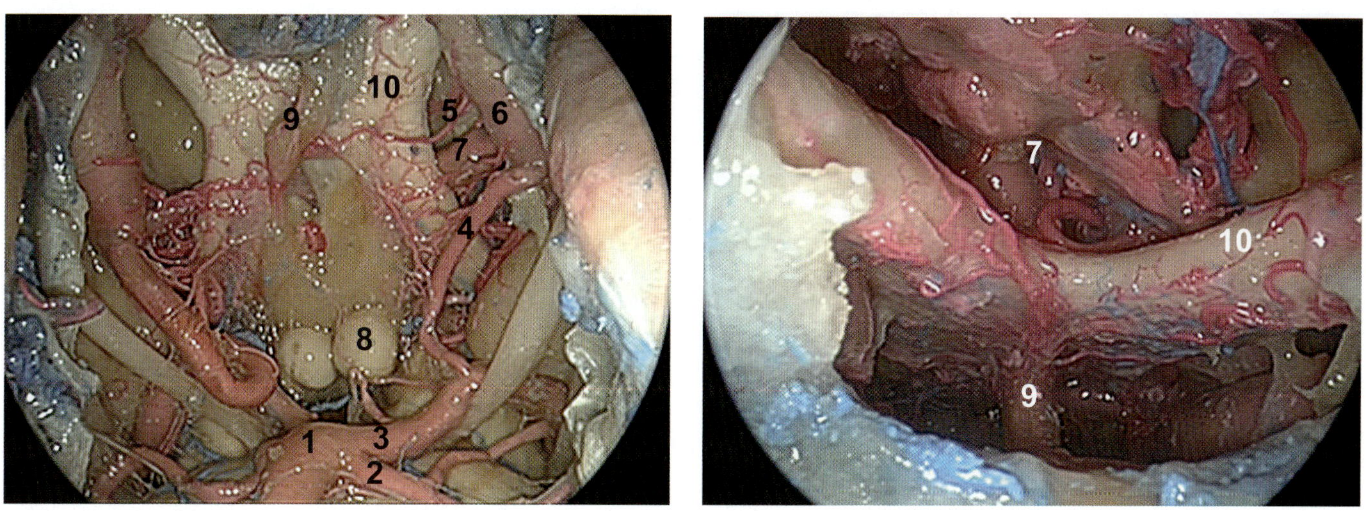

B

Fig. 2.17 **(A,B)** Suprasellar anatomy demonstrating the various neural, vascular, and cerebral anatomical units contributing to Perneczky's. triangle 1, basilar tip; 2, superior cerebellar artery; 3, posterior cerebellar artery; 4, posterior communicating artery; 5, superior hypophyseal artery; 6, supraclinoid internal carotid artery; 7, anterior cerebral artery; 8, mamillary bodies; 9, pituitary stalk; 10, optic nerves; 11, oculomotor nerve.

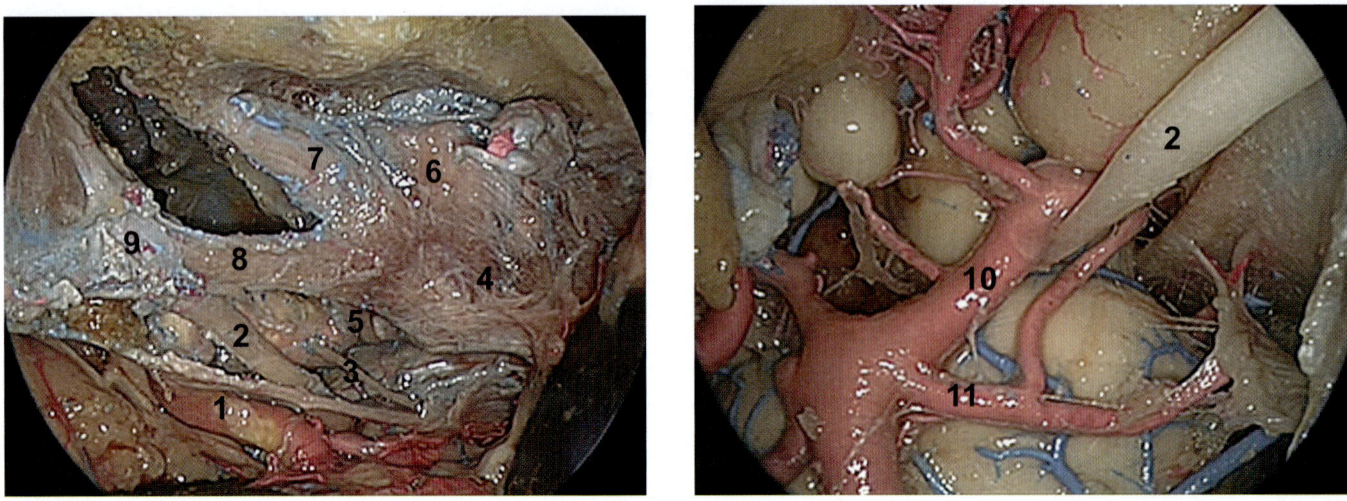

A B

Fig. 2.18 (A,B) Transnasal endoscopic suprasellar anatomy. 1, supraclinoid internal carotid artery; 2, oculomotor nerve; 3, trochlear nerve; 4, trigeminal ganglion; 5, abducens nerve; 6, VI; 7, V2; 8, V3; 9, superior orbital fissure; 10, posterior cerebral artery; 11, superior cerebral artery.

the inferior colliculus, travels contralaterally, in the ambient and crural cisterns around the midbrain, and enters the cavernous sinus behind the anterior tentorial attachment. The abducens nerve originates at the lower edge of the pons and then passes either above or below the anteroinferior cerebellar artery. It travels through the prepontine cistern to the upper border of the petrous apex to the Dorello canal, finally entering the posterior-inferior part of the cavernous sinus. The branches of the trigeminal nerve, namely the ophthalmic, maxillary, and mandibular, arise from the pons and divide at the anterior edge of the trigeminal ganglion. The ophthalmic nerve travels in the lower anterior portion of the cavernous sinus, and the maxillary nerve runs under the cavernous sinus in the lateral wall of the sphenoid sinus (**Fig. 2.18**).

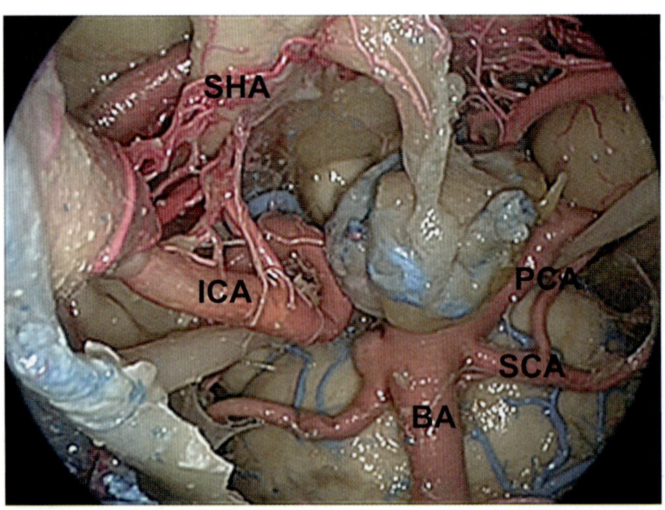

Fig. 2.19 Anterior and posterior vascular anatomy in the suprasellar region. BA, basilar artery; ICA, internal carotid artery; PCA, posterior cerebral artery; SCA, superior cerebral artery; SHA, superior hypophyseal artery.

Vascular Relationships of the Suprasellar Region

The circle of Willis and its vascular components are contained in the suprasellar region. Dissection in this area is particularly challenging, not only because of the large number of vessels that may abut a tumor, but also because of the serious consequences that accompany vascular compromise. All arteries of the circle of Willis as well as segments of the carotid and basilar systems can be seen stretched across suprasellar components of pituitary tumors. The third ventricle is closely associated with several of these vessels as well. The anterior circle of Willis, anterior cerebral, and anterior communicating arteries are adjacent to the anterior wall of the third ventricle. The posterior circle of Willis and the apex of the basilar artery are situated just inferior to the floor of the third ventricle (**Fig. 2.19**).

The internal carotid artery and its perforating branches supply the optic nerve, chiasm, optic tract, infundibulum, and floor of the third ventricle. The superior hypophyseal artery exits the carotid artery in the supraclinoid region, runs medially below the floor of the third ventricle, and connects with its counterpart on the contralateral side to form a vascular ring around the infundibulum. The ophthalmic artery, the first branch of the internal carotid artery, arises and enters the optic canal below the optic nerve. It typically arises from the supraclinoid portion of the carotid artery but sometimes (20%) comes from the

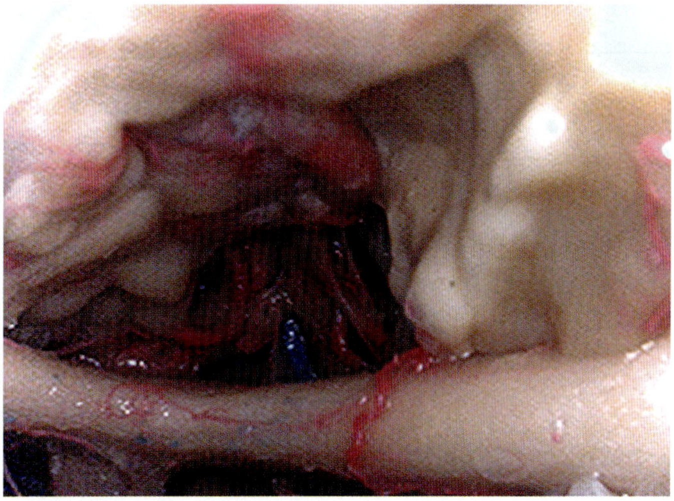

Fig. 2.20 Anterior cerebral artery circulation.

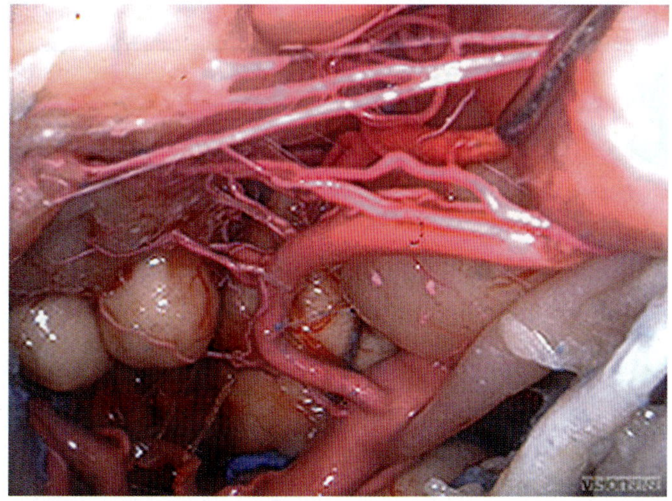

Fig. 2.21 Anterior choroidal artery.

intracavernous carotid and rarely as a branch of the middle meningeal artery.

The anterior cerebral artery comes from the internal carotid artery and runs anteromedially above the optic nerve and chiasm, connecting with its contralateral counterpart via the anterior communicating artery near the interhemispheric fissure. The confluence of the anterior communicating artery with bilateral A1 segments typically lies right above the chiasm. Shorter A1 segments are usually found above the chiasm, whereas large A1 segment are located above the optic nerves. The anterior cerebral and anterior communicating arteries give off branches that supply the hypothalamus and fornix.[5,11] (**Fig. 2.20**).

The posterior communicating artery originates from the posterior wall of the internal carotid artery and travels posteromedially below the optic tracts and floor of the third ventricle to join the posterior cerebral artery. Its branches supply the optic chiasm in addition to the thalamus, hypothalamus, and internal capsule. The anterior choroidal artery arises from the posterior aspect of the internal carotid artery above the origin of the posterior communicating artery. It travels posterolaterally below the optic tract between the uncus and cerebral peduncle and supplies the optic tract, posterior part of the third ventricle, posterior limb of the internal capsule, and medial temporal lobe structures (**Fig. 2.21**).

Venous channels in the suprasellar region are small and do not typically cause significant bleeding. The suprasellar region is usually drained by tributaries of the basal vein of Rosenthal, which is formed by a confluence of veins draining the suprasellar area. These veins travel between the midbrain and temporal lobes and form a confluence with the internal cerebral vein to form the vein of Galen.

Conclusion

Anatomical relationships in the parasellar region have been well studied and described. Endoscopic approaches to this region and the anterior skull base have encouraged surgeons to study this anatomy in a different light, emphasizing a separate subset of anatomical principles that have been extensively studied and described in the past. A thorough knowledge and command of parasellar anatomy are important for all pituitary surgeons, especially an ability to rotate these complex three-dimensional structures in the mind's eye.

References

1. Powell M, Lightman SL, Laws ER. Management of Pituitary Tumors: The Clinician's Practical Guide. Totowa, NJ: Humana Press; 2003
2. Cappabianca P, de Divitiis E. Endoscopy and transsphenoidal surgery. Neurosurgery 2004;54:1043–1048, 1048–1050
3. Rhoton AL, Natori Y. The Orbit and Sellar Region: Microsurgical Anatomy and Operative Approaches. New York: Thieme; 1996
4. Anand VK, Panje WR. Anatomy and Surgical Landmarks in Endoscopic Sinus Surgery. Practical Endoscopic Sinus Surgery. New York: McGraw-Hill, Health Professions Division; 1993
5. Rhoton AL Jr. The anterior and middle cranial base. Neurosurgery 2002;51(4, Suppl):S273–S302
6. Van Alyea OE. Nasal Sinuses—An Anatomic and Clinical Consideration, 2nd ed. Baltimore: Williams & Wilkins; 1951
7. Renn WH, Rhoton AL Jr. Microsurgical anatomy of the sellar region. J Neurosurg 1975;43:288–298
8. Anand VK, Schwartz TH. Practical Anatomy of the Sinuses and Anterior Skull Base. Practical Endoscopic Skull Base Surgery. San Diego: Plural Publishing; 2007

9. Hamid O, El Fiky L, Hassan O, Kotb A, El Fiky S. Anatomic variations of the sphenoid sinus and their impact on trans-sphenoid pituitary surgery. Skull Base 2008;18:9–15
10. Sirikci A, Bayazit YA, Bayram M, Mumbuç S, Güngör K, Kanlikama M. Variations of sphenoid and related structures. Eur Radiol 2000;10: 844–848
11. Herzallah IR, Casiano RR. Endoscopic endonasal study of the internal carotid artery course and variations. Am J Rhinol 2007;21: 262–270
12. Alfieri A, Jho HD. Endoscopic endonasal cavernous sinus surgery: an anatomic study. Neurosurgery 2001;48:827–836, discussion 836–837
13. Kassam A, Snyderman CH, Mintz A, Gardner P, Carrau RL. Expanded endonasal approach: the rostrocaudal axis. Part I. Crista galli to the sella turcica. Neurosurg Focus 2005;19:E3
14. Vescan AD, Snyderman CH, Carrau RL, et al. Vidian canal: analysis and relationship to the internal carotid artery. Laryngoscope 2007;117:1338–1342
15. Rhoton AL Jr. The sellar region. Neurosurgery 2002;51(4, Suppl):S335–S374
16. Campero A, Martins C, Yasuda A, Rhoton AL Jr. Microsurgical anatomy of the diaphragma sellae and its role in directing the pattern of growth of pituitary adenomas. Neurosurgery 2008;62:717–723, discussion 717–723
17. Yasuda A, Campero A, Martins C, Rhoton AL Jr, de Oliveira E, Ribas GC. Microsurgical anatomy and approaches to the cavernous sinus. Neurosurgery 2008; 62(6, Suppl 3):1240–1263
18. Perneczky A, Tschabitscher M, Resch KDM. Endoscopic Anatomy for Neurosurgery. Stuttgart, New York: Thieme; 1993

3 Endoscopic Equipment

Paolo Cappabianca, Luigi M. Cavallo, Felice Esposito, and Matteo G. De Notaris

The transsphenoidal midline route represents the standard approach to the pituitary and sella and is indicated for more than 95% of surgical procedures in this region. The success of the transsphenoidal route is dependent not only on its versatility as an approach to a wide variety of lesions of the sellar area but also on the following factors: (1) it is the least traumatic route to the sella; (2) it avoids any brain retraction and visible scars; (3) it provides excellent visualization of the pituitary gland and related pathology; (4) it offers a lower morbidity and mortality rate as compared with transcranial procedures; and (5) it allows a shorter hospital stay. Based on these advantages of transsphenoidal surgery in combination with the continuous search for less invasive procedures and the development of endoscopic equipment, endoscopic endonasal transsphenoidal surgery slowly and inexorably became an accepted technique in the field of pituitary surgery during the last decade of the twentieth century.[1–4]

As a result of renewed anatomic interest in both the endonasal approach and the anatomy of the skull base, endoscopy has been able to contribute to a better understanding and wider application of the transsphenoidal approach. This approach can be routinely used not only for all sellar lesions but also for extrasellar lesions, based on the increased visualization it affords. The endoscopic approach to the anterior skull base has motivated several anatomical studies and led to enhancements in a variety of procedures.[5–9] Modifications of the standard transsphenoidal approach that allow additional exposure of the perisellar areas have been used for various skull base lesions. Extended approaches, aimed not only at the pituitary, but also at extrasellar compartments, from the frontal sinus all the way down to the craniovertebral junction, have been successfully performed to provide access to a variety of lesions affecting the entire midline skull base.[10–13] Thus, endonasal approaches, once utilized for access to sellar and intra- and suprasellar subdiaphragmatic lesions only, are used today even more frequently for lesions located beyond the sella. Previously, such lesions would have been considered accessible by only transcranial approaches. An increasing number of clinical series on these extended approaches are now appearing in the literature, and guidelines for performing these techniques are being reported.[10,14–19]

Nevertheless, other factors have contributed to determine the success of the endoscopic skull base surgery. The fact that the operation itself has become increasingly simple, safe, and elegant is unimaginable without appropriate instrumentation.[20] Every operation, and every technique for each type of operation, requires a dedicated set of instruments. Endoscopic skull base surgery, as with any other type of endoscopic surgery, requires that all the instrumentation and tools—endoscope, camera, light source, monitor, videorecording systems, drills, etc.—be of the best quality possible and be dedicated to this type of operation. The instruments form a sort of chain, where each link must be strong enough to perform its role in the operation; otherwise the chain will break and the surgery will not be successful.

The Dedicated Operating Room

The operating room itself can be considered a surgical instrument (**Fig. 3.1**). An integrated operating room helps to optimize teamwork and improve patient care.[10,21] In the operating room, all of the equipment, such as the cold light source, video camera, monitor, and video recording system, are placed ergonomically behind the head of the patient and in front of the operating surgeon, who is at the right side of the patient. The anesthesiologist is positioned with his or her equipment at the left side of the patient at the level of the head. The second surgeon is at the left side of the patient, and the scrub nurse is positioned at the level of the patient's legs.

The main characteristics of this operating room are (1) compartmentalization of sterile and nonsterile activities, (2) fluidity of the workflow during the procedure, and (3) optimal access to the patient in case of emergency. The operating room control interface is user friendly, and its use creates a great sense of camaraderie among surgeons, anesthesiologists, and nurses.

Thanks to communication technology, the operating room may become a world surgical amphitheater, in that the Internet allows the real-time, two-way transmission of digital encrypted data throughout the world.

During surgical procedures the archiving system is an efficient and inexpensive mechanism for storing and analyzing neurosurgical images. All patient data collected during the operation are transmitted and stored for future reference; they are easily accessible, strictly confidential, and manipulation safe.

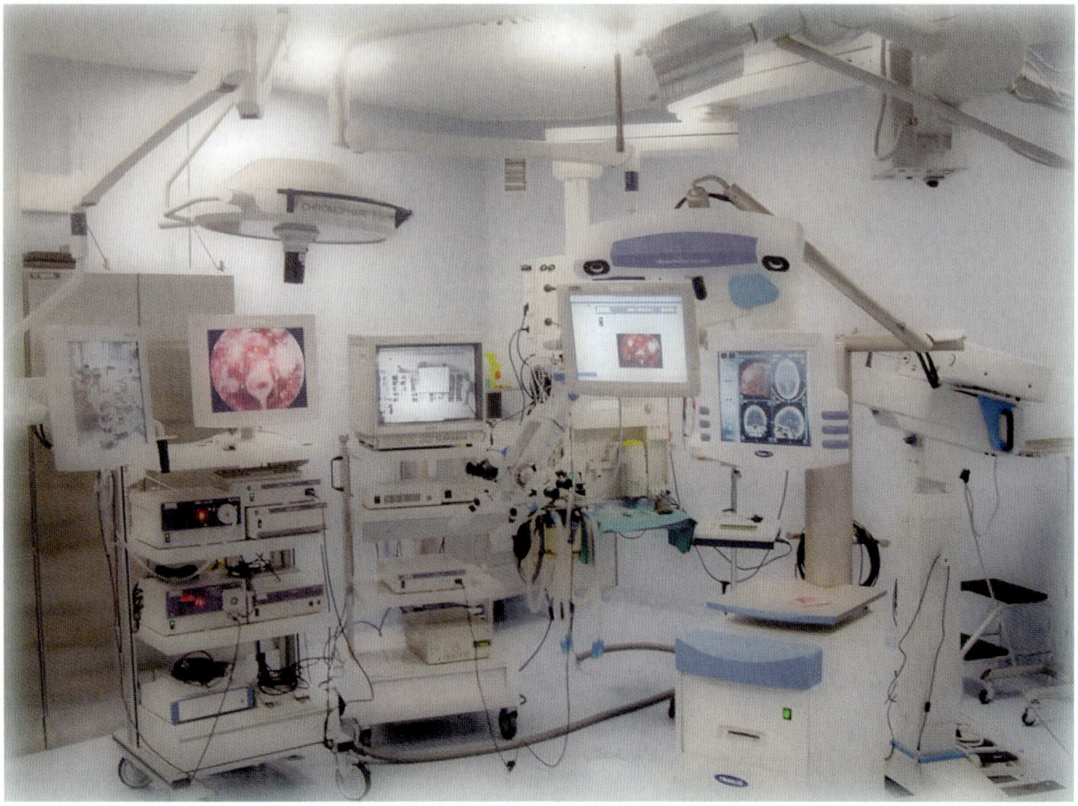

Fig. 3.1 The integrated operating room (OR1; Karl Storz, Tuttlingen, Germany) currently used at the Division of Neurosurgery of the Università degli Studi di Napoli Federico II.

The Endoscope

There could not be any endoscopic surgery without the endoscope. Such a tool permits access to deep anatomic structures in a minimally invasive manner. It enables the visualization of deep, hidden structures in the brain and transmits clear and usable images to the surgeon. It increases the precision of the surgery and permits the surgeon to differentiate tissues so that selective removal of the lesion can be achieved.[20–22]

In general, endoscopes are classified as either fiberoptic endoscopes (fiberscopes) or rod-lens endoscopes. Endoscopes specifically designed for neuroendoscopy can be classified into four types: (1) rigid fiberscopes, (2) rigid rod-lens endoscopes, (3) flexible endoscopes, and (4) steerable fiberscopes.[20,21,23] These different endoscopes have different diameters, lengths, optical quality, and number and diameter of working channels, all of which vary with size. The choice between them should be made on the basis of the surgical indication and personal preference of the surgeon.

For endoscopic skull base surgery, the best endoscopes are rigid rod-lens scopes. Their main advantage is the better quality of vision as compared with other types of scopes. They enable the surgeon to remain oriented because of the panoramic view and permit the other instruments to be inserted alongside it. Rod-lens endoscopes consist of three main parts: a mechanical shaft, glass fiber bundles for light illumination, and optics (objective, eyepiece, relay system). The angle of view of rod-lens ranges from 0 to 120 degrees, according to the objective, but an angled objective of more than 30 degrees is used only for diagnostic or visualizing purposes. The most frequently used angles are 0, 30, and 45 degrees. The 0-degree objective provides a frontal view of the surgical field and minimizes the risk of disorientation. It is used during the majority of the operation. The advantages of the 30-degree angle is that this type of endoscope, through the rotation of the lens, increases the surface area of the field of view. Moreover, visualization of the instruments is improved as they converge toward the center of image, whereas with the 0-degree objective the instruments remain in the periphery of the image.

The endoscope is used through a sheath, which is connected to a cleaning system. The irrigation system permits

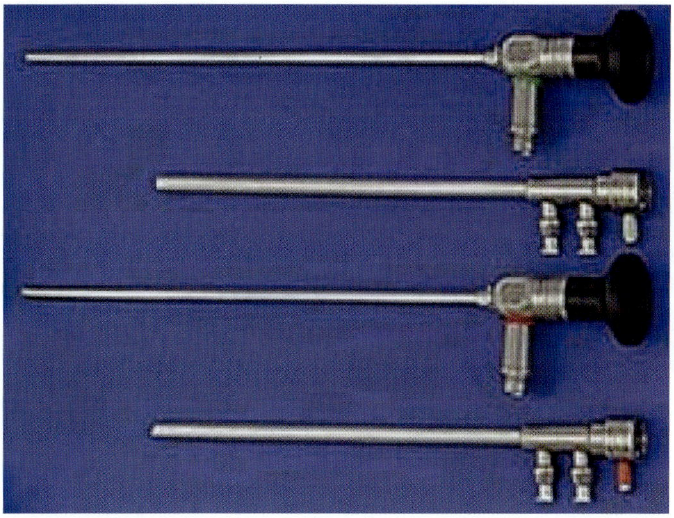

Fig. 3.2 Rigid rod-lens 4-mm endoscope without working channels used during the endoscopic endonasal transsphenoidal surgery. The length of the endoscope is 18 or 30 cm (Karl Storz, Tuttlingen, Germany).

cleaning and defogging of the distal lens, thus avoiding the repeated insertion and removal of the endoscope from the nostril. The endoscopes used for endonasal surgery are without any working channel (diagnostic endoscopes), and the other instruments are inserted into the same nostril, slid alongside the sheath, or inserted into the contralateral nostril. The diameter of rod-lens endoscopes varies between 1.9 and 10 mm, but for endonasal surgery usually only endoscopes with a diameter of 4 mm are used (**Fig. 3.2**). In selected patients with narrow nostrils and in children, a 2.7-mm endoscope can be used. The endoscope in skull base surgery can be used free-hand or fixed to a scope holder. During the first step of the operation (the approach itself), it is better to use the endoscope free-hand, so that the surgeon can dynamically handle the various instruments while creating the working space for the further steps of the procedure. The endoscope can then either continue to be used free-hand or be fixed to a scope holder. For the free-hand technique, the scope is used in a dynamic fashion and the surgeon continuously receives feedback about the anatomy and depth of the operative field based on the in-and-out movements of the scope. If a scope holder is used, a variety of systems exist. Variables include a steerable or extendable arm and a rigid or jointed arm that can be straight, curved, or pneumatic. With such devices, the endoscope is fixed in a particular position, and the surgeon can use both hands to manipulate the surgical instrumentation. Another possibility is to have the endoscope held by an assistant. With this method the dynamic movements of the scope are preserved and, at the same time, the surgeon can simultaneously use two instruments either in the same nostril or in both nostrils.

The Video Camera and Monitor

Although the surgeon can theoretically look directly into the ocular lens (proximal lens) of the endoscope, the operation cannot be easily and safely performed in this manner.[24] In fact, if the surgeon had to remain in a fixed position, surgical movements would be impaired. To properly maneuver the instruments under fine control, the endoscope is connected to a dedicated video camera, and the endoscopic images are projected onto a monitor placed in front of the surgeon. Additional monitors can be placed in varying locations in the operating room, as well as outside in the hallways or adjacent rooms, to permit other members of the team to watch the surgery.

Several types of endoscopic video cameras are available, the most common of which utilize a 3-CCD (charge-coupled device) sensor. Although the 1-CCD cameras process all three fundamental colors in one chip, the 3-CCD ones have a separate chip for each color (red, green, blue; RGB) and provide better color separation, more brilliant colors, and a sharper image with higher contrast.[25] Buttons located on the camera control the focus and the zoom. Optical zoom is preferable because it enlarges the image using the same number of pixels, whereas the electronic zoom increases the size of each pixel, which degrades the definition of the image. Most modern endoscopic cameras are analogue. This means that the signal is transmitted to a central processing unit, which outputs the signals in RGB, S-video, or Composite video formats. Digital 3-CCD endoscope cameras are available, which produce the highest quality images that can be directly connected to video recorders for high-quality video reproduction.

The images produced by the endoscope camera are displayed on one or more monitors. These need to have a high-resolution screen to support the signal quality arising from the camera. The monitors most commonly used in endoscopic surgery have a minimum horizontal resolution of 750 lines, to visualize all the details of the endoscopic images.

A further improvement of the resolution of both the video cameras and the monitors is represented by the high-definition television technology, which is ready for the future three-dimensional (3D) endoscopes. As a matter of fact, the continuous improvements in endoscopic image quality offer excellent visualization of the operative field, of the lesion, and of its relationships with the surrounding anatomical structures. A full high-definition (HD) 16:9 flat monitor (1080p60) (**Fig. 3.3A**) needs to be coupled with the HD camera (**Fig. 3.3B**) to visualize the HD images.

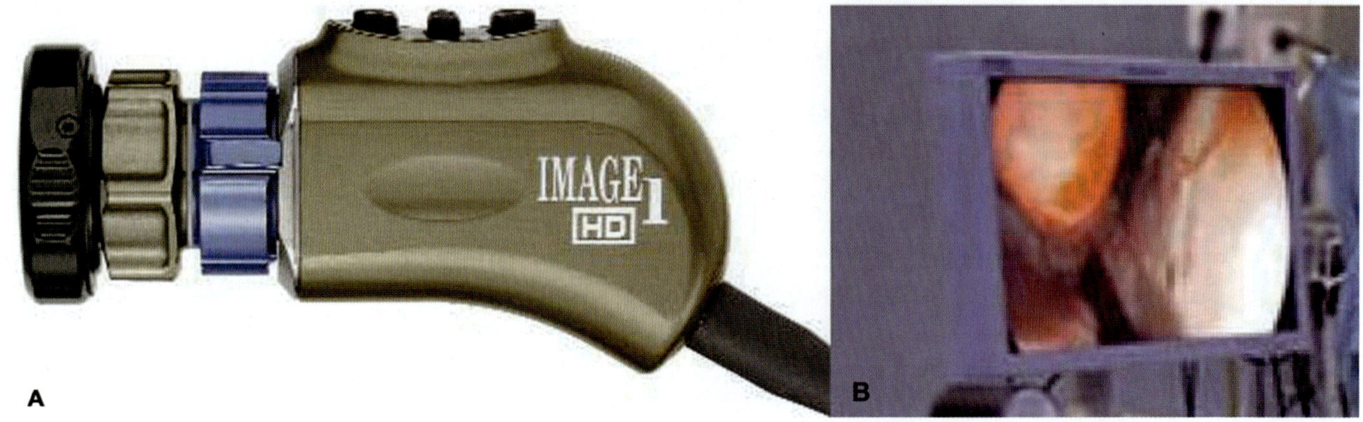

Fig. 3.3 **(A)** HD camera. **(B)** Full high-definition (HD) 16:9 flat monitor (1080p60). (Karl Storz, Tuttlingen, Germany).

The Light Source

The endoscope transmits cold light, which arises from a source inside the surgical field through a connecting cable made of glass fibers. Currently in endoscopic surgery, xenon light sources are used that have spectral characteristics similar to sunlight, with a color temperature of approximately 6000 kelvin (K), which is "whiter" than the classic halogen light (3400 K).[22] The power of the unit is commonly 300 watts. The flexible connecting cable is made of a bundle of glass fibers that brings the light to the endoscope, virtually without dispersion of visible light. Furthermore, the heat (composed by infrared light) is poorly transmitted by the glass fibers, thus reducing the risk of burning the tissues.

Video Documentation

Documentation and storage of intraoperative images and movie clips are of increasing importance for education and documentation. Although video recording is not mandatory, having the possibility to document either still images or video clips of the surgical procedure is very important for a number of reasons: (1) to review the operation, and, if any mistakes are made, learn how to avoid them in the future; (2) to obtain images for publication or produce video clips to teach residents, courses attendees, etc.; (3) to store images in an electronic library; and (4) to use the material for legal purposes.

Several systems are available to document endoscopic surgical operations. Any one of several film or digital cameras, analogue or digital VCRs, mass memory, or CD- or DVD-based systems can store and even improve the images coming from the video camera and prepare the video material for postprocessing. Such systems can be connected to dedicated devices to route the images or videos for a complete digital exchange, for computer or video streaming or teleconferencing, or for e-learning, e-teaching, or tele-counseling. Furthermore, it is possible for the modern integrated operating rooms to share digital images and video by simply pressing a touch screen, which can even be done by the surgeon while operating.

The Neuronavigator System

The neuronavigator consists of a personal computer, a multi-joint sensing arm, and an image scanner. The 3D coordinates of the arm tip are always monitored by the computer and are automatically translated into computed tomography/magnetic resonance imaging (CT/MRI) coordinates and finally displayed with a cursor on the CT/MRI images on the computer screen. The basic function of the navigator is to obtain the location of the arm tip within a surgical field and to translate it into the CT/MRI coordinates. The patient's head should initially be related to the CT/MRI coordinates. The relationship is established using a set of fiducial points on the patient's head.

Preoperative CT/MRI is taken with small metal or oil balls taped on the patient's forehead. After the introduction of general anesthesia, the patient's head is firmly held by a three-pin head holder, as in conventional craniotomy. The navigator arm is then secured to the head holder. The locations of the skin markers are automatically registered to the computer. The location of the navigator tip is thereafter automatically converted into the CT/MRI coordinates and projected onto the corresponding CT/MRI slice on the computer screen represented by cross-shaped cursors. The system thus provides information on the location of the instruments in terms of CT/MRI coordinates, which guides the surgeon during the operation.

In endoscopic endonasal skull base surgery, image-guided neuronavigation systems are very useful for intraoperative identification of the limits of the lesion and of the bony, vascular, and nervous structures, especially if they are encased by the tumor.[10] In some select cases, the classic landmarks for endoscopic transsphenoidal surgery (sellar floor, clival indentation, carotid and optic nerve protuberances, opticocarotid recess) are not easily identifiable, and neuronavigation can help to maintain the surgeon's orientation even in the presence of distorted anatomy (**Fig. 3.4**). However, the use of such devices requires the head of the patient to be fixed in the three-pin skeletal fixation headrest to render the head of the patient fixed with the reference system. Some authors use the three-pin headrest not fixed to the surgical table, but rather the head is actually placed in the horseshoe headrest.[26] The neuronavigation systems and the panoramic view provided by the endoscope also make it possible to do without the use of fluoroscopy, thus avoiding unnecessary radiation exposure to the patient and the surgical team.

Bleeding Control

One of the most cumbersome problems in endoscopic surgery is the control of bleeding. Monopolar coagulation is easy because it can be simply performed inside the nasal cavity with the use of monopolar sticks, and it is usually quite effective. Some monopolars are incorporated with a

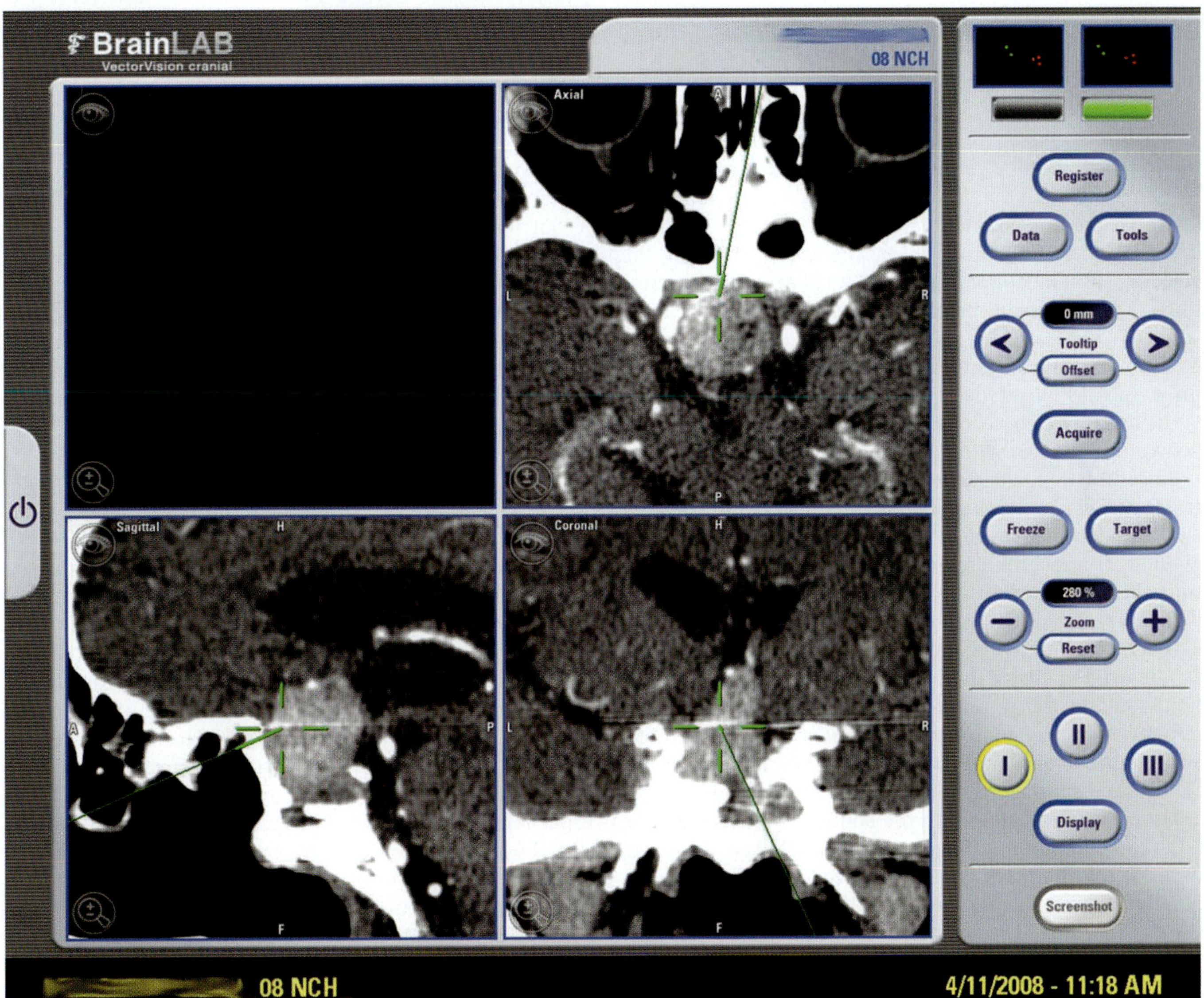

Fig. 3.4 Neuronavigation system used in selected pituitary surgery cases or in extended endoscopic endonasal operations (courtesy of BrainLAB AG GmBH, Feldkirchen, Germany).

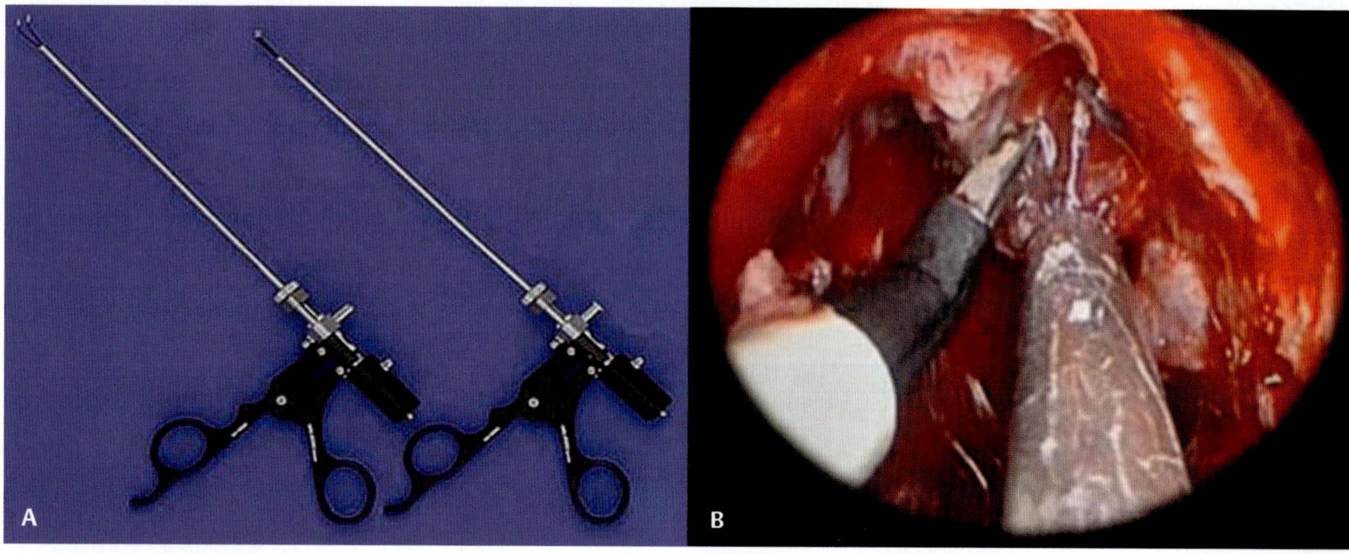

Fig. 3.5 (A,B) Endonasal dedicated Kassam's bipolar forceps (Karl Storz, Tuttlingen, Germany).

suction cannula to aspirate the smoke during coagulation, to maintain a clear surgical field. However, monopolar cautery does not prevent late rebleeding (usually after 7 to 15 days). Once the scar produced by the cautery falls off, the bleeding (usually of the mucosa or small arterial branches) starts again.[27] Furthermore, monopolar coagulation must be avoided to prevent damaging the olfactory fibers in the nasal mucosa, which is close to major neurovascular structures, such as on the posterior wall of the sphenoid sinus, in the intradural space, or in proximity to nerve or vascular bony protuberances within the sphenoid sinus.

In contrast, bipolar forceps represent the most adaptive and functional tool available to the neurosurgeon. They not only provide bipolar coagulation, but also constitute the main instrument of dissection. This feature particularly suits them for opening arachnoid planes, separating membranes, grasping small tumor tissue from the normal brain parenchyma, and dissecting blood vessels. The bipolar unit can be used to coagulate in areas where unipolar coagulation would be dangerous, for instance, near neurovascular structures. In general, bipolar coagulation is preferable, either alone or in association with hemostatic agents. The use of the microsurgical bipolar forceps, developed for the microscope, is not feasible with the endoscope. Consequently, different endonasal bipolar forceps have been designed, with various diameters and lengths, that have proven to be quite effective in bipolar control of bleeding. Endoscopic surgery requires bipolar forceps with special features: (1) they have to be easily introduced in the nasal cavity; (2) the tips of the forceps have to be adequately isolated; and (3) they must be safe. For the purposes of endonasal endoscopic surgery, the bipolar forceps has the same shape as forceps with ring handles, like scissors. The movement of the handles causes the tips to open and close and, eventually, to coagulate (**Fig. 3.5**).

Furthermore, new coagulating instruments, either monopolar and bipolar, based on radiofrequency waves have been proposed in such types of operations (Elliquence, Oceanside, NY); they have the advantages that the spatial heat dispersion is minimal, with consequent minimal risk of heating injury to the neurovascular structures.[10] Besides, the radiofrequency bipolar forceps do not need to be used with irrigation or to be cleaned every time.

Drills

High-speed, low-profile drills may be very helpful for opening the bony structures to gain access to the dural space.[26,28] They are specifically designed for endonasal use and have some special characteristics: they are low profile and also long enough but not too bulky, so they can be easily used together with the endoscope (Anspach Inc., Palm Beach Gardens, FL). The combined use of such drills and endonasal bony rongeurs has proven to be effective and timesaving during the extended approaches to the skull base, especially for access to the suprasellar or retroclival regions (**Fig. 3.6**).

Recently, a specifically designed endonasal transsphenoidal handpiece was introduced for the ultrasonic bone curette (Sonopet; Miwatec, Tokyo, Japan) (**Fig. 3.7**), which is very low profile and also quite safe because it removes the bone structures with precision but, at the same time, it respects the soft tissues, thus lowering the risks of injury to the neurovascular structures that may be close to the bone structure being removed. In our experience it has proven

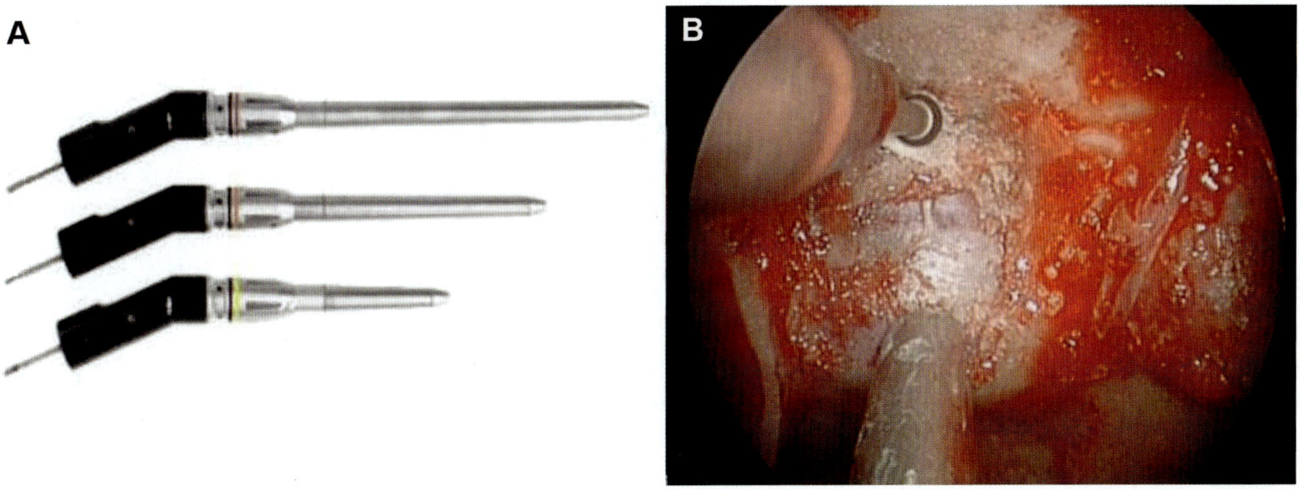

Fig. 3.6 **(A,B)** Low-profile dedicated endonasal high-speed drill with an extra-long handpiece (Anspach Inc., Palm Beach Gardens, FL).

to be useful during the removal of the tuberculum sellae in case of a prefixed chiasm, where it removes the bone but leaves soft tissues, such as the dura and the chiasm.

The Micro-Doppler Probe

Prior to opening the dura mater and whenever the surgeon thinks it is appropriate (especially while working very close to vascular structures), it is of the utmost importance to use the micro-Doppler probe to insonate the major arteries.[26,29–31] The use of such a device should be recommended every time a sharp dissection is made, to minimize the risk of injury to either the carotid or the basilar artery or to the other vascular structures that may be close or even compressed by the lesion. It is particularly useful while operating in the suprasellar space, inside the cavernous sinus or in the retroclival prepontine area.

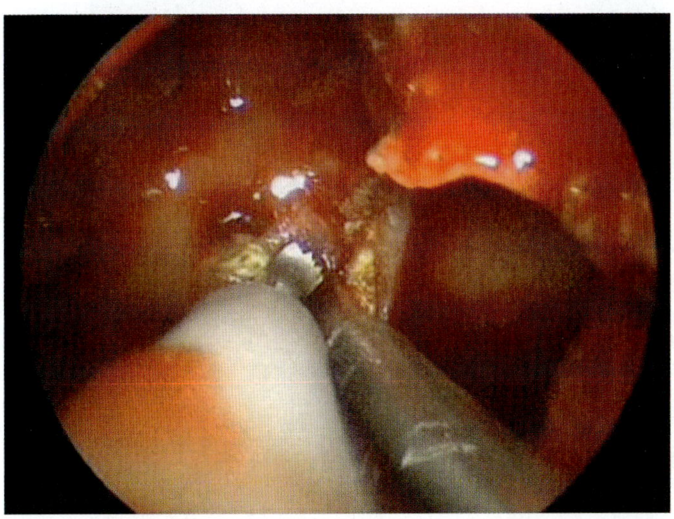

Fig. 3.7 Ultrasonic bone curette with endonasal low-profile handpiece, useful for the selective bone removal (Sonopet, Miwatec, Tokyo, Japan).

Surgical Instruments

Because of the unique environment created by the endoscopic technique, the instruments specifically conceived for use with the operative microscope are not optimally designed.[2,20,21,23,32] This is due to two peculiarities of the endoscopic approach: (1) the absence of the nasal speculum and (2) the panoramic view afforded by the endoscope. The absence of the nasal speculum (or transsphenoidal retractor) makes the approach less traumatic to the nasal mucosa and architecture.[33] On the other hand, the corridor for the surgical tools, through one or both nostrils, is narrower than during the microsurgical procedure, based on the lack of tissue spreading by the retractor. In fact, the absence of a fixed tunnel provided by the speculum is an advantage in that the surgeon has a wider angle in which to maneuver the surgical tools. With regard to the second point, the panoramic view, while the microscope produces magnification from a distant lens and light is transmitted from the lamp of the microscope to the surgical field through the speculum's blades, the vision provided by the endoscope is maintained completely inside the surgical field. Ideally, the endoscope acts like a virtual third eye for the surgeon that can direct its gaze directly to where the instruments are working at any particular moment. However, the instruments must be inserted in the nasal cavity by feel and memory, unless the endoscope is removed and inserted every time a different instrument is used. Furthermore, the wider field of view provided by the endoscope not only of the sellar cavity but also of the supra- and parasellar areas (including the clivus and planum sphenoidale, cribriform plate, pterygomaxillary fossa, and cervicomedullary junction) increases the indications for the endoscopic approach to the entire midline skull base, thus demanding new surgical instruments to effectively maneuver under these varied conditions and locations.[10,34]

Since the introduction of the standard endoscopic endonasal transsphenoidal approach for the treatment of lesions within the sella, new instruments have been designed that meet the following criteria[20–22,32]:

- Move easily and safely in a limited surgical corridor
- Be well balanced and ergonomic for safe handling, while avoiding any interference between the surgeon's hands, the endoscope, and other instruments that may be present in the same nostril
- Enable the surgeon to work in every visible zone of the surgical field provided by the endoscope

The bayoneted instruments used for microsurgical approaches are designed to avoid any interference between the surgeon's hands and the lens of the microscope. The goal is to avoid interference with the coaxial vision of the surgical field. These tools are not useful for the endoscopic technique and may even be dangerous. For the endoscopic approach, the instruments need to be inserted along the same axis as the endoscope and need to maintain the same position with respect to the endoscope for their entire length. Because of their fulcrum, the bayoneted tools developed for the microscope can potentially deviate in their direction and cross over the field of view of the endoscope, which can make the movements unsafe. New straight, low-profile instruments have been developed as adjuncts to other tools commonly used in endoscopic nasal and sinus surgery (elevators, unipolar electrodes, bipolar microforceps, nasal scissors and forceps, intranasal drills, and bone punches, among others). Straight instruments are designed specifically for endoscopic endonasal surgery, in particular for removal of the lesion in and around critical neurovascular structures. Straight curettes and dissectors with various tips and diameters, variably angled in the frontal and sagittal planes, with a length between 15 and 25 cm, maintain the same direction from the point of entrance in the nostril to the tip (i.e., if the tool is inserted on the left of the scope, it maintains the left position until its tip passes the tip of the scope and becomes visible). To manipulate the tools safely, the instrument is heavier in its proximal half so that the center of gravity of the instrument lies within the surgeon's hand for better equilibrium.

Because the surgical procedure is entirely endonasal, the instruments are inserted without direct visual control. In particular, the insertion of the blades for dural opening can potentially tear the nasal mucosa. To minimize this risk, new lancets with a retractable blade have been developed; they are inserted inside the nostril with the blade retracted within a sheath[2,20,35] (**Fig. 3.8**). The blade is then extracted when the tip of the lancet becomes visible to the endoscope, thus avoiding accidental damage to invisible nasal structures alongside the endoscope. In addition, to minimize the continuous exchange of instruments and the risk of mucosal tearing, double-function curettes have been developed, which allow curettage and suction at the same time[6,16] (**Fig. 3.9**). They combine the action of the curette in removing the pathologic tissue with that of the aspirator. Angled suction cannulas have been developed with lateral fenestrations or

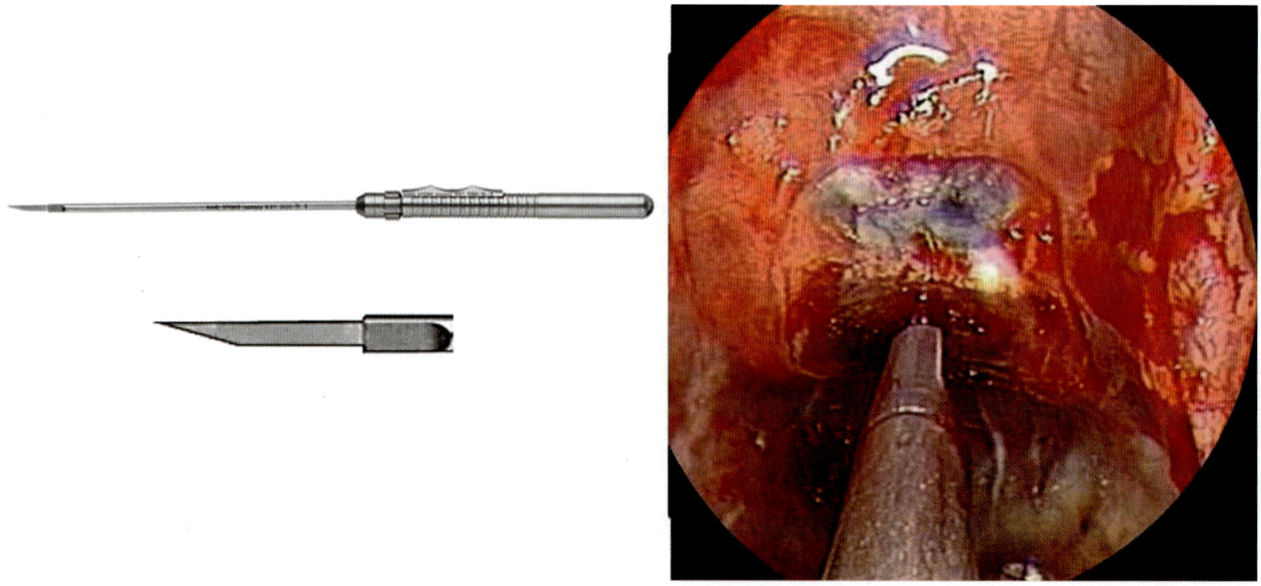

A B

Fig. 3.8 (A,B) Scalpel with retractable blade useful to avoid nasal mucosa injury during endonasal surgery (Karl Storz, Tuttlingen, Germany).

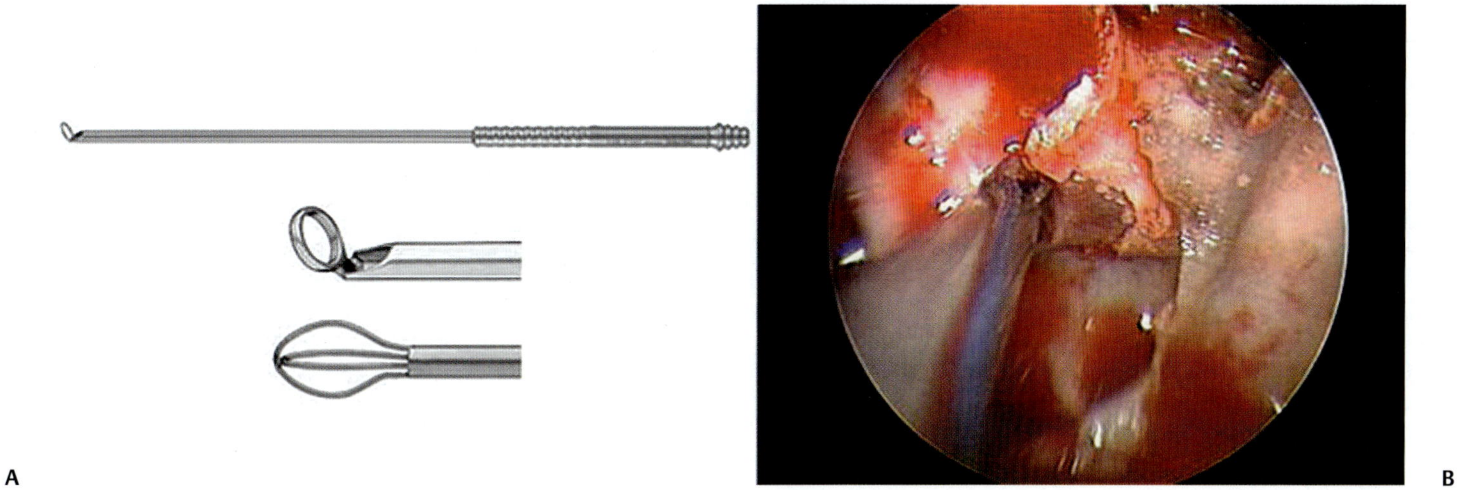

Fig. 3.9 **(A,B)** Double-function instrument (suction and curettage) facilitating two actions with one tool (Karl Storz, Tuttlingen, Germany).

with angled tips for suctioning in areas of the surgical field visible only with angled endoscopes, not otherwise reachable with regular cannulas. These are particularly useful in removing tumors located inside the cavernous sinus, specifically pituitary adenomas, particularly if they are soft.

Instruments for the Enucleation of Tumors

The best instrument for tumor enucleation is the suction apparatus. For slightly firmer tumors that are more resistant, the best technique is to grasp a portion of tumor with a ring-tipped forceps or fork, or even a biopsy rongeur in the left hand—for a right-handed surgeon—and to apply gentle traction, while using dissectors in the right hand to help free and finally lift away a section of tumor. A selection of biopsy rongeurs in two different lengths (long or short) and with a variety of jaw sizes is available. A large, rigid tumor can be excised with scissors, with the bipolar, or with monopolar loop attachment.

The loop for the monopolar electrode is available in a variety of sizes and permits rapid debulking of hard tumors. Recently, we began using the radiofrequency monopolar ball electrode (Elliquence, Oceanside, NY). This instrument uses radiofrequency power to vaporize the tumor, thus obtaining a Cavitron ultrasonic surgical aspirator (CUSA)-like effect, which is particularly useful in central debulking of meningiomas, especially if they are of firm consistency, before starting the dissection of its capsule from the surrounding neurovascular structures (**Fig. 3.10**).

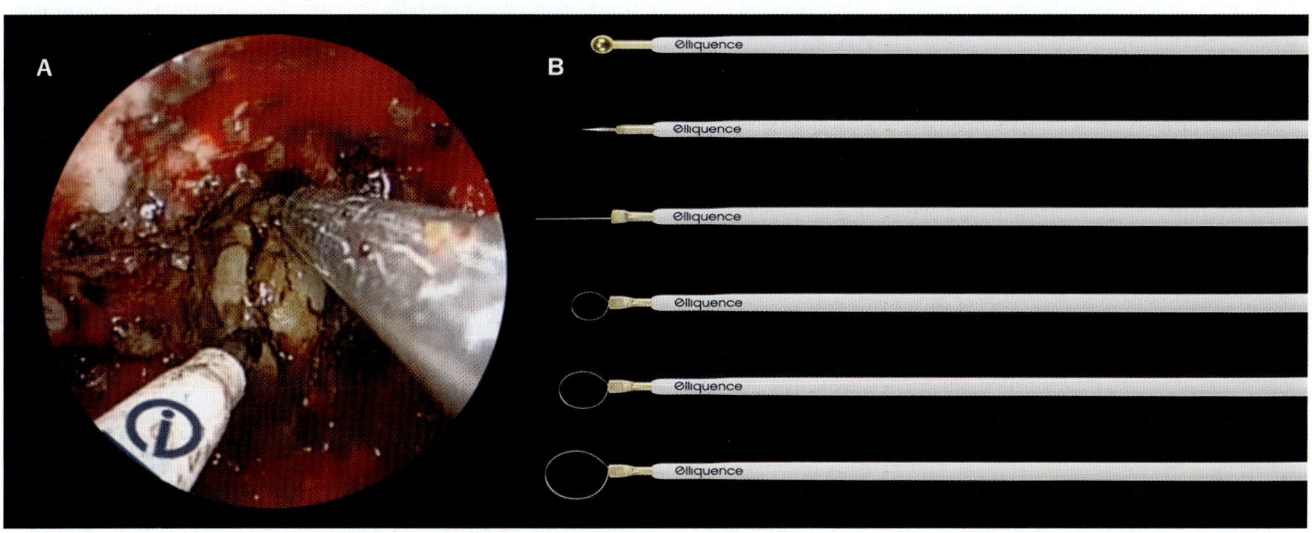

Fig. 3.10 **(A)** Radiofrequency monopolar coagulation obtaining a Cavitron ultrasonic surgical aspirator (CUSA)-like function during the debulking of a fibrous lesion (meningioma) (Elliquence, Oceanside, NY). **(B)** The different tips of the radiofrequency monopolars that can be used to produce the CUSA-like function.

For the debulking of softly to moderately firm tumor, ultrasonic aspirator systems have proven to be helpful in open cranial surgery. These systems rely on a titanium shaft that moves axially at ultrasonic speeds to emulsify tissue 1 to 2 mm from the tip. It supplies continuous irrigation and suction to aspirate the emulsified tissue. Nevertheless, the ultrasonic aspirators with handpieces and tips for use in endonasal surgery were too bulky to be used together with the endoscope inserted in the nostril. Very recently, specifically designed endonasal transsphenoidal tips were introduced for the ultrasonic aspirator (Sonopet; Miwatec, Tokyo, Japan), which is very low profile and can easily be inserted together with the endoscope, as with any other surgical instrument, and can be quite useful in tumor debulking.

Conclusion

New dedicated instruments have greatly contributed to the evolution of endoscopic endonasal transsphenoidal surgery and have permitted its progressive extension from the sella to the entire midline skull base. All such technical innovations are continuously evolving, as are the techniques to which they are dedicated.

References

1. Cappabianca P, Cavallo LM, de Divitiis E. Endoscopic endonasal transsphenoidal surgery. Neurosurgery 2004;55:933–940, discussion 940–941
2. Cappabianca P, Cavallo LM, Esposito F, de Divitiis E. Endoscopic endonasal transsphenoidal surgery: procedure, endoscopic equipment and instrumentation. Childs Nerv Syst 2004;20:796–801
3. Cappabianca P, de Divitiis O, Maiuri F. Evolution of transsphenoidal surgery. In: de Divitiis E, Cappabianca P, eds. Endoscopic Endonasal Transsphenoidal Surgery. Vienna, New York: Springer; 2003:1–7
4. Carrau RL, Jho HD, Ko Y. Transnasal-transsphenoidal endoscopic surgery of the pituitary gland. Laryngoscope 1996;106:914–918
5. Cavallo LM, Cappabianca P, Galzio R, Iaconetta G, de Divitiis E, Tschabitscher M. Endoscopic transnasal approach to the cavernous sinus versus transcranial route: anatomic study. Neurosurgery 2005;56(2, Suppl):379–389, discussion 379–389
6. Cavallo LM, de Divitiis O, Aydin S, et al. Extended endoscopic endonasal transsphenoidal approach to the suprasellar area: anatomic considerations—part 1. Neurosurgery 2007;61:ONS24–ONS34
7. Cavallo LM, Messina A, Cappabianca P, et al. Endoscopic endonasal surgery of the midline skull base: anatomical study and clinical considerations. Neurosurg Focus 2005;19:E2
8. de Notaris M, Esposito I, Cavallo LM, et al. Endoscopic endonasal approach to the ethmoidal planum: anatomic study. Neurosurg Rev 2008;31:309–317
9. Solari D, Magro F, Cappabianca P, et al. Anatomical study of the pterygopalatine fossa using an endoscopic endonasal approach: spatial relations and distances between surgical landmarks. J Neurosurg 2007;106:157–163
10. Cappabianca P, Cavallo LM, Esposito F, de Divitiis O, Messina A, de Divitiis E. Extended endoscopic endonasal approach to the midline skull base: the evolving role of transsphenoidal surgery. In: Pickard JD, ed. Advances and Technical Standards in Neurosurgery. Vienna: Springer-Verlag; 2007:1–48
11. Kassam A, Snyderman CH, Mintz A, Gardner P, Carrau RL. Expanded endonasal approach: the rostrocaudal axis. Part I. Crista galli to the sella turcica. Neurosurg Focus 2005;19:E3
12. Kassam A, Snyderman CH, Mintz A, Gardner P, Carrau RL. Expanded endonasal approach: the rostrocaudal axis. Part II. Posterior clinoids to the foramen magnum. Neurosurg Focus 2005;19:E4
13. Kassam AB, Gardner P, Snyderman C, Mintz A, Carrau R. Expanded endonasal approach: fully endoscopic, completely transnasal approach to the middle third of the clivus, petrous bone, middle cranial fossa, and infratemporal fossa. Neurosurg Focus 2005;19:E6
14. de Divitiis E, Cappabianca P, Cavallo LM, Esposito F, de Divitiis O, Messina A. Extended endoscopic transsphenoidal approach for extrasellar craniopharyngiomas. Neurosurgery 2007;61(5, Suppl 2):219–227, discussion 228
15. de Divitiis E, Esposito F, Cappabianca P, Cavallo LM, de Divitiis O. Tuberculum sellae meningiomas: high route or low route? A series of 51 consecutive cases. Neurosurgery 2008;62:556–563, discussion 556–563
16. Gardner PA, Kassam AB, Snyderman CH, et al. Outcomes following endoscopic, expanded endonasal resection of suprasellar craniopharyngiomas: a case series. J Neurosurg 2008;109:6–16
17. Kassam A, Thomas AJ, Snyderman C, et al. Fully endoscopic expanded endonasal approach treating skull base lesions in pediatric patients. J Neurosurg 2007;106(2, Suppl)75–86
18. Schwartz TH, Fraser JF, Brown S, Tabaee A, Kacker A, Anand VK. Endoscopic cranial base surgery: classification of operative approaches. Neurosurgery 2008;62:991–1002, discussion 1002–1005
19. Snyderman CH, Kassam AB. Endoscopic techniques for pathology of the anterior cranial fossa and ventral skull base. J Am Coll Surg 2006;202:563
20. Cinalli G, Cappabianca P, de Falco R, et al. Current state and future development of intracranial neuroendoscopic surgery. Expert Rev Med Devices 2005;2:351–373
21. Cappabianca P, Cavallo L, de Divitiis E. Endoscopic Pituitary and Skull Base Surgery. Anatomy and Surgery of the Endoscopic Endonasal Approach. Tuttlingen, Germany: EndoPress; 2008
22. Leonhard M, Cappabianca P, de Divitiis E. The endoscope, endoscopic equipment and instrumentation. In: de Divitiis E, Cappabianca P, eds. Endoscopic Endonasal Transsphenoidal Surgery. Vienna, New York: Springer; 2003:9–19
23. Cappabianca P, Cinalli G, Gangemi M, et al. Application of neuroendoscopy to intraventricular lesions. Neurosurgery 2008;62(Suppl 2):575–597, discussion 597–598
24. Tasman AJ, Stammberger H. Video-endoscope versus endoscope for paranasal sinus surgery: influence on stereoacuity. Am J Rhinol 1998;12:389–392
25. Tasman AJ, Feldhusen F, Kolling GH, Hosemann W. Video-endoscope versus endoscope for paranasal sinus surgery: influence on visual acuity and color discrimination. Am J Rhinol 1999;13:7–10
26. Dusick JR, Esposito F, Kelly DF, et al. The extended direct endonasal transsphenoidal approach for nonadenomatous suprasellar tumors. J Neurosurg 2005;102:832–841
27. Cavallo LM, Briganti F, Cappabianca P, et al. Hemorrhagic vascular complications of endoscopic transsphenoidal surgery. Minim Invasive Neurosurg 2004;47:145–150

28. Esposito F, Becker DP, Villablanca JP, Kelly DF. Endonasal transsphenoidal transclival removal of prepontine epidermoid tumors: technical note. Neurosurgery 2005;56(2, Suppl):E443, discussion E443
29. Arita K, Kurisu K, Tominaga A, et al. Trans-sellar color Doppler ultrasonography during transsphenoidal surgery. Neurosurgery 1998; 42:81–85, discussion 86
30. Dusick JR, Esposito F, Malkasian D, Kelly DF. Avoidance of carotid artery injuries in transsphenoidal surgery with the Doppler probe and micro-hook blades. Neurosurgery 2007;60(4, Suppl 2):322–328, discussion 328–329
31. Yamasaki T, Moritake K, Hatta J, Nagai H. Intraoperative monitoring with pulse Doppler ultrasonography in transsphenoidal surgery: technique application. Neurosurgery 1996;38:95–97, discussion 97–98
32. Cappabianca P, Alfieri A, Thermes S, Buonamassa S, de Divitiis E. Instruments for endoscopic endonasal transsphenoidal surgery. Neurosurgery 1999;45:392–395, discussion 395–396
33. Cappabianca P, Cavallo LM, Colao A, de Divitiis E. Surgical complications associated with the endoscopic endonasal transsphenoidal approach for pituitary adenomas. J Neurosurg 2002;97:293–298
34. de Divitiis E, Cappabianca P, Cavallo LM. Endoscopic transsphenoidal approach: adaptability of the procedure to different sellar lesions. Neurosurgery 2002;51:699–705, discussion 705–707
35. Cappabianca P, de Divitiis O, Esposito F, Cavallo L, de Divitiis E. Endoscopic skull base instrumentation. In: Anand V, Schwartz T, eds. Practical Endoscopic Skull Base Surgery. San Diego: Plural Publishing; 2007:45–56

4 Preoperative Endocrine Evaluation

John C. Ausiello and Pamela U. Freda

The preoperative evaluation of a patient with a pituitary tumor or sellar mass should involve the combined efforts of a neurosurgeon and an endocrinologist.[1] The first priority is to assess the stability of the patient from a neurologic perspective to gauge the urgency with which surgery should be undertaken. This task can be accomplished with a history and physical examination, coupled with a pituitary-cut magnetic resonance imaging (MRI) with gadolinium to evaluate the size and anatomical location of the tumor. In most patients with acute neurologic compromise or acute visual loss due to chiasmal involvement of the mass, emergent surgery should be pursued, irrespective of the tumor etiology. A possible exception to this rule is a patient with a macroprolactinoma, because such patients can have rapid improvement in visual field loss with dopamine agonist therapy. The majority of sellar masses, however, are diagnosed in neurologically stable patients, and it is the preoperative endocrine evaluation of these cases that is the focus of this chapter.

From an endocrine perspective, the preoperative evaluation of a patient with a known pituitary or sellar mass has two essential goals: to determine the functionality of the tumor and to assess the integrity of critical hormonal axes. Hormone-producing pituitary masses include prolactinomas, adrenocorticotropic hormone (ACTH)-secreting tumors (Cushing's disease), growth hormone (GH)-secreting tumors (acromegaly), thyroid-stimulating hormone (TSH)-secreting tumors, and gonadotropin (luteinizing hormone [LH] or follicle-stimulating hormone [FSH])–secreting tumors (**Table 4.1**). Many patients

Table 4.1 Clinical Characteristics and Initial Laboratory Evaluations for Secretory Pituitary Adenomas

Tumor Type	Clinical Signs and Symptoms	Laboratory Testing
Prolactin-secreting (prolactinoma)	Oligo- or amenorrhea	Prolactin level (at dilutions)—persistently elevated
	Impaired libido	Rule out medication-induced and other causes of hyperprolac tinemia
	Infertility	
	Galactorrhea	Consider stalk compression versus prolactinoma etiology (see text)
ACTH-secreting (Cushing's disease)	Central obesity	24-hour UFC—elevated
	Supraclavicular/dorsocervical fat pads	Overnight (1 mg) dexamethasone suppression test—cortisol ≤1.8 µg/dL excludes Cushing's
	Thin skin, bruising, striae	Nighttime salivary cortisol—elevated
	Proximal muscle weakness	ACTH level—normal or elevated
	Hypertension, diabetes	
GH-secreting (acromegaly)	Acral enlargement	IGF-1—elevated above age-adjusted normal range
	Coarsening of facial features	GH suppression during an OGTT (criteria see text)
	Hyperhidrosis	
	Snoring, sleep apnea	
	New hypertension or DM	
TSH-secreting	Hyperthyroidism symptoms	TSH—normal or high (not suppressed)
	Weight loss, tremor, sweating	Free thyroxine (FT_4)—elevated
	Goiter	
Gonadotropin	Rare clinical features	LH and FSH—circulating level may be high
		α-Subunit—circulating level may be high

Abbreviations: ACTH, adrenocorticotropic hormone; DM, diabetes mellitus; FSH, follicle-stimulating hormone; GH, growth hormone; IGF, insulin-like growth factor; LH, luteinizing hormone; OGTT, oral glucose tolerance test; TSH, thyroid-stimulating hormone; UFC, urine free cortisol.

Table 4.2 Routine Initial Laboratory Evaluation in a Patient with a Pituitary or Sellar Mass

Prolactin (at dilutions)
Cortisol (a.m.)
ACTH
IGF-1, GH
TSH, FT_4
LH, FSH
α-subunit
Testosterone (males)
Serum sodium level

Abbreviations: ACTH, adrenocorticotropic hormone; FSH, follicle-stimulating hormone; FT_4, freethyroxine; GH, growth hormone; IGF-1, insulin-like growth factor-1; LH, luteinizing hormone; TSH, thyroid-stimulating hormone.

with a hormonally active tumor, with the exception of those with a gonadotropin-secreting tumor, present with clear signs and symptoms of hormone hypersecretion, making the history and physical examination an important component of the initial preoperative evaluation. However, some patients may present with more subtle findings that are not immediately attributable to the hormone excess. Therefore, additional endocrine laboratory studies should be performed preoperatively to confirm the diagnosis of a suspected functional mass or to detect a clinically silent tumor. At our institution, our preoperative testing typically includes measurements of serum levels of prolactin and cortisol, plasma ACTH, and serum free thyroxine (T_4), TSH, LH, FSH, GH, and insulin-like growth factor-1 (IGF-1) and in some cases α-subunit (**Table 4.2**).

Among the hyperfunctional tumors, excluding or diagnosing a prolactinoma preoperatively is particularly important because most can be managed with dopamine agonists, thus obviating the need for surgery.[2] The remaining hormonally active pituitary tumors are typically treated with surgery if specific clinical, visual, and neurologic features of the patient are present, although it is important to recognize that some hormone-secreting tumors are clinically silent (typically the gonadotropin-secreting tumors). If circulating levels of none of the aforementioned hormones are elevated, the tumor may be a nonsecreting pituitary adenoma, which is often managed with surgery as well. Thus, preoperative knowledge of the tumor type is beneficial, as it may impact the preoperative, perioperative, and postoperative management of the patient.[3]

All patients, regardless of the tumor type, require preoperative assessment of the integrity of pituitary function to exclude partial or complete hypopituitarism (**Table 4.3**). With regard to anterior pituitary function, it is most important preoperatively to ensure the adequacy of the adrenal and thyroid axes, because untreated adrenal insufficiency or hypothyroidism can be clinically significant and potentially life threatening in the perioperative period. Evaluations for deficiencies in the remaining anterior pituitary hormone axes can be pursued after surgery.[3] Posterior pituitary dysfunction most commonly manifests itself in the form of diabetes insipidus (DI), which is suggested by the history and physical examination. Preoperative DI is extremely uncommon in patients with pituitary tumors, and its presence should raise the suspicion for another etiology of the sellar mass, such as a craniopharyngioma or an infectious or inflammatory lesion.[4]

This chapter describes the endocrinologic characterization of the nature of the pituitary tumor and the evaluations that should be undertaken to screen for hypopituitarism and the need for perioperative hormone replacement therapy.

Hormone-Secreting Pituitary Tumors

Prolactinomas

The most common pituitary tumors are prolactinomas accounting for approximately 40% of all adenomas.[5] Presenting symptoms of prolactinomas vary and often differ between men and premenopausal women. A man with a prolactinoma often presents with symptoms of gonadal dysfunction, such as decreased libido, impotence, or infertility, or with neurologic or visual symptoms because the tumors tend to be macroadenomas by the time medical care is sought.[5] Among premenopausal women, symptoms of gonadal dysfunction typically bring them to medical attention earlier when their tumors are microadenomas. Up to 90% of premenopausal women present with oligo/amenorrhea and up to 80% with galactorrhea.[5] In contrast, postmenopausal women may not come to medical attention until symptoms of a macroadenoma are present, such as a headache, visual disturbances, or other neurologic sequelae.[5] Given this variability in clinical presentation, it is imperative to measure a prolactin level in all patients with pituitary masses prior to pursuing surgery, especially because the vast majority of prolactinomas can be managed medically.[2]

In interpreting the prolactin level, it is important to note that the differential diagnosis of hyperprolactinemia remains broad. Prolactin can be physiologically elevated in pregnancy or during the postpartum period if a woman is nursing.[6] A pathologic elevation of prolactin can occur from the use of prescription medications, including neuroleptics, antidepressants, metoclopramide, methyldopa, reserpine, and verapamil, or from the use of illicit drugs such as cocaine or opiates.[6] Finally, hyperprolactinemia can occur in the setting of cirrhosis, renal failure, or hypothyroidism, or it can occur idiopathically or in the setting of nonpituitary lesions or pituitary adenomas other than prolactinomas that involve the hypothalamus or hypothalamic-pituitary stalk.[6]

The presence of an adenoma on MRI in the setting of a sustained elevation of serum prolactin in a patient for whom secondary causes of hyperprolactinemia have been

Table 4.3 Preoperative Assessment and Management of Pituitary Dysfunction in Patients with a Pituitary or Sellar Mass

	Clinical Signs and Symptoms	Laboratory Testing	Treatment
Anterior Pituitary Insufficiency			
Secondary adrenal insufficiency	Anorexia, weight loss, postural hypotension	Cortisol (a.m.)—low ACTH—normal or low	Hydrocortisone 15–25 mg/day (divided into two doses) Consider if cortisol <10 µg/dL or clinical picture suggestive of AI[33] Perioperative stress steroids for all patients
Central hypothyroidism	Fatigue, dry skin, bradycardia Constipation Delayed relaxation DTRs	Free thyroxine—low TSH—normal or low	Weight-based thyroxine replacement*
Gonadal insufficiency	Oligo- or amenorrhea Decreased libido Hypoestrogenemia symptoms Infertility	LH, FSH—normal or low Testosterone (men)—low Prolactin—check for elevation	Can be treated preoperatively if desired but not required
Growth hormone deficiency	Typically evaluated postoperatively[33]		
Posterior Pituitary Insufficiency			
Vasopressin deficiency (diabetes insipidus)	Polyuria, polydipsia Rare in adenomas	History and exam Dilute urine, high volume	DDAVP nasal spray 10 µg once or twice daily Mild, may be maintained on fluids as wanted or needed fluids
	Consider nonpituitary mass etiology	Serum sodium—hypernatremia possible Serum osmolarity—may increase Water deprivation test**	

*After adrenal insufficiency excluded or treated if diagnosed.
**May not be necessary in a patient with symptoms of DI and a hypothalamic, stalk, or sellar lesion.
Abbreviations: ACTH, adrenocorticotropic hormone; AI, adrenal insufficiency; DDAVP, deamino-8-D-arginine vasopressin; DTR, deep tendon reflex.

excluded is consistent with a prolactinoma. Typically, a single measurement of prolactin is sufficient for diagnosis, but ideally blood should be drawn at least 1 hour after the patient's awakening or eating, and excessive venipuncture stress should be avoided.[5] Recent guidelines for the diagnosis and management of prolactinomas suggest that prolactin levels greater than 150 µg/L are very suggestive of a prolactinoma and levels greater than 250 µg/L are suggestive of a prolactin-secreting macroadenoma.[5] Prolactin levels less than 150 µg/L are seen in patients with microprolactinomas, as well as in those with stalk compression from any pituitary or sellar mass, making this distinction difficult. Definitive proof of a prolactinoma comes from the demonstration of a clinical response to a dopamine agonist because biopsy is not routinely pursued. A trial of a dopamine agonist in unclear cases may be informative because a prolactinoma should regress in size, whereas a nonsecreting mass would remain unchanged. Close follow-up of such patients with endocrinologic assessments and serial MRI should be undertaken.

In addition to the challenges discussed above, on occasion, prolactin levels can be reported incorrectly as low in the setting of a large prolactinoma. This phenomenon, the "hook effect," is well documented and is secondary to antibody saturation by the high prolactin concentration in a immunoradiometric assay, which leads to artificially low prolactin values. To address this possibility, dilutions of the patient's serum to 1:100 should be performed on all patients with large tumors but normal to mildly elevated prolactin levels.[5] Finally, GH and IGF-1 levels should be assessed in all subjects in whom a prolactinoma is being considered. Approximately 20% of patients with acromegaly have elevations in prolactin,[7] making it necessary to rule out this condition in patients with an elevated prolactin level. For patients with a co-secreting tumor, definitive therapy is generally focused on the GH-secreting component.

Once the diagnosis is confirmed, most prolactinomas can be medically managed with bromocriptine or cabergoline. Indications for surgery include failure of medical therapy to normalize prolactin levels when hyperprolactinemia is clinically significant, intolerance of medical therapy, visual field or other neurologic deficits that do not respond to medical therapy, or the presence of apoplexy with neurologic symptoms.[5]

Cushing's Disease

The possibility of an ACTH-secreting pituitary tumor leading to Cushing's disease should be considered in all patients presenting with a pituitary tumor. The evaluation for Cushing's should begin with a complete history and physical examination. Patients with hypercortisolism in general (including Cushing's disease) may present with a variety of signs and symptoms, including the nonspecific features of hypertension, fatigue, irritability, depression, weight gain, and new-onset or worsening of existing diabetes. More specific features of hypercortisolism include abnormal fat accumulation, particularly in the supraclavicular fossae, dorsocervical region, and centrally, as well as proximal muscle weakness, thin skin, bruising, and purple striae.[8] A wide spectrum in the severity of these clinical manifestations at presentation makes screening often necessary.[9]

If a clinical suspicion of Cushing's disease emerges, further laboratory evaluation should be pursued. A random elevated serum cortisol is not sufficient to confirm a diagnosis because the stress from venipuncture alone may increase cortisol levels.[7] Instead, screening is typically performed with one of three tests: a 24-hour urine free cortisol (UFC) level, a dexamethasone suppression test (DST), or a nighttime salivary cortisol level.[9] A 24-hour UFC level provides a reflection of the free cortisol circulating in the blood, and therefore its use is not hindered by conditions affecting cortisol-binding globulin (CBG) levels.[9] A single assessment of 24-hour UFC levels, however, may not be sufficient, given the presence of mild Cushing's disease in some patients[10] and the intermittent nature of hypercortisolemia in other patients.[11] Recent guidelines recommend checking up to three 24-hour UFCs in patients for whom clinical suspicion is high and in whom the first test is normal. If all three tests are normal, then Cushing's is unlikely, assuming the glomerular filtration rate (GFR) is greater than 30 mL/min.[9] Interpretation of the results of a 24-hour UFC should also consider the assay methodology used, as newer methods of high-performance liquid chromatography (HPLC) in tandem with mass spectroscopy appear to have the best specificity.[11] Using the HPLC assay, a level greater than 50 µg/24 hours is typically considered elevated.[12]

Screening for Cushing's disease with a DST is also commonly undertaken. One method is the overnight suppression test, which involves the administration of 1 mg of dexamethasone at 11 p.m. followed by a measurement of cortisol at 8 a.m. the next morning. The 48-hour test, still performed at some centers,[9] requires the administration of 0.5 mg of dexamethasone every 6 hours for 2 days, with cortisol levels drawn at the beginning and end of the test at 9 a.m. The latter test is more cumbersome but also more specific.[11] A cortisol value less than 1.8 µg/dL is considered normal for either test.[9,11] Unfortunately, the test characteristics of the DST are affected by numerous concomitant medical conditions. Apparent failure to suppress can occur in patients who have either decreased dexamethasone absorption or increased hepatic clearance of dexamethasone (secondary to hepatic effects of concomitant medications) or in patients receiving estrogen therapy from increased levels of CBG.[9,11,12] Additionally, false-positive tests may be seen in patients with obesity, chronic illness, major depression, or other psychiatric illnesses.[12] Screening for Cushing's with nighttime salivary free cortisol levels has been shown in repeated studies to be an excellent substitute for measurement of nighttime serum cortisol levels.[12] Patients with true Cushing's syndrome have elevated nighttime cortisol levels and failure of normal diurnal variation in these levels. Different assay methods exist for measurement of salivary free cortisol, and proper interpretation of the results requires use of assay specific normative cutoffs. A recent review suggested that a level >350 ng/dL using a radioimmunoassay (RIA) is strongly suggestive of Cushing's syndrome, and a level <150 ng/dL is not suggestive of the condition, with intermediate levels prompting further testing.[12] Although there is debate about the optimal screening test for Cushing's syndrome, as no one test is 100% accurate, there is growing support for the use of nighttime salivary cortisol levels as the initial screening tool followed by a 24-hour UFC or suppression test for possible confirmation, given the simplicity of the nighttime test coupled with its reasonable sensitivity and specificity levels.[12,13] It should also be recognized that positive screening tests can be seen in patients with pseudo-Cushing's syndrome due to depression or alcohol abuse. Each of the options discussed above remains viable screening tests as long as the limitations of each are recognized.

If biochemical screening suggests Cushing's syndrome, first an ACTH level should be drawn, followed by further biochemical confirmation of the disease, and then an investigation into the differential diagnosis of Cushing's syndrome should be undertaken. Normal to elevated ACTH levels are seen in ACTH-dependent Cushing's syndrome due to an ACTH-secreting pituitary adenoma, Cushing's disease, or the ectopic ACTH syndrome. The degree of ACTH elevation is not specific enough to distinguish among these etiologies. Some corticotroph tumors are also clinically silent, with or without plasma ACTH elevations. Such tumors may have a clinically more aggressive phenotype. A macroadenoma in the setting of an elevated ACTH or biochemical evidence of

Cushing's is typically sufficient evidence to pursue surgery. However, in patients with microadenomas, because of the high prevalence of incidental microadenomas in the general population, further dynamic biochemical testing is often undertaken. In patients with clear ACTH-dependent Cushing's syndrome but equivocal dynamic testing for Cushing's disease, or in patients whose MRI studies are inconclusive, evaluation should proceed to inferior petrosal sinus sampling with corticotropin-releasing hormone (CRH) administration to confirm the pituitary source prior to surgical intervention. A lengthy discussion of preoperative evaluation of Cushing's disease is beyond the scope of this chapter, but decisions regarding further diagnostic testing and therapeutic options (including the need for surgery) should involve input from an endocrinologist.

Acromegaly

All patients undergoing evaluation of a pituitary mass should be screened for a GH-secreting tumor. Although most patients with GH-secreting tumors typically present with some signs and symptoms of GH/IGF-1 excess because of the long delay from disease onset to clinical recognition, earlier stage disease, prior to development of obvious clinical manifestations, can be detected with biochemical testing.[14] The most common presenting features of acromegaly are changes in facial features, typically coarsening, and enlargement of the hands and feet due to soft tissue swelling. Other manifestations include headache, arthralgias, jaw prognathism and bite changes, arthritis, sleep apnea, diabetes mellitus, and hypertension.[15] Patients should be screened for a GH-secreting pituitary tumor with a measurement of a GH and serum IGF-1 level. Elevation of random GH level is not specific for acromegaly, but a very high or low level can be helpful in directing the need for further evaluation. Elevation of the serum IGF-1 level is an excellent marker for detecting even subtle degrees of GH excess.[16] In interpreting IGF-1 levels, however, factors that may affect them need to be considered. IGF-1 levels decline with increasing age and thus must be interpreted in comparison to well-characterized age-adjusted normative ranges. Nutrient deprivation and liver disease can also lower IGF-1 levels. IGF-1 levels can be somewhat higher in hyperthyroidism and lower in hypothyroidism. Aside from acromegaly, IGF-1 levels are rarely above normal except in pregnancy and during adolescence.[16] Documentation of IGF-1 elevation should be followed by assessment of GH suppression after an oral glucose load of 75 or 100 g.[15,16] In many commercially available GH assays, suppression of GH to less than 1 µg/L in conjunction with a normal IGF-1 level should exclude GH excess. However, with highly sensitive and specific growth hormone assays, GH levels can be less than 1 µg/L in patients with newly diagnosed acromegaly; in these cases IGF-1 levels will also be consistently elevated.[17]

Once acromegaly is identified, both surgical and medical therapeutic options for primary therapy are available. Surgery is the initial therapy of choice in nearly all patients and clearly in any patient with a microadenoma or a macroadenoma and compressive symptoms. However, there remains some debate about the role of primary medical therapy for patients with macroadenomas that are not likely to be completely resected with surgery. The role of primary medical therapy has been supported by retrospective cross-sectional data demonstrating similar biochemical responses to octreotide therapy in 26 patients who received it as primary therapy, and 81 patients who received it following unsuccessful surgery or radiotherapy.[18] The authors of a second study found long-term primary medical therapy (up to 9 years) with somatostatin analogues in 67 patients to be effective.[19] Thus, in selected patients, primary medical therapy may be reasonable, but this decision should be considered on an individual patient basis. Factors that should be considered in making this decision include the surgical risks to the patient, the experience of the neurosurgeon, the tumor size and location, and the preference of the patient. For most patients we favor surgical debulking, even if not curative, because additional therapeutic modalities are typically more feasible or effective following surgery. In particular, radiotherapy becomes more feasible following surgical debulking, somatostatin analogue efficacy is increased in this setting,[20] and GH-receptor antagonist (pegvisomant) therapy can be administered more safely once the threat of compression of surrounding structures is reduced.

Thyroid-Stimulating Hormone–Secreting Tumors

Thyroid-stimulating hormone (TSH)-secreting tumors are rare, constituting fewer than 1% of all pituitary adenomas in one published series.[21] Patients with TSH-secreting pituitary tumors typically present with large tumors at diagnosis, causing symptoms of hyperthyroidism, such as weight loss, heat intolerance, palpitations, diarrhea, increased perspiration, hair loss, and tremors. In a series of 25 patients with TSH-secreting adenomas, 22 had mild (eight patients) or severe (14 patients) hyperthyroidism.[22] In a patient with a pituitary mass, a TSH-secreting tumor is suggested by a nonsuppressed TSH level (it may be normal or elevated), accompanied by an elevated free thyroxine level and clinical evidence of hyperthyroidism.

Hyperthyroidism needs to be recognized and treated preoperatively because untreated hyperthyroidism during surgery increases the risk for intraoperative complications, including arrhythmias. Hyperthyroidism should be treated with beta-blockers and, if time permits (i.e., it is an elective surgery), antithyroid medication.[7] In addition, some studies suggest that somatostatin analogues decrease tumor size and suppress TSH production.[21,23] As a result, somatostatin analogues have been used successfully prior to surgery[24] or in the place of surgery in a patient for whom surgery poses a high risk.[25] These data have led some authors to suggest that somatostatin analogues may be used effectively in lieu of surgery in select patients.[7]

Gonadotropin-Secreting Tumors

Many clinically nonfunctioning tumors are gonadotropin cell in origin but are diagnosed as such only with immunohistochemical staining. Some of these tumors do secrete gonadotropins, but rarely do they produce clinical manifestations. Nevertheless, preoperative measurements of LH, FSH, and an α-subunit (some tumors produce only this subunit) can be informative and help guide postoperative assessments. If a pathology analysis reveals tumor cells of gonadotroph origin and preoperative levels are elevated, postoperative measurement of LH and FSH can be used to assess for surgical cure and for the possibility of tumor recurrence.

Assessment of Pituitary Function

General Principles

Assessment of pituitary function is a critical part of the preoperative evaluation of a patient with a pituitary or sellar mass given the risks of partial or complete hypopituitarism. These risks appear to be increased in patients with macroadenomas or pituitary apoplexy at the time of presentation.[3,26] Of the anterior pituitary hormonal axes, the two that are most important to assess preoperatively are the adrenal and thyroid axes because deficiencies in either of them can increase surgical risk and perioperative morbidity. In addition to anterior pituitary dysfunction, some sellar masses, in particular those that are nonpituitary in origin, can cause disruption of vasopressin secretion, leading to diabetes insipidus. In general, the preoperative evaluation of anterior pituitary function requires the measurement of pituitary and target gland hormones, whereas the evaluation of posterior pituitary function often is accomplished with a thorough history and physical examination.

Pituitary–Adrenal Axis Assessment

Patients with a pituitary or sellar mass should be assessed for signs and symptoms suggestive of secondary adrenal insufficiency, such as weakness and fatigue, hypotension, abdominal pain, nausea and vomiting, or hyponatremia. These findings, however, are not specific to adrenal insufficiency, so biochemical assessment of adrenal function with baseline and in some cases dynamic testing is needed. The optimal test to establish the integrity of adrenal function preoperatively is debated and can depend on the clinical picture of the patient and other pituitary function.

The cosyntropin stimulation test has become the standard test for assessment of primary adrenal insufficiency, but its results may not be definitive for secondary adrenal insufficiency. Most authors accept a criterion of a peak cortisol after 250 µg of cortrosyn of greater than 18 to 20 µg/dL to be indicative of normal adrenal function.[27,28] If the peak cortisol response is low, it can be confirmatory of secondary adrenal insufficiency, but if normal, it does not necessarily exclude recent onset of secondary adrenal insufficiency because the adrenal glands in these patients may still respond to pharmacologic ACTH stimulation. In a study of 62 patients with a normal cosyntropin stimulation test 1 week after transsphenoidal surgery, 44% subsequently failed a stimulation test 1 to 3 months later, highlighting the limitations of this test in early secondary adrenal insufficiency.[29] Assessment of pituitary-adrenal reserve with the insulin tolerance test (ITT) can also be undertaken. Considered by many to be the gold standard for assessment of this axis, insulin-induced hypoglycemia stimulates the entire hypothalamic-pituitary axis, but its use is limited because it is labor intensive, it can be unpleasant for the patient, and it remains contraindicated in elderly patients and in patients with coronary artery disease or seizure disorders.[28]

Therefore, at many centers, including ours, the assessment of pituitary-adrenal function preoperatively is typically begun with measurement of a morning cortisol level. Numerous studies, mostly in the post-transsphenoidal surgery setting, have attempted to determine what cortisol levels signify adrenal sufficiency or deficiency. In one retrospective study of 193 patients with various hypothalamic or pituitary pathologies who all underwent an ITT, baseline cortisol levels greater than 469.2 nmol/L (17 µg/dL) predicted a normal ITT response, and those less than 110.4 nmol/L (4.0 µg/dL) predicted an abnormal response.[30] A review of the subject found similar levels for each cutoff, with a cortisol greater than 450 nmol/L (16 µg/dL) considered sufficient and a level less than 100 nmol/L (3.6 µg/dL) considered deficient.[31] However, the authors of another study assessing postoperative cortisol levels in patients with normal preoperative adrenal function found that levels as low as 270 nmol/L (9.8 µg/dL) typically signified preservation of the adrenal axis.[32] Thus, there is considerable debate in the literature about what constitutes a normal morning cortisol level, and practice patterns vary from institution to institution. We prescribe glucocorticoid replacement therapy preoperatively always in patients with morning cortisol levels ≤5 µg/dL and usually in those patients with levels less than 270.6 nmol/L (10 µg/dL), especially if the patient has laboratory evidence of other hypopituitarism. For replacement doses in patients who are not stressed, we favor hydrocortisone at doses of 15 to 25 mg per day and aim for the lowest dose, 10 mg in the morning and 5 mg in the evening, so long as the patient feels well. For patients with morning cortisol levels greater than 270.6 nmol/L (10 µg/dL) we typically administer glucocorticoid therapy only during periods of stress, which would include surgery. We assess pituitary adrenal function again postoperatively in all patients.[33]

At many centers, all patients scheduled to undergo transsphenoidal pituitary surgery are administered stress-dose glucocorticoid therapy perioperatively with either hydrocortisone or dexamethasone. We typically administer dexamethasone perioperatively in all patients regardless of preoperative adrenal function. We prefer dexamethasone because, although it suppresses the hypothalamic-pituitary axis, it does not interfere with determination of cortisol levels in the cortisol assay when adrenal function may need to be reassessed postoperatively. The decision to continue or stop replacement therapy postoperatively is based on cortisol levels, preoperative function, and the patient's clinical picture.[33] Patients with preoperative adrenal insufficiency are continued on replacement therapy and reassessed at a follow-up visit. In other patients, however, glucocorticoids are tapered quickly after surgery and adrenal function is assessed. However, this strategy is not universally employed, as some authors argue that patients undergoing selective adenomectomy who do not have evidence of secondary adrenal insufficiency preoperatively (defined as a peak cortisol >496.8 nmol/L [18 µg/dL] following administration of 250 µg of cosyntropin), do not need to receive steroids during surgery.[31] In a study of 83 patients without preoperative adrenal insufficiency (ITT cortisol peak >510.6 nmol/L [18.5 µg/dL] and rise >270.6 nmol/L [10 µg/dL]), perioperative glucocorticoids were held and only one subject subsequently developed adrenal insufficiency postoperatively.[34] It should be noted that this study's population was atypical for a transsphenoidal surgery cohort, as it was composed of many females with prolactinomas and microadenomas, but it does suggest that universal glucocorticoid coverage during surgery for a pituitary mass may not be necessary.

Pituitary–Thyroid Assessment

A preoperative assessment of the thyroid axis is necessary to rule out significant hypothyroidism prior to surgery. Patients with severe hypothyroidism who undergo surgery are at increased risk for perioperative morbidity and mortality.[35] Signs and symptoms associated with hypothyroidism include fatigue, weight gain, cold intolerance, constipation, bradycardia, dry skin, and delayed relaxation of the deep tendon reflexes.

To detect hypothyroidism in this setting, it is important to measure a free thyroxine (FT_4) level in addition to a TSH. Measurement of TSH alone can be misleading in patients with hypopituitarism as it may be low, "normal," or even high. It has been shown that patients with hypopituitarism may secrete a form of TSH that is biologically inactive but still detectable on immunoassay.[36] Thus, thyroid function tests in secondary hypothyroidism typically show a low FT_4 level in the setting of a normal or low TSH level. If central hypothyroidism is documented, replacement therapy with T_4[37] should begin in the preoperative period.[2,38] Thyroid replacement, however, needs to be preceded by assessment of adrenal function and replacement of glucocorticoids. In a recently published study, weight-based dosing (1.6 µg/kg) with a target FT_4 level toward the upper end of normal was shown to be optimal.[39]

Additional Pituitary Hormones

A preoperative assessment of the remaining hypothalamic/anterior pituitary axes is much less critical. Hypogonadism in both men and women carries significant long-term risks, but the immediate concerns of such deficiencies are minimal, and preoperative replacement can be undertaken if desired, but it is not necessary. Some prefer to delay the institution of male gonadal steroid replacement, in particular, until the postoperative period, given the possibility of spontaneous recovery of this axis. Long-term risks associated with adult GH deficiency exist as well, but the short-term risks have not been reported, rendering preoperative GH therapy unnecessary. Nevertheless, documentation of these deficiencies preoperatively can be undertaken if desired and may help guide postoperative management, as these preoperative deficiencies do not commonly resolve.[3]

Posterior Pituitary Function

Patients under evaluation for a pituitary or sellar mass should be assessed for disturbances of posterior pituitary function. Pituitary adenomas very rarely lead to DI preoperatively, but this condition is much more common with nonpituitary lesions that involve the sellar region. Therefore, documented DI preoperatively should raise the suspicion of a nonpituitary etiology of the sellar mass, such as a craniopharyngioma, inflammatory, infectious, or metastatic process.[4,7] All patients should be questioned about a history of excess urination or thirst, especially craving of cold liquids. The hallmark of DI is the development of large volumes of dilute urine, typically greater than 3 L/day with a low urine osmolality, and the gold standard for diagnosis remains the water deprivation test.[40] However, excess thirst and the presence of dilute polyuria with frequent nocturia (every 1 to 2 hours) in the setting of a known sellar mass is often sufficient to make the diagnosis of DI in the absence of a formal water deprivation test.[7]

In the perioperative setting it is often sufficient to manage DI, in patients who are awake and alert, by ensuring access to free water coupled with close monitoring as DI is typically transient.[2] However, if urine output becomes excessive (especially at night, preventing sleep) or it significantly exceeds fluid intake, causing hypernatremia, then medical therapy becomes necessary.[41] As such, in patients with impaired thirst or altered mental status, DI needs to be recognized quickly and treated promptly to prevent adverse outcomes associated with the development of hypernatremia. When medical therapy is required, a synthetic analogue of antidiuretic hormone, deamino-8-D-arginine vasopressin (DDAVP), which acts at V2 receptors, is the treatment of choice. It can be administered as needed in response to symptoms consistent with DI, either subcutaneously 1 to 2 μg[42,43] or intranasally 10 μg if the nasal packs are removed. If patients have been diagnosed with DI preoperatively, on the day of surgery they can be administered their usual DDAVP and normal saline intraoperatively along with close monitoring of fluid status and serum sodium levels.

Conclusion

The preoperative evaluation of any patient with a pituitary or sellar mass requires the input from a multidisciplinary team that includes a neurosurgeon and an endocrinologist. The workup should begin with a rapid assessment of the stability of the patient's neurologic status. An acute impairment in neurologic status or significant vision loss should prompt immediate surgery in most patients. In the remaining cases, which constitute the majority, the preoperative evaluation includes an assessment of the hormonal activity of the tumor and an assessment of residual pituitary function. These goals can typically be accomplished with a thorough history and physical examination coupled with a series of baseline laboratory assessments of pituitary function. Through such a rigorous clinical and laboratory assessment, most issues encountered can be safely and adequately addressed prior to pituitary surgery, thus facilitating the preoperative, perioperative, and postoperative care of the patient with a pituitary or sellar mass.

Acknowledgments

This work was funded in part by National Institutes of Health (NIH) grants R01 DK 064720 and K24 DK 073040 to the second author, and a Genentech Center for Clinical Research Center Fellowship Grant to the first author.

References

1. Inder WJ, Alford FP. Pituitary masses: the importance of a multidisciplinary approach. Med J Aust 2007;187:522–523
2. Nemergut EC, Dumont AS, Barry UT, Laws ER. Perioperative management of patients undergoing transsphenoidal pituitary surgery. Anesth Analg 2005;101:1170–1181
3. Vance ML. Perioperative management of patients undergoing pituitary surgery. Endocrinol Metab Clin North Am 2003;32:355–365
4. Freda PU, Post KD. Differential diagnosis of sellar masses. Endocrinol Metab Clin North Am 1999;28:81–117, vi
5. Casanueva FF, Molitch ME, Schlechte JA, et al. Guidelines of the Pituitary Society for the diagnosis and management of prolactinomas. Clin Endocrinol (Oxf) 2006;65:265–273
6. Molitch ME. Pathologic hyperprolactinemia. Endocrinol Metab Clin North Am 1992;21:877–901
7. Vance ML. Treatment of patients with a pituitary adenoma: one clinician's experience. Neurosurg Focus 2004;16:E1
8. Nieman LK, Ilias I. Evaluation and treatment of Cushing's syndrome. Am J Med 2005;118:1340–1346
9. Arnaldi G, Angeli A, Atkinson AB, et al. Diagnosis and complications of Cushing's syndrome: a consensus statement. J Clin Endocrinol Metab 2003;88:5593–5602
10. Kidambi S, Raff H, Findling JW. Limitations of nocturnal salivary cortisol and urine free cortisol in the diagnosis of mild Cushing's syndrome. Eur J Endocrinol 2007;157:725–731
11. Newell-Price J, Bertagna X, Grossman AB, Nieman LK. Cushing's syndrome. Lancet 2006;367:1605–1617
12. Castro M, Moreira AC. Screening and diagnosis of Cushing's syndrome. Arq Bras Endocrinol Metabol 2007;51:1191–1198
13. Gross BA, Mindea SA, Pick AJ, Chandler JP, Batjer HH. Diagnostic approach to Cushing disease. Neurosurg Focus 2007;23:E1
14. Sakharova AA, Dimaraki EV, Chandler WF, Barkan AL. Clinically silent somatotropinomas may be biochemically active. J Clin Endocrinol Metab 2005;90:2117–2121
15. Melmed S. Medical progress: acromegaly. N Engl J Med 2006;355: 2558–2573
16. Freda PU. Current concepts in the biochemical assessment of the patient with acromegaly. Growth Horm IGF Res 2003;13:171–184
17. Freda PU, Reyes CM, Nuruzzaman AT, Sundeen RE, Bruce JN. Basal and glucose-suppressed GH levels less than 1 microg/L in newly diagnosed acromegaly. Pituitary 2003;6:175–180
18. Newman CB, Melmed S, George A, et al. Octreotide as primary therapy for acromegaly. J Clin Endocrinol Metab 1998;83:3034–3040
19. Cozzi R, Montini M, Attanasio R, et al. Primary treatment of acromegaly with octreotide LAR: a long-term (up to nine years) prospective study of its efficacy in the control of disease activity and tumor shrinkage. J Clin Endocrinol Metab 2006;91:1397–1403
20. Colao A, Attanasio R, Pivonello R, et al. Partial surgical removal of growth hormone-secreting pituitary tumors enhances the response to somatostatin analogs in acromegaly. J Clin Endocrinol Metab 2006;91:85–92
21. Socin HV, Chanson P, Delemer B, et al. The changing spectrum of TSH-secreting pituitary adenomas: diagnosis and management in 43 patients. Eur J Endocrinol 2003;148:433–442
22. Brucker-Davis F, Oldfield EH, Skarulis MC, Doppman JL, Weintraub BD. Thyrotropin-secreting pituitary tumors: diagnostic criteria, thyroid hormone sensitivity, and treatment outcome in 25 patients followed at the National Institutes of Health. J Clin Endocrinol Metab 1999;84:476–486
23. Erem C, Hacihasanoglu A, Sari A, Onder Ersöz H, Ukinç K, Fidan S. A rare case and a rapid tumor response to therapy: dramatic reduction in tumor size during octreotide treatment in a patient with TSH-secreting pituitary macroadenoma. Endocrine 2004;25:141–145
24. Iglesias P, Díez JJ. Long-term preoperative management of thyrotropin-secreting pituitary adenoma with octreotide. J Endocrinol Invest 1998;21:775–778

25. Foppiani L, Del Monte P, Ruelle A, Bandelloni R, Quilici P, Bernasconi D. TSH-secreting adenomas: rare pituitary tumors with multifaceted clinical and biological features. J Endocrinol Invest 2007;30:603–609
26. Vance ML. Hypopituitarism. N Engl J Med 1994;330:1651–1662
27. Grinspoon SK, Biller BM. Clinical review 62: laboratory assessment of adrenal insufficiency. J Clin Endocrinol Metab 1994;79:923–931
28. Oelkers W. Adrenal insufficiency. N Engl J Med 1996;335:1206–1212
29. Klose M, Lange M, Kosteljanetz M, Poulsgaard L, Feldt-Rasmussen U. Adrenocortical insufficiency after pituitary surgery: an audit of the reliability of the conventional short Synacthen test. Clin Endocrinol (Oxf) 2005;63:499–505
30. Erturk E, Jaffe CA, Barkan AL. Evaluation of the integrity of the hypothalamic-pituitary-adrenal axis by insulin hypoglycemia test. J Clin Endocrinol Metab 1998;83:2350–2354
31. Inder WJ, Hunt PJ. Glucocorticoid replacement in pituitary surgery: guidelines for perioperative assessment and management. J Clin Endocrinol Metab 2002;87:2745–2750
32. Auchus RJ, Shewbridge RK, Shepherd MD. Which patients benefit from provocative adrenal testing after transsphenoidal pituitary surgery? Clin Endocrinol (Oxf) 1997;46:21–27
33. Ausiello JC, Bruce JN, Freda PU. Postoperative assessment of the patient after transsphenoidal pituitary surgery. Pituitary 2008;11: 391–401
34. Hout WM, Arafah BM, Salazar R, Selman W. Evaluation of the hypothalamic-pituitary-adrenal axis immediately after pituitary adenomectomy: is perioperative steroid therapy necessary? J Clin Endocrinol Metab 1988;66:1208–1212
35. Connery LE, Coursin DB. Assessment and therapy of selected endocrine disorders. Anesthesiol Clin North Am 2004;22:93–123
36. Persani L, Ferretti E, Borgato S, Faglia G, Beck-Peccoz P. Circulating thyrotropin bioactivity in sporadic central hypothyroidism. J Clin Endocrinol Metab 2000;85:3631–3635
37. Arafah BM. Medical management of hypopituitarism in patients with pituitary adenomas. Pituitary 2002;5:109–117
38. Schneider HJ, Aimaretti G, Kreitschmann-Andermahr I, Stalla GK, Ghigo E. Hypopituitarism. Lancet 2007;369:1461–1470
39. Slawik M, Klawitter B, Meiser E, et al. Thyroid hormone replacement for central hypothyroidism: a randomized controlled trial comparing two doses of thyroxine (T4) with a combination of T4 and triiodothyronine. J Clin Endocrinol Metab 2007;92:4115–4122
40. Lamberts SW, de Herder WW, van der Lely AJ. Pituitary insufficiency. Lancet 1998;352:127–134
41. Nemergut EC, Zuo Z, Jane JA Jr, Laws ER Jr. Predictors of diabetes insipidus after transsphenoidal surgery: a review of 881 patients. J Neurosurg 2005;103:448–454
42. Dumont AS, Nemergut EC II, Jane JA Jr, Laws ER Jr. Postoperative care following pituitary surgery. J Intensive Care Med 2005;20: 127–140
43. Loh JA, Verbalis JG. Diabetes insipidus as a complication after pituitary surgery. Nat Clin Pract Endocrinol Metab 2007;3:489–494

5 Radiographic Evaluation of Pituitary Tumors

Prashant Raghavan and C. Douglas Phillips

Magnetic resonance imaging (MRI) has established itself as the primary imaging modality in the evaluation of the pituitary gland over the last three decades. The superb contrast and excellent spatial resolution of MRI have resulted in its becoming the sole pituitary imaging technology, except when there are contraindications or in instances where bony detail or information regarding the presence of intralesional calcification is needed. Plain film radiography and catheter angiography have markedly limited roles in the evaluation of pituitary pathology.

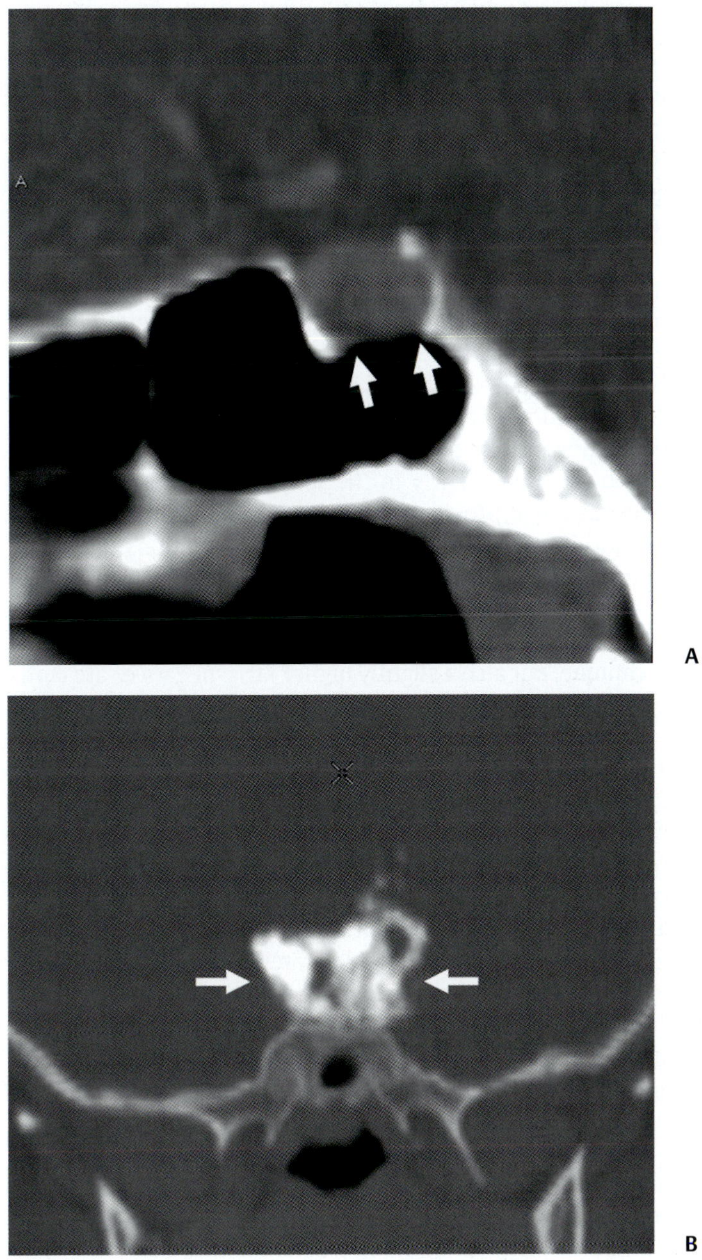

Fig. 5.1 **(A)** Sagittal reformatted computed tomography (CT) image shows erosion of sellar floor caused by microadenoma (*arrows*). **(B)** A densely calcified component of an adamantinomatous craniopharyngioma is evident (*arrows*).

Computed Tomography

The role of computed tomography (CT) in the evaluation of pituitary glandular disorders is largely limited to circumstances in which MRI is contraindicated. The CT protocol at our institution for evaluation of the sella is a 0.625-mm helical acquisition following the intravenous (IV) administration of a bolus of contrast media. This data set allows detailed coronal, sagittal, and, if necessary, oblique reformatted images. In an early study of the role of CT in the evaluation of pituitary lesions, Webb et al[1] concluded that although CT and MRI were comparable in their ability to detect macroadenomas, MRI offered superior characterization of lesional morphology and surrounding structures. However, CT may provide complementary information on surrounding osseous structures, such as the integrity of the sellar floor,[2] and it can confirm calcification in an existing lesion (**Fig. 5.1**).

Magnetic Resonance Imaging

To effectively identify and characterize pituitary abnormalities, an MRI examination must consist of high-resolution noncontrast and contrast-enhanced sequences. Fat-suppression techniques may be useful in the evaluation of the postoperative sella but have not been used routinely. At our institution, a complete sella MRI examination consists of noncontrast sagittal and coronal fast spin echo (SE) T1-weighted sequences, a coronal T2-weighted sequence, postcontrast coronal and sagittal T1-weighted sequences, and a postcontrast spoiled gradient sequence, the value of which is discussed below. The precise specifications of MRI protocols vary among scanners, but the objective of providing images with high spatial and contrast resolution is achieved by a combination of thin (3-mm) slices, a small field of view, and a fine matrix size[3] to produce images with very small voxels. The coronal noncontrast T1-weighted and T2-weighted images are first reviewed for any abnormalities. It is often possible to identify microadenomas on these images, particularly if narrow window settings are used. The administration of IV gadolinium-based contrast at 0.1 mmol/kg is required to clearly establish the presence of most lesions and define their margins. Several studies have established that IV contrast leads to increased lesional detection.[3] However, recent awareness of the risk of nephrogenic systemic fibrosis with gadolinium-based contrast agents has led to a greater degree of prudence in its use. Contrast can be avoided if a lesion is depicted clearly on noncontrast images, and if not identified, administration of half of the standard dose (0.05 mmol/kg)[4] may be a useful strategy. The scan should be performed immediately after the contrast injection when not utilized in a dynamic technique. Studies have shown that normalization of pituitary adenomas and normal gland may occur with further delays in imaging.[3]

Although SE sequences are the mainstay of sellar imaging, volumetric spoiled gradient echo sequences have been shown to be of value in the detection of small microadenomas, particularly in the setting of Cushing's disease. This sequence provides thinner slices, yields better spatial resolution, and enables multiplanar reformations to be performed as the voxel sizes are nearly isotropic.[5] Patronas et al[6] demonstrated a higher sensitivity for detection of adrenocorticotropic hormone (ACTH) microadenomas with this technique, but also a slightly higher false-negative rate compared with SE imaging.

Dynamic contrast MRI performed immediately after the administration of a bolus of IV contrast may be used as a problem-solving technique when regular imaging is inconclusive, but it is used as a routine imaging tool at some institutions. This technique is based on the principle that lesion conspicuity may be maximized by scanning immediately after administration of contrast, when the lesion and the gland demonstrate differential rates of enhancement due to the differences in their blood supply. A series of coronal T1-weighted images are rapidly acquired through the gland, with a temporal resolution of 1 to 2 seconds being achievable with modern scanners. The source of an adenoma's blood supply determines when the lesion is most conspicuous. Some are most evident on the unenhanced images and fade on the enhanced images. Others are most evident 30 to 50 seconds after contrast administration and others 1 to 2 minutes later. Addition of a dynamic MRI sequence may increase lesion detection by 10%. It may also be beneficial to add a sagittal acquisition to the standard coronal dynamic study.[5,7]

Normal Imaging Anatomy

The pituitary gland exhibits great variability in its dimensions. As a rule of thumb, as measured on a coronal image, the height of the gland is 6 mm in infants and children, 8 mm in men and postmenopausal women, 10 mm in women of childbearing age, and 12 mm in pregnancy and the postpartum state (Elster's rule of 6, 8, 10, 12).[8] In the peripartum period, the gland may demonstrate a prominent superiorly convex contour.

The adenohypophysis on MRI is usually isointense to brain but may appear slightly hyperintense on T1-weighted sequences in pregnant or postpartum women. The neonatal anterior pituitary may be substantially hyperintense on T1-weighted images. This is due to lactotroph hyperplasia and increased protein synthesis. The neurohypophysis is uniformly hyperintense on T1-weighted images (**Fig. 5.2**). The reason for this "bright spot" has not precisely been determined but is believed to be due to neurophysin, the vasopressin-associated carrier protein. Other contenders include vasopressin itself and phospholipid vesicles that contain vasopressin. The "ectopic" neurohypophysis refers to the displacement of the neurohypophyseal bright spot into the stalk or hypothalamus proximal to the site of stalk injury or disease. The bright spot may be absent in central diabetes insipidus, but it may also not be seen in a small percentage of the normal population (**Fig. 5.3**). The infundibulum demonstrates a tapered configuration and enhances homogeneously. A normal stalk is less than 4 mm thick. On postcontrast images, the gland enhances homogeneously. On dynamic images, a centrifugal pattern of enhancement from the stalk and posterior pituitary to the central and then peripheral adenohypophysis is observed.[5,9]

The optic chiasm is consistently demonstrable above the gland on all sequences. The cavernous sinuses are seen as paired parasellar heterogeneous structures. The larger sinusoids within them may appear as flow voids but will enhance following gadolinium administration. The lateral dural reflection of these sinuses is easily visualized, but demonstration of the thin medial dural walls is often problematic. Although the cranial nerves that traverse the lateral walls may be seen on coronal T2-weighted images, the performance of a high-resolution heavily T2-weighted three-dimensional sequence may be the best way to consistently demonstrate them.[10] The cavernous internal carotid artery is easily seen as a flow void (**Fig. 5.2**).

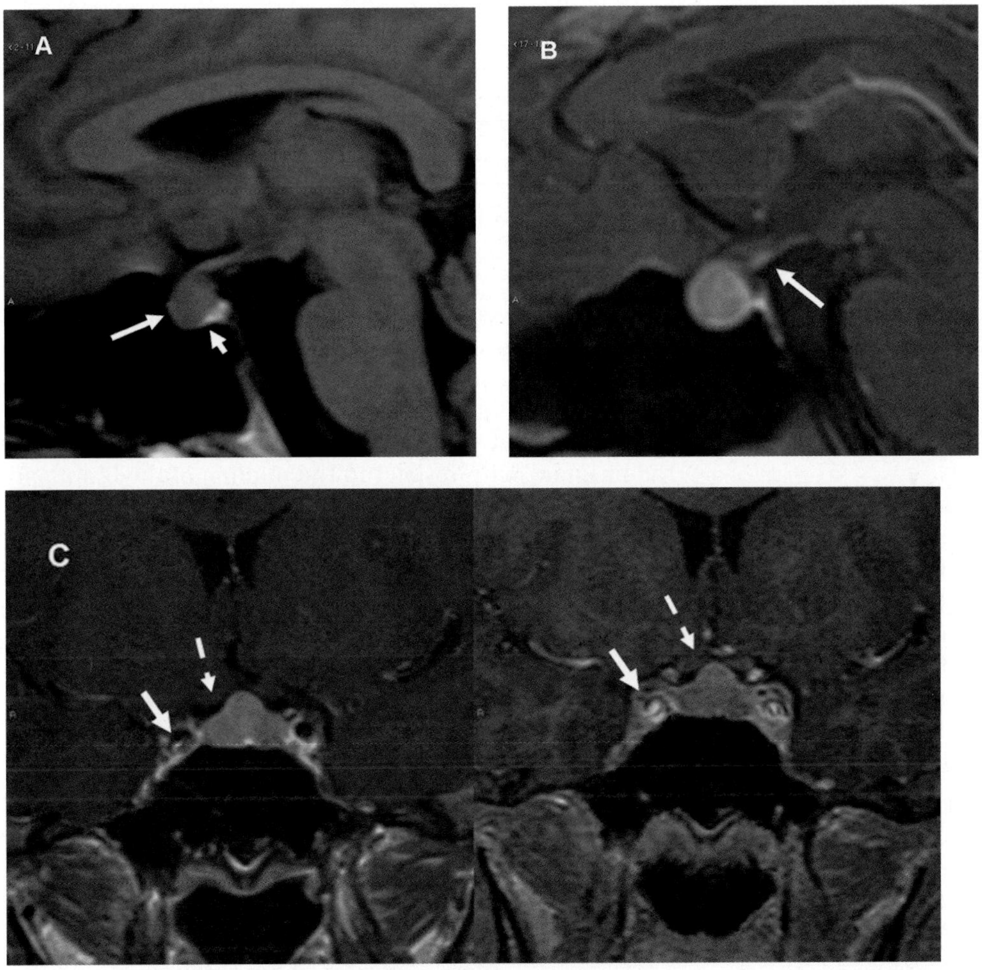

Fig. 5.2 **(A)** Normal magnetic resonance imaging (MRI) anatomy. Isointense adenohypophysis and hyperintense neurohypophysis (*long* and *short arrows*, respectively) are clearly identified on the sagittal unenhanced T1-weighted image. **(B)** Enhancement and tapered appearance of stalk are evident (*arrows*). **(C)** Postcontrast coronal T1-weighted and spoiled gradient (SPGR) images are shown. Note more homogeneous enhancement pattern in the former. The convex superior contour of the gland is normal in this 22-year-old woman. Cavernous internal carotid arteries (*solid arrows*) and optic chiasm (*dashed arrows*) are seen.

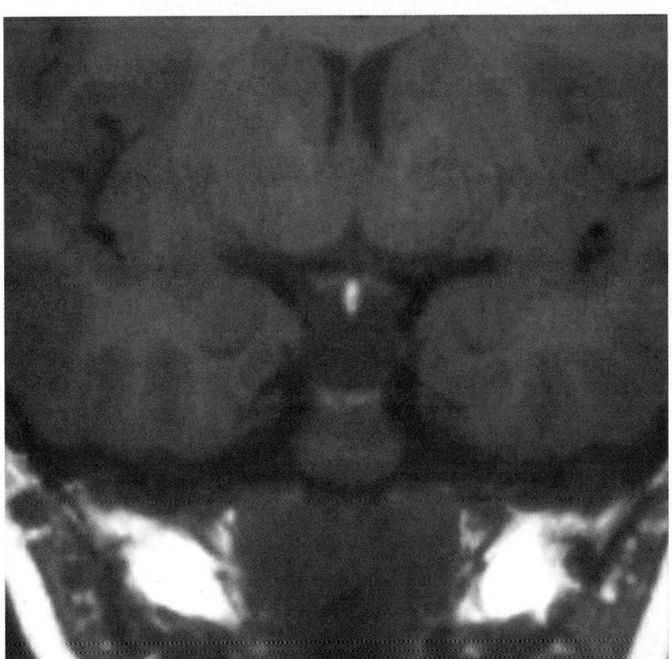

Fig. 5.3 Ectopic neurohypophysis. Transection of infundibulum has resulted in displacement of a "bright spot" of neurohypophysis into the proximal infundibulum.

Imaging of Pituitary Pathology

Tumors

Microadenomas

T1-weighted coronal sequences are best suited for the identification of microadenomas. Most (80–85%) are hypointense with respect to the remainder of the gland on T1-weighted images. The minority that are isointense are usually evident on postcontrast images. A small fraction are hyperintense due to intratumoral hemorrhage. The appearance on T2-weighted images is more variable and, in general, these lesions are less well seen[5,11] (**Fig. 5.4**).

There is no defining imaging characteristic that enables easy distinction between the different types of microadenomas. However, the distribution of these lesions tends to reflect the distribution of the cell of origin. For example, ACTH-, thyroid-stimulating hormone (TSH)–, and luteinizing hormone/follicle-stimulating hormone (LH/FSH)–producing adenomas tend to occupy the central gland, whereas prolactinomas and growth hormone (GH)–producing adenomas prefer the glandular periphery. GH–producing adenomas have been noted to demonstrate a predilection for infrasellar extension. T2 hypointensity may indicate that a microadenoma is of the densely granulated GH-producing type.[12] The smallest microadenomas are often those that produce ACTH.

A deformity of the glandular contour, in the absence of signal abnormality, may indicate the presence of an underlying microadenoma that may reveal itself on postcontrast imaging. Deviation of the infundibulum, however, is a poor radiographic sign. The infundibulum may be deviated without evidence of underlying pathology in cases of developmental asymmetry of the sellar floor or on occasion be deviated toward a lesion. The high incidence of infundibulum deviation in the normal population has been attributed to developmental lateral eccentricity of the pituitary with respect to the midline of the brain and also is due to an ontogenic eccentric insertion of the stalk off the midline in some people. Stalk deviation, therefore, should not be used to support or refute the presence of a microadenoma.[13]

Most microadenomas enhance to a lesser degree than a normal gland after administration of gadolinium-based contrast. A dynamic method, as described earlier, may be required in those instances when standard MRI is equivocal. Some authors advocate the routine incorporation of a dynamic study into their pituitary protocol. We have rarely found this necessary. As described earlier, a postcontrast

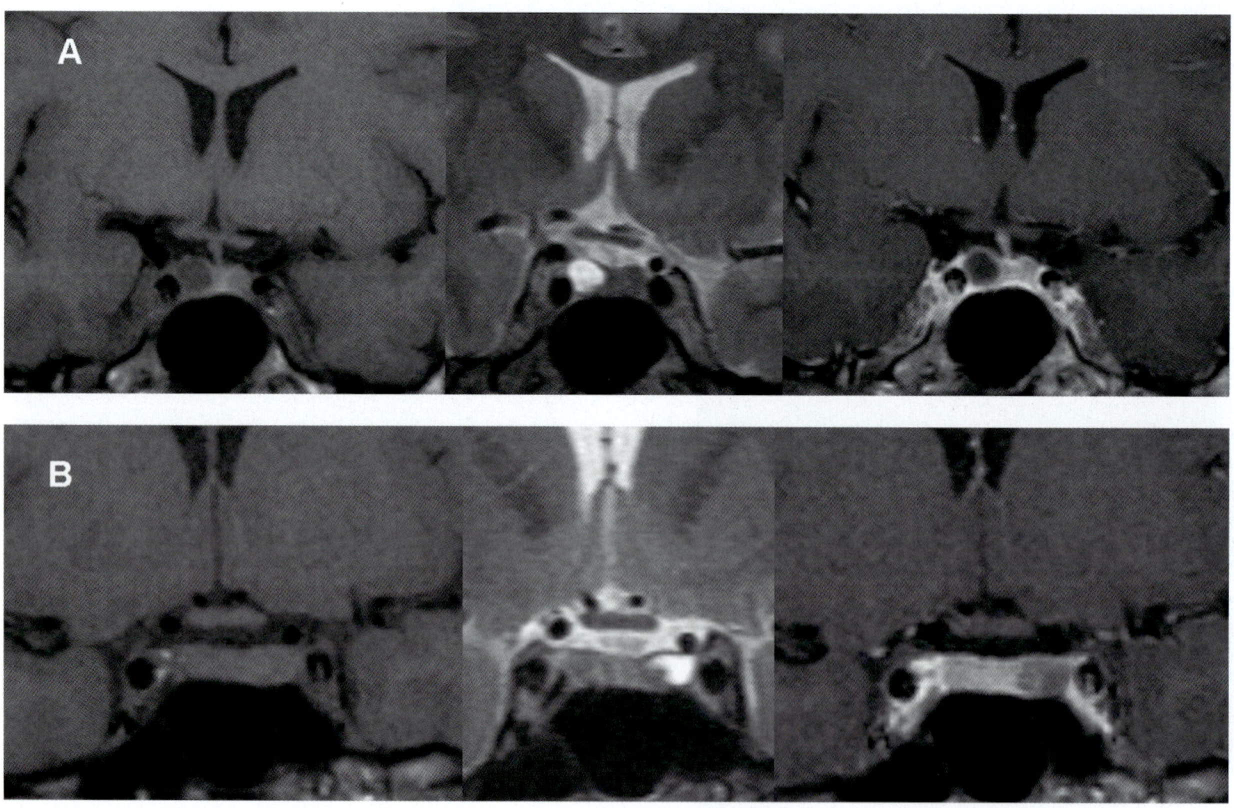

Fig. 5.4 **(A)** Typical microadenoma. This prolactinoma is hypointense on T1-weighted image (*left*), hyperintense on T2-weighted image (center) and does not enhance with contrast (right). **(B)** Adenoma is isointense on T1-weighted imaging (left) and is evident only on T2-weighted (*center*) and postcontrast sequences (*right*).

spoiled gradient (SPGR) sequence may be useful to reveal small microadenomas not demonstrated on enhanced SE T1-weighted images (**Fig. 5.5**). The utility of delayed post-contrast imaging, performed 30 to 60 minutes after administration of contrast, where contrast accumulates within the adenoma and has washed out from the normal gland, has also been described.[3] This may occasionally allow distinction of otherwise undiscovered adenomas.

Excellent correlation exists between MRI and intraoperative findings of microadenomas. The high accuracy reported in multiple early studies evaluating the role of MRI has not been refuted. Although the detection of small lesions remains occasionally problematic, the addition of SPGR sequences and the high signal-to-noise ratio obtainable with high field strength MRI units have proven to be extremely beneficial (**Fig. 5.6**). In circumstances where all noninvasive approaches fail to depict a lesion, the presence of which is strongly suspected clinically, inferior petrosal sinus (IPS) sampling may be necessary. The IPS may be safely catheterized in up to 98% of cases with a complication rate less than 1%. It is an extremely sensitive, specific, and accurate test for diagnosing Cushing's disease and distinguishing that entity from ectopic ACTH syndrome[14] (**Fig. 5.7**).

It must be noted, however, that not all small intraglandular lesions are microadenomas. Small Rathke's cleft and pars intermedia cysts may resemble adenomas, especially when filled with proteinaceous fluid. A focal susceptibility artifact in the gland adjacent to the site of insertion of the sphenoid sinus septum may simulate a lesion[15] (**Fig. 5.8**). An expanded posterior clinoid process may also simulate a lesion due to volume averaging. The pituitary gland may have small microinfarctions that could potentially mimic adenomas.

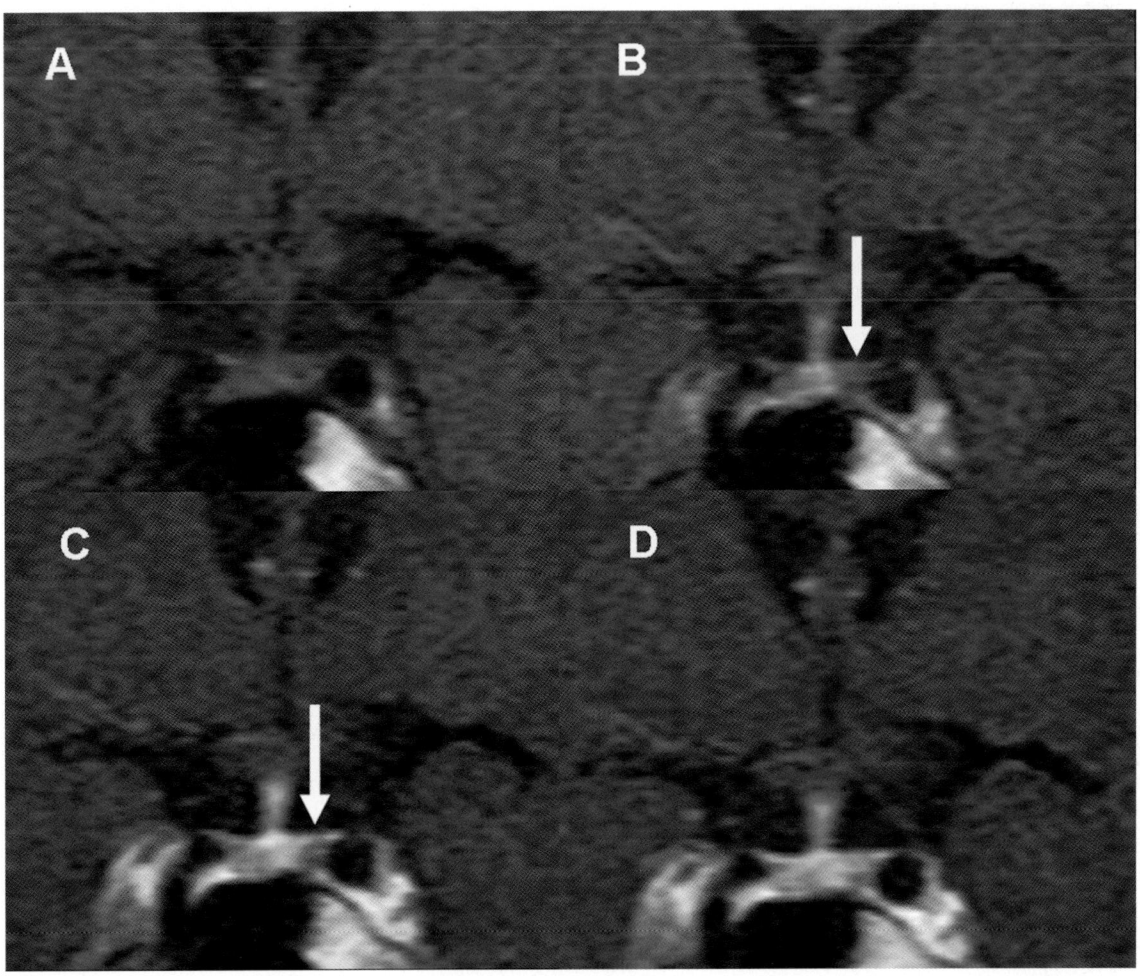

Fig. 5.5 **(A–D)** Dynamic MRI. On initial unenhanced image, no evidence of microadenoma is seen. On subsequent images, obtained 13 seconds apart, a small peripherally located hypoenhancing adenoma is identified on left side (*arrows*). **(D)** The adenoma is barely discernible and is near isointense with the remainder of gland.

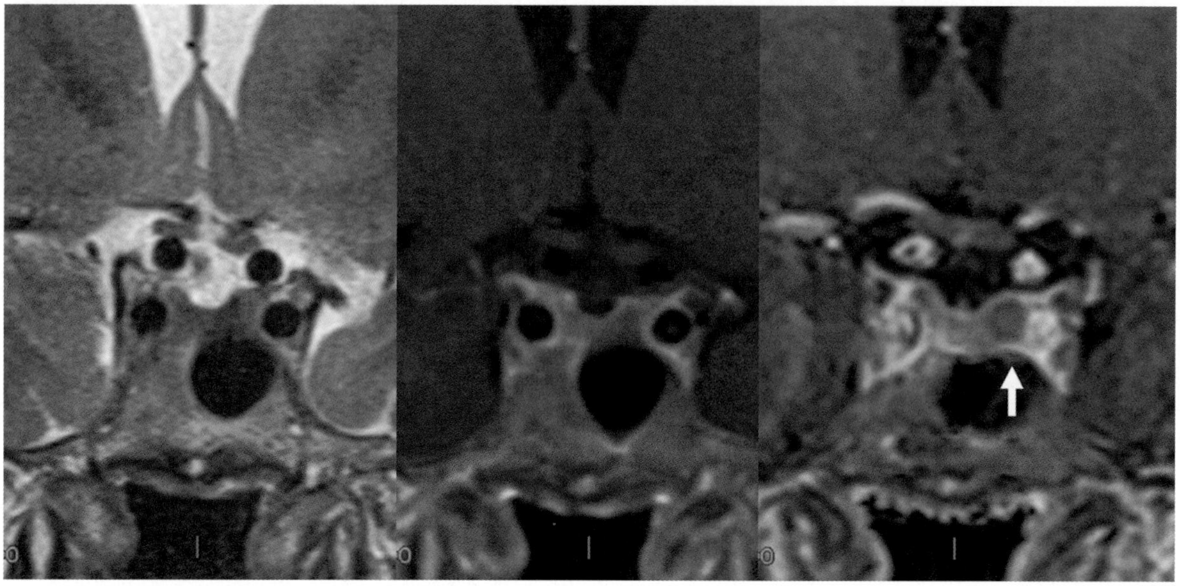

A–C

Fig. 5.6 Microadenoma are best demonstrated on spoiled gradient (SPGR) imaging. Adrenocorticotropic hormone–producing microadenoma is nearly imperceptible on the T2-weighted **(A)** and postcontrast T1-weighted spin-echo image **(B)**. It is most conspicuous on the postcontrast SPGR image **(C)** (*white arrow*).

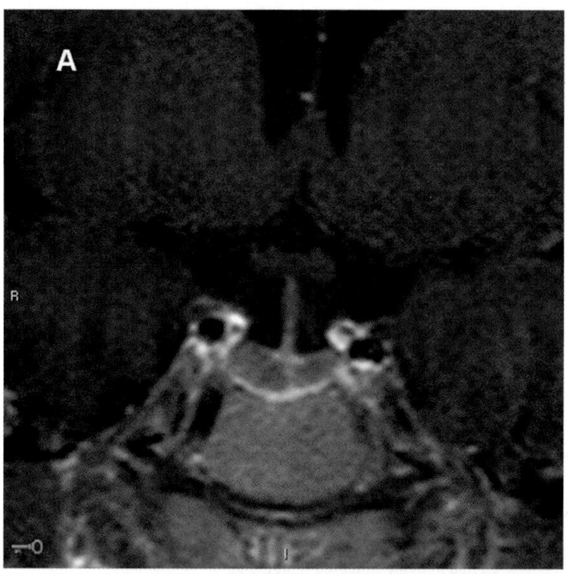

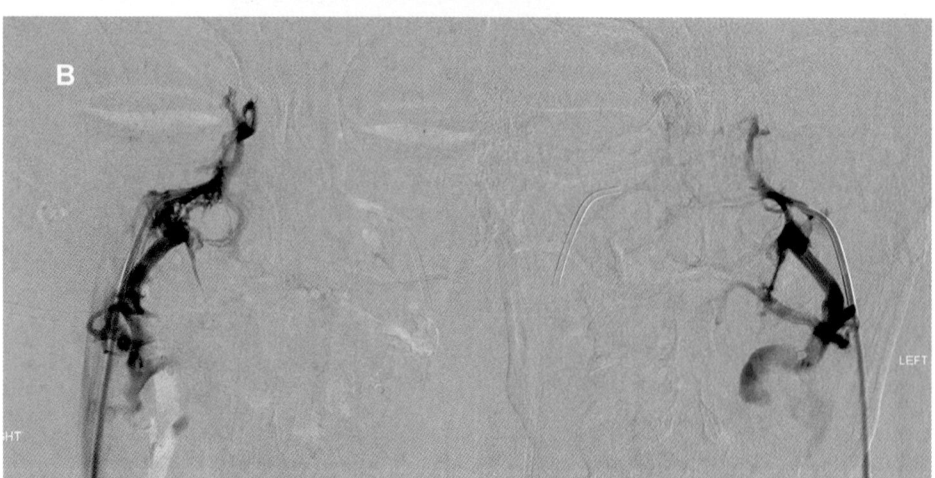

Fig. 5.7 **(A)** Inferior petrosal sinus sampling. No definite evidence of adenoma was identified on coronal postcontrast image. **(B)** Inferior petrosal sinus sampling of a lateralized adenoma (*right*), where, in retrospect, subtle contour abnormality is visible in A.

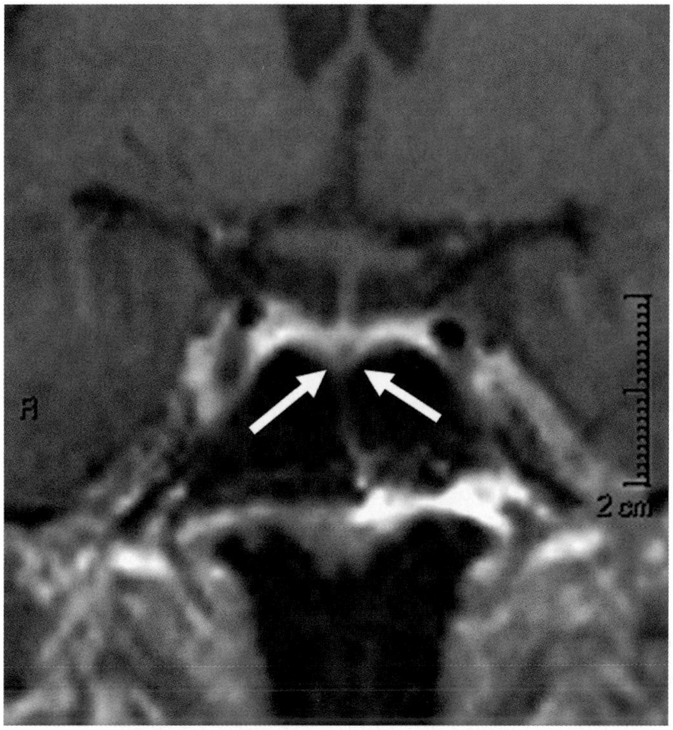

Fig. 5.8 Pituitary pseudolesion. The small focus of central glandular hypointensity (*arrows*) is a susceptibility artifact at the site of sphenoid sinus septal insertion and should not be mistaken for a microadenoma.

Macroadenomas

The imaging diagnosis of macroadenomas is straightforward and is based on two key findings: origin of the lesion from the pituitary gland, and expansion of the sella (**Fig. 5.9**). When one establishes the pituitary gland as the source of the lesion, the differential diagnosis is narrow. Expansion of the sella is not a feature of more aggressive processes that can occur in this region, such as metastases, infection, or inflammation. Macroadenomas are very variable in their signal intensity and enhancement pattern. Often these lesions are hypointense on T1-weighted images and exhibit greater variability on T2-weighted images. T1 hyperintensity may be due to intratumoral hemorrhage, occasionally after bromocriptine therapy.[16] Liquefactive change may result in macroadenomas appearing very bright on T2-weighted images. MRI has been used to predict the consistency of macroadenomas in an aim to assist surgical planning. It has been postulated that T2 hyperintense adenomas and those that demonstrate low apparent diffusion coefficient (ADC) values on diffusion-weighted imaging (DWI) may be amenable to suction due to their soft consistency. Results with T2 signal intensity have been inconsistent and DWI may hold greater promise in this regard.[17,18]

Macroadenomas that extend into the suprasellar cistern often assume a snowman configuration due to a constriction produced by the diaphragma sellae. The relationship of the optic apparatus and these lesions is easily established on

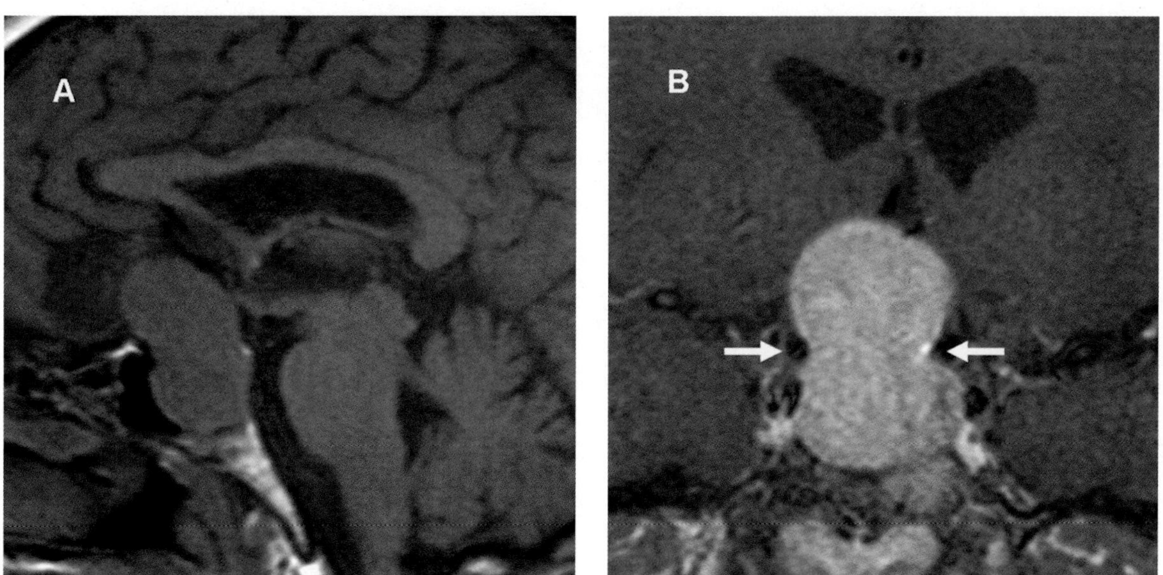

Fig. 5.9 **(A)** Typical macroadenoma. Expansion of the sella is evident. **(B)** Homogeneously enhancing macroadenoma demonstrates a typical "snowman" configuration, with the waist at diaphragma sellae (*arrows*).

MRI. The presence of optic nerve T2 hyperintensity due to edema has been correlated with the degree of visual impairment and may be reversible.[19] Rarely hemorrhage into the optic tracts may follow apoplexy.[20] Although subtle bony changes may be inapparent on MRI, extension into the sphenoid sinus or clival marrow is easily discernible. The diagnosis of cavernous sinus invasion is often problematic. This is due to the inability of MRI to confidently demonstrate the delicate medial dural wall. The only reliable indicator of cavernous sinus involvement is the presence of tumor on both sides of the intracavernous internal carotid artery (ICA) (**Fig. 5.10**). Several authors have proposed an array of MRI criteria for cavernous sinus invasion, such as the degree of circumferential arterial encasement, the relationship between the tumor and lines drawn through and tangential to the supraclinoid and intracavernous ICAs, and the involvement of certain venous compartments around the ICA, among others, with none proving to be consistently reliable. For instance, in a study by Vieira et al,[21] encasement of the intracavernous ICA of 30% or more was reliably correlated with intraoperative findings of invasion. However, Cottier et al[22] reported a corresponding value of 67% or greater to reliably predict invasion. Despite the high frequency of cavernous sinus invasion, constriction of an encased ICA is uncommon. This is of diagnostic importance, as meningiomas in the same location tend to constrict the arterial lumen. However, exceptions to the rule do exist (**Fig. 5.10**). True pituitary carcinomas are uncommon and are indistinguishable on MRI from macroadenomas, unless foci of metastatic disease are evident. Rarely, subarachnoid space seeding of benign macroadenomas occurs[23] (**Fig. 5.11**).

Nonadenomatous Pituitary/Sellar Neoplasms

Tumors of Pituicyte Origin

Pituicytoma and granulosa cell tumors are uncommon primary pituitary neoplasms. Neither of these has a

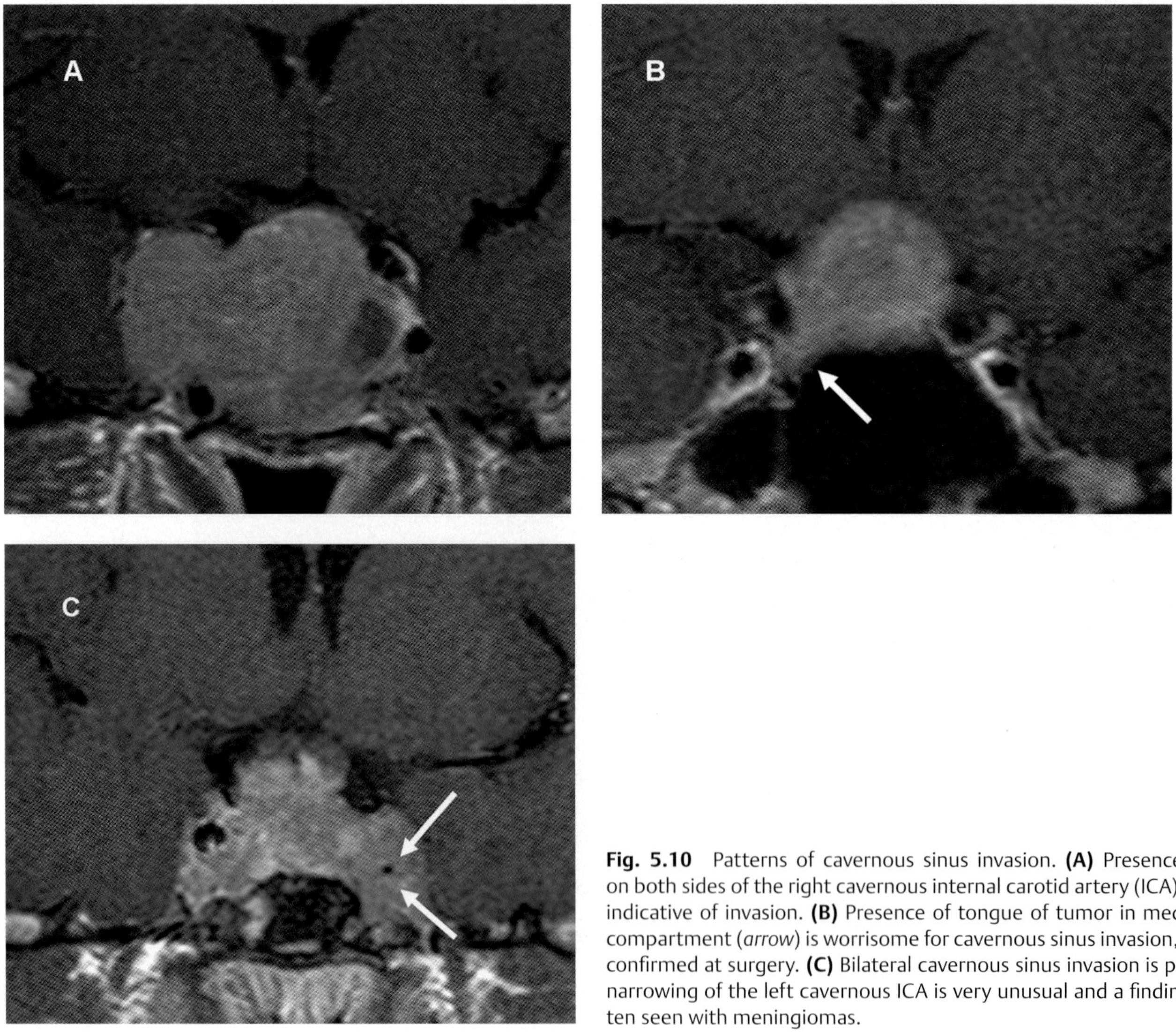

Fig. 5.10 Patterns of cavernous sinus invasion. **(A)** Presence of tumor on both sides of the right cavernous internal carotid artery (ICA) is strongly indicative of invasion. **(B)** Presence of tongue of tumor in medial venous compartment (*arrow*) is worrisome for cavernous sinus invasion, which was confirmed at surgery. **(C)** Bilateral cavernous sinus invasion is present, but narrowing of the left cavernous ICA is very unusual and a finding more often seen with meningiomas.

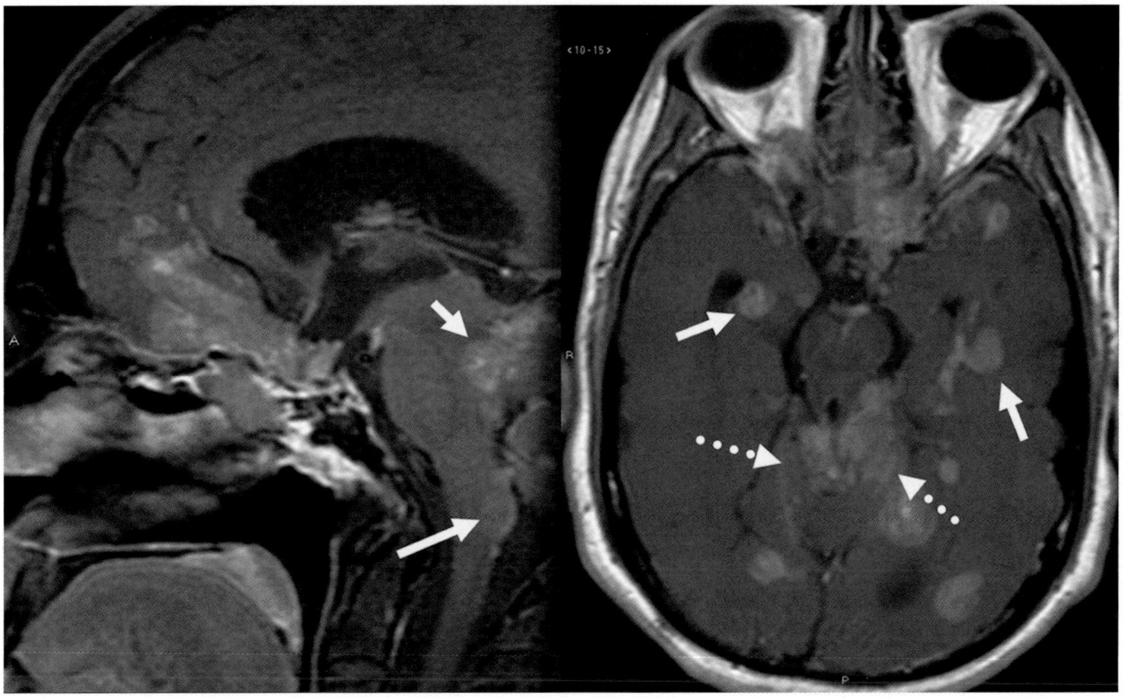

Fig. 5.11 Pituitary carcinoma. Irregular mass is seen in the sella and suprasellar cistern invading the third ventricle. Innumerable parenchymal (*arrows*) and ependymal metastatic deposits are present. Leptomeningeal metastatic deposits coat the cerebellar folia (*dotted arrows*).

characteristic imaging appearance (**Fig. 5.12**). They resemble macroadenomas on imaging but may have a greater tendency to occupy the posterior gland because of their origin from pituicytes in the neurohypophysis. As a result, the bright spot is often ectopic. These tumors are also hypervascular.[24] True astrocytomas may also arise from the neurohypophysis. Thickening of the stalk may be an important clue to the diagnosis of the uncommon tumors.[25]

Tumors Secondarily Involving the Sella and Pituitary Gland

Uncommonly, the pituitary may be the locus for the metastatic disease. A metastatic deposit does not expand the sella and may actually destroy it and thus be distinguished from macroadenoma (**Fig. 5.13**). About 1 to 5% of patients with systemic malignancy, usually lung or breast cancers, may harbor metastasis to the pituitary, with a higher number

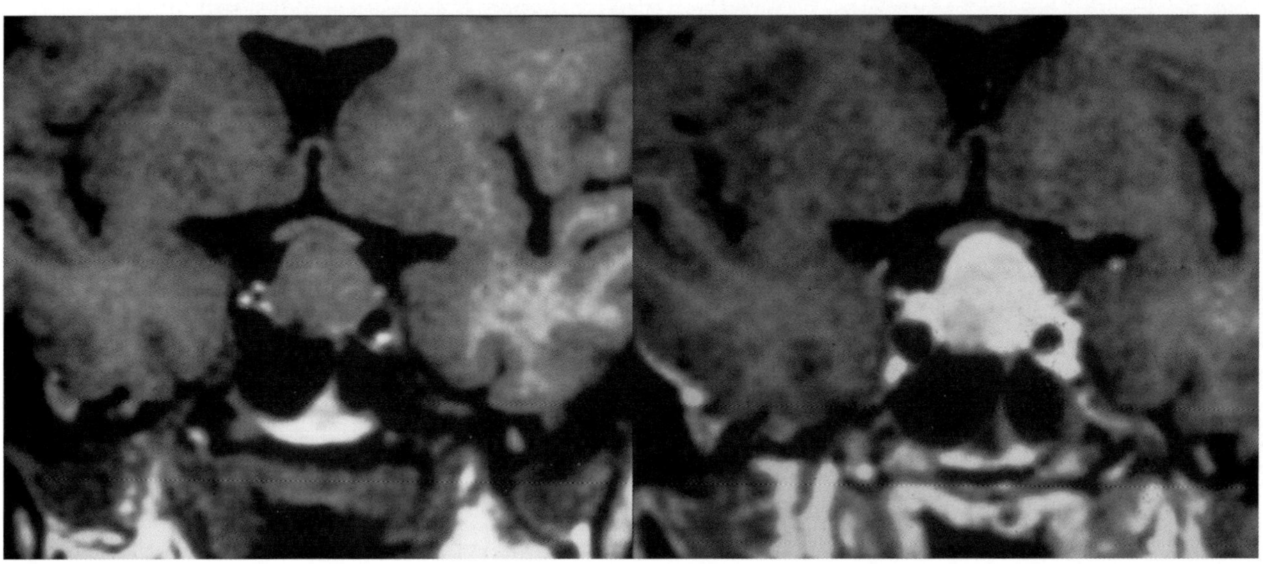

Fig. 5.12 **(A,B)** Granular cell tumor. The lesion is indistinguishable from a macroadenoma. **(B)** Note the intense enhancement on the postcontrast image.

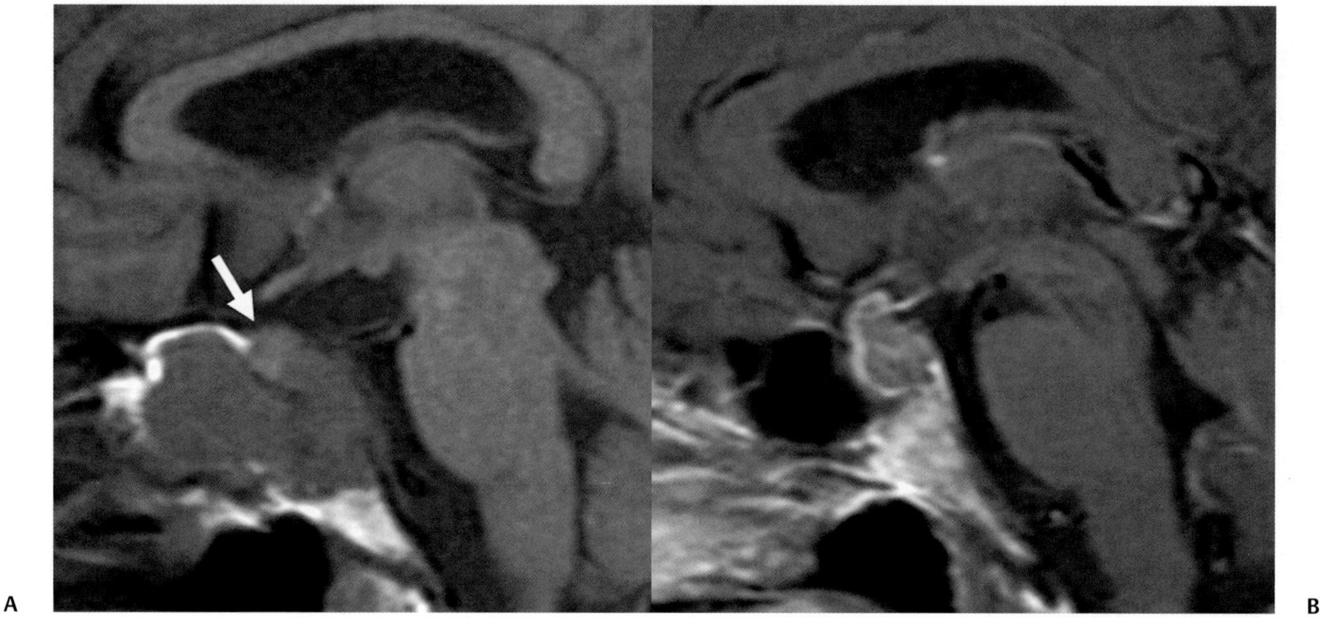

Fig. 5.13 Examples of metastatic disease. **(A)** A destructive lesion engulfs the pituitary gland (*arrow*), representing a metastatic deposit from a primary intestinal carcinoid tumor. **(B)** A mass replaces the pituitary gland without sellar expansion. This is proven to be a metastatic lesion from a breast primary.

being reported in autopsy series. The gland may be engulfed by metastatic deposits to the sphenoid bone or the adjacent dura.[5] Lymphomas of the pituitary gland are extremely rare and may be of the B- or T-cell variety. These have a tendency to be hypointense on T2-weighted images due to high nuclear-to-cytoplasmic ratio. About 1.4% of systemic leukemia patients have pituitary involvement[26] (**Fig. 5.14**). Langerhans cell histiocytosis may affect the infundibulum in up to 50% of cases when intracranial involvement is present. The occurrence of stalk thickening and enhancement

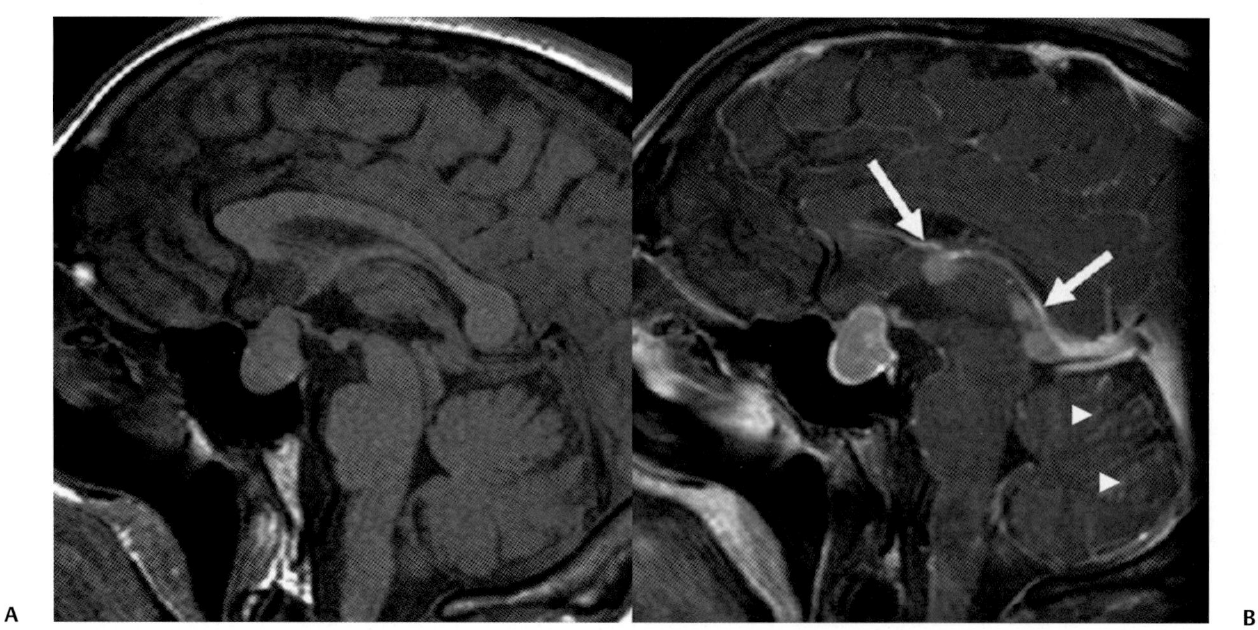

Fig. 5.14 **(A)** Pre- and **(B)** postcontrast sagittal T1-weighted images. An enhancing pituitary mass represents an acute lymphocytic leukemic deposit. Numerous ependymal deposits in third ventricle (*arrows*) and diffuse leptomeningeal infiltration in posterior fossa (*arrowheads*) are evident.

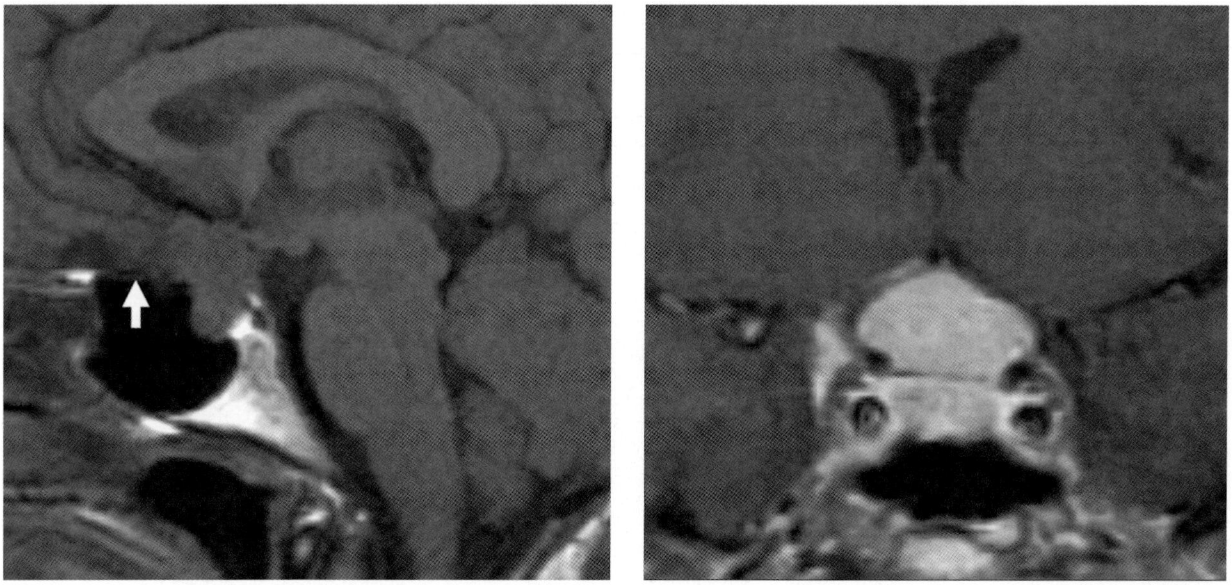

A B

Fig. 5.15 Diaphragma sellae meningioma. **(A)** Sagittal unenhanced image shows the lesion is predominantly suprasellar in location and extends anteriorly along the planum sphenoidale (*arrow*). **(B)** The lesion enhances intensely.

in conjunction with calvarial bone lesions, pineal and choroids plexus involvement, and parenchymal changes in the white and gray matter (dentate nuclei) should suggest the diagnosis.[5]

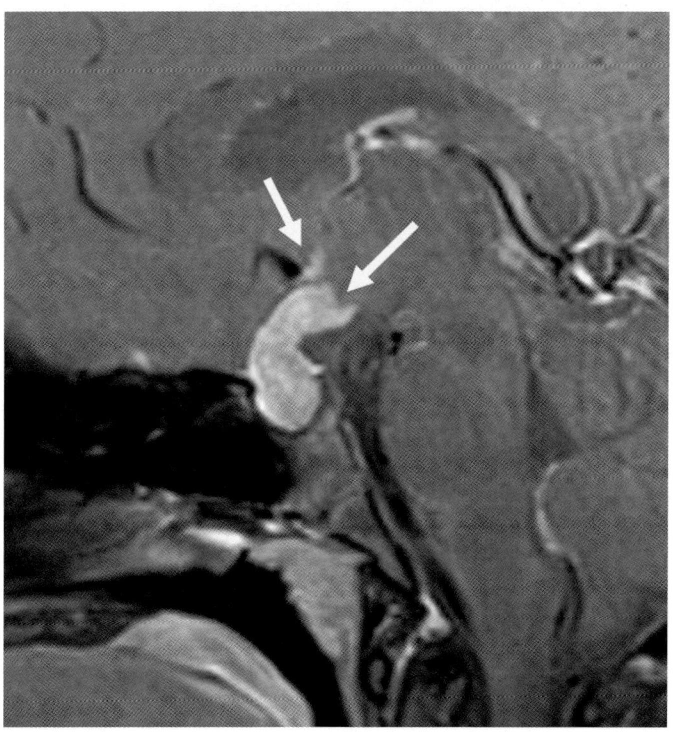

Fig. 5.16 Germinoma. The lesion involves the pituitary gland, thickens the stalk, and extends into the supraoptic and infundibular recesses (*arrows*). These findings would be atypical for macroadenoma. Note the lack of sellar expansion.

Tumors arising from the skull base such as chordomas and chondrosarcomas may secondarily involve the pituitary gland. Meningiomas arising from the diaphragma sellae, cavernous sinus dura, clinoid processes, and optic nerve sheaths may project into the sella. The identification of these lesions as being discrete from the pituitary gland is the key to their diagnosis. This may on occasion be difficult, and meningiomas that involve the sella or suprasellar cistern may be indistinguishable from macroadenomas (**Fig. 5.15**).

Germ Cell Tumors

Approximately 20% of intracranial germinomas occur in the suprasellar cistern (**Fig. 5.16**). These may arise de novo in this region or may represent metastases from a pineal or third ventricular primary. A midline suprasellar enhancing solid lesion involving the infundibulum or hypothalamus in a young patient is most likely a germinoma. The presence of a coexistent pineal lesion virtually ensures this diagnosis. Teratomas may contain foci of fat or calcification. There is also the entity of the "occult neurohypophyseal germinoma," wherein a germinoma in a young patient presenting with diabetes insipidus may be inapparent or subtle on an initial MRI only to reveal itself on a follow-up study.[27]

Craniopharyngioma

Most craniopharyngiomas occur in the suprasellar cistern but may extend into the sella. The two distinct forms of craniopharyngioma, the adamantinomatous and papillary varieties, differ not only in their clinical and pathologic manifestations but also in their imaging characteristics. The adamantinomatous variety seen in children is usually composed of a readily identifiable cystic component containing T1 hyperintense fluid due to the presence of cholesterol and a heterogeneously enhancing solid component that is often densely calcified or sometimes ossified (**Fig. 5.17**). This finding is better demonstrated on CT. These tumors are more likely to be adherent to surrounding structures, encase the adjacent vasculature, and invade adjacent brain, explaining a higher rate of postoperative

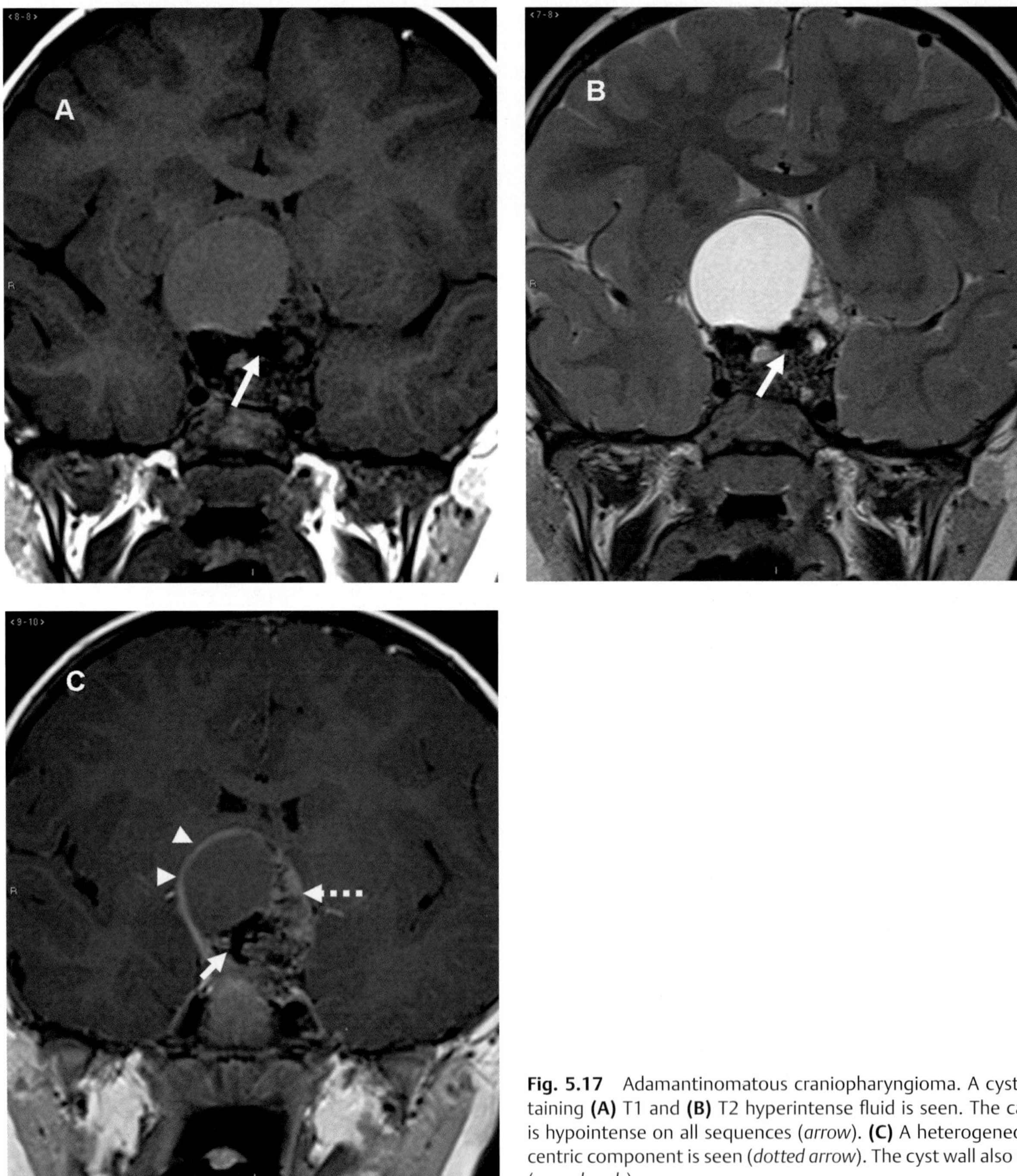

Fig. 5.17 Adamantinomatous craniopharyngioma. A cystic component containing **(A)** T1 and **(B)** T2 hyperintense fluid is seen. The calcified component is hypointense on all sequences (*arrow*). **(C)** A heterogeneously enhancing eccentric component is seen (*dotted arrow*). The cyst wall also enhances smoothly (*arrowheads*).

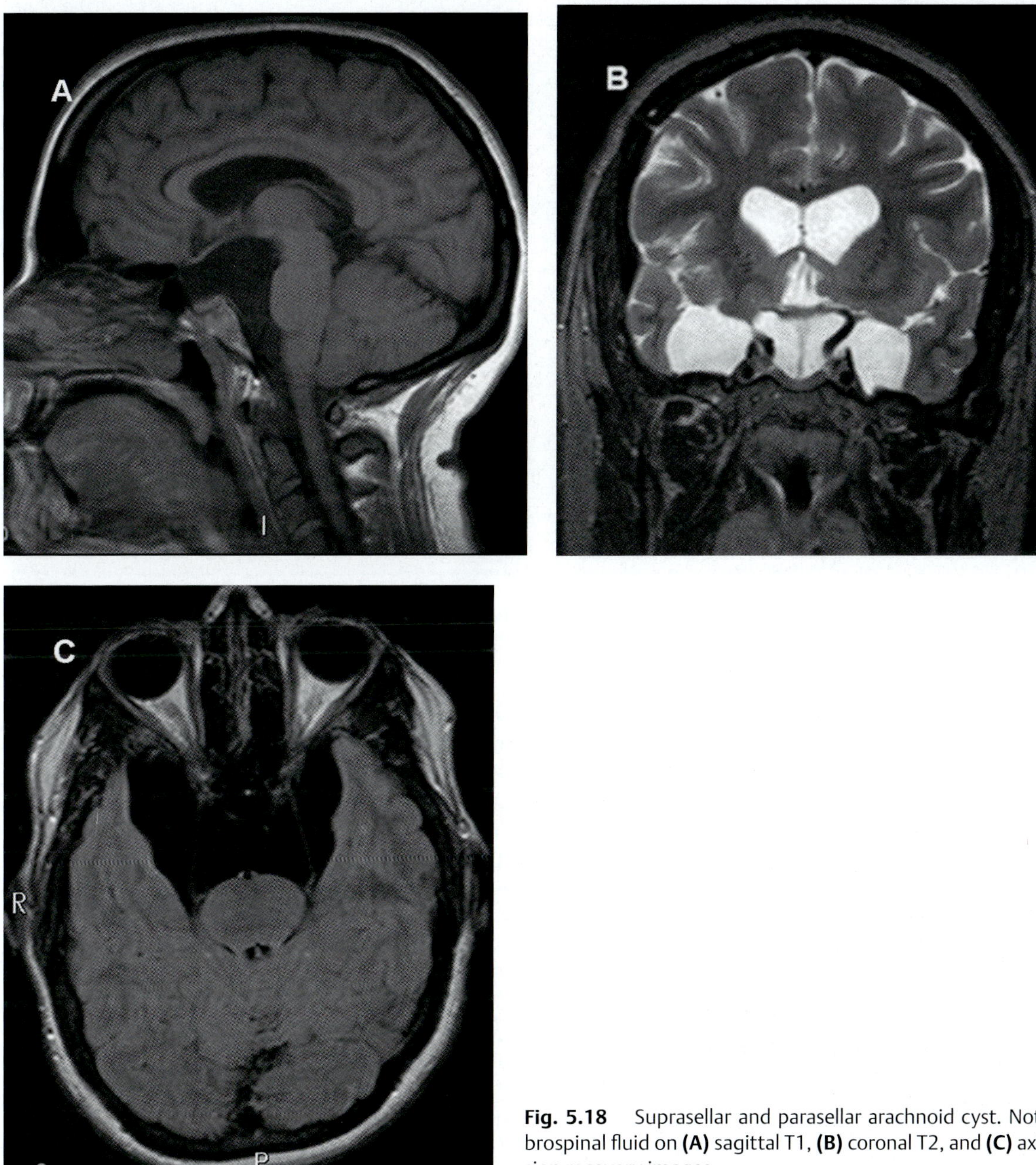

Fig. 5.18 Suprasellar and parasellar arachnoid cyst. Note isointensity with cerebrospinal fluid on **(A)** sagittal T1, **(B)** coronal T2, and **(C)** axial fluid-attenuated inversion recovery images.

recurrence. The papillary variety, on the other hand, presents most commonly as a solidly enhancing suprasellar lesion. These tumors are less likely to calcify or contain large cysts. Cysts, when present, contain fluid that is hypointense on T1-weighted images.[28]

Cystic Sellar Lesions

Arachnoid cysts of the suprasellar cistern arise from failure of perforation of the embryonic membrane of Liliequist. These cysts contain fluid that is isointense to cerebrospinal fluid (CSF) on all sequences with complete suppression of fluid signal on fluid-attenuated inversion recovery (FLAIR) images (**Fig. 5.18**). Epidermoid cysts demonstrate slightly increased signal with respect to CSF due to the presence of keratin and desquamated material. The key to their diagnosis is the lack of suppression of signal on FLAIR images and hyperintensity on DWI. The presence of T1 hyperintensity due to the presence of fat is a useful clue to the diagnosis of dermoid cysts (**Fig. 5.19**). Both dermoid and epidermoid cysts may rupture to produce chemical

A–C

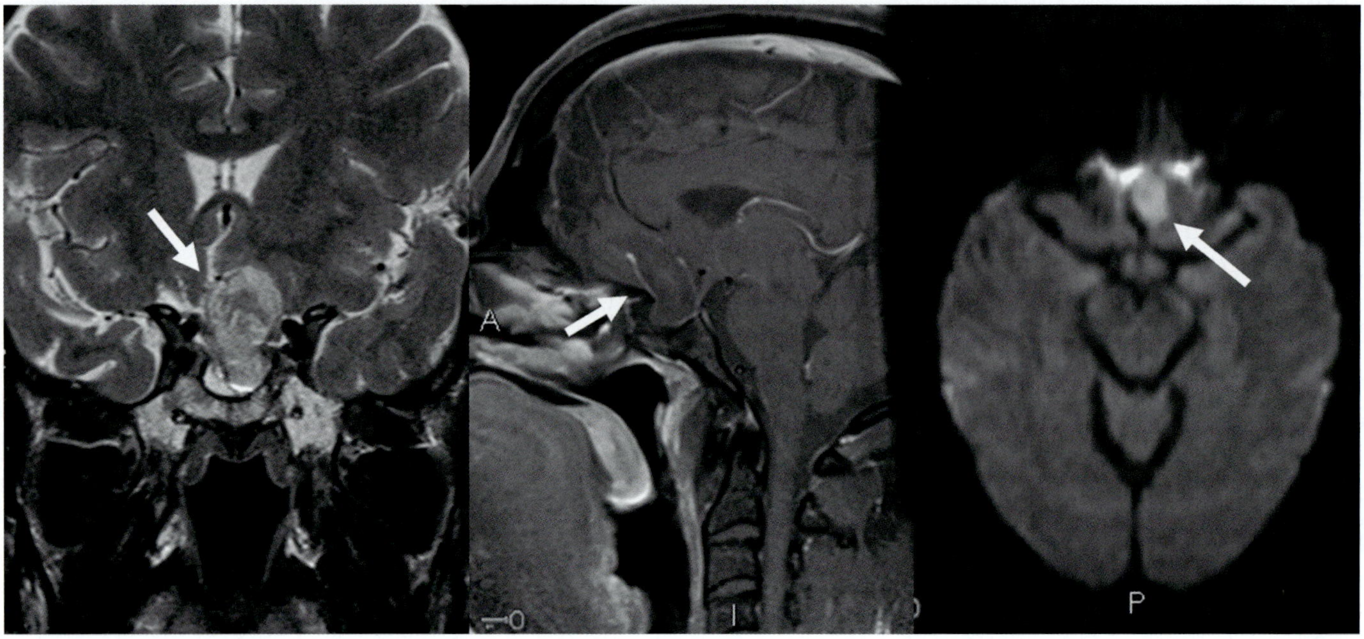

Fig. 5.19 Sellar-suprasellar epidermoid. **(A)** The presence of complex fluid on coronal T2-weighted image. The lack of enhancement on the **(B)** sagittal postcontrast image and hyperintensity on the **(C)** diffusion-weighted imaging are characteristic.

meningitis.[29] Rathke's cleft cysts, derived from the epithelium of Rathke's pouch, may occupy the sella, suprasellar cistern, or both. They may rarely be located entirely within the sphenoid sinus. Most are small but, when large, may be indistinguishable from cystic macroadenomas or craniopharyngiomas. There is great variability in the signal intensity of cyst contents, depending on the protein concentration. However, the presence of a low T2 signal nonenhancing intracystic mural nodule is specific for this entity. The nodule is composed of desquamated cellular debris[30,31] (**Fig. 5.20**).

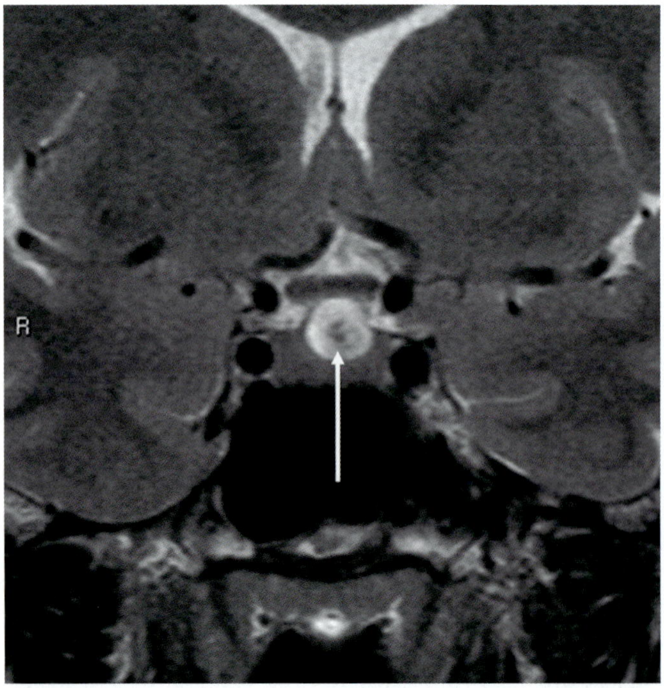

Fig. 5.20 Rathke's cleft cyst. A hypointense nodule (*arrow*) on a coronal T2-weighted image (left) and the lack of enhancement (right) are typical.

Infectious and Inflammatory Conditions

Infection

Primary infectious disorders of the pituitary gland are exceedingly rare. Hypophysitis may be bacterial or fungal in origin. Rarely, tuberculosis or syphilis may affect the gland. Pituitary abscesses, usually due to gram-positive cocci, may be caused either by hematogenous seeding or direct extension from a sphenoid sinus, cavernous sinus, or meningeal source, or a contaminated CSF fistula. Preexisting surgery, an underlying pituitary lesion, and an immunocompromised state are risk factors. Although a peripherally enhancing pituitary mass in the appropriate clinical setting should suggest an abscess, the imaging characteristics are very variable (**Fig. 5.21**). The coexistence of meningitis, sphenoid sinusitis, and intralesional gas or fluid levels is a useful clue.[32]

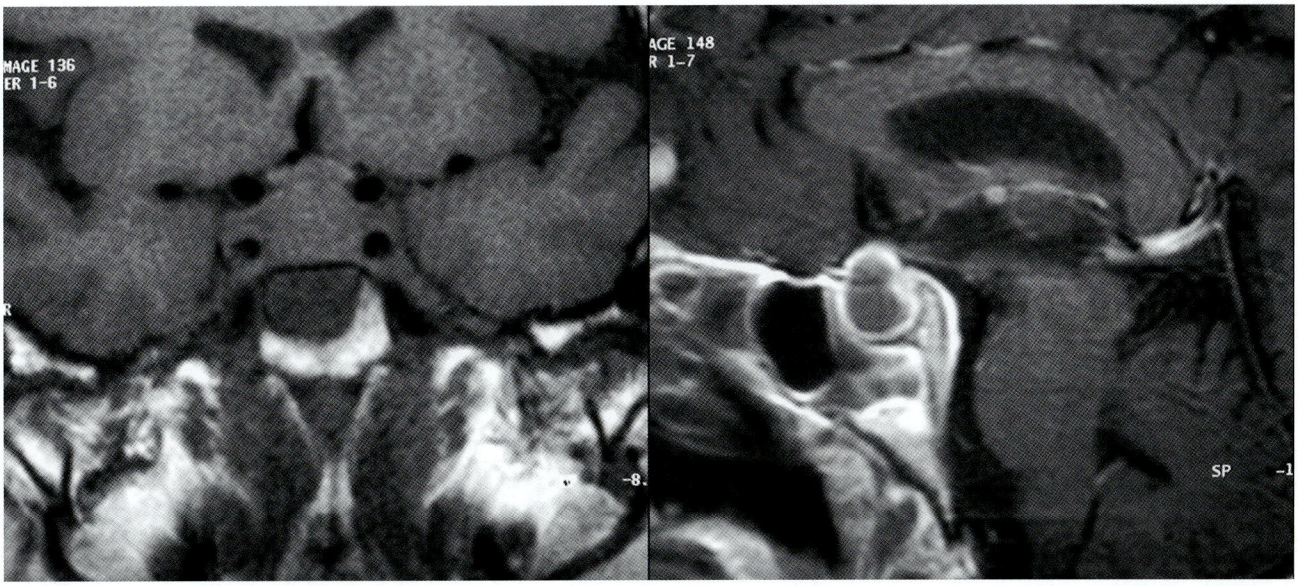

A B

Fig. 5.21 Pituitary bacterial abscess. **(A)** On this unenhanced image, the lesion simulates a macroadenoma. **(B)** The postcontrast image demonstrates peripheral enhancement. (Images courtesy of Wendy Smoker, MD)

Noninfectious Inflammatory Conditions

Lymphocytic adenohypophysitis (LAH, with or without infundibular involvement) and lymphocytic infundibuloneurohypophysitis (LIN) are autoimmune disorders with relatively distinct clinical presentations. LAH is most commonly encountered in postpartum women and presents with variable degrees of pituitary insufficiency, whereas LIN presents in middle-aged patients with diabetes insipidus and only rarely has been reported in the postpartum state.[33] LAH on MRI manifests as diffuse enhancement of the adenohypophysis with or without stalk involvement and may be indistinguishable from pituitary hyperplasia or an adenoma. Involvement of the stalk would not be a feature of either pituitary hyperplasia or adenomas and, when present should point to an alternative diagnosis (**Fig. 5.22**). Local

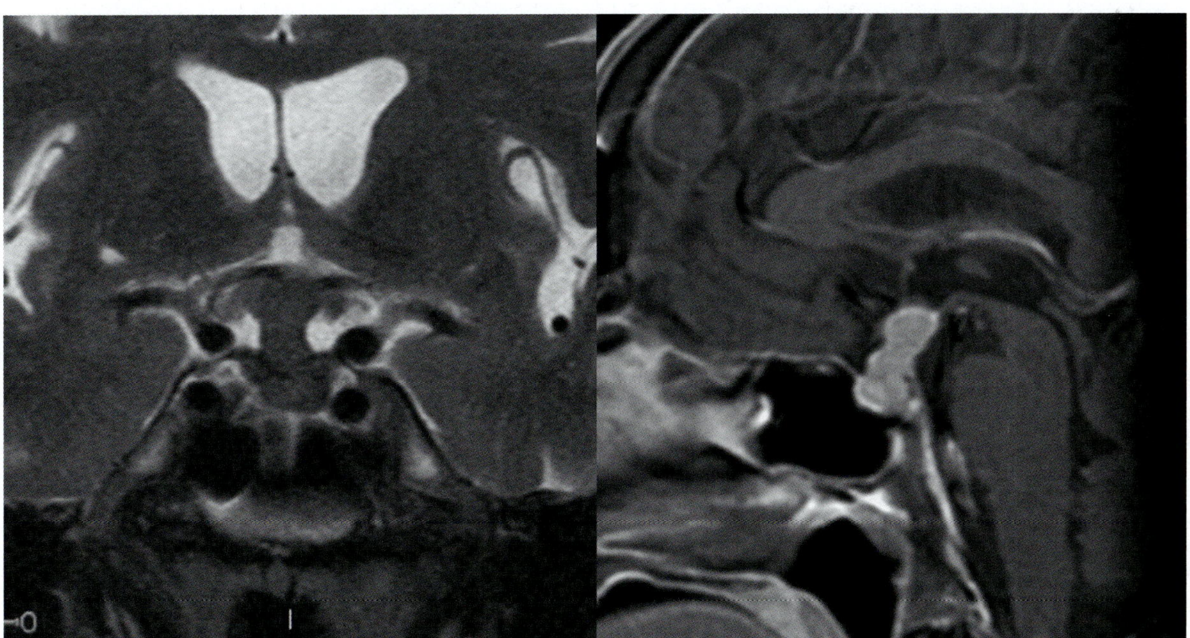

A B

Fig. 5.22 Lymphocytic adenohypophysitis with infundibular involvement. Involvement of the entirety of the pituitary with thickening and enhancement of stalk is evident on coronal T2-weighted **(A)** and sagittal postcontrast T1-weighted **(B)** images. Again, note the lack of sellar expansion.

meningeal thickening and, rarely, cavernous sinus involvement have been reported.[34] Findings that should suggest LAH over an adenoma include a relationship to pregnancy, a lower pituitary volume, a greater degree of enhancement, little to no sellar expansion, loss of the posterior pituitary bright spot, and thickening of the stalk.[35] LIN, on the other hand, presents as nonspecific stalk thickening and enhancement. Granulomatous hypophysitis occurs in middle-aged women and is indistinguishable from LAH. Xanthomatous hypophysitis may present as a cystic pituitary mass.[36] Sarcoidosis and Wegener's granulomatosis may also affect the pituitary gland. There are no MRI characteristics that enable a specific diagnosis.

Miscellaneous Conditions

The "Empty" Sella

An "empty" sella is usually a consequence of a developmental defect in the diaphragma sellae that has resulted in herniation of arachnoid and CSF into the sella. It may represent an incidental finding but may also be a consequence of chronic raised intracranial pressure as in pseudotumor cerebri. In the latter setting, it may reverse with treatment.[37] In symptomatic patients, it may be distinguished from an intrasellar arachnoid cyst by the lack of deformation of the pituitary stalk.

Intracranial Hypotension

The clinical syndrome of postural headache due to intracranial hypotension may be associated with an enlarged, superiorly convex pituitary gland (**Fig. 5.23**). This is believed to result from venous engorgement and hyperemia surrounding the gland and must not be mistaken for hyperplasia or an adenoma. The presence of findings such as smooth thickening and enhancement of the convexity dural, subdural effusions, and sagging of the brain leading to effacement of the suprasellar cisterns and tonsillar descent enable the correct diagnosis to be made.[38]

Pituitary Apoplexy

Apoplexy may be spontaneous but may also be precipitated by systemic illnesses or the use of bromocriptine or anticoagulants.[39] It may occur as an acutely symptomatic event or more often detected incidentally. The appearance of hemorrhage is highly variable on MRI and depends on the age of the blood products present. The occurrence of T1 hyperintensity in a macroadenoma is usually indicative of hemorrhage. Blood-fluid levels may also be seen due to a hematocrit effect (**Fig. 5.24**). An infarcted macroadenoma may demonstrate a complete rim of peripheral enhancement. In the acute stage, an infarct may be detectable as hyperintensity on diffusion-weighted imaging.[40]

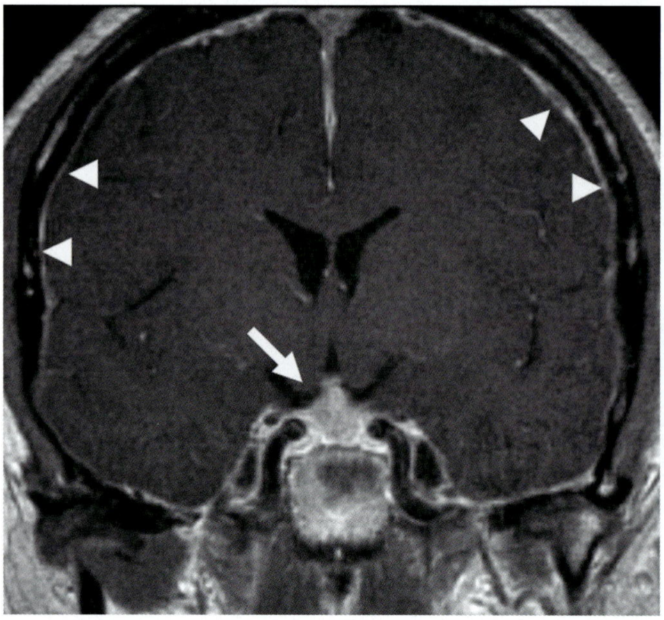

Fig. 5.23 Intracranial hypotension. The pituitary gland is prominent (*arrow*). Diffuse dural enhancement over convexities (*arrowheads*) and "sagging" suprasellar structures are clues to diagnosis.

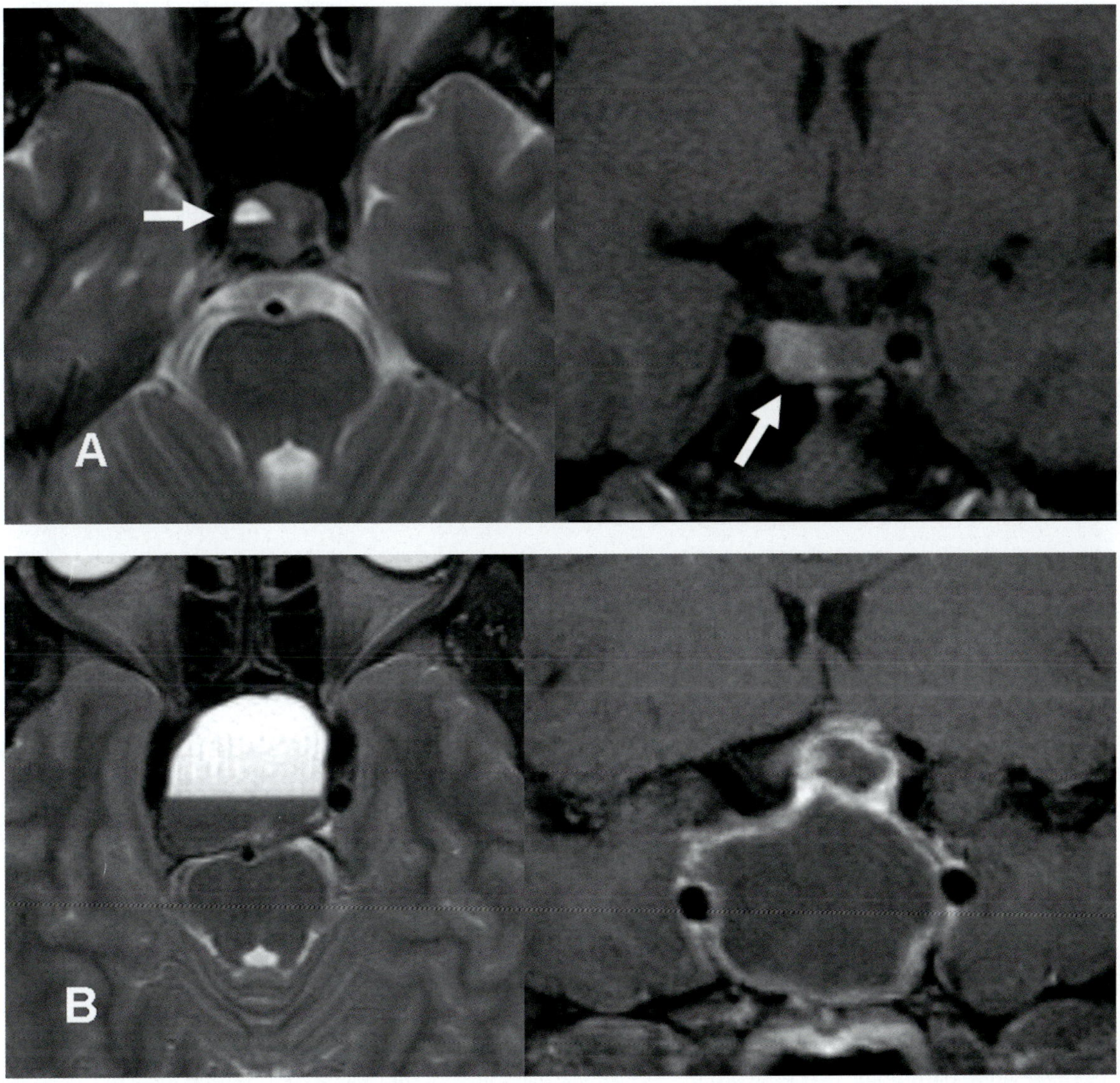

Fig. 5.24 **(A)** Hemorrhage into a pituitary adenoma after bromocriptine therapy. This early posttreatment study shows a low blood–fluid level on T2-weighted image (*left*) and the presence of T1 hyperintensity on the unenhanced image (*right*). **(B)** Patient presented with acute panhypopituitarism and vision loss. Hemorrhage into the lesion is evidenced by gross enlargement of the blood–fluid level and rim enhancement on T2-weighted (*left*) and enhanced T1-weighted (*right*) images.

The Postoperative Sella

Interpretation of MRI studies after transsphenoidal or open surgery is often challenging for the neuroradiologist. The contents of a postoperative sella may include any combination of fat packing, Gelfoam (Upjohn Company, Kalamazoo, MI), fluid, hemorrhage, residual native gland, and residual tumor (**Fig. 5.25**). The T1 hyperintensity of fat and the use of fat-suppressed sequences make recognition of fat packing fairly straightforward. Gelfoam is more variable in its signal intensity but most often demonstrates a T1 and T2 hypointense core. Both fat packing and Gelfoam tend to involute with time. Some surgeons use methylmethacrylate to fill the postoperative cavity, which will be uniformly hypointense on all sequences. Homogeneously enhancing tissue into which the stalk inserts represents the residual native gland. Residual tumor and granulation tissue may be indistinguishable. The only true sign of the presence of tumor is the demonstration of lack of resolution or actual increase in size on follow-up imaging.[5]

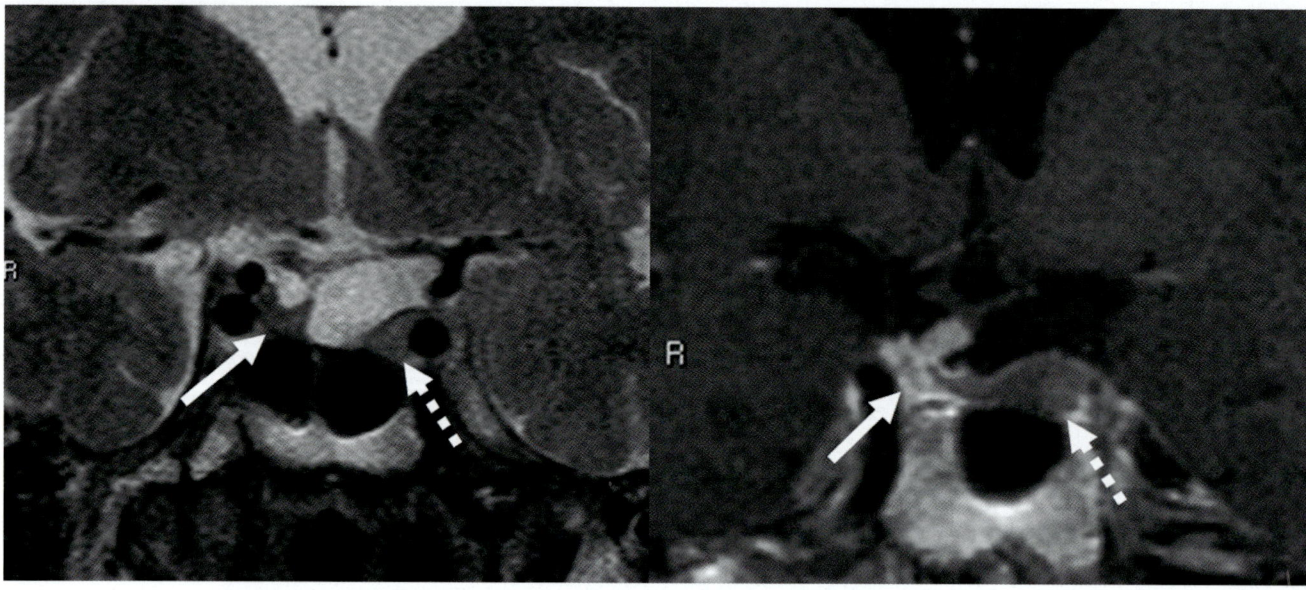

A B

Fig. 5.25 Postoperative sella. **(A)** Coronal T2-weighted image demonstrates intrasellar soft tissue on either side of the midline (*arrow*). **(B)** The stalk inserts into the homogeneously enhancing focus (*arrow*), which represents residual native pituitary gland. Relatively hypoenhancing soft tissue (*dotted arrow*) was a recurrent tumor.

■ Conclusion

Magnetic resonance imaging remains the mainstay of imaging for the pituitary gland and parasellar region. The superior contrast resolution of this technique has led to it supplanting CT in nearly all circumstances. It has a high sensitivity for the detection microadenomas and provides excellent characterization of the morphology of macroadenomas. Neuroradiologists must be aware of the diverse pathologic processes that can afflict the sella and must keep in mind the underlying clinical scenario when provide their interpretation.

References

1. Webb SM, Ruscalleda J, Schwarzstein D, et al. Computerized tomography versus magnetic resonance imaging: a comparative study in hypothalamic-pituitary and parasellar pathology. Clin Endocrinol (Oxf) 1992;36:459–465
2. Davis PC, Hoffman JC Jr, Spencer T, Tindall GT, Braun IF. MR imaging of pituitary adenoma: CT, clinical, and surgical correlation. AJR Am J Roentgenol 1987;148:797–802
3. Dwyer AJ, Frank JA, Doppman JL, et al. Pituitary adenomas in patients with Cushing disease: initial experience with Gd-DTPA-enhanced MR imaging. Radiology 1987;163:421–426
4. Davis PC, Gokhale KA, Joseph GJ, et al. Pituitary adenoma: correlation of half-dose gadolinium-enhanced MR imaging with surgical findings in 26 patients. Radiology 1991;180:779–784
5. Symons SP, Aviv RI, Montanera WJ, Kucharczyk W. The sella turcica and parasellar region. In: Atlas SW, ed. Magnetic Resonance Imaging of the Brain and Spine, Vol 2. Philadelphia: Lippincott Williams & Wilkins; 2008:1120
6. Patronas N, Bulakbasi N, Stratakis CA, et al. Spoiled gradient recalled acquisition in the steady state technique is superior to conventional postcontrast spin echo technique for magnetic resonance imaging detection of adrenocorticotropin-secreting pituitary tumors. J Clin Endocrinol Metab 2003;88:1565–1569
7. Gao R, Isoda H, Tanaka T, et al. Dynamic gadolinium-enhanced MR imaging of pituitary adenomas: usefulness of sequential sagittal and coronal plane images. Eur J Radiol 2001;39:139–146
8. Elster AD. Imaging of the sella: anatomy and pathology. Semin Ultrasound CT MR 1993;14:182–194
9. Korogi Y, Takahashi M. Current concepts of imaging in patients with pituitary/hypothalamic dysfunction. Semin Ultrasound CT MR 1995;16:270–278
10. Yagi A, Sato N, Taketomi A, et al. Normal cranial nerves in the cavernous sinuses: contrast-enhanced three-dimensional constructive interference in the steady state MR imaging. AJNR Am J Neuroradiol 2005;26:946–950
11. Kucharczyk W, Davis DO, Kelly WM, Sze G, Norman D, Newton TH. Pituitary adenomas: high-resolution MR imaging at 1.5 T. Radiology 1986;161:761–765
12. Hagiwara A, Inoue Y, Wakasa K, Haba T, Tashiro T, Miyamoto T. Comparison of growth hormone-producing and non-growth hormone-producing pituitary adenomas: imaging characteristics and pathologic correlation. Radiology 2003;228:533–538
13. Ahmadi H, Larsson EM, Jinkins JR. Normal pituitary gland: coronal MR imaging of infundibular tilt. Radiology 1990;177:389–392
14. Miller DL, Doppman JL. Petrosal sinus sampling: technique and rationale. Radiology 1991;178:37–47

15. Elster AD. Sellar susceptibility artifacts: theory and implications. AJNR Am J Neuroradiol 1993;14:129–136
16. Yousem DM, Arrington JA, Zinreich SJ, Kumar AJ, Bryan RN. Pituitary adenomas: possible role of bromocriptine in intratumoral hemorrhage. Radiology 1989;170(1 Pt 1):239–243
17. Bahuleyan B, Raghuram L, Rajshekhar V, Chacko AG. To assess the ability of MRI to predict consistency of pituitary macroadenomas. Br J Neurosurg 2006;20:324–326 http://dx.doi.org/10.1080/02688690601000717
18. Pierallini A, Caramia F, Falcone C, et al. Pituitary macroadenomas: preoperative evaluation of consistency with diffusion-weighted MR imaging—initial experience. Radiology 2006;239:223–231
19. Tokumaru AM, Sakata I, Terada H, Kosuda S, Nawashiro H, Yoshii M. Optic nerve hyperintensity on T2-weighted images among patients with pituitary macroadenoma: correlation with visual impairment. AJNR Am J Neuroradiol 2006;27:250–254
20. Kim HJ, Cho WH. Optic tract hemorrhage after pituitary apoplexy. AJNR Am J Neuroradiol 2007;28:141–142
21. Vieira JO Jr, Cukiert A, Liberman B, Liberman B. Evaluation of magnetic resonance imaging criteria for cavernous sinus invasion in patients with pituitary adenomas: logistic regression analysis and correlation with surgical findings. Surg Neurol 2006;65:130–135, discussion 135
22. Cottier JP, Destrieux C, Brunereau L, et al. Cavernous sinus invasion by pituitary adenoma: MR imaging. Radiology 2000;215:463–469
23. O'Brien DP, Phillips JP, Rawluk DR, Farrell MA. Intracranial metastases from pituitary adenoma. Br J Neurosurg 1995;9:211–218
24. Gibbs WN, Monuki ES, Linskey ME, Hasso AN. Pituicytoma: diagnostic features on selective carotid angiography and MR imaging. AJNR Am J Neuroradiol 2006;27:1639–1642
25. Shah B, Lipper MH, Laws ER, Lopes MB, Spellman MJ Jr. Posterior pituitary astrocytoma: a rare tumor of the neurohypophysis: a case report. AJNR Am J Neuroradiol 2005;26:1858–1861
26. Kaufmann TJ, Lopes MBS, Laws ER Jr, Lipper MH. Primary sellar lymphoma: radiologic and pathologic findings in two patients. AJNR Am J Neuroradiol 2002;23:364–367
27. Kato T, Sawamura Y, Tada M, et al. Occult neurohypophyseal germinomas in patients presenting with central diabetes insipidus. Neurosurg Focus 1998;5:e6
28. Sartoretti-Schefer S, Wichmann W, Aguzzi A, Valavanis A. MR differentiation of adamantinous and squamous-papillary craniopharyngiomas. AJNR Am J Neuroradiol 1997;18:77–87
29. Osborn AG, Preece MT. Intracranial cysts: radiologic-pathologic correlation and imaging approach. Radiology 2006;239:650–664
30. Byun WM, Kim OL, Kim D. MR imaging findings of Rathke's cleft cysts: significance of intracystic nodules. AJNR Am J Neuroradiol 2000;21:485–488
31. Megdiche-Bazarbacha H, Ben Hammouda K, Aicha AB, et al. Intrasphenoidal rathke cleft cyst. AJNR Am J Neuroradiol 2006;27:1098–1100
32. Vates GE, Berger MS, Wilson CB. Diagnosis and management of pituitary abscess: a review of twenty-four cases. J Neurosurg 2001;95:233–241 http://dx.doi.org/10.3171/jns.2001.95.2.0233
33. Panicker HK, Janicic N, Nguyen D, Verbalis J. Presumed infundibuloneurohypophysitis: unusual presentation in a postpartum patient. AJNR Am J Neuroradiol 2005;26:357–359
34. Melgar MA, Mariwalla N, Gloss DS, Walsh JW. Recurrent lymphocytic hypophysitis and bilateral intracavernous carotid artery occlusion. an observation and review of the literature. Neurol Res 2006;28:177–183
35. Gutenberg A, Larsen J, Lupi I, Rohde V, Caturegli P. A radiologic score to distinguish autoimmune hypophysitis from nonsecreting pituitary adenoma preoperatively. AJNR Am J Neuroradiol 2009;30:1766–1772
36. Cheung CC, Ezzat S, Smyth HS, Asa SL. The spectrum and significance of primary hypophysitis. J Clin Endocrinol Metab 2001;86:1048–1053
37. Zagardo MT, Cail WS, Kelman SE, Rothman MI. Reversible empty sella in idiopathic intracranial hypertension: an indicator of successful therapy? AJNR Am J Neuroradiol 1996;17:1953–1956
38. Alvarez-Linera J, Escribano J, Benito-León J, Porta-Etessam J, Rovira A. Pituitary enlargement in patients with intracranial hypotension syndrome. Neurology 2000;55:1895–1897
39. Biousse V, Newman NJ, Oyesiku NM. Precipitating factors in pituitary apoplexy. J Neurol Neurosurg Psychiatry 2001;71:542–545
40. Rogg JM, Tung GA, Anderson G, Cortez S. Pituitary apoplexy: early detection with diffusion-weighted MR imaging. AJNR Am J Neuroradiol 2002;23:1240–1245

6 Indications for Surgery on Pituitary Tumors: An Endocrinologist's Perspective

David L. Kleinberg and Pietro Ameri

Until 1970, only surgery or radiation therapy was available for the treatment of pituitary tumors. But four findings led to considering medical therapy as a further option: (1) prolactin existed in humans as a molecule separate from growth hormone[1]; (2) hyperprolactinemia caused sexual dysfunction, infertility, and galactorrhea; (3) many pituitary adenomas hypersecreted prolactin[2]; and (4) bromocriptine was effective in lowering serum prolactin and improving sexual function.[3] Only later was it discovered that shrinkage of prolactin-secreting pituitary tumors could be expected in response to bromocriptine and that withdrawal of medication was associated with tumor enlargement.[4,5] The concept that medical therapy might be an alternative to surgery and radiotherapy was subsequently extended to other functioning pituitary adenomas, including growth hormone (GH)-secreting[6] and thyroid-stimulating hormone (TSH)-secreting tumors.[7] Although progress regarding medical treatment of Cushing's disease is being made, this disorder and nonfunctioning pituitary adenomas are still the purview of neurosurgeons in most situations.

Expertise of Pituitary Surgeons

The best results of surgery for pituitary tumors are achieved when surgeons are highly experienced and focused in resection of pituitary lesions. In a study by Gittoes et al,[8] the outcome of surgical removal of pituitary adenomas by the transsphenoidal approach was better when a specific dedicated neurosurgeon performed the surgery, in contrast to when it was performed by one of eight otherwise excellent colleagues who had less experience in pituitary disease. The dedicated surgeon accomplished a cure rate of 86% for microadenomas and 52% for macroadenomas. In contrast, the success rates for the other eight neurosurgeons were 54% and 30%, respectively. That this was the experience in a single surgery unit indicates that the cure rates of a particular surgeon, in contrast to those of a specific medical center, should be quoted. This book discusses success rates of surgery by the endoscopic route, which may further help in the optimal choice of the neurosurgeon. It is not clear whether a direct comparison of the different surgical approaches will help identify one as being better than the others.[9]

What Constitutes a Pituitary Tumor?

Pituitary tumors are found in 11% of autopsies,[10] and they stain for prolactin in 46% of cases. They may also come to attention during imaging of the head for unrelated reasons. In one study, 10% of 100 normal volunteers had magnetic resonance imaging (MRI) findings indicative of microadenomas, ranging from 3 to 6 mm in diameter.[11] When a tumor is incidentally found, it requires a full endocrine evaluation and at minimum periodic radiologic follow-up.[12] In a survey of 248 patients with pituitary incidentalomas followed for a mean period of 26.9 months, 46.4% of the pituitary masses were nonfunctioning adenomas and only 20% of them were found to increase in size.[13] Thus, incidentalomas infrequently require therapy.

Pituitary adenomas are also brought to attention because of endocrine dysfunction or tumor mass effect. These frequently require treatment. When considering whether a patient with a pituitary adenoma should be treated medically, surgically, or not at all, it is important to evaluate its size, invasiveness, effects on adjacent structures, and secretory activity, as well as the function of the remaining normal pituitary tissue (**Table 6.1**).

Specific Types of Pituitary Tumors

Functioning Pituitary Tumors

Prolactin-Secreting Tumors

The great majority of prolactin-secreting tumors are responsive to dopamine agonists, whether they are micro- or macroadenomas. Dopamine agonists not only normalize serum prolactin values, which can reverse the associated sexual dysfunction, galactorrhea, and osteopenia, but also reduce adenoma size. Tumor shrinkage is due to a reduction in cell cytoplasm, nucleus, and nucleolus.[14–16] Even with large invasive adenomas, medication should be the first-line therapy, as it often improves vision and other mass effects. It was initially shown that tumors that shrank in response to bromocriptine would regrow with discontinuation of the drug.[5] They often do, but many, especially microadenomas, do not recur after withdrawal of dopamine agonist therapy.[17] Taken

Table 6.1 Characteristics of Pituitary Tumors that May Require Therapeutic Intervention

Effects of Pituitary Tumors	Related Clinical Features
Hypersecretion of prolactin **Hypersecretion of GH** **Hypersecretion of ACTH** **Hypersecretion of TSH**	**Sexual dysfunction, galactorrhea, reduced bone mineral density** **Features of acromegaly** **Features of Cushing's syndrome** **Features of hyperthyroidism (with measurable TSH)**
Increase in intrasellar pressure **Compression of surrounding normal pituitary tissue** **Compression of pituitary stalk**	**Headache** **Hypopituitarism** **Hyperprolactinemia**
Acute hemorrhagic infarction	**Pituitary apoplexy, hypopituitarism**
Pressure on optic chiasm	**Visual field defects**
Invasion of cavernous sinus	Rare cranial nerve deficit (most often no clinical sequelae)
Invasion of temporal or frontal lobe	Seizures, changes in personality, anosmia, hydrocephalus
Download invasion	CSF leakage, pharyngeal obstruction, meningitis
Pituitary infection	Meningitis, pituitary abscess

Abbreviations: ACTH, adrenocorticotropic hormone; CSF, cerebrospinal fluid; GH, growth hormone; TSH, thyroid-stimulating hormone.
Note: Features in bold are most frequently observed.

together, these authors and most pituitary endocrinologists consider dopamine agonists the therapy of choice for prolactinomas.[18]

Bromocriptine has been employed since the early 1970s and is very effective in reducing serum prolactin, normalizing gonadal function, and shrinking tumors. Its use is somewhat limited by side effects including postural hypotension, gastrointestinal disturbances, and poor tolerability in some. Moreover, it must be administered up to three times a day. In contrast, cabergoline can be given weekly, is better tolerated, and can be used in higher doses for tumors that are relatively resistant. In recent years it has been associated with cardiac valve thickening and regurgitation when used in much higher doses, as in Parkinson's disease.[19] The bulk of evidence, however, suggests that doses necessary to treat prolactinomas do not cause cardiac problems.

We believe that surgery should be considered in patients who are completely resistant to or intolerant of dopamine agonists, personally choose surgery, or have macroadenomas and want to prevent the development of visual problems during pregnancy.

Resistance to Dopamine Agonists

Dopamine agonists act by binding to dopamine receptors in prolactin-producing adenoma cells. Therefore, these drugs need available dopamine receptors to be effective. In general, patients resistant or relatively resistant to therapy with dopamine agonist have some reduction in the number of receptors available (**Fig. 6.1**). However, "resistance" is a relative term. In the literature it generally refers to failure to normalize prolactin in response to 15 mg of bromocriptine daily. If this definition were applied to all patients with macroprolactinomas, many would be considered resistant. In practice, patients with very high levels of serum prolactin do not always achieve complete normalization of prolactin. Nevertheless, they experience considerable tumor shrinkage, reduction in tumor mass effects, and normalization of previous deficiencies in other pituitary hormones. They may even have some restoration of sexual function. Therefore, we would not consider these patients fully resistant to dopamine agonist therapy even though they may require steroid hormone replacement or fertility treatment if pregnancy is desired. In contrast, rare individuals may present tumor growth despite prolactin being suppressed,[20] whereas others benefit through either tumor shrinkage or reduction in serum prolactin, but not both. Some prolactin-secreting tumors grow in spite of treatment with dopamine agonists. These include nonmalignant and rare malignant prolactinomas. Under these circumstances, therapeutic considerations should include surgery, radiation therapy, chemotherapy, or a combination.

Prolactinomas and Pregnancy

The normal pituitary gland enlarges during pregnancy as a result of proliferation of pituitary lactotroph cells. Pituitary adenomas can also grow in response to pregnancy-related hormones. An enlarged pituitary tumor or gland can impair vision if it impinges on the optic chiasm. Fortunately, microadenomas rarely damage visual tract during pregnancy.[21] Only 1.4% of patients with microadenomas develop visual abnormalities during pregnancy, whereas 16% of patients

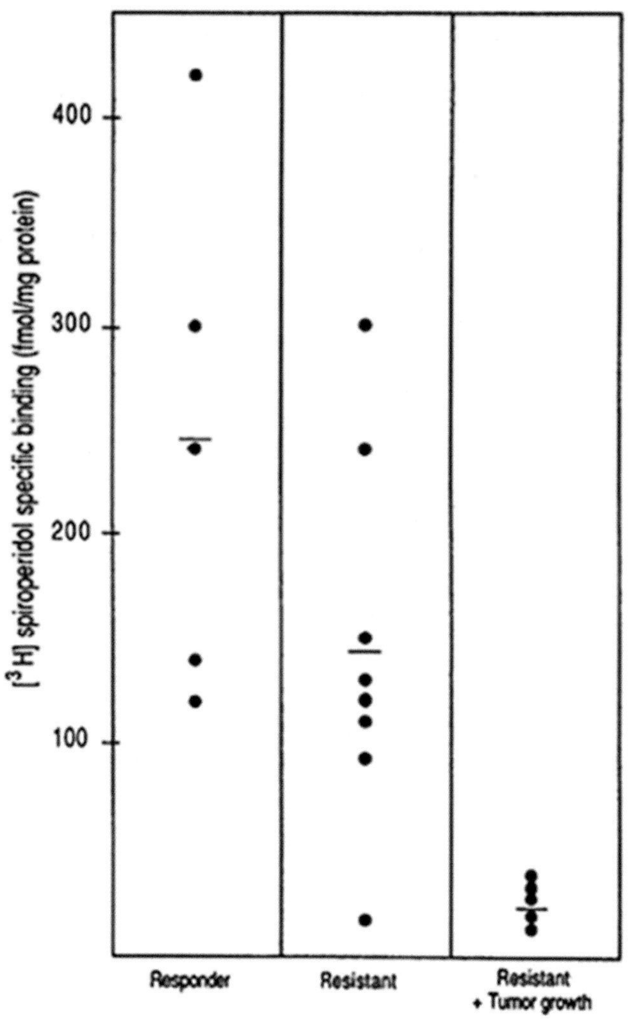

Fig. 6.1 Binding of dopamine agonist to dopamine receptors according to the sensitivity of prolactinomas to the drug. (From Pellegrini I, Rasolonjanahary R, Gunz G, et al. Resistance to bromocriptine in prolactinomas. J Clin Endocrinol Metab 1989;69:500–509)

with macroadenomas do.[10] Therefore, when a woman has a pituitary tumor in close proximity to the optic chiasm or a macroadenoma, the risk of experiencing visual disturbances in pregnancy should be considered. Even with a microadenoma we recommend visual field tests before and during pregnancy. Some patients with macroadenomas select prophylactic surgery prior to pregnancy, whereas others prefer undergoing treatment with dopamine agonist if it becomes necessary during the course of pregnancy. If the latter choice is taken, responsiveness to dopamine agonists should be determined before proceeding with a pregnancy.

Malignant Prolactinomas

Only 40 cases of malignant prolactinomas have been described. The diagnosis is made when there is evidence of metastasis outside the pituitary region. These tumors rarely respond to dopamine agonists and usually require combination therapy including debulking surgery, radiation therapy, and chemotherapy with temozolomide[22] or other agents.

Growth Hormone–Secreting Tumors

Acromegaly leads to severe comorbidities and increased mortality, especially in patients who develop diabetes or heart disease.[10] Even mild and relatively asymptomatic disease can cause long-term consequences. Thus, therapy is indicated in virtually all patients. The aims of treatment are to control tumor growth, normalize growth hormone (GH) and insulin-like growth factor-1 (IGF-1) levels, prevent or treat comorbidities, diminish mortality, and improve quality of life. Although medications that inhibit GH secretion or block its action are available and usually fulfill at least some goals of therapy, they are not as universally effective as are dopamine agonists in the treatment of prolactinomas. Therefore, if surgery is likely to cure acromegaly by complete resection of the adenoma, it becomes the treatment of choice.

When GH-secreting tumors are large and invasive, which the majority are, they may not be curable by surgery. However, surgery usually decreases serum GH concentrations, even in patients with large adenomas. Pituitary surgeons more often than not recommend surgery whether or not the disease will be cured. The rationale they espouse is that lowering serum GH by reducing tumor burden makes patients more responsive to medications or other treatments. The endocrinology community is divided regarding the relative roles of primary medical therapy versus debulking followed by medical therapy. Unfortunately, there are no authoritative randomized controlled trials that can provide conclusive data regarding the best indications for each treatment option.

We subscribe to removing well-defined, noninvasive tumors if possible, with medical treatment for those that are not cured by surgery. Patients with invasive tumors are presented with the options of surgical debulking or trying somatostatin analogues. We usually do not recommend treatment with pegvisomant, primarily because it does not reduce tumor size. Recently, several investigators have proposed the combined use of somatostatin analogues and pegvisomant.[23] We also do not suggest medical therapy prior to surgery, as this scenario is not supported by the literature. However, there is no contraindication to this strategy.

When considering surgery versus medication, the potential effects on endocrine and nonendocrine comorbidities must be taken into consideration. Many patients with acromegaly have sexual dysfunction; galactorrhea, goiter, and other thyroid disorders; and impaired glucose tolerance. Reduction in serum GH and IGF-1 can reverse sexual dysfunction, impaired glucose tolerance, and perhaps galactorrhea. Often effective treatment also reduces the severity of sleep apnea, carpal tunnel syndrome, sweating, oily skin and acne, and other nonendocrine aspects of the disease. Interestingly, when therapy lowers GH and IGF-1 levels to or very close to the normal range, life expectancy is improved. Regardless of the treatment modality, when GH and IGF-1 are normalized, improvement can be expected.

Adrenocorticotropic Hormone–Secreting Tumors

If an obvious ectopic source of adrenocorticotropic hormone (ACTH) is not present, 90 to 95% of patients with hypercortisolism and elevated serum ACTH levels have Cushing's disease. Because most cases of Cushing's disease are caused by discrete ACTH-producing corticotroph adenomas, selective adenomectomy is the treatment of choice.[24] Patients should be referred to the neurosurgeon after a careful endocrine workup has proved the presence of excess cortisol secretion together with inappropriately high ACTH values. As pituitary corticotroph tumors may be small, MRI fails to identify them in up to 40% of cases.[25] When pituitary imaging is negative or inconclusive and when biochemical and radiologic results are discordant, bilateral inferior petrosal sinus sampling (BIPSS) should be performed. In 193 patients with Cushing's disease operated on by one experienced pituitary neurosurgeon between 1987 and 2005, BIPSS was used only in cases with clinical and biochemical features inconsistent with Cushing's disease (e.g., inadequate suppression on high-dose dexamethasone suppression test) or with negative or equivocal pituitary imaging. In a retrospective review, the remission and recurrence rates were comparable in the BIPSS versus no-BIPSS groups. Moreover, no cases of missed diagnosis were observed among the patients who had not undergone BIPSS.[26]

The remission rate after transsphenoidal surgery for Cushing's disease critically depends on the neurosurgeon's experience and is approximately 80%.[26] If the disease persists or recurs, repeat pituitary surgery should be first considered, even though the eventual decision must be individualized. Although the risk of failure to achieve remission is 3.7 times higher than for first surgery,[27] repeat pituitary surgery for persistent or recurrent Cushing's disease can still be successful in 50 to 70% of patients.[24] External-beam radiotherapy and stereotactic radiosurgery can be an alternative to second surgery or can be used if repeat surgery is unsuccessful. As discussed in other chapters of this book, the effects of radiation therapy are not immediate, and medications are necessary to control cortisol levels during the first years after irradiation of the pituitary gland.[28] Bilateral adrenalectomy provides immediate control of hypercortisolism, but it is associated with the need of lifelong glucocorticoid and mineralocorticoid replacement therapy and the risk of developing Nelson's syndrome.

Drugs that directly inhibit adrenal steroidogenesis (ketoconazole and metyrapone) can be used in preparation for pituitary surgery, awaiting the effects of radiation therapy, or as a palliative treatment.[24] In recent years, a somatostatin analogue capable of binding to four of the five somatostatin receptor subtypes has been found to affect the pituitary tumor, lower ACTH and cortisol concentrations, and improve symptoms and signs of Cushing's disease in some patients.[29] However, this treatment is still investigational and as yet unproven.

Thyroid Stimulating Hormone–Secreting Tumors

Thyroid-stimulating hormone–secreting adenomas are rare and represent from 0.58 to 2.8% of pituitary tumors.[10] They present with symptoms and signs of hyperthyroidism or tumor mass effect.[7] Most are macroadenomas and a subset co-secrete other hormones, especially GH. Not infrequently hyperthyroidism lasts for a long time before diagnosis, because it is initially thought to be Graves' disease and treated accordingly. Although surgery is often recommended as primary therapy, cure is accomplished by highly qualified surgeons in less than 50% of cases. Patients, particularly those with uncontrolled hyperthyroidism, are at increased risk for thyroid storm or mortality perioperatively. For this reason, control of hyperthyroidism must be achieved prior to surgery.

Although standard treatment for hyperthyroidism such as radioactive iodine or antithyroid medications can be helpful, a rebound is often observed because of increased tumor TSH production, secondary to the inhibition of the remaining negative feedback of thyroid hormones on thyrotroph cells. Octreotide can control hyperthyroidism and also reduce the size of the TSH-secreting adenoma by a direct effect on it. Even though data are limited because of the rarity of these tumors, a schema of possible treatment paradigms is proposed in **Fig. 6.2**.

Nonfunctioning Pituitary Tumors

Nonfunctioning adenomas are the second most common pituitary tumors after prolactinomas, with a prevalence of 25 to 35%. Although they are referred to as "nonfunctioning," they do produce hormones that are detectable in culture and by immunohistochemistry.[30] Most nonfunctioning adenomas are immunoreactive for gonadotrophins or their subunits, which disclose their origin from gonadotroph cells. In rare cases, the secretion of luteinizing hormone (LH) or follicle-stimulating hormone (FSH) may be sufficient to elevate serum levels and cause an endocrine syndrome. Nonfunctioning or "silent" corticotroph adenomas (ACTH-positive) can be also observed and are thought to be more aggressive than tumors that arise from gonadotrophs. They are almost always macroadenomas and exhibit cavernous sinus or bony invasion in approximately 50% of cases.[10]

Nonfunctioning pituitary adenomas come to attention because of mass effects, including pituitary failure, or are

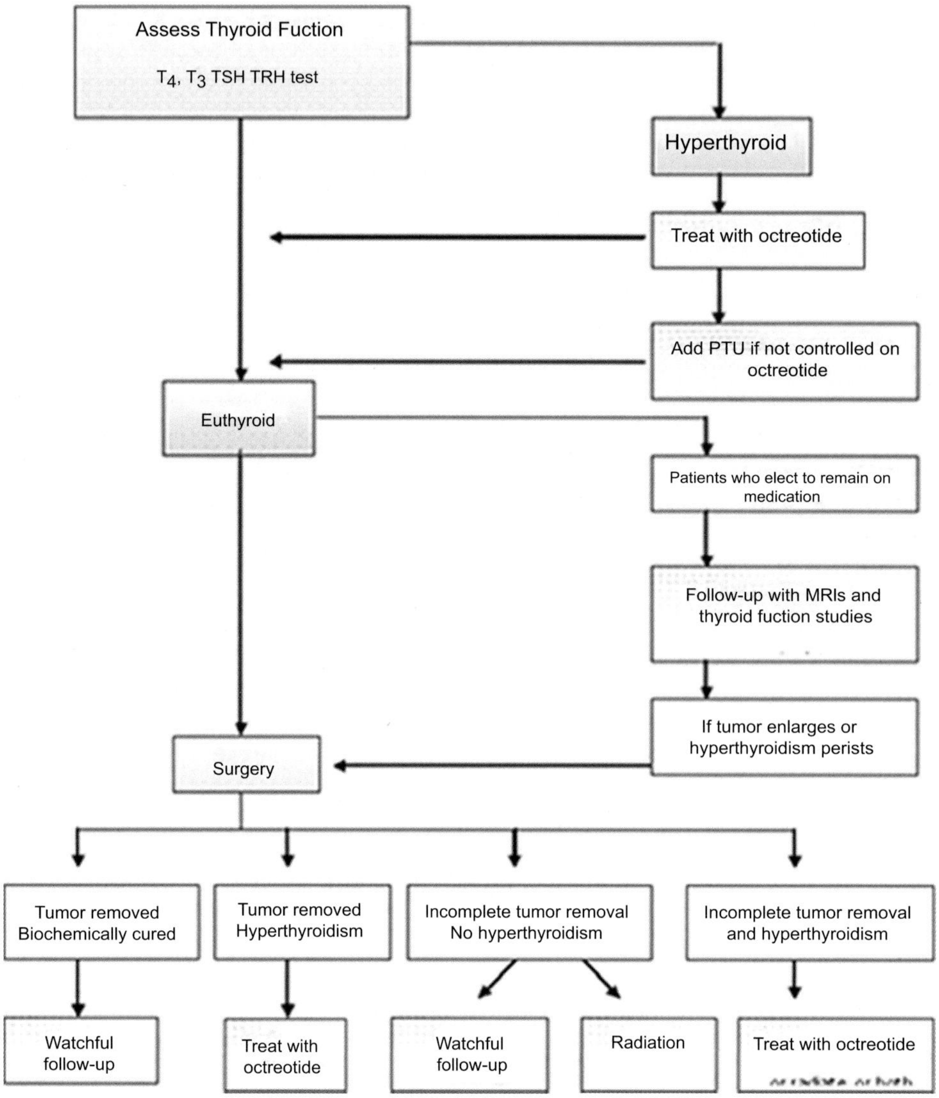

Fig. 6.2 Schema for treatment of thyroid-stimulating hormone (TSH)-secreting pituitary tumors. MRI, magnetic resonance imaging; PTU, propylthiouracil; T_3, triiodothyronine; T_4, thyroxine; TRH, thyrotropin-releasing hormone. (From Melmed S, Kleinberg D. Anterior pituitary. In: Kronenberg HM, Melmed S, Polonsky KS, Larsen PR, eds. Williams Textbook of Endocrinology. Philadelphia: Saunders Elsevier; 2008;234.)

discovered incidentally. They can also present with the acute symptoms and signs of pituitary apoplexy if they bleed and infarct. Because they have often been present for many years when finally identified, by the time of diagnosis they are frequently associated with deficiency in one or more pituitary hormones.[31–34] In patients with nonfunctioning pituitary tumors, the prevalence of GH, gonadotropin, ACTH, and TSH deficiency has been estimated to be 77 to 88%, 61 to 87%, 19 to 53%, and 18 to 43%, respectively.[31] Hyperprolactinemia has been reported in 25.3 to 38.5%.[34,35]

At present there are no effective medical therapies for nonfunctioning adenomas. If treatment is necessary, surgery and/or radiotherapy are options. Other chapters in this volume describe techniques and the relative effectiveness of the various forms of pituitary surgery. If nonfunctioning pituitary tumors are not completely resected, approximately 30 to 40% regrow. Therefore, postoperative follow-up MRI is important. The decision to administer radiation therapy should be taken by the pituitary team. If adjunctive radiotherapy is used after surgery, the recurrence rate is lower, but the incidence of hypopituitarism and other side effects is increased.

Impact of Surgery on Pituitary Function

An expanding adenoma causes a decrease in blood flow to the anterior pituitary, both directly, through the mechanical compression of portal vessels and the pituitary stalk, and indirectly, by raising the intrasellar pressure.[36] This leads to an interruption of the delivery of hypothalamic hormones to the adenohypophysis and, secondarily, to ischemia of pituitary cells, with resultant pituitary insufficiency. Even though these events can occur in the presence of functioning pituitary adenomas, they are more frequently observed with nonfunctioning tumors.[33]

If pituitary tissue is still viable, surgical removal of the adenoma and decompression of the pituitary gland can lead to recovery, or at least improvement, of pituitary function. In two large series including 721 and 491 nonfunctioning tumors, resolution of secondary hypogonadism, adrenal insufficiency, and hypothyroidism was observed after pituitary surgery in 15.9 to 32.8%, 40.8 to 41.6%, and 33.9 to 35.7% of patients, respectively.[32,34] Surgery can also be effective in reversing hypopituitarism associated with functioning adenomas, whose tendency to recover has been reported to be higher than for nonfunctioning pituitary tumors.[33] Significant factors determining postoperative restoration of adenohypophyseal function are no visible tumor remnants on imaging studies and no surrounding tissue invasion by the adenoma, as assessed by both the neurosurgeon and the pathologist.[33] It is unclear whether the size of a tumor may influence the likelihood of reversing hypopituitarism by means of surgery.[33,34] Preoperative hyperprolactinemia has been proposed as an indicator of the presence of enough viable tissue to recover pituitary function.[34,37] A similar value has been also attributed to TSH response to stimulation with thyrotropin-releasing hormone,[37] but this test is not routinely performed any longer.

Although surgery can rescue pituitary hormone secretion, it can also damage nontumoral pituitary tissue during manipulation of the gland. Therefore, hypopituitarism can also be a result of pituitary surgery. Highly variable percentages of new postoperative deficiencies of one or more pituitary axes have been reported,[31,32,34] probably because of differences in the duration of follow-up after surgery and in the criteria adopted to define a given hormone deficiency.

Depending on the clinical circumstances, we suggest retesting of pituitary function prior to starting postoperative replacement therapy, to identify those patients who recover and thus do not need any substitution treatment. Nevertheless, delaying the beginning of adrenal steroid replacement requires particular caution.

Nontumoral Hyperprolactinemia in Patients with Pituitary Adenomas

The presence of hyperprolactinemia in patients with pituitary adenomas is not always caused by hypersecretion of prolactin by the tumors themselves. In fact, it can be secondary to the interruption of the delivery of hypothalamic dopamine to the adenohypophysis due to increased intrasellar pressure and compression of the pituitary tissue and stalk.[36] Surgical decompression of the sella turcica often reverses nontumoral hyperprolactinemia.[34,37]

Assuming that patients with pituitary adenomas and elevated prolactin concentrations have a prolactinoma may lead to misdiagnosis and inappropriate treatment. Therefore, it is important to determine whether hyperprolactinemia is of tumoral or nontumoral origin. Interpreting the serum levels of prolactin can predict the presence of a prolactinoma, especially a macroadenoma. Virtually all macroprolactinomas raise serum prolactin values to at least 200 ng/mL. In a series of 96 men and women with prolactinomas, serum prolactin correlated with tumor size. Men had larger tumors (89% macroadenomas) and a mean serum prolactin value of 2789 ng/mL, whereas women (71% of whom had microadenomas) had a mean prolactin concentration of 292 ng/mL.[38] However, even an elevation of prolactin above 200 ng/mL does not ensure that tumoral lactotroph cells secrete the hormone. Atypical antipsychotics, such as risperidone, can increase prolactin to over 200 ng/mL,[39] and so can physiologic effects of pregnancy or stress.[18] In our opinion, a serum prolactin of 500 ng/mL can be interpreted as pathognomonic of a macroprolactinoma.

In contrast, microprolactinomas can be the source of even marginally elevated prolactin levels, which can be sufficient to cause decrease libido and sexual dysfunction in men. On the other hand, microprolactinomas can also raise serum prolactin to very high values. The presence of a small pituitary tumor and any increase in prolactin concentrations should alert the physician to determine whether the patients will benefit from therapy with dopamine agonists. However, these drugs are sometimes not necessary despite prolactin being elevated. For example, when menopause occurs, many women can stop therapy without adverse effects.

Drugs or medical conditions (e.g., renal disease or primary hypothyroidism) that can induce hyperprolactinemia should be always carefully excluded, to avoid incorrectly relating a nonfunctioning microadenoma to a rise in prolactin levels due to extrapituitary causes.

References

1. Frantz AG, Kleinberg DL. Prolactin: evidence that it is separate from growth hormone in human blood. Science 1970;170:745–747
2. Antunes JL, Housepian EM, Frantz AG, et al. Prolactin-secreting pituitary tumors. Ann Neurol 1977;2:148–153
3. Boyd AE III, Reighlin S. Editorial: Galactorrhea-amenorrhea, bromergocryptine, and the dopamine receptor. N Engl J Med 1975; 293:451–452
4. Thorner MO, Martin WH, Rogol AD, et al. Rapid regression of pituitary prolactinomas during bromocriptine treatment. J Clin Endocrinol Metab 1980;51:438–445
5. Thorner MO, Perryman RL, Rogol AD, et al. Rapid changes of prolactinoma volume after withdrawal and reinstitution of bromocriptine. J Clin Endocrinol Metab 1981;53:480–483
6. Besser GM, Wass JAH. Somatostatin octapeptide analogue (octreotide) in the medical management of acromegaly. Adv Biosci 1988;69: 221–225
7. Beck-Peccoz P, Brucker-Davis F, Persani L, Smallridge RC, Weintraub BD. Thyrotropin-secreting pituitary tumors. Endocr Rev 1996; 17:610–638

8. Gittoes NJ, Sheppard MC, Johnson AP, Stewart PM. Outcome of surgery for acromegaly—the experience of a dedicated pituitary surgeon. QJM 1999;92:741–745
9. Tabaee A, Anand VK, Barron Y, et al. Endoscopic pituitary surgery: a systematic review and meta-analysis. J Neurosurg 2009;111:545–554
10. Melmed S, Kleinberg D. Anterior pituitary. In: Kronenberg HM, Melmed S, Polonsky KS, Larsen PR, eds. Williams Textbook of Endocrinology. Philadelphia: Saunders Elsevier; 2008:155–261
11. Hall WA, Luciano MG, Doppman JL, Patronas NJ, Oldfield EH. Pituitary magnetic resonance imaging in normal human volunteers: occult adenomas in the general population. Ann Intern Med 1994; 120:817–820
12. Molitch ME. Pituitary incidentalomas. Endocrinol Metab Clin North Am 1997;26:725–740
13. Sanno N, Oyama K, Tahara S, Teramoto A, Kato Y. A survey of pituitary incidentaloma in Japan. Eur J Endocrinol 2003;149:123–127
14. Barrow DL, Tindall GT, Kovacs K, Thorner MO, Horvath E, Hoffman JC Jr. Clinical and pathological effects of bromocriptine on prolactin-secreting and other pituitary tumors. J Neurosurg 1984;60:1–7
15. Bassetti M, Spada A, Pezzo G, Giannattasio G. Bromocriptine treatment reduces the cell size in human macroprolactinomas: a morphometric study. J Clin Endocrinol Metab 1984;58:268–273
16. Saitoh Y, Mori S, Arita N, et al. Cytosuppressive effect of bromocriptine on human prolactinomas: stereological analysis of ultrastructural alterations with special reference to secretory granules. Cancer Res 1986;46:1507–1512
17. Colao A, Di Sarno A, Cappabianca P, Di Somma C, Pivonello R, Lombardi G. Withdrawal of long-term cabergoline therapy for tumoral and nontumoral hyperprolactinemia. N Engl J Med 2003;349:2023–2033
18. Casanueva FF, Molitch ME, Schlechte JA, et al. Guidelines of the Pituitary Society for the diagnosis and management of prolactinomas. Clin Endocrinol (Oxf) 2006;65:265–273
19. Zanettini R, Antonini A, Gatto G, Gentile R, Tesei S, Pezzoli G. Valvular heart disease and the use of dopamine agonists for Parkinson's disease. N Engl J Med 2007;356:39–46
20. Kupersmith MJ, Kleinberg DL, Warren FA, Budzilovitch G, Cooper P. Growth of prolactinoma despite lowering of serum prolactin by bromocriptine. Neurosurgery 1989;24:417–423
21. Kupersmith MJ, Rosenberg C, Kleinberg D. Visual loss in pregnant women with pituitary adenomas. Ann Intern Med 1994;121:473–477
22. Lim S, Shahinian H, Maya MM, Yong W, Heaney AP. Temozolomide: a novel treatment for pituitary carcinoma. Lancet Oncol 2006;7:518–520
23. Neggers SJ, de Herder WW, Janssen JA, Feelders RA, van der Lely AJ. Combined treatment for acromegaly with long-acting somatostatin analogs and pegvisomant: long-term safety for up to 4.5 years (median 2.2 years) of follow-up in 86 patients. Eur J Endocrinol 2009;160:529–533
24. Biller BM, Grossman AB, Stewart PM, et al. Treatment of adrenocorticotropin-dependent Cushing's syndrome: a consensus statement. J Clin Endocrinol Metab 2008;93:2454–2462
25. Testa RM, Albiger N, Occhi G, et al. The usefulness of combined biochemical tests in the diagnosis of Cushing's disease with negative pituitary magnetic resonance imaging. Eur J Endocrinol 2007;156: 241–248
26. Jehle S, Walsh JE, Freda PU, Post KD. Selective use of bilateral inferior petrosal sinus sampling in patients with adrenocorticotropin-dependent Cushing's syndrome prior to transsphenoidal surgery. J Clin Endocrinol Metab 2008;93:4624–4632
27. Patil CG, Veeravagu A, Prevedello DM, Katznelson L, Vance ML, Laws ER Jr. Outcomes after repeat transsphenoidal surgery for recurrent Cushing's disease. Neurosurgery 2008;63:266–270, discussion 270–271
28. Vance ML. Cushing's disease: radiation therapy. Pituitary 2009;12: 11–14
29. Boscaro M, Ludlam WH, Atkinson B, et al. Treatment of pituitary-dependent Cushing's disease with the multireceptor ligand somatostatin analog pasireotide (SOM230): a multicenter, phase II trial. J Clin Endocrinol Metab 2009;94:115–122
30. Saccomanno K, Bassetti M, Lania A, Losa M, Faglia G, Spada A. Immunodetection of glycoprotein hormone subunits in nonfunctioning and glycoprotein hormone-secreting pituitary adenomas. J Endocrinol Invest 1997;20:59–64
31. Dekkers OM, Pereira AM, Roelfsema F, et al. Observation alone after transsphenoidal surgery for nonfunctioning pituitary macroadenoma. J Clin Endocrinol Metab 2006;91:1796–1801
32. Losa M, Mortini P, Barzaghi R, et al. Early results of surgery in patients with nonfunctioning pituitary adenoma and analysis of the risk of tumor recurrence. J Neurosurg 2008;108:525–532
33. Webb SM, Rigla M, Wägner A, Oliver B, Bartumeus F. Recovery of hypopituitarism after neurosurgical treatment of pituitary adenomas. J Clin Endocrinol Metab 1999;84:3696–3700
34. Nomikos P, Ladar C, Fahlbusch R, Buchfelder M. Impact of primary surgery on pituitary function in patients with non-functioning pituitary adenomas—a study on 721 patients. Acta Neurochir (Wien) 2004;146:27–35
35. Karavitaki N, Thanabalasingham G, Shore HC, et al. Do the limits of serum prolactin in disconnection hyperprolactinaemia need re-definition? A study of 226 patients with histologically verified non-functioning pituitary macroadenoma. Clin Endocrinol (Oxf) 2006;65:524–529
36. Arafah BM. Medical management of hypopituitarism in patients with pituitary adenomas. Pituitary 2002;5:109–117
37. Arafah BM. Reversible hypopituitarism in patients with large nonfunctioning pituitary adenomas. J Clin Endocrinol Metab 1986; 62:1173–1179
38. Delgrange E, Trouillas J, Maiter D, Donckier J, Tourniaire J. Sex-related difference in the growth of prolactinomas: a clinical and proliferation marker study. J Clin Endocrinol Metab 1997;82:2102–2107
39. Smith S, Wheeler MJ, Murray R, O'Keane V. The effects of antipsychotic-induced hyperprolactinaemia on the hypothalamic-pituitary-gonadal axis. J Clin Psychopharmacol 2002;22:109–114

7 Indications for Surgery on Pituitary Tumors: A Neurosurgeon's Perspective

Rudolf Fahlbusch and Vincenzo Paternó

Historical Development

Historically, the development of indications for surgery in pituitary tumors can be divided into three phases. The first phase started around 1900 with the development of the surgical approaches. The transcranial approach appeared first and was favored by Victor Horsley (1889) and Fedor Krause (1900), followed by the transsphenoidal approach, favored by Hermann Schloffer (1907) and Harvey Cushing (1909).[1]

The second phase was mainly concerned with clinical findings. The indications for surgery were the patient's symptoms, especially ophthalmologic deterioration. The endocrinological classification and indications for surgery were developed much later, in the 1960s, when assessment of hormone levels became possible. At the same time, the introduction of the microscope into the neurosurgical operating room made selective adenomectomy possible, as defined by Jules Hardy for the transsphenoidal approach,[2] and further fostered by the subsequent development of computed tomography (CT) and magnetic resonance imaging (MRI).[3,4]

The third phase was characterized by improvements in surgical accuracy starting in the 1990s with the introduction of the endoscope and later the introduction of neuronavigation[5–7] and intraoperative MRI.[7–9] In parallel, alternative endocrinologic medical treatment was developed, especially antiproliferative treatment, first with a dopamine agonist for prolactinomas and later with somatostatin analogues for acromegaly.[10–12]

Indications for Surgery

Assessing the patient's appropriateness for surgery for pituitary tumors begins with a multidisciplinary evaluation of the symptoms, conducted by the primary care physician, a neurosurgeon, an endocrinologist or neuroendocrinologist, a neuroradiologist, an ophthalmologist, and radiologist. The pituitary gland's anatomy and function are assessed. The surgeon and endocrinologist evaluate the pituitary lesion. Indications for surgery for pituitary tumors, such as pituitary adenomas, depend on the functional symptoms and the imaging results. It is mandatory to assess the patient's endocrinologic function before recommending surgery.

A pituitary adenoma originates from the pituitary gland and first causes endocrine symptoms, such as hormonal excess or a partial pituitary insufficiency.

Ophthalmologic symptoms develop when the optic chiasm is contacted and compressed by the tumor. Oculomotor nerve disturbance occurs when the tumor is growing into the cavernous sinus. In addition to the endocrinologic and ophthalmologic indications for surgery, an important indication occurs in cases of suprasellar development when obstruction of the foramen of Monro in turn obstructs the hydrocephalus.

Initial symptoms may be subclinical and thus must be elucidated with sophisticated endocrine function tests, and ophthalmologic and neuroradiologic examinations.

Surgery for a primary adenoma has to be weighed against other treatment options, mainly medical antiproliferating treatment and, more rarely, x-knife/radiotherapy (RT). Surgery may be selected as an alternative treatment when primary medical treatment for a hormonally active adenoma has failed. Surgery may also be indicated for tumor recurrences or progressive growth of residual tumor.

Patient Symptoms

Many patients with a pituitary lesion appear healthy on physical examination. The pituitary adenoma is discovered only as an incidental finding when an MRI is performed (see Incidentaloma, below).

Headache is not a typical presenting symptom for a pituitary adenoma, but it is one of the main reasons why patients undergo a screening MRI. The sellar space is quite small and a lesion of any size may produce or exacerbate headaches. Acute headache occurs in pituitary apoplexy, and chronic headache occurs in transitory acromegaly or is due to an obstructive hydrocephalus (tumor blockage of the foramen of Monro). Periorbital headache occurs when the cavernous sinus is compressed or invaded by pituitary tumors. There is only one indication for surgery to relieve an isolated headache that is not necessarily accompanied by other symptoms: Rathke's pouch cyst can cause frontal or midline headache, and thus it is the only indication for surgery in patients with no endocrinologic deficit or ophthalmologic indication.[13]

Assessment of ophthalmologic symptoms entails evaluating visual acuity, visual fields, and ocular motility in a patient harboring a macroadenoma that contacts or compresses the optic chiasm or invades the cavernous sinus or sinuses.

Ophthalmologic disturbance of the optic nerves, optic chiasm, or oculomotor nerves is an indication for surgery. Evidence of an ophthalmologic or visual defect is a cause for concern and may require urgent tumor resection to decompress the involved structures. Compression of the optic chiasm may cause a mild deficit or complete bitemporal hemianopia. Tumor invasion into the cavernous sinus may generate a clinical picture that suggests involvement of one or more of the associated cranial nerves.[14–16]

Chiasma compression syndrome is characterized by a visual field defect followed by loss of visual acuity and then optic nerve atrophy. The visual field defect starts with central or paracentral scotomas followed by upper temporal defects and finally nasal field defects. The differential diagnosis for primary optic diseases includes glaucoma. The diagnosis may be difficult to make in the early stage of the tumor.

Homonymous hemianopia occurs in lateralized suprasellar tumor development when the optic tract is compressed; temporal hemianopia develops in symmetric suprasellar extension. Double vision occurs when the abducent and oculomotor nerves that are localized in the lateral part of the cavernous sinus are damaged acutely or chronically.[17]

Endocrinologic Deterioration

Two endocrinologic scenarios should been evaluated in cases of a pituitary tumor, pituitary insufficiency, or pituitary hyperfunction. The patient's signs and symptoms guide physicians in choosing which laboratory tests should been performed to determine the correct diagnosis by assessing the pituitary and target gland hormones in both the basal and dynamic states.[4,14,15]

As an initial endocrine screen, done in the morning under fasting conditions, basal serum measurements should be performed for the following hormones: prolactin (PRL), growth hormone (GH), insulin-like growth factor-1 (IGF-1), luteinizing hormone (LH), follicle-stimulating hormone (FSH), testosterone and estrogen, thyroid-stimulating hormone (TSH), free triiodothyronine (FT_3) and free thyroxine (FT_4), and cortisol. Then, additional provocative, dynamic, and special hormonal assays may be indicated to define precisely a specific endocrinopathy.

If no local facility exists to perform these studies, the blood can be sampled and stored at 4°C in the refrigerator and sent later that day or the next day to a specialized laboratory.

Pituitary insufficiency is usually a chronic process, associated with both large and small tumors. A macroadenoma contained within a normal-sized sella can cause hypogonadism, and if the tumor grows within the sella compartment it will cause total anterior pituitary insufficiency. In cases of intra- and suprasellar growth, sometimes moderate anterior pituitary (AP) insufficiency can occur, depending on the compressive effect of the tumor on the pituitary body and its stalk. Hypothalamic compression can lead to tertiary AP insufficiency.

Secondary hypogonadotropic hypogonadism (HH) is defined by absent or decreased functions of the male testes or the female ovaries. HH is caused by a lack of the gonad-stimulating pituitary hormones FSH and LH, which is associated with a decrease in the gonadal hormones testosterone and estrogen.

In addition to hyposomatotropism (GH deficiency can be assessed by insulin-induced hypoglycemia), secondary hypogonadism is the most sensitive indicator of early partial pituitary insufficiency.

The majority of patients with HH secondary to such tumors have multiple pituitary hormone deficiencies in addition to gonadotropin deficiency. In adults, prolactinomas are the most frequent cause of HH and may do so by either interfering with gonadotropin-releasing hormone (GnRH) secretion, or, in the case of macroadenomas, by local destruction and compression of the gonadotrophs. Hyperprolactinemia causes altered dopaminergic function, which has been shown to reduce GnRH messenger RNA (mRNA) levels and decrease serum levels of LH, FSH, and testosterone. Although men with hyperprolactinemia may develop galactorrhea, it occurs less frequently than in women, presumably due to the lack of stimulation by estrogen and progesterone. Clinically, men with hypogonadism may experience a loss of libido or impotence and may have soft and small testes. Loss of secondary sexual hair development starts in the pubic area, followed by thinning in the axilla and facial beard. Fine wrinkling of the facial skin is characteristic and is likely to be a result of both a testosterone and GH deficiency. In children, craniopharyngioma is the most common tumor resulting in HH and is often associated with growth retardation, visual field defects, and diabetes insipidus.

Secondary hypothyroidism occurs in about half of the patients with AP insufficiency. Clinically, the patients complain of fatigue, weakness, weight gain or increased difficulty losing weight, dry hair, rough pale skin, hair loss, cold intolerance, muscle cramps and frequent muscle aches, constipation, depression, irritability, memory loss, and decreased libido. The patient may have any number of these symptoms, and they will vary with the severity of the thyroid hormone deficiency and the length of time the body has been deprived of the proper amount of hormone.

Secondary adrenal insufficiency is caused by lack of production of adrenocorticotropic hormone (ACTH) in the pituitary gland. Patients may show symptoms of hypoglycemia, dehydration, weight loss, and disorientation. They may also experience adynamia, weakness, tiredness, dizziness, low blood pressure with orthostatic hypotension, muscle aches, nausea, vomiting, and diarrhea. These symptoms may develop gradually and insidiously. Addison's can present with tanning of the skin, which may be patchy or evenly distributed all over the body. In some cases a person with normally light skin may be mistaken for another race with darker pigmentation. Characteristic sites of tanning are skin creases (e.g., of the hands) and the inside of the cheek (buccal mucosa). Goiter and vitiligo may also be present.

Secondary hypoadrenalism can be reliably diagnosed, in the absence of acute ACTH deficiency or glucocorticoid use, by means of the short ACTH dynamic test (Synacthen test). Partial ACTH deficiency may prevent involution of the adrenal cortex and preserve the cortisol response to ACTH stimulation. A normal cortisol response in the short ACTH test does not therefore exclude the possibility of clinically relevant ACTH deficiency.

The second mode of presentation involves pituitary hyperfunction, which leads to several characteristic hypersecretory states. Because as many as 70% of pituitary adenomas are endocrinologically active, the presence of a hypersecretory endocrine state is the most common mode of presentation. Excessive secretion of PRL, GH, ACTH, and, rarely, TSH results in the amenorrhea-galactorrhea syndrome, acromegaly, or gigantism, Cushing's disease, and secondary hyperthyroidism, respectively.

Prolactinomas are pituitary adenomas that secrete PRL, leading to excessive hyperprolactinemia. Female patients with prolactinomas may present with the classic amenorrhea/galactorrhea syndromes. Two thirds of prolactinomas occur in females, and one third occur in men. Men rarely present with galactorrhea but rather with loss of libido and impotency. PRL secretion is enhanced by estrogens and inhibited by dopamine, which is synthesized within the hypothalamus and transported to the pituitary gland via the portal vessels within the pituitary stalk. This information is essential for understanding the differential diagnosis of hyperprolactinemia.

Hyperprolactinemia can also occur if the transport of dopamine to the pituitary gland is confined to the pituitary stalk by an inflammatory lesion or a compressive lesion such as an intra- and suprasellar tumor, which are mainly nonfunctioning pituitary adenomas. In this case, moderate hyperprolactinemia, with PRL levels below 150 ng/mL (five- to sevenfold elevation of normal values), is found. Furthermore, other factors such as drugs can cause hyperprolactinemia, too. Spontaneous or expressible galactorrhea may occur with an elevated PRL level; however, the absence of galactorrhea does not exclude the presence of hyperprolactinemia.

In cases of diagnosed prolactinoma, medical treatment is generally the first option. The primary goal of therapy in patients with prolactinomas is to normalize the PRL levels and to restore gonadal function. A first-generation dopamine agonist is bromocriptine, and second-generation dopamine agonists are cabergoline and quinagolide. More than 90% of patients respond to this treatment with a reduction in the serum PRL level; approximately 70% experience normalization, but a smaller number of patients experience impressive tumor shrinkage.

Surgery is mandatory in patients who do not respond to a dopamine agonist (PRL is not normalized, the tumor does not shrink, and pituitary insufficiency does not improve); in patients who experience intolerable side effects; in cases of cystic prolactinoma (no shrinkage of cyst); and in patients who wish to become pregnant (in cases of microadenoma).[10,18]

Acromegaly is the most clear-cut of the hypersecreting pituitary endocrinopathies. Patients may experience symptoms of the disease for several years before diagnosis. Their history includes enlargement of the hands, feet, and facial bones; increased spacing between the teeth; coarse facial features, including an enlarged nose, lips, tongue, and jaw (prognathism); joint pain; sleep apnea; excessive sweating; and skin tags. These changes are gradual, and thus their appearance may not be noticed by the patient or family members or may be attributed to aging.

Growth hormone suppression during oral glucose tolerance testing (OGTT) and elevated IGF-1 levels document active acromegaly. GH levels are suppressed below 1 μg/L in normal people, and levels higher than this cutoff are confirmatory of acromegaly. Patients with the rarer "burned-out" acromegaly, arising after spontaneous hemorrhages into the tumor, must be excluded from pituitary surgery, but they may present with various symptoms that are indications for other treatments. After surgical or medical treatment of the adenoma, GH levels during OGTT and IGF-1 levels are reassessed. A significant proportion (approximately 30%) of patients present diverging findings, either having elevated GH levels and a normal IGF-1 or vice versa. Other dynamic tests, besides OGTT, for the diagnosis and monitoring of acromegaly are not helpful. Assays for GH and IGF-1 are changing, and absolute levels must be treated with circumspection because of the different assays involved.

In approximately 20% of acromegaly patients, there is coexpression of GH and PRL.[11] Other pituitary hormones have to be assessed to address the secretory effects of the tumor as well as the mass effect of the tumor on the normal pituitary gland.

Transsphenoidal surgery is the treatment of choice, especially for intrasellar microadenomas, noninvasive macroadenomas (i.e., those without cavernous sinus or bone invasion), and when the tumor is causing compression symptoms. In patients with intrasellar microadenomas, surgical removal provides biochemical control with normalization of IGF-1 in 75 to 95% of patients[12,19] HQ. Control rates are lower in patients with noninvasive macroadenomas, but even in these cases surgical removal provides biochemical control, with normalization of IGF-1 in 40 to 68% of patients.[12,20] In patients who do not have a visual loss, medical therapy with a somatostatin analogue has been recommended as primary therapy, and the effects of presurgical treatment with a SRL on surgical outcome and postoperative complications (heart failure, sleep apnea, or diabetes mellitus) have been assessed in many studies.[11,12,20,21] Some authors have also concluded that pretreatment with an SRL can improve normalization of GH and IGF-1 after surgery and shorten the duration of hospitalization.[12,22] Medical treatment before surgery is certainly not contraindicated, but there is currently insufficient evidence to recommend it for improved surgical outcome or reduced postoperative complications.[12]

Complete surgical removal of GH-secreting tumors results in hormonal control of acromegaly and improvement of soft tissue changes. In experienced hands, complications of transsphenoidal surgery in acromegaly are rare, including transient oculomotor palsies, deterioration of vision, carotid artery injury, and epistaxis (occurring in less than 1% of patients).[12]

Cushing's disease (CD) defines a state of hypercortisolism caused by an ACTH-secreting pituitary adenoma. These tumors represent approximately 10 to 12% of all pituitary adenomas and are seen predominantly in women, with a female-to-male ratio of 8:1.

Clinical features include facial plethora, supraclavicular fat deposition, posterior cervical fat, acanthosis nigricans, acne, hirsutism, thin skin, ecchymoses, and violaceous striae; the last feature is present in only 50% of patients, and its absence does not exclude the presence of the syndrome. Those patients usually experience weight gain, fatigue, sleeping difficulties, irritability, depression, memory loss, difficulty with concentrating, muscle weakness, bone fractures, or osteoporosis. Development of diabetes or worsening of diabetes control and development of hypertension or worsening of treated hypertension are common features in patients with CD. When CD is suspected, either a dexamethasone suppression test (administration of dexamethasone and frequent determination of cortisol and ACTH level) or a 24-hour urinary measurement for cortisol offers equal detection rates.

The 2-mg dexamethasone suppression test overnight (from 10 p.m. to 9 a.m.) documents Cushing's syndrome (CS) when serum cortisol levels >2 mg/dL.

Central ACTH-dependent CD is documented by an 8-mg dexamethasone suppression test overnight, when 50% of the original serum cortisol level is suppressed. Furthermore, under fasting conditions the ACTH or cortisol level can be stimulated sufficiently. The rare ectopic ACTH syndrome, with an ACTH level of 120 to 150 pg/mL, has to been excluded by additional ACTH sampling at different areas of the body by venous catheterization.

There is no effective medical therapy to reduce pituitary ACTH production or decrease tumor size. Surgery is the treatment of choice for CD, in which medical management is invariably suboptimal. In the hands of an experienced neurosurgeon, selective transsphenoidal adenomectomy offers remission rates between 70 and 80%, with mortality and mobility rates less than 2%.[23,24] The absence of hypocortisolism postoperatively should prompt a reassessment of the diagnosis, evaluation of potential confounding elements, and consideration of repeated surgery. If the surgery is not successful, pituitary irradiation should be considered.[13,24]

In thyroid-stimulating hormone (TSH)-oma, overproduction of TSH can cause hyperthyroidism. TSH is increased and can be stimulated by thyrotropin-releasing hormone (TRH). T_3 and T_4 can be in the upper normal range or even slightly elevated. TSH-secreting pituitary tumors represent approximately 2% of all pituitary adenomas.

Pituitary Apoplexy

Pituitary apoplexy is an uncommon but well-described clinical syndrome resulting from pituitary hemorrhage or infarction, almost invariably occurring in the presence of an adenoma.[10] Hemorrhage may also occur in the absence of clinical features or with a subacute course, but the term *apoplexy* is properly reserved for those cases with the abrupt onset of typical symptoms and signs. In general, delayed surgical intervention is reasonable, while at first the disturbed electrolyte water balance has to be stabilized, especially the frequently observed hyponatremia; furthermore, "acute" secondary hypoadrenalism has to be replaced by >100 mg cortisol per day before surgery can be performed. The recovery or restoration of any ophthalmologic deficits will not be adversely impacted by delayed surgery awaiting stable endocrine and metabolic conditions.

Urgent surgical decompression of the sellar contents is still advocated by some authors, although the majority recommend delayed conservative therapy in certain situations.[25]

Nonfunctioning Adenoma, Craniopharyngioma, Rathke Cyst, and Infiltrative Disease

There are no effective medical therapies for these diseases. Resection is the primary therapy. Because these lesions often cause loss of pituitary function, it is vital to identify the need for glucocorticoid (steroid), thyroid hormone, and vasopressin (desmopressin acetate) replacement before surgery to minimize the risk of intraoperative and postoperative complications. Diabetes insipidus should be anticipated postoperatively if there is involvement of the pituitary stalk or the hypothalamus. The need for gonadal steroid and GH replacement therapy should be evaluated after surgery.

Incidentaloma

Pituitary incidentalomas are, by definition, asymptomatic or nontypically symptomatic masses or lesions that are discovered incidentally, usually by an MRI performed to evaluate unrelated disorders (such as head trauma), to determine cancer staging, or to assess headaches and dizziness. In some series of incidentalomas, headache was the most common reason for performing imaging studies.[26]

Once the pituitary incidentaloma has been discovered, management begins with observation and then progresses to conservative treatment and finally surgical treatment. Management should be guided by two questions:

1. Is the tumor hormonally active? Are there clinical symptoms for acromegaly or CD? A careful history and physical examination may reveal overlooked symptoms or signs of hypersecretion of a specific hormone, which can be evaluated in detail to establish the diagnosis. After the type and the degree of hormone excess has been evaluated by sophisticated endocrine tests, treatment is indicated in nearly all cases.
2. Does the lesion cause a mass effect or pituitary insufficiency? These factors should be documented.

There are two published series of incidentaloma. Arita et al[27] report that approximately 20% of cases could become symptomatic during 5-year follow-up and that the size of the incidentaloma could increase in approximately 40% (42 patients in their study). Significant growth of a pituitary incidentaloma is an indication for surgery to prevent pituitary insufficiency.[16,27] Karavitaki et al[28] observed 40 patients with a minimum follow-up of 42 months in 60 microadenomas; only 12.5 of the tumors were growing. However, in 24 macroadenomas, 50% of the tumors were growing, causing visual field defects in 57% of patients and documented chiasma contact in 21%. For the microadenomas, watchful waiting is recommend, whereas for the macroadenomas early surgery should be considered.[27,28]

In the absence of hypersecretion, hypopituitarism, or visual field defects, periodic MRI screening for enlargement should be performed in 6 months, then yearly for 5 years, and then every 2 to 3 years if the patient is stable.

Radiologic Considerations

Hypointensive areas on the MRI that are close to the wall of the cavernous sinus can be due to a partial volume effect caused by the adjacent carotid artery mimicking a pituitary microadenoma.

Microadenomas are defined as >10 mm in the longest diameter, but if the diameter is <3 mm, they generally cannot be detected by MRI.

Surgical Approaches

The goal of surgery is selective tumor removal: relief of the tumor, reduction of hormone hypersecretion to normal levels, preservation, recovery of normal pituitary function, improvement of visual disturbance, and prevention of complications. Removal of a pituitary lesion by an experienced pituitary neurosurgeon[29] offers the best possibility of achieving these goals, which are most likely accomplished in a patient with a smaller lesion. Surgery is very effective in relieving the mass effect; however, most patients harboring a large and especially invasive lesion will require additional treatment to produce hormonal remission and prevent regrowth of the residual tumor. Some will require hormone replacement therapy to reestablish a normal hormonal balance.

Surgery is also the first-line treatment of giant pituitary adenomas, with the exception of most prolactinomas, which can be effectively treated with dopamine agonists.

Transsphenoidal Pituitary Surgery

About 90% of pituitary adenomas, and especially all intra- and suprasellar symmetrically developed, and intra- and parasellar developed tumors (with focal cavernous sinus invasion) should be approached transsphenoidally.

Suprasellar tumor parts descend into the sella turcica in the majority of cases.[30] Valsalva maneuvers conducted by the anesthesiologist will transiently raise the intracranial pressure and cause inferior displacement of the mass, which may facilitate tumor removal. Parasellar extensions of pituitary tumors, however, are more difficult to manage because the microscope has limited lateral visualization. Given the proximity of the optic nerves, optic chiasm, carotid arteries, and cavernous sinuses to the sella, blind curettage of any tumor remnants extending beyond the limits of the sella is potentially dangerous.

The standard microscope-based transsphenoidal approach is limited in its ability to remove those tumors, which are developed outside the sella in two thirds of patients, as well as large parasellar tumors with general cavernous sinus invasion and large suprasellar tumors without chiasma syndrome and an irregular shape, demonstrating invasive tumor growths and the absence of a capsule.

Patients with extrasellar extensions of tumor into the anterior (subfrontal), middle, and posterior (retrosellar) cranial fossae must be considered for two-stage procedures. In these cases a primary transsphenoidal approach serves to debulk as much of the tumor as possible from below, whereas a secondary operation via a frontolateral transcranial approach allows total resection of tumor remnants.[31]

Such improvisation allows complete surgical removal of extensive lesions with minimal morbidity.

Transcranial Surgery

In many larger asymmetric tumors, with significant suprasellar, parasellar, retrosellar, and subfrontal extension, transcranial approaches may be indicated. They offer a high probability of safe, complete or near-complete, tumor removal. Often a transcranial method will be reserved for the second stage of a two-stage operation. The primary procedure is performed via microscopic- or endoscopic-assisted exposure of the sella turcica in which the bulk of the tumor is removed transsphenoidally. Residual tumor is then targeted in a subsequent transcranial exploration.

The transcranial approach is well suited to the management of other lesions affecting the parasellar areas that tend to spread regionally, including chordomas, craniopharyngiomas, meningiomas, and vascular lesions.[14]

Endoscopy

Pure endoscopic or endoscopic-assisted transsphenoidal surgery offers an "around the corner" paramount view into the cavernous sinus, as well as below the descending diaphragma sellae with its folds that may harbor residual tumor.[32]

The extended endoscopic transsphenoidal approach is also indicated and superior to the pure microscopic approach for all lesions infiltrating the clivus area (chordoma, special adenoma).

Drilling the tuberculum sella will help to remove midsized craniopharyngiomas via the transsphenoidal approach.

Additional Radiation and Medical Treatment

Radiation treatment (stereotactic, fractionated, gamma-knife, or proton-beam) of the pituitary is commonly used as an adjunctive treatment after incomplete tumor resection. In patients with a large tumor in whom the resection is incomplete, RT reduces the risk of enlargement of residual tumors and offers the possibility of permanent control of hormone hypersecretion. No form of radiation delivery is immediately effective to reduce hormone hypersecretion. To overcome the delayed RT effect, patients should be treated medically to control the disorder. For acromegaly, this treatment includes somatostatin analogues (lanreotide or long-acting-release Sandostatin) or the GH receptor antagonist pegvisomant (Somavert).

Patients with persistent hyperprolactinemia should be treated with a dopamine agonist (cabergoline, bromocriptine, quinagolide, or pergolide). There is no effective treatment to reduce ACTH production in patients with CD; however, medical therapy with ketoconazole is very effective in reducing transitory adrenal cortisol production and at consequently controlling CD. In a patient treated medically to control the disease while awaiting the effects of radiation therapy, the medication should be discontinued periodically (usually every 6 months) to determine whether the radiation treatment has become effective and whether there is any new pituitary hormone deficiency.

Recurrence

True tumor recurrence discovered on a postoperative MRI in active adenomas, even with normalization of hormonal excess, is an indication for reoperation.

Although successful surgical treatment has been performed and no tumor was seen on MRI, and hormonal excess was eliminated, there is a lifelong risk of tumor recurrence. Regardless of the tumor type, recurrence occurs in 12 to 16% of patients within 10 years after surgery. Thus, any patient with a pituitary tumor requires lifelong follow-up review and appropriate endocrinologic and anatomical studies. Symptomatic recurrence in a patient with a hypersecretory tumor is straightforward and is confirmed by measurement of the appropriate hormone followed by an MRI study. In patients with a nonsecretory tumor, MRI studies should be performed annually for the first 5 years after surgery. If there is no recurrence or growth of residual tumor, the neuroimaging interval may be increased to every 2 years. A pituitary adenoma may recur even 20 or more years after surgery; thus, all patients should be observed throughout life. Other long-term management issues include determining the ongoing need for hormone replacement therapy, particularly in patients who have received pituitary radiation treatment and regular monitoring for adequacy of therapy.

Timing plays an important role in recurrences. Similar to incidentalomas, all hormonally active adenomas must treated urgently. In invasive adenoma, the tumor-growth time plays a determining role. Surgery should be performed at the latest when ophthalmologic symptoms and new endocrinologic deterioration occur.

With respect to the low complication rate of reoperation in experienced hands, surgery of recurrence is indicated when significant tumor growth is documented and functional disturbance can be expected.

In CD, reoperation of suspicious adenomas, mainly developed in the same location, as at first surgery, should be performed as soon it is safe to do so.[23] However, inactive adenomas can be observed for some time. Continued growth, even above the sella entrance, close to the optic nerve and the onset of deterioration of pituitary function are indications for surgery.

RT offers the possibility of tumor control but it induces anterior pituitary insufficiency in the majority of patients years after treatment.

References

1. Cushing HW. The basophil adenomas of the pituitary body and their clinical manifestations (pituitary basophilism). Bulletin of the Johns Hopkins Hospital, Baltimore 1932;50:137–195
2. Hardy J. Transsphenoidal microsurgery of the normal and pathological pituitary. Clin Neurosurg 1969;16:185–217
3. Johnson MR, Hoare RD, Cox T, et al. The evaluation of patients with a suspected pituitary microadenoma: computer tomography compared to magnetic resonance imaging. Clin Endocrinol (Oxf) 1992;36:335–338
4. Kaye TB, Crapo L. The Cushing syndrome: an update on diagnostic tests. Ann Intern Med 1990;112:434–444
5. Elias WJ, Chadduck JB, Alden TD, Laws ER Jr. Frameless stereotaxy for transsphenoidal surgery. Neurosurgery 1999;45:271–275, discussion 275–277
6. Kawamata T, Iseki H, Shibasaki T, Hori T. Endoscopic augmented reality navigation system for endonasal transsphenoidal surgery to treat pituitary tumors: technical note. Neurosurgery 2002;50:1393–1397
7. Schulder M, Sernas TJ, Carmel PW. Cranial surgery and navigation with a compact intraoperative MRI system. Acta Neurochir Suppl (Wien) 2003;85:79–86
8. Nimsky C, von Keller B, Ganslandt O, Fahlbusch R. Intraoperative high-field magnetic resonance imaging in transsphenoidal surgery of hormonally inactive pituitary macroadenomas. Neurosurgery 2006;59:105–114, discussion 105–114
9. Schwartz TH, Stieg PE, Anand VK. Endoscopic transsphenoidal pituitary surgery with intraoperative magnetic resonance imaging. Neurosurgery 2006;58(1, Suppl):ONS44–ONS51, discussion ONS44–ONS51
10. Kreutzer J, Buslei R, Wallaschofski H, et al. Operative treatment of prolactinomas: indications and results in a current consecutive series of 212 patients. Eur J Endocrinol 2008;158:11–18
11. Losa M, Mortini P, Urbaz L, Ribotto P, Castrignanó T, Giovanelli M. Presurgical treatment with somatostatin analogs in patients with acromegaly: effects on the remission and complication rates. J Neurosurg 2006;104:899–906
12. Melmed S, Colao A, Barkan A, et al; Acromegaly Consensus Group. Guidelines for acromegaly management: an update. J Clin Endocrinol Metab 2009;94:1509–1517
13. Madhok R, Prevedello DM, Gardner P, Carrau RL, Snyderman CH, Kassam AB; Clinical article. Endoscopic endonasal resection of Rathke cleft cysts: clinical outcomes and surgical nuances. J Neurosurg 2010;112:1333–1339
14. Aron DC, Tyrrell JB, Wilson CB. Pituitary tumors. Current concepts in diagnosis and management. West J Med 1995;162:340–352
15. Vance ML. Treatment of patients with a pituitary adenoma: one clinician's experience. Neurosurg Focus 2004;16:E1
16. Serhal D, Weil RJ, Hamrahian AH. Evaluation and management of pituitary incidentalomas. Cleve Clin J Med 2008;75:793–801
17. Kreutzer J, Fahlbusch R. Diagnosis and treatment of pituitary tumors. Curr Opin Neurol 2004;17:693–703
18. Casanueva FF, Molitch ME, Schlechte JA, et al. Guidelines of the Pituitary Society for the diagnosis and management of prolactinomas. Clin Endocrinol (Oxf) 2006;65:265–273
19. Buchfelder M, Schlaffer S. Surgical treatment of pituitary tumours. Best Pract Res Clin Endocrinol Metab 2009;23:677–692
20. Colao A, Ferone D, Cappabianca P, et al. Effect of octreotide pretreatment on surgical outcome in acromegaly. J Clin Endocrinol Metab 1997;82:3308–3314
21. Abe T, Lüdecke DK. Effects of preoperative octreotide treatment on different subtypes of 90 GH-secreting pituitary adenomas and outcome in one surgical centre. Eur J Endocrinol 2001;145:137–145
22. Jho HD, Carrau RL. Endoscopic endonasal transsphenoidal surgery: experience with 50 patients. J Neurosurg 1997;87:44–51
23. Hofmann BM, Hlavac M, Martinez R, Buchfelder M, Müller OA, Fahlbusch R. Long-term results after microsurgery for Cushing disease: experience with 426 primary operations over 35 years. J Neurosurg 2008;108:9–18
24. Fahlbusch R, Buchfelder M, Müller OA. Transsphenoidal surgery for Cushing's disease. J R Soc Med 1986;79:262–269
25. Verrees M, Arafah BM, Selman WR. Pituitary tumor apoplexy: characteristics, treatment, and outcomes. Neurosurg Focus 2004;16:E6
26. Molitch ME. Pituitary tumours: pituitary incidentalomas. Best Pract Res Clin Endocrinol Metab 2009;23:667–675
27. Arita K, Tominaga A, Sugiyama K, et al. Natural course of incidentally found nonfunctioning pituitary adenoma, with special reference to pituitary apoplexy during follow-up examination. J Neurosurg 2006;104:884–891
28. Karavitaki N, Collison K, Halliday J, et al. What is the natural history of nonoperated nonfunctioning pituitary adenomas? Clin Endocrinol (Oxf) 2007;67:938–943
29. Ciric IS, Zhao J. Transsphenoidal microsurgery: past, present and future. Expert Rev Anticancer Ther 2006;6(Suppl 9):S75–S78
30. Kanter AS, Dumont AS, Asthagiri AR, Oskouian RJ, Jane JA Jr, Laws ER Jr. The transsphenoidal approach. A historical perspective. Neurosurg Focus 2005;18:e6
31. Nomikos P, Fahlbusch R, Buchfelder M. Recent developments in transsphenoidal surgery of pituitary tumors. Hormones (Athens) 2004;3:85–91
32. Cappabianca P, Cavallo LM, Colao A, et al. Endoscopic endonasal transsphenoidal approach: outcome analysis of 100 consecutive procedures. Minim Invasive Neurosurg 2002;45:193–200

8 Histology of Pituitary Tumors

Theresa Scognamiglio and Ehud Lavi

Normal Pituitary Gland

The human pituitary gland is a small bean-shaped organ located at the base of the brain and is situated within the confines of the sella turcica. It measures 10 mm in length, 5 to 10 mm in height, and 10 to 15 mm in width and has an average weight of 600 mg. The pituitary gland on average weighs more in females and increases in weight during pregnancy.[1] Considered the master endocrine organ, it functions along with the hypothalamus in the regulation of other endocrine organs. The pituitary is attached to the hypothalamus by the pituitary stalk and is composed of two anatomical and functionally distinct parts: the anterior lobe (adenohypophysis) and the posterior lobe (neurohypophysis).

The anterior lobe is embryologically derived from Rathke's pouch and constitutes the majority of the gland (80%). It consists of three components: the pars distalis, pars intermedia, and pars tuberalis. The pars distalis constitutes the majority of the anterior lobe, and histologically five different cell types can be identified in the pars distalis: growth hormone (GH)-producing somatotrophs; prolactin (PRL)-producing lactotrophs; corticotrophs (adrenocorticotropic hormone [ACTH], pro-opiomelanocortin [POMC], melanocyte-stimulating hormone, endorphins, and lipotrophins); thyrotrophs (thyroid-stimulating hormone [TSH]); and gonadotrophs (follicle-stimulating hormone [FSH], luteinizing hormone [LH]).

Various transcription factors control the development of the anterior pituitary. The identification of these transcription factors has enabled further classification of pituitary tumors and has provided an explanation for adenomas with multiple hormone production. Three main pathways of cell differentiation have been defined in the anterior pituitary. The expression of T-pit, which binds to corticotrophin upstream transcription-binding element (CUTE) proteins, is involved in the differentiation of ACTH-producing corticotrophs. The cytodifferentiation of gonadotrophs requires the expression of steroidogenic factor (SF)-1, GATA-2, and members of the *Lhx* gene family. Cells that express Pit-1 can develop into somatotrophs, lactotrophs, mammosomatotrophs, or thyrotrophs.[2,3]

The posterior pituitary comprises the remaining 20% of the gland and is composed of the infundibulum, pituitary stalk, and pars nervosa. It consists of pituicytes (modified glial cells) and axonal processes arising from the supraoptic and paraventricular nuclei in the hypothalamus. It is embryologically derived from an outpouching of the floor of the third ventricle. Antidiuretic hormone (vasopressin) and oxytocin are produced in the neuronal bodies of these nuclei and are stored in axon terminals in the posterior pituitary.

The pituitary has a dual circulation—a portal and an arterial system. The internal carotid artery gives rise to the superior, middle, and inferior hypophyseal arteries, which supply the gland. The infundibulum of the neurohypophysis is supplied by the superior hypophyseal artery, which forms the portal system of the pituitary. Direct blood supply to the anterior pituitary comes from the middle hypophyseal artery, whereas the pars nervosa is supplied by the inferior hypophyseal artery. Venous drainage is mainly to the internal jugular.

Surgical Pathology Approach to the Diagnosis of Pituitary Adenoma

The surgical pathologist often encounters several challenges during the process of diagnosing pituitary adenomas. In intraoperative consultations the main challenge is distinguishing between pituitary tissue and other lesions (**Table 8.1**) that are in the differential diagnosis for masses in the pituitary region. This is particularly important in cases where the distinction is between a tumor and an inflammatory condition, which may affect the surgeon's decision about the continuation of the operation. The recognition of a neuroendocrine cell versus features specific for the other lesions is essential. Both smear preparations and frozen sections are helpful for providing information on cellular morphology and architecture.

The next challenge is to distinguish between normal pituitary and adenoma. On cytologic preparations, abundant cellularity usually favors adenoma. On both cytologic and histologic preparations, cytologic monomorphism, uniform cytoplasmic staining quality, occasional multinucleate or pleomorphic cells, prominent nucleoli, and mitotic figures are all indicative of adenomas. Histologically, the presence of acinar or small-cluster architecture with delicate fibrous septa and variability in the cytologic staining pattern are indicative of a normal pituitary tissue. The effacement of the acinar pattern and replacement by a sheet-like morphology lacking organized fibrous septa, the presence of papillary morphology or a sinusoidal architecture, with or without

Table 8.1 Sellar Region Masses

Tumors/masses of Pituitary Origin	**Metastatic/Hematopoietic Tumors**
Tumors of adenohypophyseal origin	Carcinoma
Pituitary adenoma	Lymphoma
Intrasellar gangliocytoma	Plasmacytoma
Spindle cell oncocytoma	Leukemias
Pituitary carcinoma	**Cysts/hamartomas/malformations/vascular**
Tumors of neurohypophyseal origin	Rathke's cleft cyst
Pituicytoma (glioma)	Arachnoid cyst
Granular cell tumor	Epidermoid, dermoid, teratomatous cysts
Adenohypophyseal hyperplasia	Hamartomas
Primary nonpituitary tumors	Aneurysms
Craniopharyngioma	Cavernous hemangioma
Germ cell tumors	Arteriovenous malformation
Meningioma	**Inflammatory conditions**
Chordoma	Lymphocytic hypophysitis
Gliomas	Langerhans cell histiocytosis
Schwannoma	Sarcoidosis
Paraganglioma	Other granulomatous conditions
Tumors of mesenchymal origin	Mucocele
Sarcomas (osteo-, chondro-, leiomyo-, rhabdomyo-, fibro-, etc.)	Pyogenic/infectious abscess
Solitary fibrous tumors/hemangiopericytoma (HPC)	
Lipoma	
Chondroma	
Giant cell tumor of bone	

pseudo-rosette formation are indicative of a pituitary adenoma. Additional challenges facing the pathologist are cases of previously treated adenomas that may present excessive fibrous deposition and cases of pituitary apoplexy in which infarcted, hemorrhagic, nonviable tissue is predominantly seen. Occasionally, hypoxic damage in a pituitary adenoma may produce small cells with pyknotic nuclei resembling lymphocytes, which may be confused with lymphocytic hypophysitis.

In permanent sections the diagnosis is usually made by routine hematoxylin and eosin (H&E) staining, assisted by immunohistochemistry of the antibodies against the six hormones (PRL, GH, ACTH, TSH, LH, and FSH) in addition to synaptophysin (with or without chromogranin). The immunohistochemical staining may be useful for both diagnostic purposes (for example, distinguishing between a pituitary adenoma and a metastatic carcinoma, or between nonneoplastic pituitary, normal, or hyperplastic versus adenoma), and for providing useful information to the endocrinologist (for example, distinguishing between PRL-secreting adenoma versus PRL elevation in a nonfunctional adenoma due to compression of the stalk). The addition of synaptophysin with or without chromogranin might be useful for the diagnosis of adenomas that do not stain with any hormonal product (about one fourth to one third of all adenomas). Occasionally, reticulin staining can be helpful in distinguishing between adenomas and normal pituitary.

Primary Tumors of Adenohypophysial Cells

Most pituitary tumors that arise in the anterior pituitary are benign (pituitary adenomas). Pituitary carcinomas represent a small proportion of pituitary lesions.

Pituitary Adenomas

The majority of pituitary tumors are pituitary adenomas, which constitute approximately 10 to 25% of all intracranial tumors.[4,5] Although most of these tumors arise in the sella turcica, some may be ectopic.[6] It has been reported that up to 27% are incidental findings (incidentalomas) found at the time of autopsy or during radiologic studies for other reasons.[5,7] These incidental tumors are usually hormonally inactive or slow growing without mass effect.

There are no currently reliable markers to predict behavior in adenomas. Proliferation markers such as K_i-67/Mib-1, proliferating cell nuclear antigen (PCNA), and DNA topoisomerase IIα have been suggested as useful parameters.[8–10] Growth factors and receptor expression,[11–13] in addition to oncogene and tumor suppressor gene alterations,[14,15] have been evaluated as potential prognostic markers.[2,16] DNA ploidy does not predict tumor prognosis or recurrence.[17]

Pituitary adenomas are most commonly found in adults, with the peak occurrence in the fourth to sixth decade. They are uncommon in children, representing approximately 2 to 6% of all intracranial tumors.[18–20] The majority of pituitary adenomas are functioning in children, with nonfunctioning tumors being rare. Some authors have found that tumors in children are larger, more aggressive, and more invasive.[19]

Although the majority of lesions occur in isolation (sporadic), a small percentage is associated with multiple endocrine neoplasia (MEN) type 1. Multiple adenomas have been reported in less than 1% of patients at autopsy and are very rare in surgical specimens.[21]

The pathogenesis and development of these tumors is not well understood, although several factors have been implicated.[3] They lack mutations in well-known tumor suppressor genes and oncogenes.[22]

Several classification systems are used for pituitary adenomas. Functional, anatomical, and histologic classifications have been employed. In the functional classification system, tumors are classified according to their in vivo hormonal activity and are either functioning or nonfunctioning (silent [no clinical symptoms] or hormone negative [immunohistochemical and ultrastructurally negative for hormone]). Anatomical or radiographic classification differentiates tumors according to their size and degree of local invasion. Morphologic classification uses a combination of conventional cytoplasmic staining, immunohistochemical detection of tissue antigens, and ultrastructural evaluation. Immunohistochemical detection of hormone content with the addition of immunohistochemical detection of other markers of cell differentiation such as transcription factors and cytokeratins can also be useful in classifying pituitary adenomas. Histologic (acidophil, basophil, chromophobe) and ultrastructural classifications are not commonly used. The most effective classification scheme is clinicopathologic and combines both morphologic and clinical features of the tumors.

Functioning Somatotroph Adenomas

Functioning somatotroph adenomas are derived from somatotrophs, which produce GH. They represent 10 to 15% of all adenomas.[1]

Pathology

Grossly, these tumors are located in the lateral wing of the pituitary. Microadenomas tend to be well demarcated, whereas macroadenomas, which represent the majority of GH-producing adenomas, commonly show suprasellar or lateral extension.[3]

Densely Granulated Somatotroph Adenomas

These tumors consist of acidophilic cells arranged in a trabecular, sinusoidal, or diffuse growth pattern (**Fig. 8.1**). They show strong diffuse reactivity for GH and nuclear staining for Pit-1. Perinuclear positivity for low molecular weight cytokeratin is seen, whereas there is variable staining for the α-subunit of glycoproteins. Ultrastructurally, the cells resemble normal somatotrophs. They have rough endoplasmic reticulum arranged in arrays and well-formed Golgi complexes.

Numerous dense secretory granules measuring 150 to 600 nm are present.

Sparsely Granulated Somatotroph Adenomas

These tumors are composed of chromophobic cells in a solid growth pattern. The cells show prominent nucleoli and nuclear pleomorphism. Positivity for low molecular weight cytokeratin in a juxtanuclear pattern highlights the characteristic

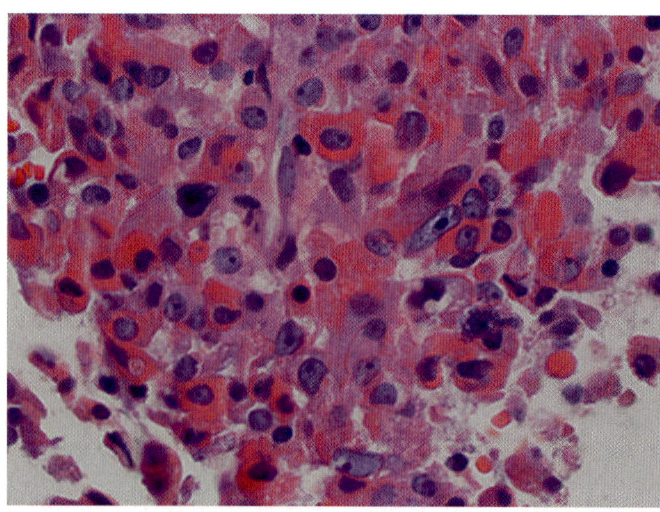

Fig. 8.1 Acidophilic, densely granulated, somatotroph adenoma with nuclear pleomorphism (×400).

fibrous body seen in these adenomas. There is weak immunoreactivity for GH. Nuclear reactivity for Pit-1 is seen, whereas there is occasional immunoreactivity for the α-subunit of glycoproteins. Ultrastructurally, the nuclei are eccentric and pleomorphic. The rough endoplasmic reticulum can be poor to well developed. Juxtanuclear whorls of intermediate filaments representing the fibrous body are seen. Secretory granules are sparse and measure 100 to 250 nm.

Mammosomatotroph Adenomas

These tumors are composed of uniform cells with chromophobic appearance, with or without slight acidophilia, arranged in a solid or diffuse pattern. These tumor cells produce both GH and PRL and this tumor is the most common cause of gigantism.[1] The tumor cells are strongly reactive for GH with variable reactivity for α-subunit and PRL.[1] Perinuclear positivity for low molecular weight cytokeratin is seen. There is strong Pit-1 nuclear positivity and rare positivity for the β-subunit of TSH. Ultrastructurally, the tumor cells resemble densely granulated somatotrophs. Secretory granules in these tumors can measure up to 1000 nm and have mottled cores. Misplaced exocytosis, which is a classic feature seen in prolactinomas, is identified in these adenomas.

In a small number of these tumors, mature somatotrophs and lactotrophs are identified with GH and PRL immunostaining localized to each individual cell type. These tumors have been referred to as mixed somatotroph-lactotroph adenomas.

Functioning Lactotroph Adenomas

These adenomas produce PRL and are derived from the lactotroph cells of the adenohypophysis.

Pathology

Most arise in the lateral or posterior pituitary. Macroadenomas tend to be more aggressive lesions and may invade into the dura and nasal sinuses.

Sparsely Granulated (Chromophobe) Lactotroph Adenomas

These are the most common variant of lactotroph adenomas. They are composed of chromophobic or slightly acidophilic large cells with indistinct cell borders and irregular nuclei with prominent nucleoli. The tumor cells can show a papillary, trabecular, or solid growth pattern. Calcifications in the form of psammoma bodies may be occasionally seen. Less frequently amyloid may be identified.

There is strong staining for PRL in the Golgi region (globular juxtanuclear pattern), and the cells are periodic acid-Schiff (PAS) negative. Ultrastructurally, there is prominent rough endoplasmic reticulum arranged in parallel arrays or concentric whorls (Nebenkern formations), large Golgi complex with immature granules, and sparse electron-dense granules measuring 150 to 300 nm. Misplaced lateral cell wall exocytosis is characteristic.

Densely Granulated Lactotroph Adenomas

These are the less common variant of the lactotroph adenoma, which is composed of acidophil cells. Unlike the Golgi staining seen in sparsely granulated tumors, PRL staining in these tumors is diffuse and cytoplasmic. Ultrastructurally, there are abundant rough endoplasmic reticulum, numerous secretory granules measuring up to 700 nm, and misplaced exocytosis.

Acidophil Stem Cell Adenomas

Acidophil adenomas are composed of large chromophobic cells with a slightly acidophilic cytoplasm secondary to mitochondria accumulation. There is strong diffuse PRL staining, with weak or negative immunoreactivity for GH. Ultrastructurally, numerous enlarged mitochondria characteristic of this adenoma are identified. In addition, fibrous bodies (juxtanuclear bundles of cytokeratin intermediate filaments) and misplaced exocytosis can be seen. There are sparse secretory granules measuring 150 to 200 nm.

Functioning Thyrotroph Adenomas

These are pituitary adenomas producing TSH and originating from the thyrotroph cells.

Pathology

When these tumors are microadenomas they can be localized to the mucoid wedge of the anterior pituitary. However, most are macroadenomas with no specific localization.

These tumors have a solid or sinusoidal growth pattern and are composed of chromophobic cells with indistinct cell borders and variable pleomorphism. Stromal fibrosis is not uncommon, and psammoma bodies may be seen.

There is variable staining for β-TSH and the α-subunit. Strong cytoplasmic staining for PAS is seen. Ultrastructurally, there are abundant rough endoplasmic reticulum with prominent spherical Golgi bodies within long interdigitating cell processes. Secretory granules measuring 150 to 250 nm are identified along the cell membrane.

Functioning Corticotroph Adenomas

These adenomas are pituitary tumors derived from corticotrophs, and they produce ACTH.

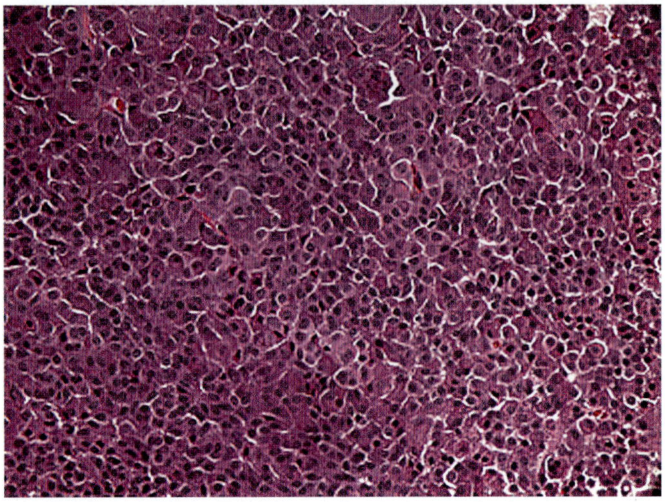

Fig. 8.2 Basophilic densely granulated, corticotroph pituitary adenoma (×200).

Pathology

Most of these tumors are microadenomas with no predominant localization in the pituitary.

Densely Granulated Corticotroph Adenomas

These are the most common type of corticotroph adenoma, and they are composed of basophilic cells in a sinusoidal pattern (**Fig. 8.2**). There is strong PAS-positive cytoplasmic staining. Strong immunoreactivity for ACTH and β-endorphins is seen. There is immunoreactivity for low molecular weight cytokeratins. Ultrastructurally, there are large polygonal cells with nucleoli in contact with the inner nuclear membrane. The cells have prominent rough endoplasmic reticulum, spherical Golgi complexes, and perinuclear intermediate filaments. Secretory granules are numerous and range in size from 150 to 450 nm.

Sparsely Granulated Corticotroph Adenomas

These tumors are composed of chromophobic cells. They have negative or focal positivity for PAS. There is weak staining for ACTH and β-endorphins. Immunoreactivity for low molecular weight cytokeratins is identified. The secretory granules are scant and there are less well developed organelles.

Crooke's Cell Adenoma

In general, Crooke's hyaline, which is seen in normal corticotrophs in response to glucocorticoid excess, is rarely seen in adenomas (**Fig. 8.3**). These adenomas are usually associated with Cushing's syndrome, with nonfunctioning tumors being uncommon.[23] Marked cytologic and nuclear atypia can be seen. A study of 36 Crooke's cell adenomas suggests that these adenomas are more aggressive than the typical corticotroph adenomas.[24] The tumor cells show peripheral positivity with PAS staining, which represents ACTH in secretory granules at the cell periphery or in the perinuclear region.

Functioning Gonadotroph Adenomas

These are pituitary adenomas derived from the gonadotroph cells and produce FSH or LH.

Pathology

They are usually large macroadenomas and may show areas of hemorrhage and necrosis.

They are composed of chromophobic cells arranged in trabecular, papillary, and sinusoidal pattern (**Fig. 8.4**). Oncocytic change is common, and characteristic vascular pseudorosettes can be seen.[3] Focal PAS positivity is seen with variable reactivity for α-subunit, β-FSH, and β-LH. The tumor cells show strong nuclear staining for SF-1. There is variable ultrastructural morphology, with well-differentiated cells showing polarity of secretory granules, and the nucleus and poorly differentiated cells lacking polarity. Polar cells have well-developed rough endoplasmic reticulum composed of short dilated profiles with flocculent material and globular perinuclear Golgi bodies. Small secretory granules measuring up to 250 nm are distributed along the cell membrane. Nonpolar cells have variably developed rough endoplasmic reticulum and Golgi complexes.

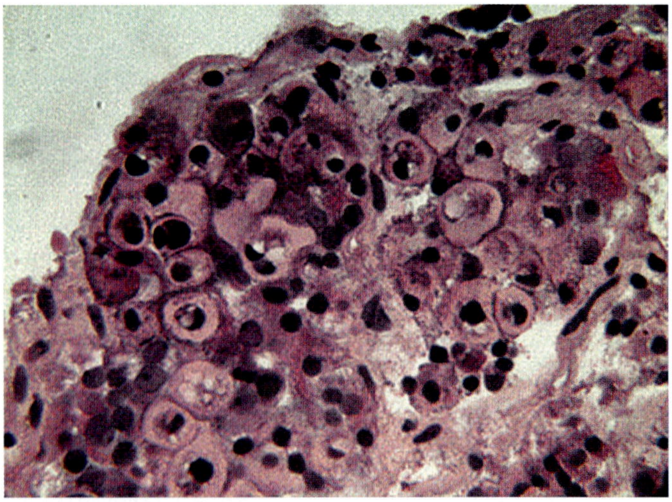

Fig. 8.3 Crooke's hyalinization in cells from a corticotroph pituitary adenoma (×400).

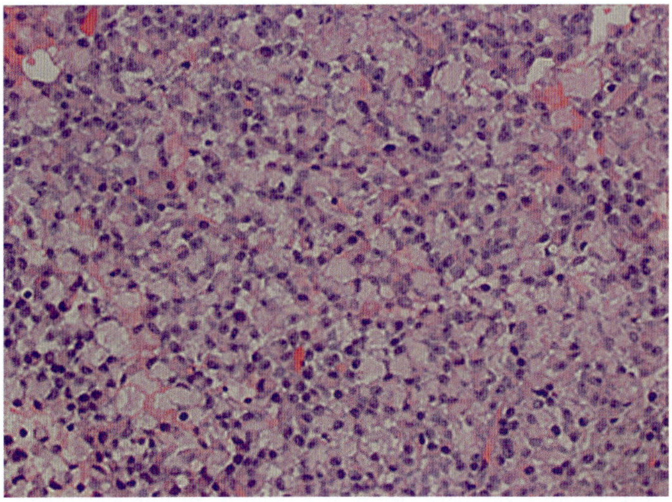

Fig. 8.4 Chromophobe, sheet-like architecture, gonadotroph pituitary adenoma (×200).

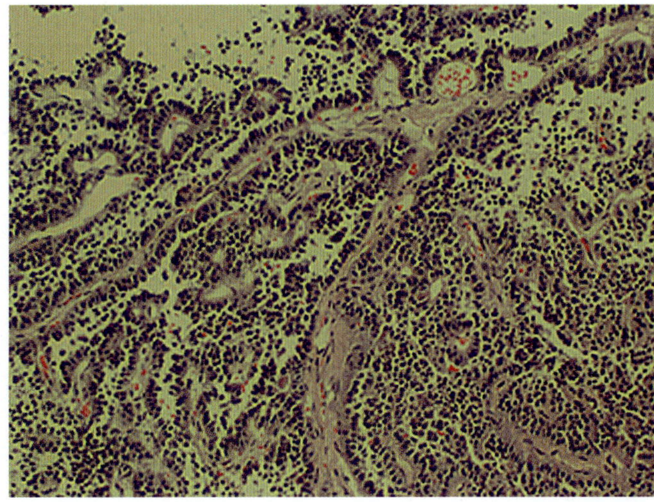

Fig. 8.5 Nonfunctional, chromophobe pituitary adenoma with papillary architecture (×200).

Clinically Nonfunctioning Pituitary Adenomas

Nonfunctioning tumors account for approximately 30% of adenomas (**Figs. 8.5** and **8.6**). These tumors have no evidence of hormonal secretion. The majority of nonfunctioning pituitary adenomas are identified as silent gonadotroph adenomas.[25]

Although increased levels of LH or FSH are not identified, frequently uncombined subunits (free α-subunit, free LH β-subunit) can be detected.[26] The identification of the transcription factors involved in the cytodifferentiation of adenohypophysis has helped further classify these tumors. Most tumors classified as null cell adenomas represent silent gonadotroph adenomas and stain with SF-1 in the absence of gonadotropin reactivity.

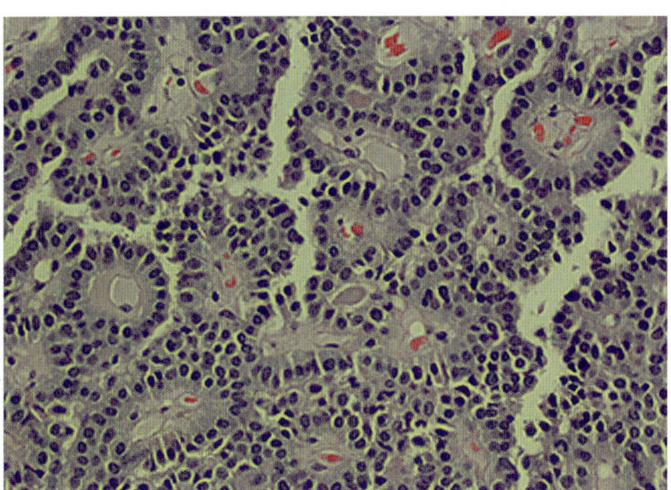

Fig. 8.6 Nonfunctional, chromophobe adenoma with pseudorosette architecture (×200).

Pathology

Silent pituitary adenomas resemble the morphology of their functioning counterparts.[1] Silent somatotroph adenomas resemble sparsely granulated somatotroph adenomas. Two types of silent corticotroph adenomas are described: type 1 resembles the functioning densely granulated corticotroph adenoma, whereas type 2 resembles the sparsely granulated corticotroph adenoma. Most oncocytomas are gonadotroph adenomas with oncocytic change, and they demonstrate SF-1 reactivity.[27]

Poorly differentiated pituitary adenomas represent adenomas that show negative staining for all hormones and other transcription factors and no ultrastructural markers.

Plurihormonal Pituitary Adenomas

Pituitary adenomas can on occasion produce more than one hormone. These tumors are rare. Most commonly these tumors produce a combination of GH and PRL, or of GH, PRL, and TSH. These hormone elaborations can be explained by the expression of Pit-1, which regulates the expression of these hormones.

Pathology

Pituitary adenomas can be divided into monomorphous plurihormonal adenomas, plurimorphous plurihormonal adenomas, and subtype 3 adenomas. Monomorphous adenomas are composed of one cell type, whereas plurimorphous are composed of two or more distinct cell types. The subtype 3 adenomas are composed of spindle cells with fibrous stroma. Ultrastructurally, they show large cells with polarized nuclei and contain spheridia (fragments of nuclear inclusions), prominent tortuous Golgi complex, abundant rough endoplasmic reticulum in continuity with tubular smooth endoplasmic reticulum, and sparse small secretory granules in cell processes.

Pituitary Carcinoma

Pituitary carcinoma is by definition a tumor that has cerebrospinal or systemic metastasis. Although pituitary adenomas may exhibit an invasive growth pattern with extension into neighboring structures, this criterion is not used for malignancy.

Clinical Features

The etiology of these lesions is unknown. Many carcinomas seem to arise in the setting of multiple recurrences of a pituitary adenoma or irradiated invasive adenomas with progression of cytologic atypia and mitotic activity.[28] Less commonly, the pituitary carcinoma is present from the onset. The prognosis is poor, with a high mortality rate.

Radiographic studies are employed to confirm the presence of metastases. Systemic metastasis is more common than craniospinal metastasis.[28] Systemic metastasis to lung, liver, lymph nodes, and bone occurs through hematogenous dissemination. Occasional cervical lymph node involvement is thought to be secondary to invasion of the skull base and soft tissues because the pituitary lacks lymphatic drainage. Metastases in the brain can be indistinguishable from secondary metastasis.[3]

Pathology

Most of these tumors are large, rapidly growing invasive lesions with extension into adjacent structures of the sellar region (dura, bone, cavernous sinus, cranial nerves).

The histopathology of pituitary carcinomas does not differ from that of pituitary adenomas. There are no histologic features that are diagnostic of carcinoma. Cellular pleomorphism, mitotic activity, necrosis, and invasion are not reliable distinguishing features and may be seen in varying degrees in pituitary adenomas. Immunohistochemical stains for synaptophysin and chromogranin are positive. Immunoreactivity for PRL and ACTH is most commonly seen in these tumors.

Various immunohistochemical studies have been performed to try to distinguish pituitary adenomas from carcinomas. Proliferation marker K_i-67 and PCNA have been studied as a potential markers for the prediction of tumor behavior; however, significant overlap exists among adenomas, invasive adenomas, and carcinomas.[29] Several other markers have been immunohistochemically evaluated including topoisomerase IIα,[10] epidermal growth factor,[30] p53,[31] p27,[32] and vascular endothelial growth factor.[33] Microvessel density is increased in carcinomas versus adenomas.[34] However, no reliable markers are available to distinguish benign from malignant.

Other Masses in the Pituitary Region

Although pituitary adenomas comprise the majority of tumors arising in and around the sellar region, other tumors are known to arise in this area and may be considered in the differential diagnosis (**Table 8.1**). Many simulate clinically and radiologically nonsecretory pituitary adenomas.

Primary Tumors of the Sella Turcica

Spindle Cell Oncocytoma

A newly recognized entity was recently included in the 2007 World Health Organization (WHO) classification of brain tumors. This is a mass originating in the adenohypophysis and composed of nests of spindle interlacing fascicles and epithelioid cells with granular eosinophilic cytoplasm. Immunohistochemically the tumor is S-100, epithelial membrane antigen (EMA), and antimitochondrial antibody 113–1 positive but negative for glial fibrillary acidic protein (GFAP), synaptophysin, cytokeratin (CK) pituitary hormones, and smooth muscle markers. The tumor is believed to be derived from the folliculo-stellate cells of the anterior hypophysis.

Pituicytoma

A pituicytoma is a rare, circumscribed mass originating from pituicytes (glial cells) in the posterior hypophysis (neurohypophysis). The tumor is composed of spindle cells arranged in interlacing fascicles in a fibrillary background. The main differential diagnosis of this tumor is pilocytic astrocytoma (there are no Rosenthal fibers or eosinophilic granular bodies in a pituicytoma) and normal posterior pituitary (the distinction can be difficult). The tumor is immunohistochemically positive for S-100 and GFAP (from faint to strong).

Craniopharyngiomas

Craniopharyngiomas are unique neoplasms of the sellar that arise from remnants of Rathke's pouch and represent 1 to 3% of all intracranial neoplasms.[35]

Although pituitary adenomas constitute the majority of sellar tumors in adults, craniopharyngiomas account for the majority of pediatric sellar tumors, with the peak incidence at 5 to 20 years of age.

Pathology

These tumors are predominantly suprasellar in location. Grossly, they are composed of solid and cystic components. The majority of tumors will have calcifications and they usually contain a thick oil-like substance. Malignant change is rare in craniopharyngiomas.[36] These tumors are composed of epithelial-lined cysts with cholesterol clefts and keratinous debris.[1] There are two defined histologic types: adamantinomatous and papillary. The more common adamantinomatous variant resembles an ameloblastoma and has a stellate appearance. The papillary variant shows pseudopapillary squamous islands without palisading.

Germ Cell Tumors

Germ cell tumors are rare tumors arising in the sellar region from residual germ cells present along the midline. Although accounting for less than 1% of all adult intracranial tumors, they represent up to 11.2%[37] of intracranial tumors in children. Germ cell tumors include germinomas, teratomas, embryonal carcinomas, endodermal sinus tumors, and choriocarcinomas. Germinomas, teratomas, and mixed germ cell tumors are the most common tumors.[1]

Gangliocytomas

These are extremely rare tumors that occur most commonly in children and young adults. They are often associated with a pituitary adenoma. Many show evidence of hormone secretion, with the most common syndromes being acromegaly/gigantism and precocious puberty.[38]

Gangliocytomas are composed of neuronal cells in neuropil background. Ganglion cells can be bi- or multinucleated with prominent nucleoli and basophilic Nissl bodies. Ganglion cells may be seen interspersed in a pituitary adenoma, or two distinct components may be identified. Immunohistochemically, the ganglion cells stain with chromogranin, synaptophysin, and neurofilaments. Expression of hypothalamic and pituitary hormones may be seen in the ganglion cells.

Gliomas

Gliomas of the sellar region are rare and include astrocytomas, oligodendrogliomas, and ependymomas.[1] They may arise after radiation therapy for pituitary adenomas, and in this setting are aggressive and rapidly lethal.[39]

Granular Cell Tumors

Granular cell tumors are tumors composed of polygonal cells with abundant granular eosinophilic cytoplasm. More common locations for this tumor include the tongue, skin, breast, and gastrointestinal tract. Less commonly, the tumor can arise in the neurohypophysis or infundibulum.

Pathology

These tumors are usually well-circumscribed unencapsulated nodular lesions with eosinophilic granular cytoplasm. The cells stain with PAS and are diastase resistant. These tumors can be S-100 negative.[40] They are considered benign tumors, although there have been rare reports of atypical or malignant granular cell tumors.[41]

Chordomas

Chordomas are rare lesions of the sella turcica. Most of these tumors occur in the parasellar or suprasellar region. They more commonly occur in the sacral region or clivus, where they can present with intracranial hypertension, pain, and oculomotor findings.[1] Hypopituitarism may be seen.[3] Chordomas are believed to arise from remnants of the notochord.[1] Although slow growing, they can be locally aggressive. A rare presentation of a chordoma with high PRL levels mimicking a prolactinoma has been reported.[42]

Chordomas are composed of characteristic physaliphorous cells. These are large polygonal cells with bubbly cytoplasm secondary to vacuoles containing neutral mucin and glycogen. The tumor cells are arranged in nests or trabeculae that lie in an abundant myxoid and mucinous matrix. In addition to physaliphorous cells, smaller stellate cells can be identified. The tumor cells stain with EMA, S-100, vimentin, and keratins.[3] The extracellular matrix stains weakly with PAS and strongly with Alcian blue.

Schwannoma

Schwannomas are exceedingly rare, with only a handful of cases reported. They can clinically and radiographically mimic pituitary adenomas.[43]

Histologically, they resemble schwannomas in other locations. The tumor is composed of spindle cells arranged in Antoni type A (compact) or Antoni type B (loose) areas. Verocay bodies and thick-walled vessels may be seen. These tumors show strong positive staining for S-100. On electron microscopy, characteristic long-spacing collagen (Luce bodies) and prominent basal lamina are identified.

Meningioma

Meningiomas are tumors that arise from the arachnoid layer of the meninges. Meningiomas occurring in this region account for approximately 20% of all meningiomas. They are more common in women than in men.[44] These tumors are usually located in the parasellar or suprasellar region, with true intrasellar lesions being rare. Meningiomas may arise after radiation therapy for pituitary adenomas.[45]

There are several variants of meningiomas, with the meningothelial, fibroblastic, and transitional variants the most common in this area.

Meningiomas stain with vimentin, EMA, and variably with S-100. Progesterone receptor staining is seen in the majority of meningiomas and less frequently estrogen.

Hematologic Tumors

The hypophysis and hypothalamus are usually secondarily involved by systemic hematologic malignancies (lymphomas, leukemias, plasmacytomas). Primary hematologic malignancies of this region are rare.[46,47]

The majority of these tumors are non-Hodgkin's lymphomas of the B-cell type, with T-cell lymphomas and natural killer (NK)/T-cell lymphomas less common.[47]

These tumors histologically resemble their systemic counterparts, and there is often subcapsular infiltration rather than intraparenchymal involvement.[1]

Langerhans' Cell Histiocytosis

This is a disorder of the histiocyte-like Langerhans' cell. It can be divided into three clinical entities: Letterer-Siwe disease, eosinophilic granuloma, and Hand-Schüller-Christian disease.

Pathology

Histologically, the Langerhans' cells are epithelioid histiocytic cells with abundant eosinophilic cytoplasm and characteristic kidney bean–shaped or indented nuclei. The background usually consists of a mixed inflammatory infiltrate of lymphocytes, eosinophils, and plasma cells. The Langerhans' cells are positive for S-100 and CD1a. Ultrastructurally, characteristic Birbeck granules can be identified.

Mesenchymal Tumors

These tumors arise from fat, cartilage, bone, connective tissue, and vessels. Lesions involving the sella turcica are rare and usually result after radiation therapy for other tumors.[48] Reported tumors have included hemangioblastoma,[49] sclerosing epithelioid fibrosarcoma,[50] chondrosarcoma,[51] fibrosarcoma,[52] leiomyoma,[53] hemangioma, glomangioma, lipoma, chondroma, giant cell tumor, and alveolar soft part sarcoma.[1]

Metastatic Tumors

Symptomatic metastases to the pituitary are relatively uncommon (3.6% of cases autopsy). Most of these are found incidentally at autopsy. Many may mimic nonfunctioning adenomas clinically and radiographically. The most common reported metastases seen are breast and lung. Less frequently reported metastases have included hepatocellular carcinoma, adenocarcinoma of the uterine cervix, pancreatic and ileal neuroendocrine tumors, adenocarcinoma of the colon, nasopharyngeal carcinomas, renal cell carcinoma, and small-cell lung carcinoma.[54–60] Pituitary apoplexy can be a rare presenting symptom.[61] Metastasis is more commonly found in the posterior pituitary rather than in the anterior pituitary, and this is a reflection of the difference in blood supply to the posterior pituitary, which receives blood directly from the carotid artery.[3] Metastases to pituitary adenomas have been reported.[62,63]

Pathology

The histology reflects the tumor of origin, and generally histology alone is sufficient in identifying the tumor. Immunohistochemical and ultrastructural studies may prove helpful in cases where the origin of the tumor is not obvious.

"Tumor-Like" Mass Lesions of the Sellar Region

Nonneoplastic condition can produce sellar masses and mimic neoplastic conditions. The recognition of these entities is extremely important for instituting the correct surgical and medical management. Inflammatory conditions exist in the sellar region; among them, the most notable is lymphocytic hypophysitis. This is considered an autoimmune condition, mostly in young women, and it can be associated with pregnancy. The condition can cause a significant enlargement of the pituitary and is often associated with elevation of PRL because of stalk compression, thus mimicking a prolactinoma. The pituitary is replaced by a sea of lymphocytes, plasma cells, eosinophils, and macrophages, destroying the architecture of the gland.

Other inflammatory conditions include granulomatous conditions such as sarcoidosis and giant cell granuloma.

Cystic lesions in the sellar region include a variety of cysts: Rathke's cleft cyst originates from Rathke's pouch and is most often composed of a uniloculated cyst with thin walls and watery to mucoid content. The lining is usually a monolayer of cuboidal to columnar cells, often ciliated. There is a debate about the relationship between this entity and craniopharyngioma, especially because some of the Rathke's cleft cysts are entirely suprasellar and some of them undergo squamous metaplasia and resemble craniopharyngioma. Other cysts include arachnoid cysts, epidermoid cysts, dermoid cysts, teratomas, and mucoceles.

References

1. Asa SL. Tumors of the Pituitary Gland, 3rd ed. Washington, DC: Armed Forces Institute of Pathology; 1998
2. Al-Shraim M, Asa SL. The 2004 World Health Organization classification of pituitary tumors: what is new? Acta Neuropathol 2006;111:1–7
3. DeLellis RA, Lloyd RV, Heitz PU, Eng C. Pathology and Genetics of Tumours of Endocrine Organs. Lyon: IARC Press; 2004
4. Ezzat S, Asa SL, Couldwell WT, et al. The prevalence of pituitary adenomas: a systematic review. Cancer 2004;101:613–619
5. Sanno N, Teramoto A, Osamura RY, et al. Pathology of pituitary tumors. Neurosurg Clin N Am 2003;14:25–39, vi vi
6. Warczyńska A, Zieliński G, Koziarski A, Podgórski JK. [Ectopic pituitary adenoma. Case report and review of literature]. Neurol Neurochir Pol 2002;36:1185–1196
7. Tomita T, Gates E. Pituitary adenomas and granular cell tumors. Incidence, cell type, and location of tumor in 100 pituitary glands at autopsy. Am J Clin Pathol 1999;111:817–825
8. Thapar K, Kovacs K, Scheithauer BW, et al. Proliferative activity and invasiveness among pituitary adenomas and carcinomas: an analysis using the MIB-1 antibody. Neurosurgery 1996;38:99–106, discussion 106–107
9. Suzuki M, Minematsu T, Oyama K, et al. Expression of proliferation markers in human pituitary incidentalomas. Endocr Pathol 2006;17:263–275
10. Vidal S, Kovacs K, Horvath E, et al. Topoisomerase IIalpha expression in pituitary adenomas and carcinomas: relationship to tumor behavior. Mod Pathol 2002;15:1205–1212
11. Wang J, Liu YS. [Expression of MMPPs and TIMP and invasiveness in pituitary adenomas]. Zhong Nan Da Xue Xue Bao Yi Xue Ban 2004;29:647–650
12. Qian ZR, Sano T, Yoshimoto K, et al. Tumor-specific downregulation and methylation of the CDH13 (H-cadherin) and CDH1 (E-cadherin) genes correlate with aggressiveness of human pituitary adenomas. Mod Pathol 2007;20:1269–1277
13. Abbass SA, Asa SL, Ezzat S. Altered expression of fibroblast growth factor receptors in human pituitary adenomas. J Clin Endocrinol Metab 1997;82:1160–1166
14. Oliveira MC, Marroni CP, Pizarro CB, Pereira-Lima JF, Barbosa-Coutinho LM, Ferreira NP. Expression of p53 protein in pituitary adenomas. Braz J Med Biol Res 2002;35:561–565
15. Saeger W. Pituitary tumors: prognostic indicators. Endocrine 2005;28:57–66
16. Asa SL. The pathology of pituitary tumors. Endocrinol Metab Clin North Am 1999;28:13–43, v–vi v–vi
17. Machado AL, Nomikos P, Kiesewetter F, Fahlbusch R, Buchfelder M. DNA-flow cytometry of 207 pituitary adenomas: ploidy, proliferation, and prognosis. J Endocrinol Invest 2005;28:795–801
18. Partington MD, Davis DH, Laws ER Jr, Scheithauer BW. Pituitary adenomas in childhood and adolescence. Results of transsphenoidal surgery. J Neurosurg 1994;80:209–216
19. Mehrazin M. Pituitary tumors in children: clinical analysis of 21 cases. Childs Nerv Syst 2007;23:391–398
20. Artese R, D'Osvaldo DH, Molocznik I, et al. Pituitary tumors in adolescent patients. Neurol Res 1998;20:415–417
21. Kontogeorgos G, Kovacs K, Horvath E, Scheithauer BW. Multiple adenomas of the human pituitary. A retrospective autopsy study with clinical implications. J Neurosurg 1991;74:243–247
22. Asa SL, Ezzat S. The pathogenesis of pituitary tumours. Nat Rev Cancer 2002;2:836–849
23. Roncaroli F, Faustini-Fustini M, Mauri F, Asioli S, Frank G. Crooke's hyalinization in silent corticotroph adenoma: report of two cases. Endocr Pathol 2002;13:245–249
24. George DH, Scheithauer BW, Kovacs K, et al. Crooke's cell adenoma of the pituitary: an aggressive variant of corticotroph adenoma. Am J Surg Pathol 2003;27:1330–1336
25. Croue A, Beldent V, Rousselet MC, et al. Contribution of immunohistochemistry, electron microscopy, and cell culture to the characterization of nonfunctioning pituitary adenomas: a study of 40 cases. Hum Pathol 1992;23:1332–1339
26. Chanson P, Brochier S. Non-functioning pituitary adenomas. J Endocrinol Invest 2005;28(11, Suppl International):93–99
27. Yamada S, Asa SL, Kovacs K. Oncocytomas and null cell adenomas of the human pituitary: morphometric and in vitro functional comparison. Virchows Arch A Pathol Anat Histopathol 1988;413:333–339
28. Pernicone PJ, Scheithauer BW, Sebo TJ, et al. Pituitary carcinoma: a clinicopathologic study of 15 cases. Cancer 1997;79:804–812
29. Turner HE, Wass JA. Are markers of proliferation valuable in the histological assessment of pituitary tumours? Pituitary 1999;1:147–151
30. Onguru O, Scheithauer BW, Kovacs K, et al. Analysis of epidermal growth factor receptor and activated epidermal growth factor receptor expression in pituitary adenomas and carcinomas. Mod Pathol 2004;17:772–780
31. Thapar K, Scheithauer BW, Kovacs K, Pernicone PJ, Laws ER Jr. p53 expression in pituitary adenomas and carcinomas: correlation with invasiveness and tumor growth fractions. Neurosurgery 1996;38:765–770, discussion 770–771
32. Lidhar K, Korbonits M, Jordan S, et al. Low expression of the cell cycle inhibitor p27Kip1 in normal corticotroph cells, corticotroph tumors, and malignant pituitary tumors. J Clin Endocrinol Metab 1999;84:3823–3830
33. Lloyd RV, Scheithauer BW, Kuroki T, Vidal S, Kovacs K, Stefaneanu L. Vascular endothelial growth factor (VEGF) expression in human pituitary adenomas and carcinomas. Endocr Pathol 1999;10:229–235
34. Vidal S, Kovacs K, Horvath E, Scheithauer BW, Kuroki T, Lloyd RV. Microvessel density in pituitary adenomas and carcinomas. Virchows Arch 2001;438:595–602
35. Alvarez M. Craniopharyngiomas. J Neurosci Nurs 2006;38:362–368
36. Kristopaitis T, Thomas C, Petruzzelli GJ, Lee JM. Malignant craniopharyngioma. Arch Pathol Lab Med 2000;124:1356–1360
37. Cho KT, Wang KC, Kim SK, Shin SH, Chi JG, Cho BK. Pediatric brain tumors: statistics of SNUH, Korea (1959–2000). Childs Nerv Syst 2002;18:30–37
38. Puchner MJ, Lüdecke DK, Saeger W, Riedel M, Asa SL. Gangliocytomas of the sellar region—a review. Exp Clin Endocrinol Diabetes 1995;103:129–149

39. Tsang RW, Laperriere NJ, Simpson WJ, Brierley J, Panzarella T, Smyth HS. Glioma arising after radiation therapy for pituitary adenoma. A report of four patients and estimation of risk. Cancer 1993;72:2227–2233
40. Vang R, Heck K, Fuller GN, Medeiros LJ. Granular cell tumor of intracranial meninges. Clin Neuropathol 2000;19:41–44
41. Kasashima S, Oda Y, Nozaki J, Shirasaki M, Nakanishi I. A case of atypical granular cell tumor of the neurohypophysis. Pathol Int 2000;50:568–573
42. Haridas A, Ansari S, Afshar F. Chordoma presenting as pseudoprolactinoma. Br J Neurosurg 2003;17:260–262
43. Whee SM, Lee JI, Kim JH. Intrasellar schwannoma mimicking pituitary adenoma: a case report. J Korean Med Sci 2002;17:147–150
44. LiVolsi VA. Endocrine Pathology. Philadelphia: Churchill Livingstone; 2002
45. Tsukamoto H, Yoshinari M, Okamura K, Ishitsuka T, Fujishima M. Meningioma developed 25 years after radiation therapy for Cushing's disease. Intern Med 1992;31:629–632
46. Quintero Wolfe S, Hood B, Barker J, Benveniste RJ. Primary central nervous system lymphoma mimicking pituitary apoplexy: case report. Pituitary 2009;12:76–79
47. Liu JK, Sayama C, Chin SS, Couldwell WT. Extranodal NK/T-cell lymphoma presenting as a pituitary mass. Case report and review of the literature. J Neurosurg 2007;107:660–665
48. Gnanalingham KK, Chakraborty A, Galloway M, Revesz T, Powell M. Osteosarcoma and fibrosarcoma caused by postoperative radiotherapy for a pituitary adenoma. Case report. J Neurosurg 2002;96:960–963
49. Goto T, Nishi T, Kunitoku N, et al. Suprasellar hemangioblastoma in a patient with von Hippel-Lindau disease confirmed by germline mutation study: case report and review of the literature. Surg Neurol 2001;56:22–26
50. Massier A, Scheithauer BW, Taylor HC, Clark C, Llerena L. Sclerosing epithelioid fibrosarcoma of the pituitary. Endocr Pathol 2007;18:233–238
51. Allan CA, Kaltsas G, Evanson J, et al. Pituitary chondrosarcoma: an unusual cause of a sellar mass presenting as a pituitary adenoma. J Clin Endocrinol Metab 2001;86:386–391
52. Lopes MB, Lanzino G, Cloft HJ, Winston DC, Vance ML, Laws ER Jr. Primary fibrosarcoma of the sella unrelated to previous radiation therapy. Mod Pathol 1998;11:579–584
53. Kleinschmidt-DeMasters BK, Mierau GW, Sze CI, et al. Unusual dural and skull-based mesenchymal neoplasms: a report of four cases. Hum Pathol 1998;29:240–245
54. Harzallah L, Migaw H, Harzallah F, Kraiem Ch. Diabetes insipidus and panhypopituitarism revealing pituitary metastasis of small cell lung carcinoma: a case report. Ann Endocrinol (Paris) 2005;66(2 Pt 1):117–120
55. Gunn GB, Villa RD, Sedler RR, Hardwicke F, Fornari GA, Mark RJ. Nasopharyngeal carcinoma metastasis to the pituitary gland: a case report and literature review. J Neurooncol 2004;68:87–90
56. Karamouzis MV, Melachrinou M, Fratzoglou M, Labropoulou-Karatza Ch, Kalofonos HP. Hepatocellular carcinoma metastasis in the pituitary gland: case report and review of the literature. J Neurooncol 2003;63:173–177
57. Salpietro FM, Romano A, Alafaci C, Tomasello F. Pituitary metastasis from uterine cervical carcinoma: a case presenting as diabetes insipidus. Br J Neurosurg 2000;14:156–159
58. Gur C, Lalazar G, Salmon A, Dubiner V, Gross DJ. Metastatic pancreatic neuroendocrine tumor presenting as a pituitary space occupying lesion: a case report. Pituitary 2008;11:293–297
59. Goglia U, Ferone D, Sidoti M, et al. Treatment of a pituitary metastasis from a neuroendocrine tumour: case report and literature review. Pituitary 2008;11:93–102
60. Tomita H, Urui S, Kokunai T, Tamaki N. [A case of metastatic tumor of the pituitary gland presenting as a subarachnoid hemorrhage]. No Shinkei Geka 2000;28:1117–1120
61. Hanna FW, Williams OM, Davies JS, Dawson T, Neal J, Scanlon MF. Pituitary apoplexy following metastasis of bronchogenic adenocarcinoma to a prolactinoma. Clin Endocrinol (Oxf) 1999;51:377–381
62. Molinatti PA, Scheithauer BW, Randall RV, Laws ER Jr. Metastasis to pituitary adenoma. Arch Pathol Lab Med 1985;109:287–289
63. Ramsay JA, Kovacs K, Scheithauer BW, Ezrin C, Weiss MH. Metastatic carcinoma to pituitary adenomas: a report of two cases. Exp Clin Endocrinol 1988;92:69–76

9 Prolactinomas and Apoplexy

Jeroen R. Coppens and William T. Couldwell

Prolactin-secreting adenomas (prolactinomas) are the most common form of secreting pituitary tumors. Among pituitary tumors, they are second in frequency only to nonfunctioning adenomas. They account for 30% of all pituitary adenomas and 50 to 60% of functional pituitary tumors. Although it has been estimated that there are 100 cases per 1 million people, the authors of more recent studies describe that number as an underestimate of the true prevalence.[1] Autopsy and radiologic studies indicate an overall prevalence of pituitary microadenomas from 10 to 25%, although most of these are thought to be insignificant.[2]

Prolactinomas present most commonly as microadenomas (<10 mm) causing a prolonged state of hyperprolactinemia. Macroadenomas (≥10 mm) also cause local mass effect on the rest of the gland as well as the adjacent structures. Prolactinomas can also be a manifestation of multiple endocrine neoplasia (MEN) type 1 syndrome or be familial.[1]

The need for surgical treatment of prolactinomas sharply declined after the U.S. Food and Drug Administration approval of bromocriptine in 1978. Medical treatment with dopamine agonists (D2 agonists) has become the mainstay for treatment of most prolactinomas, with a goal of normalizing prolactin levels as well as tumor shrinkage. Thus, the indications for treating prolactinomas surgically are evolving; these indications as well as the different surgical options available are discussed in this chapter.

Table 9.1 Clinical Manifestations of Prolactinomas

Hyperprolactinemia
Amenorrhea (female patients)
Galactorrhea
Infertility
Decreased libido
Impotence (male patients)
Osteoporosis
Delayed puberty (adolescents)
Mass effect
Headaches
Visual acuity and field impairment
Cranial nerve palsies
Hypothalamic dysfunction
Hydrocephalus
Hypopituitarism
Pituitary apoplexy

Clinical Manifestations of Prolactinomas

Patients with prolactinomas can present with the clinical sequelae of hyperprolactinemia, endocrine dysfunction, local mass effect, or pituitary apoplexy (**Table 9.1**). Despite an equal distribution of prolactinomas among men and women, women are four times more likely than men to be symptomatic. Women usually present earlier in the course of the disease, with smaller tumors at the time of diagnosis. Men's loss of libido and impotence in cases of hyperprolactinemia are more commonly missed.

Patients with prolonged hyperprolactinemic states usually seek medical attention because of the effect of the hyperprolactinemia on the gonadal function and breast tissue, with a classic presentation of amenorrhea and galactorrhea in women and loss of libido in men. Prolactin inhibits the production of gonadotropin-releasing hormone at the level of the hypothalamus, resulting in hypogonadism and infertility. Children and postmenopausal women do not develop clinical symptoms of hypogonadism. Adolescents can present with delay or failure of sexual and reproductive development. Premenopausal women usually present with galactorrhea, amenorrhea, and infertility when their use of oral contraceptive regimen has been discontinued. Approximately 5% of women with primary amenorrhea and 25% of women with secondary amenorrhea (excluding pregnancy) have a prolactinoma.[3] When galactorrhea accompanies amenorrhea, the incidence of a prolactinoma is as high as 80%.

Untreated hyperprolactinemia also leads to premature osteoporosis in both sexes secondary to the estrogen and testosterone deficiency. The osteopenia is progressive and correlates with the duration of hypogonadism. Normalization of prolactin levels halts further bone loss, and some increase of bone density is seen, but normalization to baseline values is not the norm.

Prolactinomas can also present with symptoms due to local mass effect on local structures, such as headaches, visual compromise, cranial nerve palsies, hypopituitarism, and hydrocephalus. Suprasellar extension of the tumor to the visual apparatus most commonly results in a homonymous bitemporal hemianopsia, and cranial nerve palsies occur from lateral extension into the cavernous sinus.

Pituitary apoplexy (acute hemorrhage into or infarction of the pituitary adenoma) can present with acute signs of hypopituitarism and compression of the sellar and suprasellar structures. Patients present with a sudden onset of headache, nausea, vomiting, diplopia, visual loss, or a decreased level of consciousness.[4] Signs of meningeal irritation can also be observed in cases in which the hemorrhage extends into the subarachnoid space. Pituitary apoplexy can occur in patients with a known prolactinoma or can be the cause of initial presentation of the patient.

Differential Diagnosis of the Hyperprolactinemic State

Before offering treatment to patients with hypogonadic dysfunction due to a hyperprolactinemic state, it is imperative to correctly differentiate patients who harbor a prolactinoma. The cause of hyperprolactinemia can be physiologic, pharmacologic, or pathologic (**Table 9.2**). A thyroid-stimulating hormone (TSH) level should always be measured simultaneously with a prolactin level because of the stimulatory effect of TSH on prolactin release by the pituitary gland. Lactotroph cells that secrete prolactin are stimulated by estrogen and inhibited by dopamine. Prolactin levels below 25 ng/mL in women and 20 ng/mL in men are within the normal range.

Physiologic hyperprolactinemia occurs in a variety of physical and psychological stress states, but the prolactin level rarely exceeds 40 ng/mL. It is imperative to rule out pregnancy as a cause because the prolactin level increases during the first and second trimester and peaks in the third trimester above several hundred nanograms per milliliter. Prolactin levels rapidly decrease in the postpartum period in women who do not breast-feed. In women who breast-feed, prolactin levels decrease after a few weeks despite surges after suckling. Within a few months, prolactin levels return to normal even if breast-feeding is continued.

Macroprolactin can be responsible for hyperprolactinemia in up to 20% of cases.[5] Macroprolactin, a complex of prolactin and immunoglobulins, has a longer half-life than free prolactin and may cause an increase of the total level of prolactin in the blood.[5] It is generally thought that macroprolactin does not have any biologic effect, and several laboratory tests can be used to differentiate macroprolactin from free prolactin levels.

Medications are a common cause of hyperprolactinemia, which can be seen with any agent that antagonizes dopamine receptors on lactotroph cells in the pituitary gland. Antidepressant therapies, antihypertensive drugs, and estrogen can induce hyperprolactinemia, resulting in prolactin levels in the range of 25 to 100 ng/mL. The hyperprolactinemia usually resolves in a few days to weeks after cessation of the offending medication.[6]

Primary hypothyroidism causes hyperprolactinemia in 20 to 30% of patients because of the effects of an increased

Table 9.2 Causes of Hyperprolactinemia

Physiologic
Pregnancy
Breast-feeding (suckling reflex)
Stress
Exercise
Pharmacologic
Neuroleptic medication (phenothiazines, haloperidol)
Atypical antipsychotic medications (clozapine, risperidone)
Antidepressant medication (tricyclics, monoamine oxidase inhibitors, selective serotonin reuptake inhibitors)
Antihypertensive medication (α-methyldopa, reserpine, verapamil)
Metoclopramide
H-2 blockers
Sellar/parasellar lesions
Prolactinomas
Pituitary adenomas with stalk effect
Germinomas
Craniopharyngiomas
Meningiomas
Primary empty sella syndrome
Lymphocytic hypophysitis
Histiocytosis X
Sarcoidosis
Metastasis
Other
Primary hypothyroidism
Hypothalamic dysfunction
Chronic renal failure
Liver failure
Ectopic secretion of prolactin
Seizures
Macroprolactin

thyrotropin-releasing hormone. Thyrotroph hypertrophy as well as pituitary hyperplasia may ensue and in rare cases may cause visual field defects. Correction of primary hypothyroidism leads to normalization of prolactin levels within a few months. Chronic renal failure also results in hyperprolactinemia because of a decreased renal clearance of serum prolactin.

Any mass in the sellar and suprasellar region can interrupt the dopaminergic inhibition of the lactotrophs and result in a state of hyperprolactinemia from "stalk effect." The stalk effect rarely induces prolactin levels above 150 ng/mL, although rare cases of significant elevation have been reported.[3] In some cases of acromegaly, prolactin can be co-secreted with growth hormone, and some rare cases of Cushing's disease have also been described with co-secretion of prolactin.

Most cases of hyperprolactinemia that are not related to the presence of a prolactinoma can be ruled out based on the patient's history and physical examination. In case of doubt, magnetic resonance imaging (MRI) of the pituitary with and without gadolinium enhancement is used to correlate the level of the hyperprolactinemia with the radiologic findings of an adenoma. Patients with visual loss based on physical and radiologic findings should be evaluated by formal visual field testing. All patients with radiologic signs of a pituitary adenoma should also be evaluated with a pregnancy test (in women of child-bearing age), thyroid and renal function tests, and a full evaluation of other pituitary hormones (growth hormones, insulin-like growth factor-1, fasting morning cortisol, thyroid function tests, adrenocorticotrophic hormone, luteinizing hormone, follicle-stimulating hormone, sex hormones).

Laboratory and Radiologic Correlation of Prolactin Levels

Correlating the degree of hyperprolactinemia with the radiologic findings is important to make a correct diagnosis of a pituitary prolactin-secreting adenoma. Patients with a microprolactinoma typically have prolactin levels in the range of 100 to 250 ng/mL. Patients with a macroprolactinoma typically have levels above 250 ng/mL. In cases in which a lateral extension of the tumor is seen toward the cavernous sinus, the serum prolactin level may attain a level of several thousand nanograms per milliliter. A falsely low prolactin level (25 to 150 ng/mL) is observed in some cases of large prolactin-secreting macroadenomas with very high levels of prolactin that induce a high-dose "hook effect."[7] The hook effect is observed when using radioimmunoassays with a monoclonal sandwich technique where both the capture and signal antibody become saturated. The hook effect can be overcome by performing serial dilutions of the serum samples.

Radiologic Characteristics of Prolactinomas

All patients with a suspected prolactinoma should undergo MRI scanning with and without the use of gadolinium. MRI has replaced the need for any other imaging. Coronal and sagittal views centered on the pituitary gland should be obtained. On T1 sequences obtained immediately after injection of gadolinium, pituitary adenomas including prolactinomas present as hypointense lesions compared with the rest of the normal pituitary tissue. On delayed T1 sequences after gadolinium administration, prolactinomas are hyperintense to the rest of the pituitary gland because of a washout phenomenon (**Fig. 9.1**). Small microprolactinomas may easily be missed if a dynamic study is not performed. Coronal views enable the surgeon to evaluate the anatomy of the sphenoid septa as well as the carotid arteries to ensure a transsphenoidal approach can safely be performed if surgery is contemplated.

Medical Treatment of Prolactinomas

Prolactinomas can be controlled medically with the use of dopamine agonists. These agents bind the lactotrophs on their D2 receptors and inhibit prolactin synthesis and release. Bromocriptine accomplishes tumor shrinkage and control of microprolactinomas in approximately 85% of cases.[8] Bromocriptine dosing is usually started at 1.25 to 2.5 mg per day and is slowly increased to a total dose of 5 to 10 mg per day. The initial treatment is usually started with oral intake of the medication at bedtime to limit side effects of orthostatic hypotension. Side effects are a limiting factor in 5 to 10% of cases and consist of dizziness, nausea, arrhythmias, and gastrointestinal discomfort. Cabergoline can be used as an alternative to bromocriptine because it has fewer side effects and superior efficacy (**Fig. 9.2**).[9] Overall tumor shrinkage and normalization of prolactin levels are superior to those of bromocriptine, but the cost of treatment is higher.[10] Treatment is usually started at 0.5 to 1.5 mg once or twice per week. Similar dose escalation may be necessary when treating large tumors, with subsequent decrease of the dose after tumor shrinkage has been accomplished. Cabergoline is most useful in patients who are resistant to bromocriptine or who cannot tolerate its side effects.[9] After several years of normoprolactinemia under medical treatment, an attempt at weaning the patient from dopamine agonist therapy can be accomplished, with a sustained biochemical cure in up to 38% of cases of microprolactinomas.[11] Normoprolactinemia seems to be more common after cabergoline withdrawal and has been reported in 22 to 59% of cases of microprolactinomas and in 11 to 23% of cases of macroprolactinomas.[10] Prolonged normoprolactinemia is more probable in cases in which the

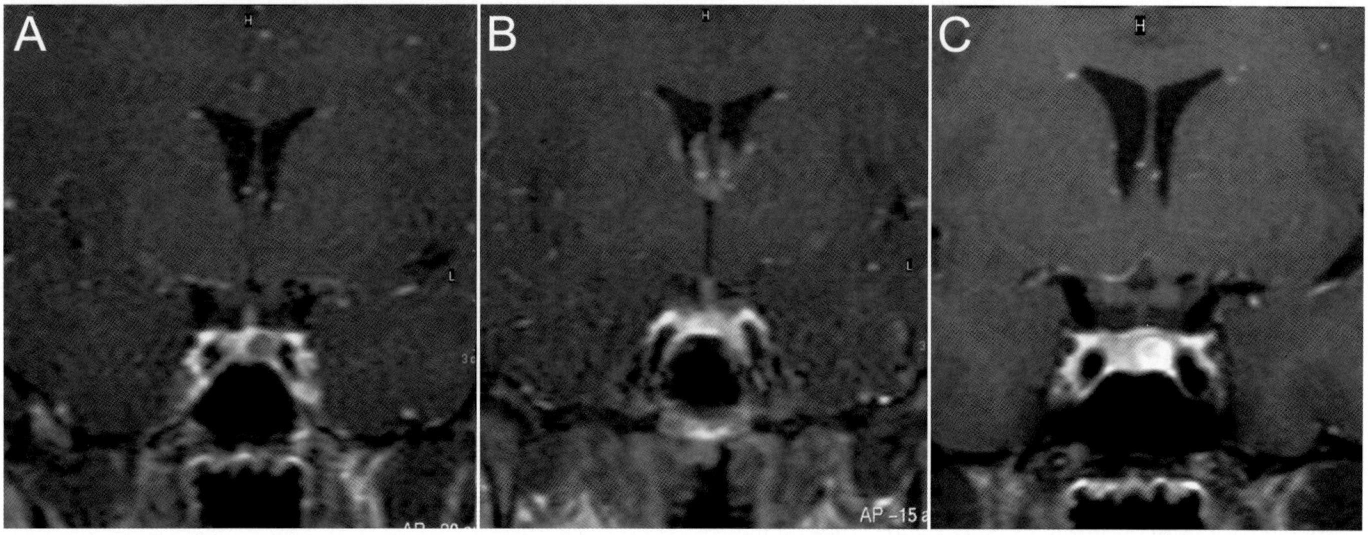

Fig. 9.1 Coronal T1-weighted MRI views of a microprolactinoma during a dynamic study. **(A)** The microprolactinoma is hypointense to the rest of the gland, which has taken up gadolinium. **(B)** The microprolactinoma is becoming isodense to the rest of the pituitary gland as the adenoma takes up gadolinium while the rest of the gland is losing the contrast agent. **(C)** The microprolactinoma is hyperintense to the gland because of delayed retention of gadolinium.

tumor disappeared on imagery during dopamine agonist treatment, in cases of microprolactinomas, and in cases of prolonged normoprolactinemia on medical treatment for at least 1 year before drug withdrawal.[10] Long-term data are not available to determine the durability of normoprolactinemia after dopamine agonist withdrawal. Recurrences of hyperprolactinemia are associated with a radiologically observable rate of tumor growth in 10% of cases of microprolactinomas.[12] Alternatives to bromocriptine and cabergoline have been developed with the use of pergolide, lisuride, and quinagolide, but the experience with these options is very limited in North America.

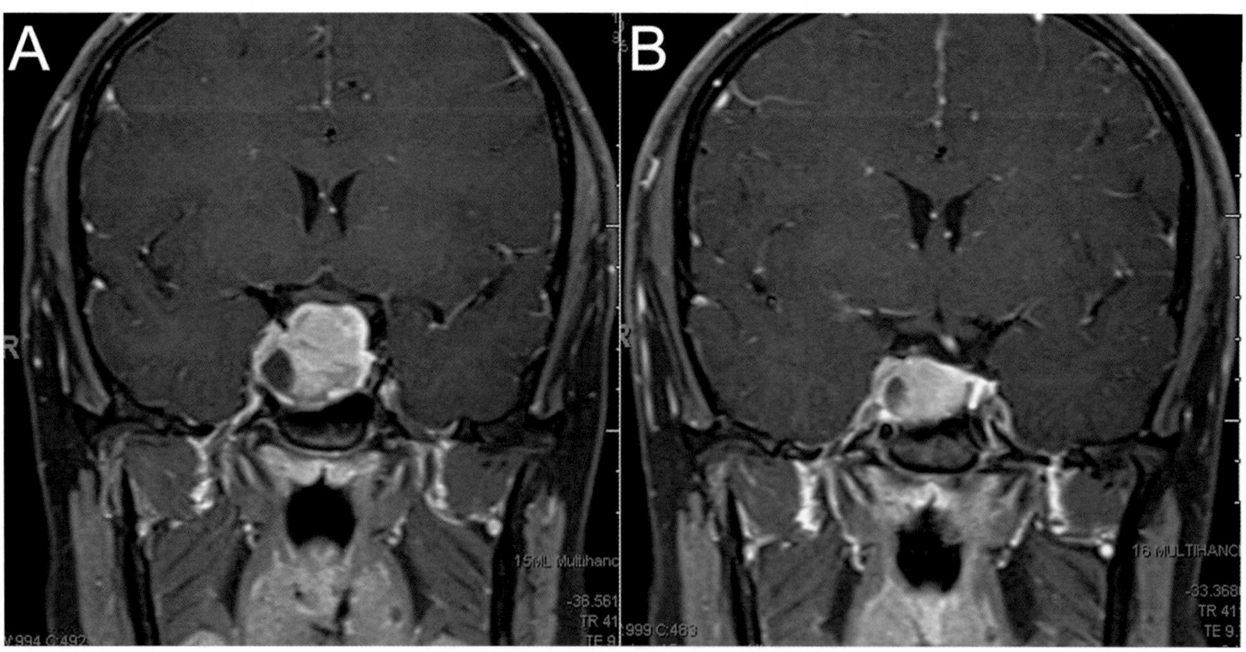

Fig. 9.2 Coronal T1-weighted MRI views with contrast. **(A)** Prolactinoma at time of diagnosis with a prolactin level of 880 ng/mL. **(B)** Treatment with cabergoline results in tumor shrinkage and a prolactin level of 15 after 4 months.

Surgical Indications for the Treatment of Prolactinomas

The surgical indications for the treatment of prolactinomas take into account the need to normalize the serum prolactin levels; to decompress the visual apparatus, cranial nerves, and the rest of the pituitary gland; and to prevent the tumor from progressing or recurring. The surgical strategy used differs depending on whether a surgical cure can be expected or the surgery is adjuvant therapy.

Surgery as a Curative Therapy

In cases of microprolactinomas that are restricted to the pituitary gland, surgery is an option for patients who fail medical treatment by remaining hyperprolactinemic. About 15% of patients undergoing medical treatment do not respond to either bromocriptine or cabergoline, with a significant decrease in prolactin levels by 6 weeks after initiation of medical therapy. Surgery is also warranted for patients who do not tolerate medical therapy because of its side effects or for young patients who do not wish to undergo lengthy (and perhaps lifelong) medical treatment.[13] Lastly, patients undergoing antipsychotic treatment may wish to undergo surgical treatment for their prolactinoma because of the risk of inducing psychotic episodes with medical therapy. Surgery can be offered as a first-line treatment in these patients who harbor a prolactinoma limited to the pituitary gland without cavernous sinus extension because of the high cure rates observed in experienced hands. The surgical goal when dealing with a microprolactinoma is a complete oncologic and endocrinologic cure.

Curative surgery for microprolactinoma is performed through a transsphenoidal route. The preoperative MRI is carefully inspected to visualize the location of the adenoma in relationship to the rest of the gland. A wide exposure of the sella is necessary to inspect the rest of the gland intraoperatively and ensure that no other disease is apparent. The adenoma is removed with great care to prevent spillage of the tumor in the sphenoid sinus or in the rest of the pituitary gland.

In cases of microprolactinomas that are limited to the pituitary gland, surgical cure rates of at least 90% have been reported by experienced surgeons.[14–16] Patients achieve normal levels of prolactin, with return of menstrual cycles in women and fertility in men. A complete cure can be identified by a prolactin level lower than 10 ng/mL on postoperative day 1.[14] Recurrence of hyperprolactinemia can occur up to 5 years after an initial transsphenoidal resection of a prolactinoma and is most likely in patients with a prolactin level greater than 10 ng/mL on postoperative day 1.[14] Recurrence can be detected by monitoring prolactin levels at 6 weeks, 3 months, 6 months, and yearly thereafter. Recurrence of hyperprolactinemia after transsphenoidal surgery is rarely radiologically accompanied by the presence of an adenoma. The best preoperative predictor for a cure after surgical removal of a microprolactinoma through the transsphenoidal approach is a preoperative prolactin level lower than 200 ng/mL.

Fewer than 10% of patients undergoing an adequate transsphenoidal resection of a microprolactinoma fail to achieve a complete cure and require medical therapy in the form of dopamine agonists to normalize their prolactin levels. Lower doses of dopamine agonists are usually necessary because patients are better able to tolerate the side effects.

Surgery as Adjuvant Therapy to Medical Therapy

The surgical treatment in cases of macroprolactinomas accomplishes full normalization of the prolactin levels in less than 50% of cases.[14] Thus, surgery should be contemplated only as an adjuvant therapy that provides cytoreduction to facilitate the effects of medical therapy.[8] Surgery therefore may be indicated in patients in whom normal levels of prolactin cannot be reached despite adequate medical therapy. Surgery is also offered in cases of tumor enlargement during medical therapy or when the side effects of medical therapy become too pronounced at higher doses. Lastly, surgery is warranted in patients who experience worsening of their visual field impairment or cranial nerve palsies that do not respond within a short period of time to high-dose dopamine agonist therapy combined with steroid therapy. Young patients who present with a cystic macroadenoma (**Fig. 9.3**) are one exception in whom surgery can be curative for a macroadenoma.

A transsphenoidal approach is the procedure of choice when resecting macroprolactinomas. The sellar floor is opened widely and posteriorly to the dorsum sellae. Resection of the adenoma with standard pituitary instruments should be started in its inferior aspect. As some tumor is debulked, it is essential to continue the dissection laterally toward the medial wall of the cavernous sinus to increase the chances of a complete resection. The superior aspect of the tumor is addressed last, as it will have a spontaneous tendency to descend in the surgical field. A Valsalva maneuver may be helpful intraoperatively to encourage descent of the tumor. Careful dissection of the tumor is then performed in its superior and anterior aspect, which corresponds to the area with the greatest potential for cerebrospinal fluid (CSF) leak in these cases. In rare cases of giant prolactinomas with involvement of the vascular structures and the sylvian fissure, a complete resection through a transsphenoidal route is not recommended because those structures are best addressed under direct microscopic vision through a subsequent craniotomy. Morbidity associated with adjuvant surgical treatment is similar to that observed in cases of microprolactinomas except for a higher risk of an intraoperative CSF leak.

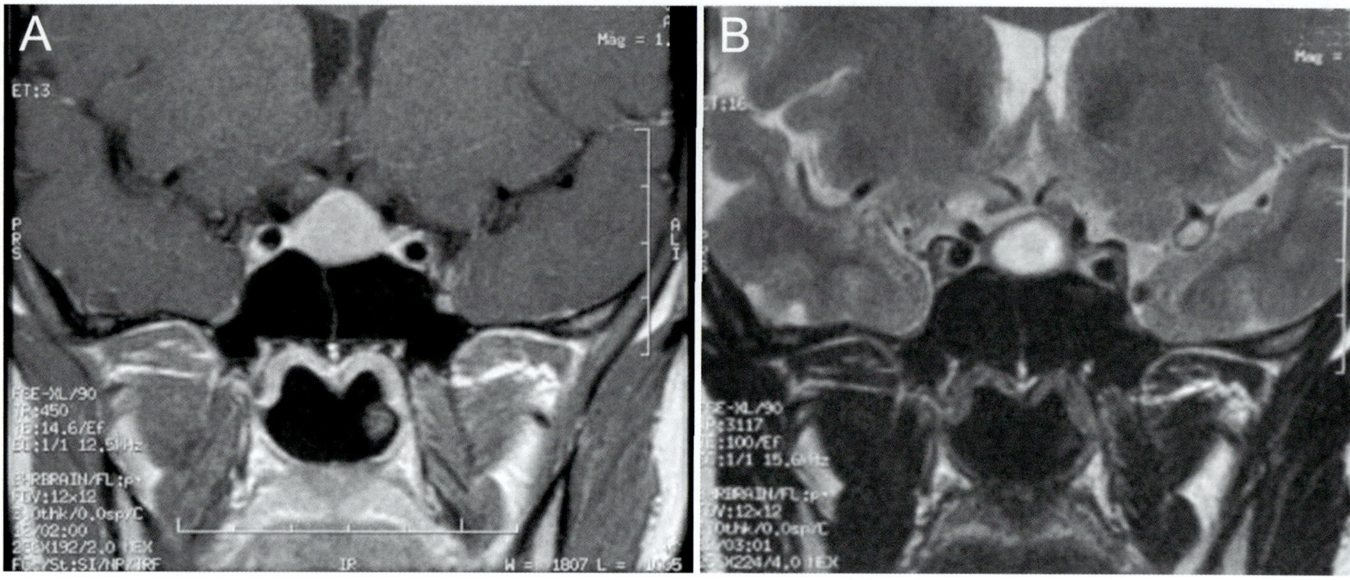

Fig. 9.3 **(A)** Coronal T1-weighted MRI view with gadolinium enhancement. **(B)** T2-weighted view of a macroprolactinoma that has become partially cystic after an episode of apoplexy.

Surgery and Pituitary Apoplexy

Patients with pituitary apoplexy who harbor a prolactinoma may present de novo or after initiation of medical therapy. Surgical considerations in these patients include the need to acutely decompress the visual apparatus and cranial nerves as well as to decompress the rest of the pituitary gland. In patients who present de novo, most surgeons recommend emergency transsphenoidal decompression with the use of glucocorticoid therapy.[17] Some cases have been described with good results with the use of bromocriptine with glucocorticoid administration.[4] In cases in which medical therapy is tried first, we recommend surgical decompression if there is worsening of visual function or if the cranial nerve palsy does not resolve within 48 hours.

In cases of pituitary apoplexy in patients who have a known prolactinoma that is under medical treatment, emergent transsphenoidal decompression with glucocorticoid administration is recommended.

Surgery as Adjuvant Therapy to Radiosurgery

In cases of prolactinomas with invasion of the cavernous sinus that remain refractory to medical therapy, we recommend surgical debulking followed by stereotactic radiosurgery. Secondarily, a hypophysopexy or pituitary transposition with interposition of a fat graft between the pituitary gland and the cavernous sinus is also performed.[18] By this procedure, the distance between the target for radiosurgery and the pituitary gland is increased, which decreases the dose of radiation delivered to the gland to limit the further risk of radiation-induced hypopituitarism.

Symptoms and Management of Pituitary Apoplexy

Pituitary apoplexy occurs when acute hemorrhage or necrosis occurs in the pituitary gland. It is most commonly seen in the setting of an underlying pituitary adenoma.[19] Clinically, apoplexy presents as an acute onset of headache, frequently coupled with nausea, vertigo, meningismus, and decreased level of consciousness. Compression of the optic apparatus and contents within the cavernous sinuses may lead to impairment of visual acuity or fields, ophthalmoplegia, Horner syndrome, facial pain, and hemiparesis. Dysfunction of the rest of the pituitary gland may lead to hypopituitarism and diabetes insipidus. The severity and level of acuity of the symptoms are highly variable, which may complicate the differentiation of apoplexy from other causes of intracranial hemorrhages, migraines, optic neuritis, carotid-cavernous fistulas, cavernous sinus thrombosis, hypertensive encephalopathy, and other causes of ophthalmoplegia.[19]

The symptoms of apoplexy may progress over a few hours to days, and failing to recognize the endocrine disturbance clearly increases the incidence and extent of morbidity.[20] Confirmation of a clinical diagnosis should consist of a full laboratory endocrinologic investigation of pituitary function as well as MRI. A computed tomography scan may miss the presence of hemorrhage in approximately 50% of cases.[21]

Clinically evident apoplexy seems to occur in less than 10% of pituitary adenomas, but subclinical apoplexy may be more prevalent, with some authors reporting an incidence of up to 28% based on histologic specimens.[22] Nearly 50% of cases of apoplexy present in patients who were known to harbor a pituitary adenoma. Men are more often affected than women (2:1 ratio), and most cases present in the fifth and sixth decade.[19] Pituitary tumor apoplexy occurs more commonly in the setting of macroadenomas than in microadenomas without preponderance for tumor type.[19] Predisposing factors are identified in 50% of cases and consist of head trauma, bromocriptine administration or withdrawal, anticoagulation, pregnancy, cardiac bypass, bowel or other surgery, atherosclerosis, diabetic ketoacidosis, estrogen therapy, radiation therapy, hypertension, and hypotension.[19]

Apoplexy can also occur independently of pituitary adenomas. Cases of apoplexy have also been reported in patients with Rathke cleft cysts, in normal pituitary tissue, and in association with empty sella turcicae. A common cause of pituitary apoplexy in developing countries is Sheehan syndrome.[23,24] The pituitary gland undergoes significant hyperplasia without a corresponding increase in the vascular supply through the portal system during pregnancy, increasing its susceptibility to ischemia. A severe episode of hypotension or hemorrhagic shock usually precedes the onset of Sheehan syndrome, but the onset has also been attributed in some cases to vasospasm, thrombosis, or vascular compression of the hypophyseal arteries. The acuity and severity of the syndrome are highly variable, and most women are diagnosed with a delayed onset of panhypopituitarism and an empty sella on MRI.[23,25]

The first step in treatment of pituitary apoplexy consists of administering hydrocortisone to prevent an adrenal crisis.[26] Adequate hormone replacement in addition to administration of glucocorticoids may also be necessary. Definitive treatment of pituitary tumor apoplexy usually consists of a transsphenoidal surgical decompression, except in cases of extensive hemispheric extension of hemorrhage or hemorrhage that could not be reached through a small diaphragma sella. Local conditions related to a poorly aerated sphenoid sinus may also prompt a craniotomy. Surgical decompression is clearly indicated in cases of visual compromise or diminished levels of consciousness.[19] A complete tumor resection may not be possible, but surgery offers the best chance of visual and endocrinologic restitution. A few authors have reported the medical management of pituitary apoplexy in cases of isolated and stable meningismus or ophthalmoplegia.[27] As discussed previously, a larger role may exist for medical management in the case of prolactinoma-related pituitary apoplexy.

Visual improvements after surgical decompression in pituitary apoplexy usually affect optic motility first followed by visual fields and acuity.[21] More than half of patients require long-term hormone replacement after surgical decompression.[21] The timing of surgical decompression from the onset of symptoms may influence the extent of endocrinologic recovery.[19]

Radiosurgery as a Primary Treatment for Prolactinomas

Radiosurgery has been used as a primary treatment when managing prolactinomas. Control rates of 40% have been reported when treating microprolactinomas primarily with radiosurgery[28,29]; however, control rates vary based on the technique used as well as the doses delivered. Delayed hypopituitarism has also been observed with varying frequency in up to 17% of cases.[28] Radiosurgery is usually reserved for elderly patients or in patients who have failed other therapies and is rarely used as a first-line therapy.

Radiosurgery is also an important tool used to control prolactinoma recurrence after surgical resection. Reduction and control of prolactin levels can be accomplished in 25 to 80% of cases.[30,31] Long-term hypopituitarism may develop and requires long-term follow-up. Normalization of the hypersecretory state is more difficult to achieve in cases of recurrent prolactinomas compared with other pituitary adenomas and may require higher doses of radiation. Concurrent treatment with dopamine agonists seems to induce some degree of radioresistance.[30,31] Radiosurgery offers faster prolactin normalization when compared with external-beam radiation with a decreased incidence of long-term hypopituitarism. Prolactin normalization seems to occur around 24 months after radiosurgery on average.[31]

Transsphenoidal Surgical Approaches for Prolactinomas

The transsphenoidal approach remains the first-line surgical treatment when dealing with pituitary adenomas, including prolactinomas. Three main variations to the approach include the sublabial transsphenoidal approach, the endonasal transsphenoidal approach, and the endonasal endoscopic transsphenoidal approach. Each of these approaches has been used successfully with low complication rates, and the endoscope can be used as an adjunct to the microscope with the first two techniques.[32] The advantages of each technique are described in later chapters.

Rarely, an extended transsphenoidal approach is necessary when dealing with macroprolactinomas that extend anteriorly along the planum sphenoidale. The extent of bony removal of the planum sphenoidale should be tailored to the extent of the disease.[33] Careful coagulation of the intercavernous sinus is necessary when performing an extended transsphenoidal resection, and the risk of a CSF leak increases. Lastly, the use of micro-Doppler ultrasound is of benefit before the opening of the dura to limit the risk of a vascular injury.

Any of the transsphenoidal approaches can be used with the adjunct of stereotaxy. The use of stereotaxy is most beneficial in cases in which the patient has undergone a previous transsphenoidal approach and the bony landmarks are absent. Stereotaxy can be useful to find the sellar floor and determine where the midline is to decrease the chance of an injury to the carotid artery in cases in which anatomical landmarks are absent or those in which the sellar floor is narrow.

Craniotomy for Prolactinomas

Craniotomies are seldom required in the treatment of prolactinomas. Subfrontal or pterional craniotomies are used most often, but their use is usually restricted to patients for whom a previous transsphenoidal approach failed. A craniotomy may be necessary as a first-line procedure in cases of kissing carotid arteries. The craniotomy is performed on the nondominant side or, in cases with visual compromise, usually on the side with worse vision. A craniotomy may also be recommended as a second-stage operation in cases of large prolactinomas extending into the sylvian fissure or the interhemispheric fissure because of the risk of vascular injury.

Intraoperative Imaging for the Surgical Treatment of Prolactinomas

In some medical facilities MRI technology is now available to perform intraoperative imaging. Different philosophies have been adopted when transposing this technology to the operating room. Fields strengths vary, and thus the quality of imaging that is available varies.

Low-field MRI machines are mobile, do not necessitate MRI-compatible instruments except in the immediate vicinity of the magnets, and are cheaper to operate than a high-field MRI machine. A high-field MRI machine has a higher imaging quality but is more cumbersome and can be operated only with MRI-compatible equipment in the room. Some high-field MRI setups require the patient to be moved to a different room to undergo the imaging. Intraoperative MRI is best suited for the surgical treatment of macroprolactinomas. The surgeon is able to verify complete tumor removal in the suprasellar space and ensure that all accessible tumor has been removed. The use of intraoperative MRI is becoming more widespread, but its cost-effectiveness has yet to be demonstrated because the use of this technology remains time-consuming and expensive. Although the use of intraoperative MRI has shown tumor residual in up to 66% of macroadenomas cases, necessitating further tumor removal,[34] published series about the use of intraoperative MRI have so far been small, and further experience is needed before definitive analysis of the technology can be made.

Invasive Prolactinomas and Pituitary Carcinomas

The vast majority of prolactinomas are benign tumors. Prolactinomas are considered invasive when extensive invasion of the skull base affects the sphenoid sinus, oropharynx, clivus, orbit, pituitary fossa, cavernous sinus, or infratemporal fossa. Invasive prolactinomas usually present with higher prolactin levels and have a more aggressive clinical course. A combination of medical and surgical treatment is usually necessary in these patients. Unfortunately, strict criteria for defining invasive prolactinomas are not universally accepted and include clinical, radiologic, and molecular markers.[35] Pituitary carcinomas are rare and are defined by the presence of cerebrospinal or extracranial metastasis. A recent review noted that a total of 48 cases have been published.[36] These carcinomas are thought to derive from a benign prolactinoma that has undergone malignant degeneration. Extracranial metastasis has been described in bones, lymph nodes, lung, liver, and ovaries. The presence of high Ki-67/MIB-1 indexes or *p53* mutations seems to indicate a higher propensity for degeneration, but this correlation has not been found in all cases.[36] The presence of cellular atypia and nuclear pleomorphism as well as an aggressive clinical course with resistance to dopamine agonists should alert the physician to the possibility of a more aggressive tumor. An atypical pituitary adenoma has been defined by the World Health Organization as a tumor having a Ki-67 labeling index >3% and a *p53* immunoreactivity >3%. Treatment of these tumors requires a combination of surgery, radiotherapy, and chemotherapy for better tumor control. Temozolomide, an alkylating agent that depletes MGMT (0-6-methylguanine-DNA methyltransferase) has been used anecdotally in some cases of invasive or malignant prolactinomas.[37] Prognosis for patients harboring atypical pituitary adenoma remains poor, with a mean survival of 8 years after diagnosis of a prolactinoma and 1 year after developing metastasis.[36]

Giant Prolactinomas

A giant prolactinoma is classified as having a diameter greater than 4 cm on imaging studies, a prolactin level over 1000 ng/mL, and clinical signs of mass effect. These tumors are rare, accounting for 0.5% of all pituitary tumors, and seem to be more common in men. They are more responsive to dopamine agonists than are regular macroprolactinomas. The prolactin levels may not correlate with size in cases of giant prolactinomas, and the physician should be alert to the possibility of a hook effect. Indications for surgery include progression of the tumor or rising prolactin levels despite medical therapy, worsening visual examination despite medical therapy, the presence or development of intratumoral hemorrhage, or the development of a CSF leak during medical therapy.[38]

Management of Prolactinomas in Pregnancy

Before pregnancy, patients are preferably treated with bromocriptine because of the larger clinical experience with the drug and the fact that it does not seem to increase the likelihood of spontaneous abortion, ectopic pregnancy, or congenital malformations.[39] Patients with known macroprolactinomas who wish to become pregnant may benefit from a surgical resection before the pregnancy. Women with a medically treated microprolactinoma can be treated with contraceptive pills to prevent pregnancy as long as the dose of estrogen is equivalent to 30 µg of ethinyl estradiol or less. A systematic recommendation cannot be made for treatment with estrogens in cases of macroprolactinomas.[40]

The most common practice in North America consists of the patient stopping the use of dopamine agonists when the pregnancy is confirmed. The patient is monitored clinically and, in case of a microprolactinoma, undergoes formal visual field testing and MRI evaluation at the appearance of any symptoms of tumor enlargement. Symptomatic tumor enlargement occurs in 0.5 to 1% of cases of microprolactinomas and 15 to 35% of cases of macroprolactinomas.[8,39] Pregnant patients who harbor a macroprolactinoma are closely monitored with formal visual field testing every 3 months during pregnancy.

Cases of symptomatic tumor enlargement during pregnancy can be treated with bromocriptine, or the patient may wish to undergo surgery in selected cases.[41] Women who wish to breast-feed postpartum should not be given dopamine agonists because the resulting decrease in prolactin will impair lactation. There is no evidence to suggest that lactation increases the tumor size.

Conclusion

Prolactinomas are the second most common form of pituitary adenomas and are categorized as either microadenomas (<10 mm) or macroadenomas (≥10 mm). Their correct diagnosis implies an elevated prolactin level with the presence of an adenoma on MRI that correlates with the patient's symptoms. Women are more commonly symptomatic and present earlier in the course of the disease with amenorrhea, galactorrhea, infertility, visual and cranial nerve dysfunction, and osteoporosis. Men more commonly present with macroadenomas, and the early signs of hypogonadism are commonly unrecognized.

Medical therapy has become the most common initial treatment, and surgery is usually reserved for cases in which the patient is resistant to medical therapy or cannot tolerate its side effects. Surgery can become emergent in cases of prolactinomas that present with apoplexy. Surgery can also be offered in young patients with microprolactinomas and preoperative prolactin levels below 200 ng/mL. Medical therapy generally consists of treatment with dopamine agonists, principally bromocriptine but also cabergoline. In some cases, the patient can be weaned from medical therapy if prolonged normoprolactinemia is maintained.

Surgery is most commonly performed through a transsphenoidal route via one of three main variations: the sublabial, endonasal, or purely endoscopic endonasal transsphenoidal techniques. The transsphenoidal techniques are performed through a microscope, endoscope, or both, depending on the surgeon's preference. These techniques can be supplemented by the use of stereotaxy as well as intraoperative imaging. Rarely, a pterional or frontobasal craniotomy is required.

The goal of surgery is dependent on the size, suprasellar or intracavernous location of the tumor, and preoperative prolactin level. Surgery can be curative in more than 90% of cases of microprolactinomas but less than 50% of cases of macroprolactinomas. Surgery is likely to be curative if the prolactin level decreases below 10 ng/mL on postoperative day 1, although if that is not the case recurrence can occur up to 5 years after surgery.

Surgery can be used in conjunction with medical therapy or radiation in cases of macroadenomas or in cases with an intracavernous component to achieve normal levels of prolactin.

Rarely, prolactinomas can be more aggressive and present as invasive prolactinomas or degenerate into carcinomas. Treatment is more difficult in these cases and commonly requires the combination of medication, surgery, and radiation.

References

1. Ciccarelli A, Daly AF, Beckers A. The epidemiology of prolactinomas. Pituitary 2005;8:3–6
2. Ezzat S, Asa SL, Couldwell WT, et al. The prevalence of pituitary adenomas: a systematic review. Cancer 2004;101:613–619
3. Weiss M. Pituitary tumors: an endocrinological and neurosurgical challenge. Clin Neurosurg 1992;39:114–122
4. Liu JK, Couldwell WT. Pituitary apoplexy: diagnosis and management. Contemp Neurosurg. 2003;25:1–6
5. Suliman AM, Smith TP, Gibney J, McKenna TJ. Frequent misdiagnosis and mismanagement of hyperprolactinemic patients before the introduction of macroprolactin screening: application of a new strict laboratory definition of macroprolactinemia. Clin Chem 2003;49:1504–1509
6. Biller BM. Diagnostic evaluation of hyperprolactinemia. J Reprod Med 1999;44(12, Suppl):1095–1099
7. Frieze TW, Mong DP, Koops MK. "Hook effect" in prolactinomas: case report and review of literature. Endocr Pract 2002;8:296–303
8. Vance ML, Thorner MO. Prolactinomas. Endocrinol Metab Clin North Am 1987;16:731–753

9. Colao A, Di Sarno A, Sarnacchiaro F, et al. Prolactinomas resistant to standard dopamine agonists respond to chronic cabergoline treatment. J Clin Endocrinol Metab 1997;82:876–883
10. Colao A, Di Sarno A, Cappabianca P, Di Somma C, Pivonello R, Lombardi G. Withdrawal of long-term cabergoline therapy for tumoral and nontumoral hyperprolactinemia. N Engl J Med 2003;349:2023–2033
11. Passos VQ, Souza JJ, Musolino NR, Bronstein MD. Long-term follow-up of prolactinomas: normoprolactinemia after bromocriptine withdrawal. J Clin Endocrinol Metab 2002;87:3578–3582
12. van't Verlaat JW, Croughs RJ, Brownell J. Treatment of macroprolactinomas with a new non-ergot, long-acting dopaminergic drug, CV 205-502. Clin Endocrinol (Oxf) 1990;33:619–624
13. Couldwell WT, Rovit RL, Weiss MH. Role of surgery in the treatment of microprolactinomas. Neurosurg Clin N Am 2003;14:89–92, vii
14. Amar AP, Couldwell WT, Chen JC, Weiss MH. Predictive value of serum prolactin levels measured immediately after transsphenoidal surgery. J Neurosurg 2002;97:307–314
15. Jane JA Jr, Laws ER Jr. The surgical management of pituitary adenomas in a series of 3,093 patients. J Am Coll Surg 2001;193:651–659
16. Wang M, Weiss M. Is there a role for surgery for microprolactinomas? Semin Neurosurg 2001;12:289–294
17. Laws ER Jr, Ebersold MJ. Pituitary apoplexy—an endocrine emergency. World J Surg 1982;6:686–688
18. Couldwell WT, Rosenow JM, Rovit RL, Benzil DL. Hypophysopexy technique for radiosurgical treatment of cavernous sinus pituitary adenoma. Pituitary 2002;5:169–173
19. Verrees M, Arafah BM, Selman WR. Pituitary tumor apoplexy: characteristics, treatment, and outcomes. Neurosurg Focus 2004;16(4): E6
20. da Motta LA, de Mello PA, de Lacerda CM, Neto AP, da Motta LD, Filho MF. Pituitary apoplexy. Clinical course, endocrine evaluations and treatment analysis. J Neurosurg Sci 1999;43:25–36
21. Bills DC, Meyer FB, Laws ER Jr, et al. A retrospective analysis of pituitary apoplexy. Neurosurgery 1993;33:602–608, discussion 608–609
22. Mohanty S, Tandon PN, Banerji AK, Prakash B. Haemorrhage into pituitary adenomas. J Neurol Neurosurg Psychiatry 1977;40:987–991
23. Keleştimur F. Sheehan's syndrome. Pituitary 2003;6:181–188
24. Sheehan H. Postpartum necrosis of the anterior pituitary. J Pathol Bacteriol. 1937;45:189–214
25. Anfuso S, Patrelli TS, Soncini E, Chiodera P, Fadda GM, Nardelli GB. A case report of Sheehan's syndrome with acute onset, hyponatremia and severe anemia. Acta Biomed 2009;80:73–76
26. Lee CC, Cho AS, Carter WA. Emergency department presentation of pituitary apoplexy. Am J Emerg Med 2000;18:328–331
27. Maccagnan P, Macedo CL, Kayath MJ, Nogueira RG, Abucham J. Conservative management of pituitary apoplexy: a prospective study. J Clin Endocrinol Metab 1995;80:2190–2197
28. Ma ZM, Qiu B, Hou YH, Liu YS. [Gamma knife treatment for pituitary prolactinomas]. Zhong Nan Da Xue Xue Bao Yi Xue Ban 2006;31: 714–716
29. Pan L, Zhang N, Wang EM, Wang BJ, Dai JZ, Cai PW. Gamma knife radiosurgery as a primary treatment for prolactinomas. J Neurosurg 2000;93(Suppl 3):10–13
30. Landolt AM, Lomax N. Gamma knife radiosurgery for prolactinomas. J Neurosurg 2000;93(Suppl 3):14–18
31. Pouratian N, Sheehan J, Jagannathan J, Laws ER Jr, Steiner L, Vance ML. Gamma knife radiosurgery for medically and surgically refractory prolactinomas. Neurosurgery 2006;59:255–266
32. Ciric I, Ragin A, Baumgartner C, Pierce D. Complications of transsphenoidal surgery: results of a national survey, review of the literature, and personal experience. Neurosurgery 1997;40:225–236, discussion 236–237
33. Liu JK, Weiss MH, Couldwell WT. Surgical approaches to pituitary tumors. Neurosurg Clin N Am 2003;14:93–107
34. Bohinski RJ, Warnick RE, Gaskill-Shipley MF, et al. Intraoperative magnetic resonance imaging to determine the extent of resection of pituitary macroadenomas during transsphenoidal microsurgery. Neurosurgery 2001;49:1133–1143, discussion 1143–1144
35. Gürlek A, Karavitaki N, Ansorge O, Wass JA. What are the markers of aggressiveness in prolactinomas? Changes in cell biology, extracellular matrix components, angiogenesis and genetics. Eur J Endocrinol 2007;156:143–153
36. Kars M, Roelfsema F, Romijn JA, Pereira AM. Malignant prolactinoma: case report and review of the literature. Eur J Endocrinol 2006;155:523–534
37. Kovacs K, Horvath E, Syro LV, et al. Temozolomide therapy in a man with an aggressive prolactin-secreting pituitary neoplasm: morphological findings. Hum Pathol 2007;38:185–189
38. Shrivastava RK, Arginteanu MS, King WA, Post KD. Giant prolactinomas: clinical management and long-term follow up. J Neurosurg 2002;97:299–306
39. Molitch ME. Pregnancy and the hyperprolactinemic woman. N Engl J Med 1985;312:1364–1370
40. Christin-Maître S, Delemer B, Touraine P, Young J. Prolactinoma and estrogens: pregnancy, contraception and hormonal replacement therapy. Ann Endocrinol (Paris) 2007;68:106–112
41. Konopka P, Raymond JP, Merceron RE, Seneze J. Continuous administration of bromocriptine in the prevention of neurological complications in pregnant women with prolactinomas. Am J Obstet Gynecol 1983;146:935–938

10 Acromegaly

Brian J. Snyder and Kalmon D. Post

Although acromegaly has been recognized as an entity for a very long time, it was first clinically described by Pierre Marie[1] in 1886. Initially acromegaly was thought to be a disease, primarily bone hypertrophy, and pituitary gland enlargement was regarded as a further manifestation of generalized bodily organ enlargement.[2,3] Massalongo[4] was the first to suggest that the pituitary gland may be the cause of the disease, and in 1900 Benda[5] postulated that the eosinic granules that were observed in the glands of acromegalics were secretory. In the same year that Massalongo first made his assertion, F. T. Paul attempted a temporal craniotomy to remove a large pituitary tumor. Although he was unsuccessful at resecting the tumor, the patient apparently did benefit from the subtemporal decompression.[6] Subsequent to this success there was an increase in transcranial approaches to the gland, but surgery was usually reserved for treatment of mass effect. In 1908 Hochenegg[7] performed the first transsphenoidal operation for acromegaly, and one year later Harvey Cushing[8] did his first transsphenoidal operation for acromegaly in the United States. The transsphenoidal approach, although initially well accepted, fell out of favor in exchange for the transcranial approaches, and due to the rather high morbidity and relatively poor results, surgical treatment of acromegaly was employed only for decompression for mass effect.[9] Most patients were treated with radiation or medical therapy. In 1963 the first growth hormone (GH) assay was developed, and it enabled the clinician to assess the treatment of the disease.[10,11] As it became apparent that the available treatments at the time were far from optimal, the time was right for the reintroduction of the transsphenoidal approach for the treatment of acromegaly. Gerard Guiout[12–14] and his pupil Jules Hardy,[15–17] incorporating the operative microscope and fluoroscopy, were the first to demonstrate the safety and efficacy of the procedure for selective resection of pituitary tumors while preserving normal pituitary gland function. Over the past several decades the techniques have been refined and the procedure has reemerged as the first-line treatment to cure GH-secreting adenomas.[18,19]

Patients with acromegaly are at significantly increased risk of morbidity and mortality compared with an age-matched population. The deleterious effects of chronic GH and its downstream hormone insulin-like growth factor-1 (IGF-1), formerly known as somatomedin C, cause damage to all of the organs in the body, and the increased risk of death is largely due to an increase in cardiovascular disease in the acromegalic population.

Presentation

Acromegaly is found in the general population at a rate of 50 to 70 cases per million with an incidence of 3 to 4 cases per million per year.[20–22] Patients typically present with the disease between ages 40 and 50. GH-secreting pituitary adenomas make up approximately 16% of surgical cases of pituitary lesions.[23] Acromegalic patients have between a 1.9- and 3.3-fold increased mortality rate.

Acromegaly is a disease of chronic overproduction of GH. In the child and preadolescent, excess GH leads to abnormally increased height and gigantism as well as organomegaly. Once the epiphyseal plates have closed, the manifestations are that of acromegaly. The consequences of GH hypersecretion are numerous. Bone and soft tissue overgrowth is almost always present. Patients may first notice changes in shoe size, ring size, and a coarsening of their facial features, with enlargement of their lips, macroglossia, a prominent brow, prognathism, and increased spaces between their teeth. A low voice is a product of laryngeal hypertrophy. Patients go on to develop skeletal abnormalities secondary to new bone growth, including vertebral body osteophyte formation leading to spinal stenosis, and bowing of the long bones. Overgrowth contributes to a significant increase in weight and stress on the joints, cartilaginous erosion, and severe osteoarthritis. Acromegaly causes numerous cardiovascular complications, such as cardiomyopathy, arrhythmias, and coronary artery disease.[24–26] Patients with acromegaly develop impaired diastolic cardiac function even in the absence of frank cardiomyopathy.[25] GH elevation contributes to markedly increased rates of diabetes and hypertension. Interestingly, patients with acromegaly less commonly present with significant panhypopituitarism than do those with nonsecreting tumors.[27] Although there is an increased frequency of hypothyroidism, patients with acromegaly are less likely to have hypothyroidism, impaired adrenal function, or hypogonadal function than similar patients with nonsecreting pituitary adenomas. This remains true even when macroadenomas are independently compared in both groups. This may be due to secondary effects of GH. IGF-1 has been observed in vitro to stimulate DNA[28,29] and thyroglobulin synthesis.[30]

The vast majority of patients presenting with acromegaly have an underlying pituitary tumor. Rarely the disease can be caused by growth hormone–releasing hormone (GHRH) elevation secondary to hypothalamic dysfunction.[31] Very rarely the disease can also be caused by ectopic release of GHRH by carcinoid or pancreatic islet tumors.[32–34] Although these are truly the exceptions, the possibility must be considered to avoid potentially unnecessary pituitary surgery. Furthermore, glands that have been biopsied under these circumstances demonstrate hyperplasia without evidence of adenomatous changes.[34] Clearly, increased stimulation of the gland by GHRH is not enough to produce an adenoma.

Mortality is significantly increased in patients with untreated or uncured acromegaly. Retrospective data from New Zealand showed a significant increase in the death rate from cardiovascular complications. Analysis revealed that there were statistically significant increases in survival with decreasing GH levels. At random GH levels of 1 µg/L, the death rate approaches that of the general population.[35] Reduction of IGF-1 to the normal range produced a mortality equivalent to that of the general population. Other studies have found that mortality approximated that of the general population when GH approached 2.5 µg/L[36] or 5 µg/L.[37] Most recent studies confirm that a lower GH is associated with a better long-term morbidity and a reduced mortality rate. Cardiomyopathy has been shown to reduce significantly when IGF-1 levels are normalized and GH levels are <1 µg/L after an oral glucose load.[25] Patients with uncured acromegaly have not only an increased cardiac risks but also an increased risk of respiratory and cerebrovascular death. These increases may not decrease fully with normalization of GH levels.[36] This is speculated to be due to the fact that some of the processes associated with acromegaly, such as diabetes and hypertension, may have already caused significant end-organ damage by the time that GH levels are normalized, so that the patient continues to experienced an increased risk of death. The association between acromegaly and malignancy is unclear. Orme et al[36] performed a large retrospective review of 1362 patients with acromegaly and found a higher than expected rate of colon cancer in patients with acromegaly but a lower than expected overall incidence of malignancy in this population. Increased colonic adenocarcinoma rates have been found in other series as well.[37–39] Other studies have failed to document this increased rate of malignancy.[35]

Reduction in morbidity and mortality relies on prompt diagnosis and early intervention and treatment.[18] Patients frequently present early to their primary care physicians with protean complaints, and it is incumbent upon physicians to recognize the disease in its earliest manifestations and refer the patient for definitive care.

Diagnosis

Growth hormone is under the control of the hypothalamic hormone GHRH. The pituitary somatotrophs and adenomas secrete multiple isoforms of GH. The predominant one is a 22-kd monomeric form accounting for approximately 50% of the circulating GH in most patients, but the other monomers are also active. Different assays have different sensitivity and specificity for the different monomers of GH. Because of this there still exists test-to-test variation until adequate standardization is employed.[40]

Hypersecretion of GH leads to increased production of IGF-1. In the past, diagnosis of acromegaly relied solely on the recognition of the constellation of physical signs and symptoms. In the 1960s the advent of radioimmunoassay allowed for the measurement of GH levels, and following that similar tests were developed to measure IGF-1 levels.[41] As these tests have been refined and their sensitivity increased, it has prompted further evaluations of what is considered "normal" levels of these hormones.[42] Accurate measurements of these biochemical markers allows for earlier diagnosis of the patient and assessment of cure.

Growth hormone has a half-life of 15 to 20 minutes and is released in a pulsatile fashion secondary to stimulation by GHRH. It is inhibited by the release of somatostatin. Acromegaly can be characterized by increased frequency of GH pulses, increased mean GH nadir, increased nonpulsatile GH fraction, and an increase in the "disorderliness" of GH release.[43–45] In the normal individual GH ranges from <0.1 to 0.2 µg/L interspersed with periods with levels as high as 20 to 30 µg/L. Although individuals with exceedingly high random levels of GH may be considered likely to have acromegaly, especially if clinically suspected, there is some limitation to interpreting a random GH sample.[41] More effective and popular is the measurement of GH levels after an oral glucose load. In the normal individual GH levels will drop significantly following ingestion of 75 to 100 g of glucose. The criteria for diagnosis of acromegaly have changed over the years. In the 1980s levels of <10 µg/L of GH on random assay were considered within normal limits,[46] and <2 µg/L after oral glucose was also considered normal.[47] Recent data have set the cutoff for a random level at 2.5 µg/L, and the cutoff for a normal suppression test at 1 µg/L.[48]

As IGF-1 is the "downstream" hormone of GH, there is reason to think that continuing to measure the IGF-1 levels may provide more reliability in the consideration of remission in the acromegalic. Up to 50% of patients with GH nadirs of <1 µg/L still have elevated IGF-1.[42] A subset of patients also exists with the obvious stigmata of acromegaly and IGF-1 elevation but with normal mean GH levels.[47] The need to measure IGF-1 levels becomes further necessary as the new competitive GH antagonist pegvisomant has been introduced, which results in *elevated* GH levels accompanied by a decrease in IGF-1 levels. IGF-1 has a significantly longer half-life, and therefore random measurement is more feasible to assess posttreatment acromegalics. Current recommendations are that IGF-1 levels be at normal age- and sex-adjusted levels to define remission. The patient's risk of mortality has been shown to approach that of the general population when the IGF-1 level is normalized.[49] However, IGF-1 levels do not increase significantly once GH levels are <20 µg/L, and because of this IGF-1 in the absence of GH measurement will not be effective in assessing partial responses to therapy when the GH levels remain high.

Because of the complementary nature of information provided by IGF-1 and GH levels, it seems prudent to continue to measure both sets of data in posttreatment patients to properly assess and manage them, and currently this remains our protocol.

Histopathology and Prognosis

Microscopically, the appearance of adenoma is very varied. Cells may be round or ovoid. They may be arranged in monotonous sheets or show acinar or papillary patterns. The nuclei may be cytologically pleomorphic with mitotic figures and a stippled chromatin appearance. Invasion of local dura may be demonstrated even in cells with bland cytologic features.[50] GH-secreting tumors can be categorized into two distinct morphologic types: densely granulated (DG) and sparsely granulated (SG) adenomas (see Chapter 6). DG cells resemble the well-differentiated somatotroph cells of the normal anterior pituitary gland, whereas in contrast the SG cells bear little resemblance to the normal GH-secreting cells.[51] SG cells have cytoplasmic cytokeratin aggregates sometimes called fibrous bodies or intracytoplasmic filamentous aggregates. The two subtypes of tumors have been reported to occur in relatively equal frequency.[52] SG adenomas tend to grow more rapidly and are more likely to be invasive at the time of diagnosis.[53]

Recent studies have suggested that the K_i-67 labeling index may predict clinical outcome in the postsurgical management of acromegalic patients, with a lower index correlating with a higher remission rate.[54]

Treatment

The goals of treatment are control of GH and IGF-1 levels such that GH levels are <1 µg/L after an oral glucose load and that IGF-1 levels are normal, adjusted for age and sex. The tumor mass needs to be removed or significantly enough reduced so that there is no chance of recurrence and so that the optic nerves are free of compression or impending threat of such.[48] It is common that acromegaly will require multimodality therapy.[55]

Surgery

Transsphenoidal microsurgery is the preferred primary treatment for acromegaly, though craniotomy rarely is indicated as a primary surgical intervention.[48,49,56–59] We prefer a transseptal endonasal approach to the sphenoid. Patients with significant bony and cartilaginous hypertrophy with small nares may provide more of a challenge for maneuvering of the instruments, but with a well-placed speculum we usually find that the nasal route still affords adequate surgical exposure of the sella and enough space to safely remove tumor. Nonetheless, we are prepared to convert to a sublabial approach should we find that the exposure is unsatisfactory for tumor resection, though we very rarely need to do this. We make no significant modifications to our standard approach to the sphenoid for acromegalics. We do not employ lumbar drainage as a standard part of our protocol. We believe that adequate exposure of the sella and surrounding structures can be afforded by the microscope or the endoscope, but there are situations where some may find the endoscope beneficial to assess for completeness of tumor resection after microscopic removal.

Surgical resection of the adenoma provides the highest hope for cure and is generally safe with acceptable morbidity.[49,56–58,60–63] As previously discussed the definition of biochemical cure in the acromegalic patients has been evolving. Older series of transsphenoidal surgery for acromegaly, which incorporated now outdated definitions of cure, may obscure the interpretation of the success of surgery for GH-secreting tumors in the literature. Early studies used GH levels of <5 µg/L or <10 µg/L as the definition of cure[58,64] When these numbers were employed, cure rates ranged between 67 and 90%.[63,65,66] Rates of cure for acromegaly by transsphenoidal surgery as defined by a GH of <5 µg/L ranged from 53[15] to 81%.[63] Abosch et al,[56] using as a definition of cure a GH of <5.0 µg/L, found a 76% remission rate. Age, tumor size, grade, and preoperative GH levels were all predictive of remission. Of the patients who were defined as being in remission, 13% nonetheless had elevated IGF-1 levels (**Table 10.1**).

Tumor size obviously influences the likelihood of remission. The odds of remission for microadenomas was found to be 3.3 times higher than the odds for macroadenomas.[49] The success rate for modern microadenoma resection alone ranges from 74 to 88%.[56,67,68] Success rates for surgery on macroadenomas are, as expected, lower than those for smaller tumors. Macrodenomas that are noninvasive have modestly lower remission rates of 67%,[68] whereas those that invade the cavernous sinus and other adjacent structures have rates as low as or lower than 30%. Further analysis revealed the rather unsurprising fact that tumors can further be subclassified beyond micro- and macroadenoma, and that increasing size correlates with decreasing success rate. Major decreases in remission exist when the tumor was invasive and >20 mm. GH rates may be predictive of the

Table 10.1 Surgical Results: Percent of Remission

Authors	Microadenoma	Macroadenoma	Total	No. of Patients
Freda et al, 1997	88	53	61	115
Laws et al, 2000	87	51	67	117
Kaltsas et al, 2001	59	26	34	67
Shimon et al, 2001	84	64	74	91
Abe and Ludecke, 2001	95	68	72	147
De et al, 2003	79	56	63	90
Beauregard et al, 2003	82	60	52	103
Nomikos et al, 2005	75	50	57	506
Trepp et al, 2005	80	39	42	69

likelihood of success. According to Shimon et al,[69] although patients with a preoperative GH level of <20 µg/L or of 20 to 50 µg/L had cure rates of 90% or 79%, respectively, those with a GH level of >50 µg/L had a cure rate of only 16%. Similarly, Freda et al[68] found 80% and 90% cure rates of micro- and macroadenomas, respectively, when the preoperative GH level was <10 µg/L, falling to 55% for tumors with a GH of 30 to 50 µg/L. No patients were cured with a preoperative GH of >200 µg/L. Because GH levels rapidly fall following resection, whereas IGF-1 can take a long time to normalize, GH levels are routinely the test of choice in the immediate postoperative period. Early GH levels can be predictive of success or failure. There is no clear cutoff on the early postoperative laboratory results to define cure, but GH levels of <2 µg/L on the first postoperative day are found to correlate with surgical success in 99% of patients.[67] GH levels of <3 µg/L predict cure in 89%,[68] whereas a GH of >5 µg/L in the early postoperative period is associated with much poorer normalization rates of IGF-1 of 0 to 21%.[58,68,70] According to Krieger et al,[67] only one of 65 patients with a GH level of >2 µg/L on postoperative day one was later determined to have a biochemical cure. Dural invasion and extrasellar extension of tumors have been associated with persistent disease.

Patients with acromegaly usually present for endocrinologic disturbances. Some patients present with visual disturbances. Most patients recover some degree of visual function following transsphenoidal surgery. The recovery of visual function relates to the time of optic nerve compression and the ability to adequately decompress the nerves in the operating room. As patients with acromegaly largely have other symptoms as well, they are more likely recognized at an earlier point in their disease. Nonetheless, some patients do present with significant nerve compression or pituitary apoplexy, leading to acute visual deterioration; 80 to 86% of patients presenting for primary surgery for visual disturbance due to various lesions of the sella typically improve postoperatively.[71,72] In one study, 75% of patients had an improved visual examination following transsphenoidal surgery for acromegaly.[61]

Some patients do not present until they are elderly; as many as 5% of patients with acromegaly present after the age of 65.[73,74] Many clinicians are tempted to steer these patients away from surgical resection because of the belief that they are unable to handle the stresses of surgery. Puchner et al[74] report very good results for patients over the age of 65 undergoing surgery for acromegaly. They report no significant perioperative morbidity and no mortality. Results of resection are extremely good. As patients can experience reversal of the effects of acromegaly within 6 months to 1 year following successful surgery, even elderly patients may benefit. These patients may experience improvement in their cardiac function, glucose tolerance, and hypertension, all of which may improve life expectancy and quality of life. Thus, many elderly patients, despite their acromegaly and its complications, are deemed to be acceptable surgical candidates.[75]

Reoperation for acromegaly is a controversial subject. Rates of surgical success are poor, probably because many patients have extensive tumor involvement that is not as likely to be amenable to curative resection. Rates of surgical success for endocrine cure range from 0 to 57%.[62,69,76] Morbidity associated with reoperation is much higher; 63% of patients develop hypopituitarism.[62] One group classified reoperative tumors according to size and invasiveness and documented significant success with the microadenomas and those that radiographically did not appear to be invasive.[76] However, the group had no successes reoperating on those tumors already deemed to be invasive. Some patients need to be reoperated on for progressive visual deterioration. Patients undergoing reoperation for impairment do not generally seem to garner as much visual improvement as those undergoing a primary operation with the same complaint.[72]

Recurrence of active acromegaly is a confusing issue. As testing becomes more sensitive, more patients are noted to have subtle signs of endocrinologic laboratory abnormality. Some patients now considered to have had a recurrence may just have had mild GH dysfunction that was not detected as abnormal by less accurate earlier tests. More contemporary literature has defined the rate of recurrence as between 1.1 and 19%.[49,56,61,68,77] Patients who experience a recurrence are typically managed in multimodality therapy with medical and radiation therapy.[56] Recently we reported on a subset of patients with normalized IGF-1 levels postoperatively but who failed to suppress to levels of <1 µg/L; five of 14 of these patients later developed evidence of elevated IGF-1.[78] This suggests a group of patients with subtle endocrinologic dysfunction that although having normal IGF-1 levels, and hence technically being in remission, probably still have some latent disease. Although no intervention is considered necessary provided the IGF-1 remains under control, this group may benefit from closer monitoring.[78,79]

Morbidity

Transsphenoidal surgery for GH-secreting tumors is very safe. In general, the morbidity associated with surgical resection of tumors in the acromegalic patient mirrors that of surgery on other tumors via the same method. However, the soft tissue, cartilaginous, and bony overgrowth associated with the disease may contribute to a narrowed surgical corridor, especially when a transnasal route is employed, making instrument manipulation even more challenging. An overall complication rate of 6.7% is reported for transsphenoidal surgery for acromegaly.[56,60] Complications reported include cerebrospinal fluid rhinorrhea in 2%, with 1.2% needing reoperation[49]; meningitis in 1[37] to 2%[63]; transient diabetes insipidus rates of up to 6.8%[49]; permanent diabetes insipidus requiring vasopressin in 1.3[37] to 10%[49]; sinusitis in 3%[74]; epistaxis[56] and new hypopituitarism variously reported in 2%,[50] 6%,[57] and 12%.[57] Nasal septal perforation occurs. Few cases of postoperative visual deterioration exist.[56] Patients are at risk for associated medical problems such as arrhythmia, deep venous thrombosis, and pneumonia. Due to the generally speedy recovery from surgery and the rapid mobilization of patients, these problems are relatively uncommon. The risks of transsphenoidal surgery as well as the likely rates of cure reported with this chapter are predicated on the procedure being done by an experienced surgeon.[80–83] Complication of surgery can be three to four times as high when performed by a surgeon less familiar with the procedure.[84,85]

Medical Therapy

Dopamine agonists, somatostatin receptor analogues, and GH receptor antagonists are the three classes of drugs used most commonly in the treatment of acromegaly. Medical therapy is almost never recommended for patients who have a potentially resectable pituitary adenoma. All of the medical treatment currently available can help control the endocrinologic manifestations of the disease and may help control tumor growth, but the effects last only as long as the patient is taking the drug. However, some patients have tumors that may not be readily surgically resected and may not be amenable to radiation therapy, and some patients might not be surgical candidates for other reasons. In this group, medical intervention has received new attention as a primary treatment modality. Furthermore, pharmaceuticals also can be of much help in pretreatment and adjuvant treatment when associated with the other modalities available.

The question of whether pretreatment with octreotide improves surgical results in macroadenomas has been studied with varying results. One recent study from Norway[86,87] suggests that 6-month pretreatment might improve surgical cure rates.

Dopamine Agonists

Dopamine agonists are orally active agents that bind to the dopamine D2 receptor in the pituitary gland and prevent it from secreting GH. The main advantage of this class of drugs is that they are orally active. However, bromocriptine has historically been used with only poor to modest success; 20% of patients taking bromocriptine have GH levels of <5 µg/L following treatment, and only 10% experience normalization of their IGF-1 levels.[88] Cabergoline is a newer agent with greater effect and a lower side-effect profile. IGF-1 normalization is seen in 35% of patients taking it for GH-secreting adenomas in the largest study to date. Dopamine agonists, however, are not well tolerated in many patients, with side effects such as nausea, vomiting, dizziness, and mood disturbances. Long-term use of cabergoline has been associated with cardiac valve dysfunction, but only with the very high dosages used in a movement disorder patient. This has not been reported with dosages used for pituitary adenomas.

Somatostatin Analogues

Somatostatin analogues inhibit the release of GH as well as other peptide hormones and neurotransmitters.[89] Synthetic analogues were developed to overcome the half-life of natural somatostatin of 1 to 3 minutes. Octreotide is a common drug used in clinical practice, though lanreotide is also commonly prescribed. Newer long-acting forms of these drugs have been developed and require injecting only every 4 to 6 weeks. Among newly diagnosed acromegalics, 38% and 33% of patients had normalization of there GH and IGF-1 levels, respectively, after 24 weeks of therapy, and a 43 to 49% shrinkage in their tumors was also observed in one study.[90] Newman et al[90] found that 73% of patients taking octreotide as primary therapy had normalization of IGF-1 by 3 years.[91] Tumor size was reduced by 10% in six of 13 patients and by

25% in three of 13; 60 to 75% of patients had improvement or resolution of symptoms 6 months following initiation of treatment.[92] Early tumor shrinkage after 3 months of octreotide predicted a better 12-month shrinkage.[93] Most patients tolerate these drugs very well. The main symptoms included abdominal discomfort and cramping. Octreotide analogues, however, increase the risk of gallbladder disease. The exact degree of this risk is unclear. Current recommendations, however, are that patients on octreotide be managed in the same fashion as any other patients with respect to their gallbladder.[94,95] Although surgery is clearly the best option if the lesion is thought to be resectable, octreotide therapy seems to be a valid adjunct to radiation for those who are not surgical candidates and in cases where the tumor is thought to be unresectable. Its equivocal results in tumor shrinkage, however, may still necessitate surgical intervention for debulking of the lesion to minimize possible visual deterioration.

Octreotide therapy previously necessitated subcutaneous injections three times daily. But now there are many years of experience with a long-acting depot form of the drug. This long-acting release form is administered once every 4 weeks. It has been found to lower GH levels equivocally to the regular octreotide preparation.[96] Other studies have shown that in a subset of these patients the drug can be dosed even less frequently than that. At 6-week intervals, 13 of 14 patients in one study continued to have GH suppression, although 30% developed elevated IGF-1 levels.[97,98]

There is great interest in the use of these drugs in the preoperative setting. Preoperative medical treatment of acromegaly has two main goals in mind: to increase the success rate of surgical resection of the tumor and to decrease the morbidity of surgery in the patient. No studies have assessed either of these questions in a blinded fashion. One study utilized 100 µg every 8 hours subcutaneously for 8 weeks prior to surgery for invasive adenomas; 60% of patients had radiographic tumor shrinkage (9–78% decrease in volume), whereas another series found significant tumor shrinkage in only 22% of patients.[99] A larger review found 23 to 100% of patients experienced radiographic tumor shrinkage of >20%.[99] Surgical cure rates in patients with macroadenomas average approximately 50% in the most experienced hands. In a review of multiple series of patients pretreated with somatostatin analogues, Melmed et al[99] found a 55 to 89% cure rate in series with *mostly* macroadenomas. Patients with acromegaly are at increased risk during anesthesia secondary to cardiac, pulmonary, and metabolic derangement[36]; 60% of mortalities in acromegaly are attributed to cardiovascular sources,[101,102] so interventions to reduce these risks may be warranted prior to anesthesia in higher risk patients. Although there are no direct data to recommend pretreatment, octreotide in controlled patients has been shown to decrease left ventricular wall mass,[103] normalize electrocardiograms in a subset of patients,[102] improve left ventricular ejection fraction,[101] decrease blood pressure,[91] and improve vocal cord elasticity and decrease its mass[104] (which may help in difficult intubations, as 10 to 30% of acromegaly patients' intubations are considered to be).[98] Patients in one series showed significantly shorter average length of stay: 5.6 versus 8.6 days postoperatively if pretreated with octreotide. The length-of-stay difference was due to a reduction in medical complications.[105]

Colao et al[106] have shown that the incidence of cardiac valve regurgitation did not change with somatostatin analogues. But improvement was seen in left ventricular hypertrophy and diastolic filling.

Pegvisomant

Pegvisomant is one of the newest options for treatment. It is a chemically engineered analogue of GH and functions at the level of the receptor as a competitive antagonist.[107] It differs from the wild-type GH by eight amino acids in the region of binding site 1, and it has a single mutation at binding site 2, preventing functional dimerization. The drug is administered as a daily subcutaneous injection. Patients on pegvisomant have a paradoxical rise in their GH levels, making IGF-1 the most important laboratory data to measure. Maximal response is seen within 2 weeks of initiation of treatment. Patients have been found to have a dose-dependent significant decrease in their IGF-1 levels (to normal in 89% of patients receiving 20 mg daily) as well as symptomatic resolution on the drug. Of note, due to its role as a GH receptor antagonist, it appears also to reverse some of the associated abnormalities of GH hypersecretion. Insulin sensitivity increases on pegvisomant, and abnormalities in cortisol metabolism are reversed.[105] Acromegalic cardiomyopathy may be improved with long-term treatment with the GH receptor antagonist.[108] Morbidity and side effects are minimal, with asymptomatic liver function test abnormalities having been reported. There are anecdotal reports of increased tumor size when taking this drug. This may be the pharmacologic GH equivalent to Nelson's syndrome. Current recommendations are that all patients taking this drug with any tumor have follow-up magnetic resonance imaging scans every 6 months to look for tumor growth.[40]

Some studies have shown that quality of life in acromegalic patients may be improved with combined therapy of somatostatin analogue treatment and pegvisomant.[109,110]

Radiation

Radiation therapy is relatively effective at treating uncured acromegaly patients. Most patients presenting for radiation have undergone microsurgery and are likely to be on a somatostatin analogue or dopamine agonist as well. Because of the significant risk of panhypopituitarism, it is not employed as a first-line treatment in general and is reserved for patients for whom surgical therapy has failed. The other main drawback of radiation therapy is that it is a gradual effect. Conventional radiotherapy is constrained by the surrounding structures, such as the optic nerves and hypothalamus.[111] Conventional radiotherapy has now largely been supplanted by stereotactic radiosurgery for these tumors. Stereotactic radiosurgery is high-precision single-session treatment delivered typically via gamma knife, proton accelerator, CyberKnife, or linear accelerator.[112]

Radiation therapy can provide very good tumor growth control of 72 to 97%.[113,114] Conventional radiation is typically given in fractions of 160 to 180 cGy four to five times a week over 5 to 6 weeks for a total dose of 40 to 50 Gy.[115] Conventional radiotherapy typically leads to a 50% decrease in GH levels by 2 years. These levels continue to fall for up to 10 years.[116,117] When fractionated radiation was employed postoperatively, 63% of patients went on to normalize IGF-1 at 6.7 years.[49] Abosch et al[56] reported that 83% of patients had disease remission as defined by a GH of <2.5 µg/L after undergoing radiation. The exact frequency of remission conferred by radiation therapy is varied in the literature and is as low as 5%.[118] This may be partially attributed to the extended period of follow-up necessary to assess the response to radiotherapy.[119] Radiotherapy effectiveness appears to be related to the pretreatment GH levels.[120]

Stereotactic radiosurgery has the advantages of greater conformality and single-session dosing relative to radiotherapy. With greater conformity to the target, a higher dose of radiation can be given to the tumor while still keeping the vital adjacent structures within acceptable dosing parameters. Radiosurgery appears to confer better rates of endocrinologic cure than does radiation therapy and may confer cure at a faster rate.[114,118,121,122] Gamma knife surgery has been shown to normalize IGF-1 levels in selected patients in rates varying from 25 to 82%.[123–126] GKS provides very good control of tumor growth with shrinkage in some patients.[127–129] GKS causes up to 90% of patients' tumors to shrink, with the majority of the remainder being stable.[122,129] The higher the dose that is given to the tumor, the greater the likelihood of success. A maximum dose of 40 Gy correlated to hormonal cure in one series.[122] Linear accelerator radiosurgery used as salvage following failed microsurgery or conventional radiation therapy results in 54% of patients in one series with normalization of their IGF-1 and GH levels defined as 2 µg/L[111]; 40% of patients were able to be withdrawn from somatostatin therapy and 30% had reduced doses. No change in tumor size was reported.[111]

Some reports suggest that octreotide may act as a radioprotectant.[122,130,131] In a subset of patients reviewed following stereotactic radiosurgery, there is marked divergence of the patients on the medication versus those not receiving it. It is possible that octreotide, by reducing the metabolic demands of the adenoma, desensitizes it to the effects of radiosurgery. This prompted the authors of this study to begin radiosurgical treatment during "gaps" in medical treatment.[130,131]

The main risks involved in radiation therapy (both conventional and the stereotactic techniques) are radiation-induced optic neuropathy and damage to the remaining pituitary gland.[129] Similar to the results for treatment, these effects continue to develop for years following treatment. Hypopituitarism is very common after radiation therapy. Depending on case series and dosing parameters, between 0 and 69% of patients need hormone replacement at 6 to 10 years following conventional radiation. Data for stereotactic radiosurgery seem to indicate a comparable trend.[132] Risk to vision, although certainly much lower than the risk of panhypopituitarism, is of much greater concern to the physician and patient. As an increasing dose of radiation appears to correlate with endocrine cure, a careful balance must be achieved. One patient in a mixed series of endocrinologically active tumors recently was reported to have gone blind with a dose of 8 to 10 cGy to the optic nerve.[122] Many centers limit the dose to the nerve at 8 cGy maximum.[133] Finally, there are reports of carotid stenosis secondary to radiation. Although most of these cases are asymptomatic and we are unaware of any cases of stroke or necessary intervention following modern radiation protocols in the acromegalic patient, as dosing regimens evolve to treat newer definitions of biochemical cure the physician must be aware of this possible sequela.

Management of Complications of Acromegaly

As has been discussed, the results of chronic GH stimulation produce disease in multiple organ systems. The best treatment option for these patients is lowering the GH and IGF-1 levels as outlined. Obviously, patients should have appropriate medical care as well while awaiting or pursuing definitive care. Aggressive management of hypertension, cardiac disease, and diabetes is necessary. Patients should have sleep studies if they demonstrate documented respiratory disease. Colonoscopy should be performed every 3 to 5 years depending on the clinical scenario.[40]

Conclusion

The current treatment paradigm for acromegaly involves a multidisciplinary approach. It is incumbent upon the patient's primary care doctor to notice the signs and symptoms of the disease early and refer the patient for definitive cure. Treatment success correlates with pretreatment GH levels. To reduce the patient's risk of mortality back to baseline levels, the IGF-1 must be normalized and the GH level must be under 1 µg/L following an oral glucose tolerance test. Surgery offers the best possible opportunity for cure (**Table 10.2**). In experienced hands with a microadenoma, cure rates approach 90%, whereas those with larger or invasive tumors do not fare quite so well. Patients who do not have full normalization of their IGF-1 level postoperatively should be considered for further therapy or reoperation. Reoperation can be considered, but rates of cure are significantly lower than in the primary surgical group. Medical therapy is successful in lowering GH and IGF-1 levels and may be employed both presurgically and postsurgically, but its effects are sustained only during the course of administration (**Table 10.3**). New long-acting depot forms of somatostatin analogues are available with equal efficacy and longer dosing intervals. The newer GH antagonist holds further promise in the medical armamentarium, but patients' GH levels can no longer be followed. Radiation is a good treatment option for patients with uncured acromegaly following surgery. The cure is slow to develop, but greater than 50% of patients may reach normalized IGF-1 levels this way. Both radiation therapy and stereotactic radiosurgery have significant risks of panhypopituitarism, necessitating hormone therapy. Similar to the prolonged time to cure, patients have a gradual onset of pituitary hormone dysfunction, should it develop.

Table 10.2 Advantages of Surgery

- Transsphenoidal surgery (TSS) provides an excellent chance of long-term cure in patients with microadenomas
- Surgery alone is also successful in most patients with noninvasive macroadenomas, but most patients with invasive macroadenomas also require adjunctive therapy
- Surgical results correlate with size of adenoma, invasiveness preoperative growth hormone (GH) level, co-secretion
- Morbidity and mortality are very low
- Recurrence rates for microadenomas and noninvasive macroadenomas <2 cm are very low
- All patients require careful long-term endocrinologic follow-up
- Surgery is still the first treatment for larger invasive tumors
- TSS offers rapid decline in GH, yielding rapid reduction of acromegaly signs and symptoms

A treatment algorithm for acromegaly is provided (**Fig. 10.1**).

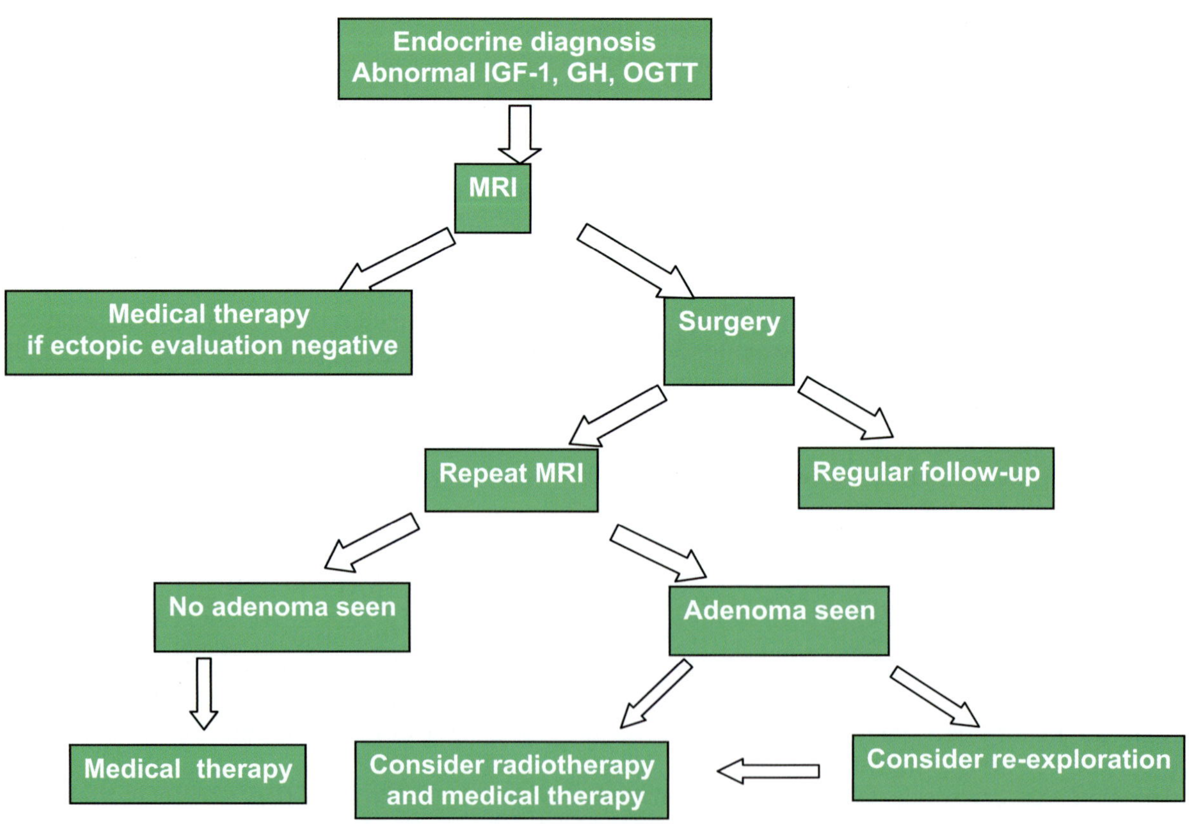

Fig. 10.1 Acromegaly algorithm.

Table 10.3 Expected Results of Surgery and Medical Treatment

- TSS can normalize GH and IGF-1 as follows:
  - In 80–90% of patients with microadenomas
  - In 50–60% of patients with macroadenomas
- Conventional fractionated radiotherapy
  - Can normalize IGF-1 in most patients but can take 10 years
- Gamma Knife
  - Appears to have shorter lag time
- Somatostatin analogues
  - Control GH and IGF-1 in approximately 50–60% of patients
  - Overall approximately 30% of patients have tumor shrinkage
- Combination of somatostatin and pegvisomant is very effective
- Multimodality therapy is often necessary to adequately control the disease

Abbreviations: GH, growth hormone; IGF-1, insulin-like growth factors - 1; TSS, transsphenoidal surgery.

References

1. Marie P. Sur deux cas d'acromegalie. Hypertrophie singuliere noncogenitale des extremites superiures, inferiures et cephalique. Rev Mens de Med 1886;297
2. Jane JA Jr, Thapar K, Laws ER Jr. Acromegaly: historical perspectives and current therapy. J Neurooncol 2001;54:129–137
3. Brigidi V. Studii anatomo-patologici sopra un uomo divenuto stranamente deforeme per cronica infermita. Arch Scuola Anat Patol Firenze 1881;65–92
4. Massalongo R. Sull'acromegalia. Riforma Med 1892;8:74
5. Benda C. Beitrage zur normalen und pathologischen histologie der menschlichen hypophysos cerebri. Klin Wochenschr 1900;26:1205
6. Caton R, Paul FT. Notes of a case of acromegaly treated by operation. BMJ 1893;2:1421–1423
7. Hochenegg J. Operat geheilte Akromegalie bei Hypophysentumor. Verh Dtsch Ges Chir 1908;37:80–85
8. Cushing H III. Partial hypophysectomy for acromegaly: with remarks on the function of the hypophysis. Ann Surg 1909;50:1002–1017
9. Henderson WR. The pituitary adenomata. A follow-up study of the surgical results in 338 cases (Dr. Harvey Cushing's series). Br J Surg 1939;26:811–921
10. Glick SM, Roth J, Yalow RS, Berson SA. Immunoassay of human graowth hormone in plasma. Nature 1963;199:784–787
11. Utiger RD, Parker ML, Daughaday WH. Studies on human growth hormone. I. A radio-immunoassay for human growth hormone. J Clin Invest 1962;41:254–261
12. Guiot G, Bouche J, Oproiu A. [Indications of the trans-sphenoidal approach to pituitary adenomas. Experience with 165 operations]. Presse Med 1967;75:1563–1568
13. Guiot G, Derome P. [Surgical approaches to hypophyseal adenomas]. Rev Otoneuroophtalmol 1974;46:337–346
14. Guiot G, Derome P. [Indications for trans-sphenoid approach in neurosurgery. 521 cases]. Ann Med Interne (Paris) 1972;123:703–712
15. Hardy J. Transsphenoidal hypophysectomy. J Neurosurg 1971; 34:582–594
16. Hardy J. [Surgery of the pituitary gland, using the trans-sphenoidal approach. Comparative study of 2 technical methods]. Union Med Can 1967;96:702–712
17. Hardy J. Transsphenoidal microsurgery of the normal and pathological pituitary. Clin Neurosurg 1969;16:185–217
18. Beauregard C, Truong U, Hardy J, Serri O. Long-term outcome and mortality after transsphenoidal adenomectomy for acromegaly. Clin Endocrinol (Oxf) 2003;58:86–91
19. Dekkers OM, Biermasz NR, Pereira AM, Romijn JA, Vandenbroucke JP. Mortality in acromegaly: a metaanalysis. J Clin Endocrinol Metab 2008;93:61–67
20. Alexander L, Appleton D, Hall R, Ross WM, Wilkinson R. Epidemiology of acromegaly in the Newcastle region. Clin Endocrinol (Oxf) 1980;12:71–79
21. Bengtsson BA, Edén S, Ernest I, Odén A, Sjögren B. Epidemiology and long-term survival in acromegaly. A study of 166 cases diagnosed between 1955 and 1984. Acta Med Scand 1988;223:327–335
22. Ritchie CM, Atkinson AB, Kennedy AL, et al. Ascertainment and natural history of treated acromegaly in Northern Ireland. Ulster Med J 1990;59:55–62
23. Mindermann T, Wilson CB. Age-related and gender-related occurrence of pituitary adenomas. Clin Endocrinol (Oxf) 1994;41:359–364
24. Colao A. Are patients with acromegaly at high risk for dysrhythmias? Clin Endocrinol (Oxf) 2001;55:305–306
25. Herrmann BL, Bruch C, Saller B, et al. Acromegaly: evidence for a direct relation between disease activity and cardiac dysfunction in patients without ventricular hypertrophy. Clin Endocrinol (Oxf) 2002;56:595–602
26. Ozbey N, Oncül A, Buğra Z, et al. Acromegalic cardiomyopathy: evaluation of the left ventricular diastolic function in the subclinical stage. J Endocrinol Invest 1997;20:305–311
27. Greenman Y, Tordjman K, Kisch E, Razon N, Ouaknine G, Stern N. Relative sparing of anterior pituitary function in patients with growth hormone-secreting macroadenomas: comparison with nonfunctioning macroadenomas. J Clin Endocrinol Metab 1995;80:1577–1583
28. Saji M, Tsushima T, Isozaki O, et al. Interaction of insulin-like growth factor I with porcine thyroid cells cultured in monolayer. Endocrinology 1987;121:749–756
29. Tramontano D, Cushing GW, Moses AC, Ingbar SH. Insulin-like growth factor-I stimulates the growth of rat thyroid cells in culture and synergizes the stimulation of DNA synthesis induced by TSH and Graves'-IgG. Endocrinology 1986;119:940–942
30. Tode B, Serio M, Rotella CM, et al. Insulin-like growth factor-I: autocrine secretion by human thyroid follicular cells in primary culture. J Clin Endocrinol Metab 1989;69:639–647
31. Ezzat S, Forster MJ, Berchtold P, Redelmeier DA, Boerlin V, Harris AG. Acromegaly. Clinical and biochemical features in 500 patients. Medicine (Baltimore) 1994;73:233–240
32. Altstadt TJ, Azzarelli B, Bevering C, Edmondson J, Nelson PB. Acromegaly caused by a growth hormone-releasing hormone-secreting carcinoid tumor: case report. Neurosurgery 2002;50:1356–1359, discussion 1360
33. Bolanowski M, Schopohl J, Marciniak M, et al. Acromegaly due to GHRH-secreting large bronchial carcinoid. Complete recovery following tumor surgery. Exp Clin Endocrinol Diabetes 2002;110:188–192
34. Ezzat S, Asa SL, Stefaneanu L, et al. Somatotroph hyperplasia without pituitary adenoma associated with a long standing growth hormone-releasing hormone-producing bronchial carcinoid. J Clin Endocrinol Metab 1994;78:555–560

35. Holdaway IM, Rajasoorya RC, Gamble GD. Factors influencing mortality in acromegaly. J Clin Endocrinol Metab 2004;89:667–674
36. Orme SM, McNally RJ, Cartwright RA, Belchetz PE; United Kingdom Acromegaly Study Group. Mortality and cancer incidence in acromegaly: a retrospective cohort study. J Clin Endocrinol Metab 1998;83:2730–2734
37. Barzilay J, Heatley GJ, Cushing GW. Benign and malignant tumors in patients with acromegaly. Arch Intern Med 1991;151:1629–1632
38. Pines A, Rozen P, Ron E, Gilat T. Gastrointestinal tumors in acromegalic patients. Am J Gastroenterol 1985;80:266–269
39. Ron E, Gridley G, Hrubec Z, Page W, Arora S, Fraumeni JF Jr. Acromegaly and gastrointestinal cancer. Cancer 1991;68:1673–1677
40. Growth Hormone Research Society; Pituitary Society. Biochemical assessment and long-term monitoring in patients with acromegaly: statement from a joint consensus conference of the Growth Hormone Research Society and the Pituitary Society. J Clin Endocrinol Metab 2004;89:3099–3102
41. Barkan AL. Biochemical markers of acromegaly: GH vs. IGF-I. Growth Horm IGF Res 2004;14(Suppl A):S97–S100
42. Freda PU, Post KD, Powell JS, Wardlaw SL. Evaluation of disease status with sensitive measures of growth hormone secretion in 60 postoperative patients with acromegaly. J Clin Endocrinol Metab 1998;83:3808–3816
43. Jaffe CA, Friberg RD, Barkan AL. Suppression of growth hormone (GH) secretion by a selective GH-releasing hormone (GHRH) antagonist. Direct evidence for involvement of endogenous GHRH in the generation of GH pulses. J Clin Invest 1993;92:695–701
44. Plotsky PM, Vale W. Patterns of growth hormone-releasing factor and somatostatin secretion into the hypophysial-portal circulation of the rat. Science 1985;230:461–463
45. Vance ML, Kaiser DL, Evans WS, et al. Pulsatile growth hormone secretion in normal man during a continuous 24-hour infusion of human growth hormone releasing factor (1–40). Evidence for intermittent somatostatin secretion. J Clin Invest 1985;75:1584–1590
46. Christy NP. Choosing the best treatment for acromegaly. [Editorial] JAMA 1982;247:1320
47. Dimaraki EV, Jaffe CA, DeMott-Friberg R, Chandler WF, Barkan AL. Acromegaly with apparently normal GH secretion: implications for diagnosis and follow-up. J Clin Endocrinol Metab 2002;87:3537–3542
48. Melmed S, Casanueva FF, Cavagnini F, et al. Acromegaly Treatment Consensus Workshop Participants. Guidelines for acromegaly management. J Clin Endocrinol Metab 2002;87:4054–4058
49. Swearingen B, Barker FG II, Katznelson L, et al. Long-term mortality after transsphenoidal surgery and adjunctive therapy for acromegaly. J Clin Endocrinol Metab 1998;83:3419–3426
50. Ellison D, et al. Neuropathology: A Reference Text of CNS Pathology, 2nd ed. New York: Mosby; 2004
51. Yamada S, Aiba T, Sano T, et al. Growth hormone-producing pituitary adenomas: correlations between clinical characteristics and morphology. Neurosurgery 1993;33:20–27
52. Horvath E, Kovacs K. Pituitary gland. Pathol Res Pract 1988;183:129–142
53. Smallman LA, Dunn PJ, Curran RC, London DR. Pituitary adenomas producing growth hormone in acromegalic patients. J Clin Pathol 1984;37:382–389
54. Fusco A, Zatelli MC, Bianchi A, et al. Prognostic significance of the Ki-67 labeling index in growth hormone-secreting pituitary adenomas. J Clin Endocrinol Metab 2008;93:2746–2750
55. Trepp R, Stettler C, Zwahlen M, Seiler R, Diem P, Christ ER. Treatment outcomes and mortality of 94 patients with acromegaly. Acta Neurochir (Wien) 2005;147:243–251, discussion 250–251
56. Abosch A, Tyrrell JB, Lamborn KR, Hannegan LT, Applebury CB, Wilson CB. Transsphenoidal microsurgery for growth hormone-secreting pituitary adenomas: initial outcome and long-term results. J Clin Endocrinol Metab 1998;83:3411–3418
57. Davis DH, Laws ER Jr, Ilstrup DM, et al. Results of surgical treatment for growth hormone-secreting pituitary adenomas. J Neurosurg 1993;79:70–75
58. Ross DA, Wilson CB. Results of transsphenoidal microsurgery for growth hormone-secreting pituitary adenoma in a series of 214 patients. J Neurosurg 1988;68:854–867
59. Nomikos P, Buchfelder M, Fahlbusch R. The outcome of surgery in 668 patients with acromegaly using current criteria of biochemical 'cure'. Eur J Endocrinol 2005;152:379–387
60. Fahlbusch R, et al. Results of surgery in acromegaly. In: Wass AH, ed. Treating Acromegaly: 100 Years On. Bristol, England: Society of Endocrinology; 1994:49–54
61. Kreutzer J, Vance ML, Lopes MB, Laws ER Jr. Surgical management of GH-secreting pituitary adenomas: an outcome study using modern remission criteria. J Clin Endocrinol Metab 2001;86:4072–4077
62. Long H, Beauregard H, Somma M, Comtois R, Serri O, Hardy J. Surgical outcome after repeated transsphenoidal surgery in acromegaly. J Neurosurg 1996;85:239–247
63. Tindall GT, Oyesiku NM, Watts NB, Clark RV, Christy JH, Adams DA. Transsphenoidal adenomectomy for growth hormone-secreting pituitary adenomas in acromegaly: outcome analysis and determinants of failure. J Neurosurg 1993;78:205–215
64. Balagura S, Derome P, Guiot G. Acromegaly: analysis of 132 cases treated surgically. Neurosurgery 1981;8:413–416
65. Baskin DS, Boggan JE, Wilson CB. Transsphenoidal microsurgical removal of growth hormone-secreting pituitary adenomas. A review of 137 cases. J Neurosurg 1982;56:634–641
66. Faglia G, Paracchi A, Ferrari C, Beck-Peccoz P. Evaluation of the results of trans-sphenoidal surgery in acromegaly by assessment of the growth hormone response to thyrotrophin-releasing hormone. Clin Endocrinol (Oxf) 1978;8:373–380
67. Krieger MD, Couldwell WT, Weiss MH. Assessment of long-term remission of acromegaly following surgery. J Neurosurg 2003;98:719–724
68. Freda PU, Wardlaw SL, Post KD. Long-term endocrinological follow-up evaluation in 115 patients who underwent transsphenoidal surgery for acromegaly. J Neurosurg 1998;89:353–358
69. Shimon I, Cohen ZR, Ram Z, Hadani M. Transsphenoidal surgery for acromegaly: endocrinological follow-up of 98 patients. Neurosurgery 2001;48:1239–1243, discussion 1244–1245
70. Kaltsas GA, Isidori AM, Florakis D, et al. Predictors of the outcome of surgical treatment in acromegaly and the value of the mean growth hormone day curve in assessing postoperative disease activity. J Clin Endocrinol Metab 2001;86:1645–1652
71. Ludecke DK, Abe T. Transsphenoidal microsurgery for newly diagnosed acromegaly: a personal view after more than 1,000 operations. Neuroendocrinology 2006;83:230–239
72. Laws ER Jr, Fode NC, Redmond MJ. Transsphenoidal surgery following unsuccessful prior therapy. An assessment of benefits and risks in 158 patients. J Neurosurg 1985;63:823–829

73. Etxabe J, Gaztambide S, Latorre P, Vazquez JA. Acromegaly: an epidemiological study. J Endocrinol Invest 1993;16:181–187
74. Puchner MJ, Knappe UJ, Lüdecke DK. Pituitary surgery in elderly patients with acromegaly. Neurosurgery 1995;36:677–683, discussion 683–684
75. Minniti G, Jaffrain-Rea ML, Esposito V, et al. Surgical treatment and clinical outcome of GH-secreting adenomas in elderly patients. Acta Neurochir (Wien) 2001;143:1205–1211
76. Abe T, Lüdecke DK. Recent results of secondary transnasal surgery for residual or recurring acromegaly. Neurosurgery 1998;42:1013–1021, discussion 1021–1022
77. Biermasz NR, van Dulken H, Roelfsema F. Ten-year follow-up results of transsphenoidal microsurgery in acromegaly. J Clin Endocrinol Metab 2000;85:4596–4602
78. Freda PU, Nuruzzaman AT, Reyes CM, Sundeen RE, Post KD. Significance of "abnormal" nadir growth hormone levels after oral glucose in postoperative patients with acromegaly in remission with normal insulin-like growth factor-I levels. J Clin Endocrinol Metab 2004;89:495–500
79. Espinosa-de-los-Monteros AL, Mercado M, Sosa E, et al. Changing patterns of insulin-like growth factor-I and glucose-suppressed growth hormone levels after pituitary surgery in patients with acromegaly. J Neurosurg 2002;97:287–292
80. Ahmed S, Elsheikh M, Stratton IM, Page RC, Adams CB, Wass JA. Outcome of transsphenoidal surgery for acromegaly and its relationship to surgical experience. Clin Endocrinol (Oxf) 1999;50:561–567
81. Bates PR, Carson MN, Trainer PJ, Wass JA; UK National Acromegaly Register Study Group (UKAR-2). Wide variation in surgical outcomes for acromegaly in the UK. Clin Endocrinol (Oxf) 2008;68:136–142
82. De P, Rees DA, Davies N, et al. Transsphenoidal surgery for acromegaly in wales: results based on stringent criteria of remission. J Clin Endocrinol Metab 2003;88:3567–3572
83. Lissett CA, Peacey SR, Laing I, Tetlow L, Davis JR, Shalet SM. The outcome of surgery for acromegaly: the need for a specialist pituitary surgeon for all types of growth hormone (GH) secreting adenoma. Clin Endocrinol (Oxf) 1998;49:653–657
84. Ciric I, Ragin A, Baumgartner C, Pierce D. Complications of transsphenoidal surgery: results of a national survey, review of the literature, and personal experience. Neurosurgery 1997;40:225–236, discussion 236–237
85. Sheaves R, Jenkins P, Blackburn P, et al. Outcome of transsphenoidal surgery for acromegaly using strict criteria for surgical cure. Clin Endocrinol (Oxf) 1996;45:407–413
86. Beckers A. Does preoperative somatostatin analog treatment improve surgical cure rates in acromegaly? A new look at an old question. J Clin Endocrinol Metab 2008;93:2975–2977
87. Carlsen SM, Lund-Johansen M, Schreiner T, et al. Preoperative Octreotide Treatment of Acromegaly study group. Preoperative octreotide treatment in newly diagnosed acromegalic patients with macroadenomas increases cure short-term postoperative rates: a prospective, randomized trial. J Clin Endocrinol Metab 2008;93:2984–2990
88. McKeage K, Cheer S, Wagstaff AJ. Octreotide long-acting release (LAR): a review of its use in the management of acromegaly. Drugs 2003;63:2473–2499
89. Bevan JS, Atkin SL, Atkinson AB, et al. Primary medical therapy for acromegaly: an open, prospective, multicenter study of the effects of subcutaneous and intramuscular slow-release octreotide on growth hormone, insulin-like growth factor-I, and tumor size. J Clin Endocrinol Metab 2002;87:4554–4563
90. Newman CB, Melmed S, George A, et al. Octreotide as primary therapy for acromegaly. J Clin Endocrinol Metab 1998;83:3034–3040
91. Ezzat S, Snyder PJ, Young WF, et al. Octreotide treatment of acromegaly. A randomized, multicenter study. Ann Intern Med 1992;117:711–718
92. Newman CB. Medical therapy for acromegaly. Endocrinol Metab Clin North Am 1999;28:171–190
93. Colao A, Pivonello R, Auriemma RS, et al. Growth hormone-secreting tumor shrinkage after 3 months of octreotide-long-acting release therapy predicts the response at 12 months. J Clin Endocrinol Metab 2008;93:3436–3442
94. Fløgstad AK, Halse J, Bakke S, et al. Sandostatin LAR in acromegalic patients: long-term treatment. J Clin Endocrinol Metab 1997;82:23–28
95. Hunter SJ, Shaw JA, Lee KO, Wood PJ, Atkinson AB, Bevan JS. Comparison of monthly intramuscular injections of Sandostatin LAR with multiple subcutaneous injections of octreotide in the treatment of acromegaly; effects on growth hormone and other markers of growth hormone secretion. Clin Endocrinol (Oxf) 1999;50:245–251
96. Biermasz NR, van den Oever NC, Frölich M, et al. Sandostatin LAR in acromegaly: a 6-week injection interval suppresses GH secretion as effectively as a 4-week interval. Clin Endocrinol (Oxf) 2003;58:288–295
97. Lucas-Morante T, García-Uría J, Estrada J, et al. Treatment of invasive growth hormone pituitary adenomas with long-acting somatostatin analog SMS 201-995 before transsphenoidal surgery. J Neurosurg 1994;81:10–14
98. Clemmons DR, Chihara K, Freda PU, et al. Optimizing control of acromegaly: integrating a growth hormone receptor antagonist into the treatment algorithm. J Clin Endocrinol Metab 2003;88:4759–4767
99. Melmed S, Ho K, Klibanski A, Reichlin S, Thorner M. Clinical review 75: recent advances in pathogenesis, diagnosis, and management of acromegaly. J Clin Endocrinol Metab 1995;80:3395–3402
100. Seidman PA, Kofke WA, Policare R, Young M. Anaesthetic complications of acromegaly. Br J Anaesth 2000;84:179–182
101. Colao A, Cuocolo A, Marzullo P, et al. Effects of 1-year treatment with octreotide on cardiac performance in patients with acromegaly. J Clin Endocrinol Metab 1999;84:17–23
102. Lim MJ, Barkan AL, Buda AJ. Rapid reduction of left ventricular hypertrophy in acromegaly after suppression of growth hormone hypersecretion. Ann Intern Med 1992;117:719–726
103. Colao A, Ferone D, Cappabianca P, et al. Effect of octreotide pretreatment on surgical outcome in acromegaly. J Clin Endocrinol Metab 1997;82:3308–3314
104. Schmitt H, Buchfelder M, Radespiel-Tröger M, Fahlbusch R. Difficult intubation in acromegalic patients: incidence and predictability. Anesthesiology 2000;93:110–114
105. Trainer PJ, Drake WM, Katznelson L, et al. Treatment of acromegaly with the growth hormone-receptor antagonist pegvisomant. N Engl J Med 2000;342:1171–1177
106. Colao A, Marek J, Goth MI, et al. No greater incidence or worsening of cardiac valve regurgitation with somatostatin analog treatment of acromegaly. J Clin Endocrinol Metab 2008;93:2243–2248
107. Paisley AN, Trainer PJ, Drake WM. The place of pegvisomant in the acromegaly treatment algorithm. Growth Horm IGF Res 2004;14(Suppl A):S101–S106

108. Pivonello R, Galderisi M, Auriemma RS, et al. Treatment with growth hormone receptor antagonist in acromegaly: effect on cardiac structure and performance. J Clin Endocrinol Metab 2007;92:476–482
109. Neggers SJ, van Aken MO, de Herder WW, et al. Quality of life in acromegalic patients during long-term somatostatin analog treatment with and without pegvisomant. J Clin Endocrinol Metab 2008;93:3853–3859
110. Neggers SJ, van Aken MO, Janssen JA, Feelders RA, de Herder WW, van der Lely AJ. Long-term efficacy and safety of combined treatment of somatostatin analogs and pegvisomant in acromegaly. J Clin Endocrinol Metab 2007;92:4598–4601
111. Swords FM, Allan CA, Plowman PN, et al. Stereotactic radiosurgery XVI: a treatment for previously irradiated pituitary adenomas. J Clin Endocrinol Metab 2003;88:5334–5340
112. Roberts BK, Ouyang DL, Lad SP, et al. Efficacy and safety of CyberKnife radiosurgery for acromegaly. Pituitary 2007;10:19–25
113. McCollough WM, Marcus RB Jr, Rhoton AL Jr, Ballinger WE, Million RR. Long-term follow-up of radiotherapy for pituitary adenoma: the absence of late recurrence after greater than or equal to 4500 cGy. Int J Radiat Oncol Biol Phys 1991;21:607–614
114. Tsang RW, Brierley JD, Panzarella T, Gospodarowicz MK, Sutcliffe SB, Simpson WJ. Role of radiation therapy in clinical hormonally-active pituitary adenomas. Radiother Oncol 1996;41:45–53
115. Jackson IM, Noren G. Role of gamma knife radiosurgery in acromegaly. Pituitary 1999;2:71–77
116. Brada M, Rajan B, Traish D, et al. The long-term efficacy of conservative surgery and radiotherapy in the control of pituitary adenomas. Clin Endocrinol (Oxf) 1993;38:571–578
117. Wass JA. Long-term effects of radiotherapy for acromegaly. Metabolism 1996;45(8, Suppl 1):107–108
118. Barkan AL, Halasz I, Dornfeld KJ, et al. Pituitary irradiation is ineffective in normalizing plasma insulin-like growth factor I in patients with acromegaly. J Clin Endocrinol Metab 1997;82:3187–3191
119. Powell JS, Wardlaw SL, Post KD, Freda PU. Outcome of radiotherapy for acromegaly using normalization of insulin-like growth factor I to define cure. J Clin Endocrinol Metab 2000;85:2068–2071
120. Littley MD, Shalet SM, Swindell R, Beardwell CG, Sutton ML. Low-dose pituitary irradiation for acromegaly. Clin Endocrinol (Oxf) 1990;32:261–270
121. Landolt AM, Haller D, Lomax N, et al. Stereotactic radiosurgery for recurrent surgically treated acromegaly: comparison with fractionated radiotherapy. J Neurosurg 1998;88:1002–1008
122. Pollock BE, Nippoldt TB, Stafford SL, Foote RL, Abboud CF. Results of stereotactic radiosurgery in patients with hormone-producing pituitary adenomas: factors associated with endocrine normalization. J Neurosurg 2002;97:525–530
123. Attanasio R, Epaminonda P, Motti E, et al. Gamma-knife radiosurgery in acromegaly: a 4-year follow-up study. J Clin Endocrinol Metab 2003;88:3105–3112
124. Ikeda H, Jokura H, Yoshimoto T. Transsphenoidal surgery and adjuvant gamma knife treatment for growth hormone-secreting pituitary adenoma. J Neurosurg 2001;95:285–291
125. Jezková J, Marek J, Hána V, et al. Gamma knife radiosurgery for acromegaly—long-term experience. Clin Endocrinol (Oxf) 2006;64:588–595
126. Vik-Mo EO, Oksnes M, Pedersen PH, et al. Gamma knife stereotactic radiosurgery for acromegaly. Eur J Endocrinol 2007;157:255–263
127. Lim YL, Leem W, Kim TS, Rhee BA, Kim GK. Four years' experiences in the treatment of pituitary adenomas with gamma knife radiosurgery. Stereotact Funct Neurosurg 1998;70(Suppl 1):95–109
128. Mokry M, Ramschak-Schwarzer S, Simbrunner J, Ganz JC, Pendl G. A six year experience with the postoperative radiosurgical management of pituitary adenomas. Stereotact Funct Neurosurg 1999;72(Suppl 1):88–100
129. Jagannathan J, Sheehan JP, Pouratian N, Laws ER Jr, Steiner L, Vance ML. Gamma knife radiosurgery for acromegaly: outcomes after failed transsphenoidal surgery. Neurosurgery 2008;62:1262–1269, discussion 1269–1270
130. Landolt AM, Haller D, Lomax N, et al. Octreotide may act as a radioprotective agent in acromegaly. J Clin Endocrinol Metab 2000; 85:1287–1289
131. Pollock BE, Jacob JT, Brown PD, Nippoldt TB. Radiosurgery of growth hormone-producing pituitary adenomas: factors associated with biochemical remission. J Neurosurg 2007;106:833–838
132. Biermasz NR, van Dulken H, Roelfsema F. Long-term follow-up results of postoperative radiotherapy in 36 patients with acromegaly. J Clin Endocrinol Metab 2000;85:2476–2482
133. Tishler RB, Loeffler JS, Lunsford LD, et al. Tolerance of cranial nerves of the cavernous sinus to radiosurgery. Int J Radiat Oncol Biol Phys 1993;27:215–221

11 Cushing's Disease

Charles A. Sansur, Stephen J. Monteith, and Edward H. Oldfield

Cushing's disease (CD) is generally recognized as being best treated with surgery. Careful preoperative assessment and good surgical technique are the most reliable methods of achieving the optimal outcome: elimination of hypercortisolism, permanent eradication of the tumor, and preservation of pituitary function while avoiding complications. Depending on the surgeon's experience and the specific characteristics of the lesion, one can often feel confident in offering the patient a likely cure while preserving normal pituitary function. If surgery alone is unsuccessful, in almost all patients hypercortisolism can be eliminated with irradiation therapy or bilateral adrenalectomy. To better convey our surgical strategy for the treatment of patients with CD, we first discuss the preoperative evaluation of patients with Cushing's syndrome, as well as the histopathologic findings that form the basis of our surgical technique.

Pathology

Cushing's disease is caused by an adrenocorticotropic hormone (ACTH)-secreting adenoma. As such, the adenomas stain for ACTH using immunohistochemistry and, as with other types of pituitary tumors, they are monoclonal in origin.[1] They disrupt the normal acinar pattern of the gland when stained for reticulin. When no definite tumor is identified at surgery and partial or total hypophysectomy is performed, the tissue specimen is examined using closely spaced sequential slices because tumors as small as 1 mm in diameter or less can be the source of CD. In the event that no tumor is found, the diagnosis of corticotroph hyperplasia is entertained if there is histologic evidence of hyperplasia, and a peripheral venous level of corticotropin-releasing hormone (CRH) is obtained to assess this possibility further. In the experience of the senior author, corticotroph hyperplasia is exceedingly rare (only two suspected, but unproven, cases from over 900 operations for CD). In the presence of sustained hypercortisolism a unique cytoplasmic staining pattern, known as Crooke's hyaline change, occurs in the normal corticotrophs of the pituitary from which ACTH production has been shut down. The "hyaline" is composed of intracytoplasmic microfilaments that do not stain for ACTH. Crooke's changes may also be found in the ACTH-staining cells of the adenoma itself.

It is important to note that pituitary adenomas compress the immediately adjacent normal anterior lobe, producing a histologic pseudocapsule, which has surgical implications. Although the presence of a histologic pseudocapsule around pituitary tumors was noted in the early 1900s, until recently the sequence of the stages of its development was unexplored. In 2006 a study reported the examination of pseudocapsule development by histologic analysis of portions of pituitary glands removed during operations for CD in patients in whom no adenoma could be identified during surgery.[2] The distribution of tumor size and its relation to the presence of a histologic pseudocapsule were examined. A multilayered reticulin capsule occurred in tumors that exceeded 2 to 3 mm in maximum diameter. For tumors 1 mm or smaller, there was no reticulin capsule. The absence of this reticulin capsule in cases of very small tumors contributes to difficulty with their identification during surgical exploration of the pituitary gland in patients with CD and negative magnetic resonance imaging (MRI). On the other hand, for lesions larger than 2 mm the presence of the pseudocapsule enveloping the adenoma contributes to the identification of microadenomas buried in the pituitary gland during surgery, even in patients with negative MRI, and allows consistency of complete tumor excision.[2–4]

Diagnosis

It is imperative to have complete and accurate diagnostic testing before surgery is considered. The most commonly used tests to detect hypercortisolism, and establish the presence of Cushing's syndrome, are serial 24-hour urine free cortisol (UFC) measurements to establish excess cortisol secretion, diurnal plasma cortisol levels, or evening salivary cortisol levels to detect loss of diurnal rhythm of cortisol secretion, and the overnight low-dose dexamethasone suppression test to detect a relative resistance to negative feedback by glucocorticoids.

The UFC measurements are assayed using a variety of techniques. The normal upper levels vary with the technique used and with the laboratory performing the assay. Hypercortisolism is associated with the loss of normal diurnal variation in cortisol secretion, which is demonstrated by obtaining morning (8 to 9 a.m.) and evening (11 p.m. to 12 midnight) plasma cortisol levels. Salivary cortisol levels are also reliably used for this purpose and are well suited for outpatient screening of adult and pediatric patients for hypercortisolism.[5] A study of more than 140 patients demonstrated a sensitivity of 93% and a specificity of 100% using this test to determine the presence of Cushing's syndrome.[6]

The low-dose (1-mg) dexamethasone suppression test is commonly used to detect abnormal regulation of cortisol secretion. The overnight test, rather than the 2-day test, is the most commonly used test today. In persons with a normal hypothalamic-pituitary-adrenal axis, morning cortisol levels are suppressed by the overnight low-dose dexamethasone suppression test (1.0 mg given the night before a morning [7 to 8 a.m.] cortisol measurement). A morning plasma cortisol level greater than 1.8 µg/dL after the bedtime (11 p.m.) administration of 1 mg of dexamethasone detects most patients with Cushing's syndrome and justifies further diagnostic evaluation.[7]

When hypercortisolism has been found, one must determine whether the process is ACTH-dependent or ACTH-independent. With Cushing's disease or ectopic ACTH secretion, the ACTH levels will be normal or elevated. In contrast, in adrenal disease, because of the negative feedback of the high cortisol levels on hypothalamic CRH production and secretion and on pituitary ACTH production and secretion, plasma ACTH is undetectable or low (<5 pg/mL) relative to the degree of glucocorticoid secretion. For this reason, these two entities are categorized as ACTH-dependent, in contrast with adrenal tumors in ACTH-independent Cushing's syndrome, as the adrenal cortical cortisol secretion is autonomous.

In patients with Cushing's syndrome the differential diagnosis of Cushing's disease from adrenal disease and ectopic ACTH secretion can be accomplished through the high-dose overnight dexamethasone suppression test. For this test, 8 mg of dexamethasone is administered orally at 11 p.m. and morning (7 to 8 a.m.) plasma cortisol measurements are obtained; suppression of morning serum cortisol of greater than 68% is required to assign a diagnosis of CD,[8,9] although greater sensitivity is obtained if more than 90% suppression is used.

The CRH stimulation test is also used to differentiate between ectopic ACTH-secretion and an ACTH-secreting pituitary tumor.[10–12] Because ACTH secreting adenomas are well-differentiated tumors derived from pituitary corticotrophs, most ACTH-secreting adenomas respond to CRH. Ectopic tumors, not being derived from pituitary tissue, do not express receptors for CRH and therefore do not respond to it. The sensitivity and specificity of the test are optimal using ≥35% for the maximum ACTH response from the 15- or 30-minute samples to indicate Cushing's disease.[13]

The presence of ACTH-dependent hypercortisolism leads to an MRI focused on the sella. In many patients with CD a high-resolution pituitary MRI will demonstrate the presence and location of a pituitary tumor. However, a negative MRI does not rule out an adenoma. The false-negative rate using the standard T1-weighted spin echo after contrast enhancement in Cushing's disease is as high as 40 to 50% at many centers (**Fig. 11.1**).[14]

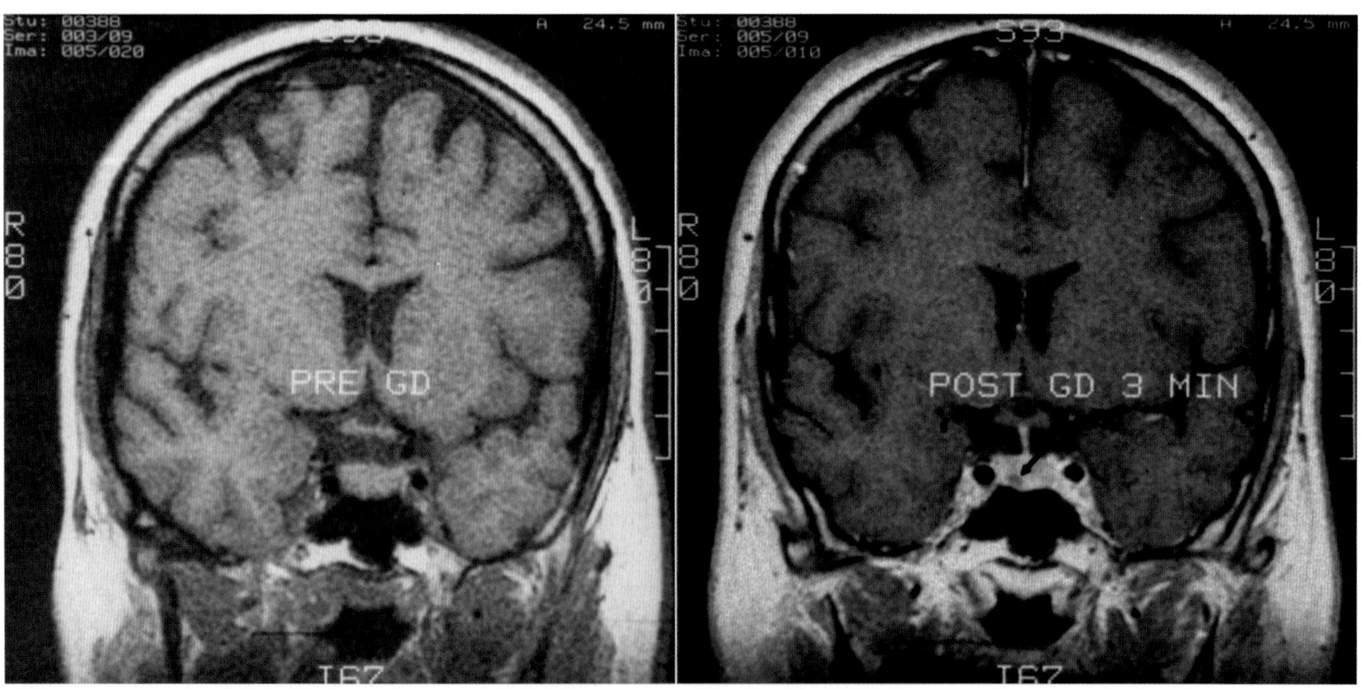

Fig. 11.1 Pre– and post–gadolinium-enhanced coronal spoiled gradient (SPGR) magnetic resonance imaging scan demonstrating an adenoma in the right anterior aspect of the pituitary gland. The SPGR technique with 1-mm cuts has improved sensitivity in finding small adenomas.

If the high-dose dexamethasone suppression test and the CRH stimulation test are consistent with CD and the pituitary MRI reveals an adenoma, no further diagnostic testing is necessary. However, if either of the provocative endocrine tests is inconsistent with CD, or the MRI does not reveal an adenoma, inferior petrosal sinus sampling (IPSS) is performed. IPSS has the greatest diagnostic accuracy of the available tests for the differential diagnosis of CD versus ectopic ACTH syndrome.[15] By placing catheters into the inferior petrosal sinuses and a peripheral vein, one can obtain simultaneous samples for central and peripheral plasma ACTH concentrations at 2 and 0 minutes before and 3, 5, and 10 minutes after intravenous CRH administration (1 µg/kg body weight). IPSS is used only in patients with confirmed hypercortisolism, as the test cannot discriminate between normal subjects and patients with CD. Because this is an invasive procedure with rare but serious associated risks,[16] it is reserved for patients in whom the results of provocative endocrine testing are conflicting or equivocal and in instances where there is no lesion found on MRI. A peak central ACTH concentration to peripheral ACTH concentration ratio of 2:1 during baseline (before CRH) or 3:1 before or after CRH is diagnostic of CD.[15] Although reports of false-negative results exist,[17] these are often due to improper placement of the catheter tips, and in our experience the diagnostic accuracy approaches 100% in patients who undergo successful sampling bilaterally. Because the accuracy of the test relies on successful placement of the catheter tips in the inferior petrosal sinuses bilaterally, venography is performed to confirm placement and evaluate the venous anatomy. It is important to note that IPSS does not reliably allow lateralization of MRI-negative adenomas, as the lateralization accuracy is only approximately 70% in patients with microadenomas identified at surgery, compromising its usefulness as a localizing measure during surgery.[15]

Imaging

Magnetic resonance imaging is the imaging modality of choice for detection of pituitary adenomas. Aside from detecting the presence of tumors and defining their anatomy, MRI provides anatomical information that is useful during the surgical approach. In particular, the anatomy of the sphenoid sinus and the parasellar anatomy, and the location of the carotid arteries can be assessed from an MRI scan. Recently the spoiled gradient recalled acquisition technique, used with 1-mm nonoverlapping slices, was shown to be more sensitive than the conventional spin echo approach (sensitivity 80% versus 49%) in detecting adenomas in patients with CD.[18] Because the sensitivity of the conventional MRI techniques (spin echo) for CD (**Fig. 11.1**) is only 50 to 75%,[19–22] many patients have a negative MRI. When interpreting the results of an MRI scan, one must keep in mind that pituitary adenomas are found incidentally in 10% of normal volunteers and in 5 to 20% of random autopsy specimens. Incidental adenomas may also be identified during surgery.[23,24] It is therefore important to establish the diagnosis of CD through endocrine testing before performing surgery.

Surgery

As discussed previously in the pathology section, the pseudocapsule can be used as a surgical capsule in the surgical treatment of microadenomas. The discussion in this section reflects the surgical technique of the senior author, which has been developed over several years of experience.

Initially a wide, bloodless exposure of the sella is established. Using a drill with a 3- to 4-mm bur, the bone covering the anterior and inferior surfaces of the sella is thinned to less than 0.5-mm thickness, and then an initial opening of the anterior face of the sella turcica (**Fig. 11.2**) is performed. In patients with a positive MRI, the initial opening is made away from the tumor, over the normal anterior lobe. A 2-mm Kerrison rongeur with a thin distal lip (0.75 mm) is used to remove the remaining thin layer of bone of the anterior sella face in small increments. The bone is removed laterally until at least 2 mm of the most medial aspect of each cavernous sinus is visible. Superiorly bone removal extends to the tuberculum sellae. Inferiorly, a disk dissector is used to separate gently the dura from the bone of the sella floor after the anterior face of the sella has been removed. The sella floor is then removed with a small pituitary rongeur. Oozing bone margins are covered with a thin layer of bone wax. Because of the very low pressure in the cavernous sinus and the smaller dural veins draining into it, the same technique, or placement of small pieces of Gelfoam soaked in thrombin, can be used successfully for any site that slowly oozes blood from the layer between the dura and bone at the margins of the bone removal. At this stage the operative field should be bloodless and should expose the entire anterior sella dura and most of the inferior dura covering the pituitary. Inspection of the dura reveals any region of invasion of the anterior or inferior dura. In cases of small tumors that reach the anterior surface of the pituitary gland, careful examination of the dural surface may provide clues to the site of the tumor. Coagulation of the dura is avoided during the exposure because it tends to adhere the dura to the underlying pituitary capsule and because coagulation produces a region of white discoloration of the pituitary capsule and the contiguous region of gland immediately beneath it, a change in color that may be misleading in the search for small, gray-white adenomas of CD. The dura is opened using a no. 15 scalpel, with care taken to make the incision completely through the dura but not to enter the capsule of the pituitary gland.

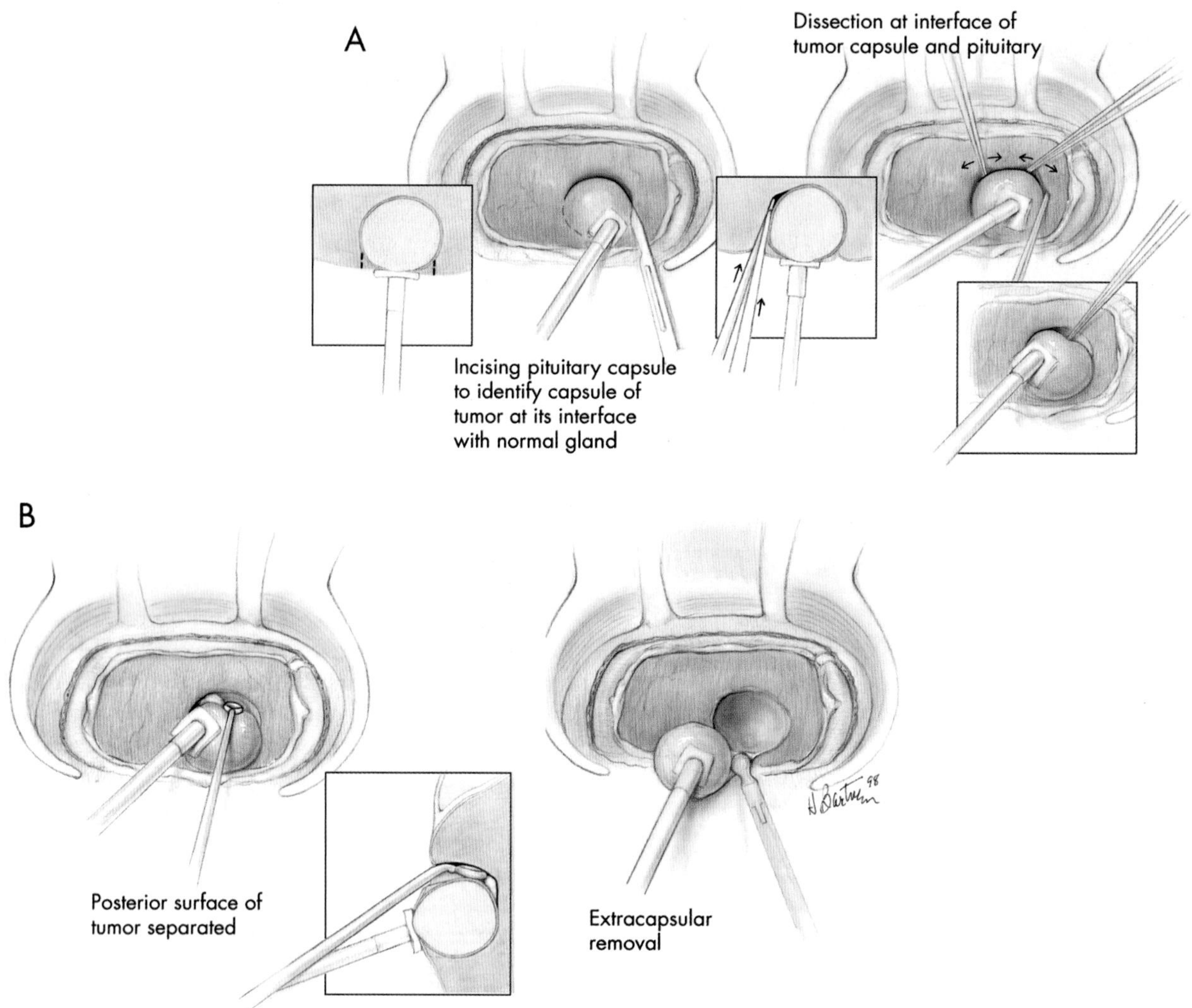

Fig. 11.2 Illustration of the surgical technique. A curvilinear incision is made through the pituitary capsule just beyond the point at which the most superficial dome of the tumor reaches the surface of the gland (**A**, *left*). This permits a thin layer of normal gland to be passed through before reaching the surgical capsule of the adenoma (*left inset*), allowing easy identification of the surgical capsule and the creation of a surgical plane of dissection at the margin of the tumor, at the interface of the normal gland and the surgical capsule of the adenoma. This interface is further defined using the tips of the bipolar forceps in a series of movements parallel to the surface of the adenoma and in the crevice between the gland and the adenoma (**B**, *right* and *center*). Gentle dissection of the interface between the adenoma and gland is continued following the curvilinear margin of the adenoma. After the most superficial portion of the tumor has been defined circumferentially, the deeper adenoma margins are defined and dissected in a similar fashion **(B)**; the posterior margin of the adenoma often requires dissection using a disk dissector and a small or medium ring curette (**B**, *center*). After the margins of the tumor have been completely dissected, to prevent rupture of the tumor the last remaining connection between the pseudocapsule of the specimen and the pituitary capsule is grasped with a small cup forceps and the tumor is removed (**B**, *right*). In cases of tumors 8 to 10 mm or less in diameter, the entire tumor can usually be shelled out of its bed in the anterior lobe as an intact specimen. Successful and complete removal leaves a smoothly lined hemispherical tissue void in the anterior lobe. (From Oldfield EH, Vortmeyer AO. Development of a histological pseudocapsule and its use as a surgical capsule in the excision of pituitary tumors. J Neurosurg 2006;104:7–19. Reprinted with permission.)

To achieve the widest available exposure, the superior margins of the incisions are extended laterally to reach the interface of the circular sinus and the medial margin of the cavernous sinus. To achieve wide exposure the cavernous sinus is often intentionally entered along the superior and lateral margin of the exposure, where the lateral aspect of the circular sinus meets the medial aspect of the superior portion of the cavernous sinus. Low-pressure venous bleeding from any opening in the cavernous sinus is controlled by simply plugging the opening with a small piece of Gelfoam moistened in thrombin. To achieve a wide exposure laterally and inferiorly, the medial inferior region of the cavernous sinus is frequently opened during the lateralmost extent of the incision, and bleeding is controlled in a similar fashion. The dura is gently and cleanly separated from the pituitary capsule by using a disk dissector in the tissue plane between these layers. This exposes the entire anterior surface of the pituitary gland with an intact pituitary capsule in a bloodless field. Similar to the pia mater, the capsule of the pituitary gland is a strong layer despite its translucent nature and, even though it is visible histologically, the capsule is invisible to the surgeon. It must be cut sharply as blunt dissection will transfer pressure to the interior of the gland and to the tumor, potentially causing the tumor to rupture.

When dealing with tumors within the gland that are visible on MRI, the initial incision is not made directly into the tumor. A curvilinear incision is made through the pituitary capsule just beyond the point at which the most superficial dome of the tumor reaches the surface of the gland. This permits the incision to pass through a thin layer of normal gland before reaching the surgical capsule of the adenoma, allowing identification of the interface between the pseudocapsule of the tumor and the surrounding anterior lobe and the creation of a surgical plane of dissection at the margin of the tumor, at the interface of the normal gland and the surgical capsule of the adenoma (the histologic pseudocapsule). This interface between the adenoma and gland is further defined using the tips of the bipolar forceps in a series of movements parallel to the surface of the adenoma and in the crevice between the gland and the adenoma. If the correct tissue plane is used, the dissection is unimpeded and the gray–white surface of the adenoma is spherical and smooth. After this interface has been clearly defined, gentle dissection of the interface between the adenoma and gland is continued following the curvilinear margin of the adenoma, and with further incisions in the capsule of the pituitary gland just beyond the tumor margin to release tension on the tumor as the dissection proceeds. A small Hardy sucker (2-mm tip) on the margin of a cotton pad is used to provide separation of the interface between the gland and the adenoma for dissection and for sponging the small amount of bleeding out of the field of view. The posterior margin of the adenoma often requires dissection using a disk dissector and a small or medium ring curette. This is performed gently; very little pressure is required if the correct tissue plane is being used, and the limited pressure that is applied is directed at the dissection plane, slightly more toward the gland than the adenoma. After the margins of the tumor have been completely dissected, to prevent rupture of the tumor, the last remaining connection between the pseudocapsule of the specimen and the pituitary capsule is grasped with a small cup forceps and the tumor is removed. In cases of tumors 8 to 10 mm or less in diameter, the entire tumor can usually be shelled out of its bed in the anterior lobe as an intact specimen. Successful and complete removal leaves a smoothly lined hemispherical tissue void in the anterior lobe.

If the tumor breaches the capsule of the pituitary gland, careful inspection of the contiguous dura is performed to ensure that dural invasion by the tumor is not overlooked. This is particularly important laterally along the medial wall of the cavernous sinus, where even small tumors may spread into the adjacent dura and cavernous sinus.

In the rare instance when an ACTH-secreting adenoma is located outside of the adenohypophysis, such as in a suprasellar or parasellar location,[25] special techniques are required. For tumors of the pituitary stalk in the suprasellar cistern, an extended transsphenoidal approach may be used.[26] With this technique, during the standard midline approach, bone removal is extended rostrally to include the tuberculum sella and the most posterior 6 to 8 mm of the planum sphenoidale. The dura superior and anterior to the gland is opened to expose the suprasellar cistern. Bleeding from the opened circular sinus is interrupted by packing it with small pieces of Gelfoam or with bipolar coagulation. Direct visual access of the pituitary stalk is thus provided.

In patients in whom a lesion is not identified on the preoperative MRI, the surgeon must explore the gland and locate the distinct encapsulated margin of the adenoma intraoperatively (**Fig. 11.3**). Coagulation of the sella dura is avoided during exposure of the pituitary because this can produce a white area on the surface of the underlying gland that may falsely suggest the presence of an adenoma. The dura is widely opened, revealing an intact pituitary capsule and the extreme lateral margins of the anterior surface. This is carefully inspected for regions of focal discoloration. The adenoma usually appears to be a gray–blue or yellow–white nodule and can be identified against the background of the anterior lobe surface whose color is orange–red. If no tumor is seen, the lateral surfaces of the anterior lobe are then inspected by passing a disk dissector outside the capsule of the pituitary, between the lateral margin of the gland and the lateral dural wall of the sella (the medial wall of the cavernous sinus). Using fine-tipped bipolar forceps, this space can be dissected superficially and then more deeply until the posterior sella has been reached. After these two tissues have been separated, small pieces of Gelfoam are packed into the intervening space to rotate the lateral surface of the pituitary anteriorly and to gently displace it medially into the surgeon's direct view. After both lateral surfaces are exposed and examined in this fashion, the inferior surface of the gland is separated from the dura. If a tumor can be identified from inspection of the surface, it is removed as described. If no tumor is identified on inspection of the superficial gland, a series of vertical incisions is then made, each of which begins 1 to 2 mm below the superior edge of the pituitary exposure and is directed downward, initially to a depth of only approximately 1 mm, and then in stages deeper through the anterior lobe until either the intermediate

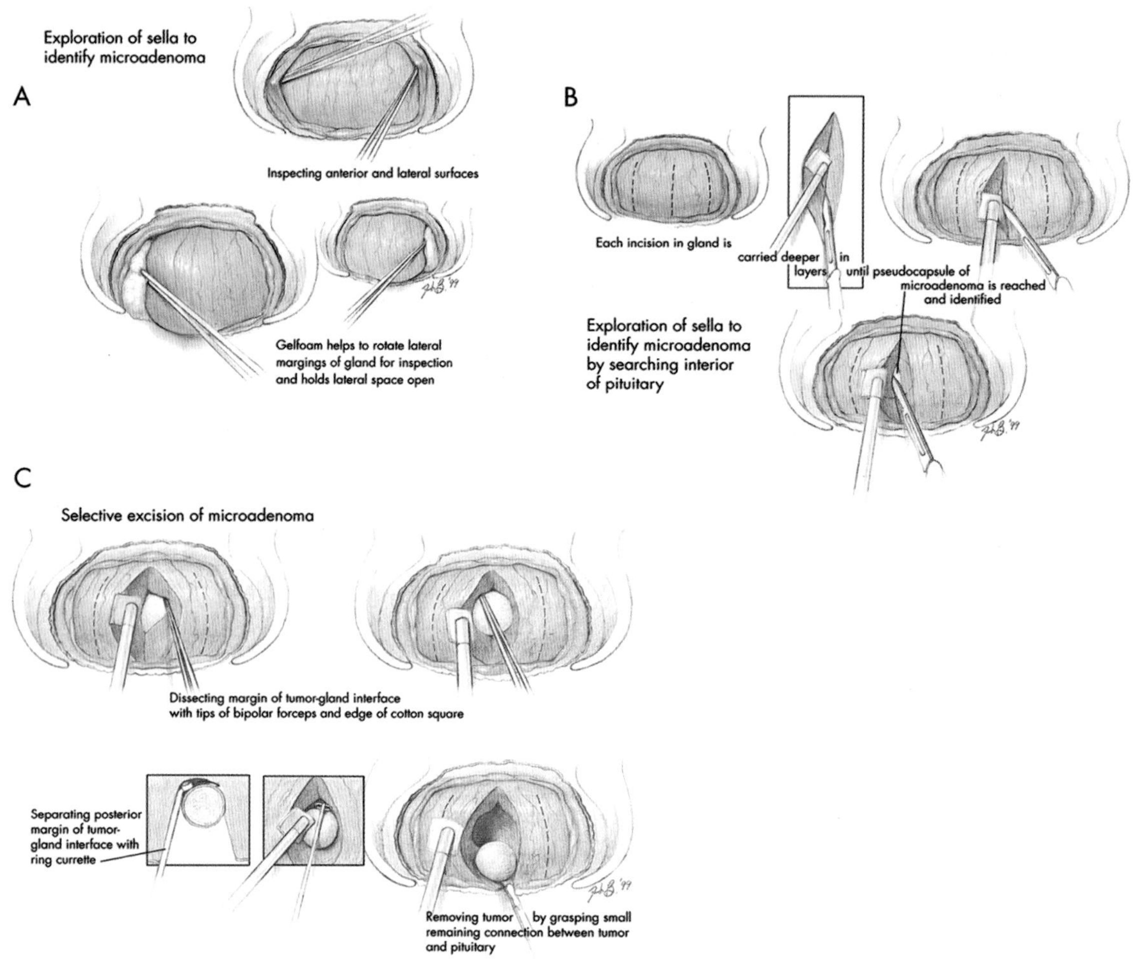

Fig. 11.3 Exploration of the pituitary gland in patients with an endocrine-active adenoma whose imaging studies appear normal. The goal of the exploration is to find and identify the distinct encapsulated margin of the adenoma. Success depends on beginning with a widely exposed, bloodless surgical field **(A)**. Coagulation of the anterior and inferior sella dura is avoided during the exposure and dural opening because it would produce a white area on the surface of the underlying gland that may falsely suggest the site of the adenoma. After widely opening the dura, which provides exposure of an intact pituitary capsule covering the anterior surface of the gland, and after exposure of the extreme lateral margins of the anterior surface, the surfaces are carefully inspected for regions of focal discoloration. The adenoma usually appears to be gray–blue or yellow–white, and can be identified against the background of the anterior lobe surface whose color is orange–pink. **(B)** If no tumor is seen, the lateral surfaces of the anterior lobe are then inspected. For this the lateral dural wall of the sella (the medial wall of the cavernous sinus) is separated from the pituitary capsule by gently passing a disk dissector between these two layers from top to bottom. The space produced provides room for dissection of the interface between the lateral pituitary capsule and the dural wall with the closed tips of a fine-tipped bipolar forceps **(B)**. Dissection is initially superficial and then progresses in stages to deeper levels until the posterior sella has been reached. After these two tissues have been separated, small pieces of Gelfoam are packed into the intervening space to rotate the lateral surface anteriorly and to gently displace it medially into the surgeon's direct view. After both lateral surfaces are exposed and examined in this fashion, the inferior surface of the gland is separated from the dura. (This is the site at which these two layers—the surface of the pituitary and the dura mater—are most tenaciously attached to each other.) If a tumor can be identified from inspection of the surface, it is removed as described in the text and the legend to **Fig. 11.2**. If no tumor is identified on inspection of the superficial gland, a series of vertical incisions is then made **(B)**, each of which begins 1 to 2 mm below the superior edge of the pituitary exposure and is directed downward, initially to a depth of only approximately 1 mm, and then in stages deeper through the anterior lobe until either the intermediate lobe or the glistening white anterior surface of the posterior lobe is reached. Because the pituitary blood supply and the delivery of hypothalamic trophic factors to the pituitary are oriented vertically, vertical incisions should be less likely to cause an infarction in a portion of the pituitary or to isolate the gland from its hypothalamic regulation. A distinct tissue capsule is the primary object of the search, with the intent to identify the margin of the tumor before entering it and spilling its contents, by using the surgical capsule of the adenoma **(B,C)**. When the surgical capsule of the adenoma is identified, the tumor is removed using dissection along the interface of the adenoma and the normal gland, as described in **Fig. 11.2**. In cases of tumors lying in the posterior portion of the anterior lobe, a 2-mm-wide slice of the anterior lobe may be removed to provide space for dissection and removal of the deep microadenoma (not shown). (From Oldfield EH, Vortmeyer AO. Development of a histological pseudocapsule and its use as a surgical capsule in the excision of pituitary tumors. J Neurosurg 2006;104:7–19. Reprinted with permission.)

lobe or the glistening white anterior surface of the posterior lobe is reached. A distinct tissue capsule is the primary object of the search, with the intent to identify the pseudocapsule of the tumor without penetrating it and spilling its contents. With the capsule exposed, the tumor is removed using dissection along the interface of the adenoma and the normal gland. In cases of tumors lying in the posterior portion of the anterior lobe, a 2-mm-wide slice of the anterior lobe may be removed to provide space for dissection and removal of the deep microadenoma.[2]

Surgical Results of Case Series Reported in the Literature

For ACTH-secreting tumors that are detected on imaging and contained within the anterior lobe of the gland, conventional microsurgical technique, in which an incision is made in the tumor and the tumor is removed from within, has been the standard treatment. Hofmann et al[27] in 2008 reported their long-term results for the microsurgical technique. They assessed their results in 426 primary operations over 35 years. Immediate remission of hypercortisolism was achieved in 292 of the 426 operations (69%). In patients in whom an adenoma was identified and removed, after selective adenomectomy the remission rate was 75.9%. This rate showed no improvement over the years. The best results were achieved in microadenomas confirmed on MRI or with positive histopathologic investigation. The recurrence rate (15%) and the complication rate (5.9%) declined over the years. If no adenoma was found, exploration of the sella turcica was performed in 45.6% of cases, with hypophysectomy in 3.5% of cases, and hemihypophysectomy in 50.9% of these patients, leading to an early remission in 37.9%. In another large series of 215 patients limited to patients with microadenomas, surgical remission was achieved in 86%.[28] The recurrence rate in the 184 patients who initially achieved remission was 25.5% at 5 years but reached 46% in patients followed up for longer than 5 years. The same study found that those patients with immediate postoperative hypocortisolemia of >2 µg/dL were 2.5 times more likely to have a recurrence than patients who had a serum cortisol ≤2 µg/dL.

Using the pseudocapsular extraction technique described for encapsulated adenomas, Oldfield's group[3] achieved 100% resolution of hypercortisolism in 261 patients prior to hospital discharge. Of the 261 patients in the study, 135 patients (52%) had a positive MRI whereas 126 patients (48%) had a normal MRI. After a mean clinical follow-up of 84 months (range 12–215 months), six patients (2.3%) had recurrence of hypercortisolism but all were successfully retreated with surgery. These results imply that the use of the pseudocapsule allows reliable identification of the tumor at surgery and for its complete excision.

Endonasal endoscopic approaches to the sella are being examined to assess their utility for resection of ACTH-secreting adenomas. Long-term results are as yet unestablished. Two recent studies using a purely endoscopic approach reported remission rates of 77 and 80%.[29,30] A recent study from the Mayo Clinic assessed whether the type of surgical approach to the sella (conventional microsurgical or endoscopic) had an affect on the surgical outcome among patients with CD.[31] In this study, they identified 42 adults with CD undergoing initial surgery for MRI-visible microadenomas and with a minimal follow-up of 3 months. They had 21 microsurgery patients and 21 endoscopic patients. There was no significant difference in complication rates for cerebrospinal fluid leak and transient diabetes insipidus in these groups or cure rate (86% initial remission; 76% relapse-included remission). We emphasize that all these series included only a small number of patients and have limited follow-up, and the recurrence rates are unknown.

Postoperative Assessment

To determine the success of surgery during the immediate postoperative period, replacement therapy is not administered, and serum cortisol levels are obtained while the patient is still hospitalized. When the cortisol level has dropped to less than 2 µg/dL, or the patient develops symptoms of hypocortisolism, patients begin to receive replacement hydrocortisone therapy. This immediate determination of surgical success provides the surgeon with the potential to offer early reoperation, if indicated.[32,33] The complete removal of the abnormal source of ACTH should produce hypocortisolism not only in the immediate postoperative period but also for several months. Because it takes several months for the hypothalamic-pituitary-adrenal axis to recover, these patients require replacement therapy for approximately 6 to 24 months. Thus, in almost all instances of successful surgery for CD, the patient will be hypocortisolemic during this period.

Without glucocorticoid replacement, the patient may develop addisonian crisis. These symptoms include lethargy, headache, anorexia, and abdominal discomfort or nausea. The patient's blood pressure is normal or even low, and patients who have previously been hypertensive may need to stop the antihypertensive medications. Similarly, because glycemic control may be restored after surgery, preoperative diabetic medications are withheld, and blood glucose is monitored in the immediate postoperative state. Patients are discharged with daily physiologic cortisol replacement, administered in the morning and the evening. A popular choice is hydrocortisone, 15 to 20 mg in the morning and 5 mg in the evening, until normal function of the hypothalamic-pituitary-adrenal axis is reestablished. The patient is told to stop taking the replacement hydrocortisone for 2 days before each return appointment so that the autonomous cortisol production can be assessed.

When patients develop a eucortisolic state immediately after surgery or within a few weeks of surgery, clinical remission is still likely. These patients must be advised, however, that recurrence of CD is more likely to occur than in patients with postoperative hypocortisolism.[34]

Early Repeat Surgery

If results of cortisol measurement shortly after surgery indicate persistent hypercortisolism, immediate repeat surgery should be considered in certain circumstances.[33] Early reoperation (within 1–6 weeks) can induce remission in many patients. However, there is an increased risk of hypopituitarism in this circumstance. The best candidates for early repeat surgery are those patients who have had incompletely resected adenomas, as evidenced by persistent hypercortisolism in the face of pathologic confirmation of an ACTH-positive adenoma. Patients who have undergone limited exploration of the pituitary and selective excision of an area that at surgery appeared to be, but proved not to have been, an adenoma also are good candidates for repeat surgery. However, patients who had an extensive exploration and partial resection of the anterior lobe are unlikely to benefit from a repeat operation if there is no ACTH-positive adenoma in the excised specimen.[33] With appropriate patient selection, early repeat surgery warrants consideration, especially when prompt control of hypercortisolism is required.

Surgical Management of Recurrent Cushing's Disease

Patients who have remission of hypercortisolism following surgery occasionally develop recurrent CD. In a report detailing the results of transsphenoidal surgery in 31 patients who had previously undergone a transsphenoidal operation and two patients who had had previous pituitary irradiation only, in 24 (73%) of the 33 patients, remission of hypercortisolism was achieved by surgery.[32] Although computed tomography imaging identified an adenoma in only three of the 33 patients, in 20 patients a discrete adenoma was identified at pituitary exploration. The incidence of remission of hypercortisolism was greatest if an adenoma was identified at surgery and the patient received selective adenomectomy (19 [95%] of 20 patients), if there was evidence at surgery or by preoperative imaging that the previous surgical exposure of the pituitary was incomplete (seven [78%] of nine patients), if an adenoma was seen on preoperative imaging (three of three patients), or if the patient had had prior pituitary irradiation without surgery (two of two patients). In contrast to the results in patients with selective adenomectomy, only five (42%) of 12 patients who received subtotal or total hypophysectomy had remission of hypercortisolism. Surgically induced hypopituitarism occurred in six (50%) of these 12 patients, but in only one (5%) of the 20 patients who underwent selective adenomectomy. Three (13%) of the 24 patients who were in remission from hypercortisolism following repeat surgery developed recurrent hypercortisolism 10 to 47 months postoperatively.

A recent report describes remission of recurrent CD by surgical treatment using the endoscopic approach in 71% of 14 patients. No patient had a relapse during a median follow-up of 24 months. Cerebrospinal fluid leakage occurred in six patients, and 11 patients required hormonal replacement therapy after surgery.[35]

It is now established that in patients with recurrent CD the recurrent adenoma is always at, or immediately contiguous to, the site of the adenoma at the original surgery.[36,37] Furthermore, the recurrent tumor usually is invading the dura, most commonly the cavernous sinus wall contiguous to the former location of the adenoma. In the series of Dickerman and Oldfield,[36] repeated surgery (44 ± 35 months after the initial surgery) in all 43 patients in whom tumor had been identified at the initial surgery, the tumor was found at the same site or contiguous to the same site. Dural invasion by an ACTH-producing tumor was identified during repeated surgery in 42 (62%) of the 68 patients reexplored after prior surgery and recurrent or persistent CD. In addition, 39 (93%) of the 42 invasive adenomas were located laterally and involved the cavernous sinus. Overall adenoma invasion of the dura mater was found in 31 (54%) of 57 microadenomas and in all 11 macroadenomas at repeated surgery. The presence of tumor was not detected in 28 of the 59 patients studied preoperatively with MRI and in none of these 59 patients was dural invasion evident on MRI. The results of this study thus established that recurrent and persistent CD consistently results from residual tumor. At repeated surgery the residual tumor can be found at, or immediately contiguous to, the site at which the tumor was originally found. Thus, unappreciated dural invasion with growth of residual tumor within the cavernous sinus dura, which frequently occurs without residual tumor or dural invasion being evident on MRI or to the surgeon during surgery, is the basis of surgical failure in many patients with CD.

Therefore, repeat transsphenoidal exploration of the pituitary and treatment limited to selective adenomectomy should be considered in patients with hypercortisolism despite previous pituitary treatment. If an adenoma is identified during surgery, the chance of remission of CD is high and the risk of hypopituitarism is low; however, if no adenoma can be found and partial or complete hypophysectomy is performed, remission of hypercortisolism is less likely and the risk of hypopituitarism is approximately 50%.

Radiation Therapy

Fractionated radiation of the sella after failed transsphenoidal surgery achieves biochemical remission in most patients (80% at 4 years).[38] Because remission is delayed 6 months to several years after radiation therapy, medical therapy is used to block adrenal production of glucocorticoids, permitting remission of the clinical syndrome of hypercortisolism until the effects of irradiation occur. Hypopituitarism is an expected side effect, but it usually occurs 5 to 10 years after treatment and does not occur in all patients. Other risks of sellar irradiation include, in decreasing likelihood, optic neuropathy, oculomotor neuropathy, and secondary neoplasia. Stereotactic radiosurgery may produce an earlier response than fractionated conventional radiation therapy and may reduce the risk of complications associated with radiation therapy. Radiosurgery of residual tumor or of the entire sella appears to be an effective treatment in about half of patients with CD in whom surgery is not curative. However, similar to fractionated therapy, biochemical remission is delayed and permanent hypopituitarism occurs in some patients.[39]

Medical Therapy

Certain drugs have the capacity to block production of biologically active cortisol by the adrenal cortex. This is helpful while awaiting the effects of pituitary irradiation or, less commonly, while awaiting surgery. Ketoconazole, which blocks steroidogenesis, is used for this purpose.[40] Its use is limited primarily by hepatic toxicity. Other side effects include reduced androgen production and gynecomastia in men and a disulfiram reaction. Metyrapone inhibits glucocorticoid and mineralocorticoid production, but its clinical usefulness is also limited by its toxicity.

Adrenalectomy

The current use of bilateral adrenalectomy is limited to patients for whom other treatments have failed. Adrenalectomy may be used instead of radiation to avoid hypopituitarism in young patients with CD refractory to surgery, or it may be combined with radiation to reduce the risk of development of Nelson's syndrome, which occurs in 10 to 20% of patients after adrenalectomy for CD.[41]

Conclusion

The optimal surgical management of CD continues to evolve. Currently, the most important predictors of success with surgery for CD are a solid diagnosis and the capacity to identify and selectively remove the adenoma at surgery. The results are often rewarding for the patient and surgeon.

References

1. Schulte HM, Oldfield EH, Allolio B, Katz DA, Berkman RA, Ali IU. Clonal composition of pituitary adenomas in patients with Cushing's disease: determination by X-chromosome inactivation analysis. J Clin Endocrinol Metab 1991;73:1302–1308
2. Oldfield EH, Vortmeyer AO. Development of a histological pseudocapsule and its use as a surgical capsule in the excision of pituitary tumors. J Neurosurg 2006;104:7–19
3. Jagannathan J, Smith R, DeVroom HL, et al. Outcome of using the histological pseudocapsule as a surgical capsule in Cushing disease. J Neurosurg 2009;111:531–539
4. Watson JC, Shawker TH, Nieman LK, DeVroom HL, Doppman JL, Oldfield EH. Localization of pituitary adenomas by using intraoperative ultrasound in patients with Cushing's disease and no demonstrable pituitary tumor on magnetic resonance imaging. J Neurosurg 1998;89:927–932
5. Gafni RI, Papanicolaou DA, Nieman LK. Nighttime salivary cortisol measurement as a simple, noninvasive, outpatient screening test for Cushing's syndrome in children and adolescents. J Pediatr 2000;137:30–35
6. Papanicolaou DA, Mullen N, Kyrou I, Nieman LK. Nighttime salivary cortisol: a useful test for the diagnosis of Cushing's syndrome. J Clin Endocrinol Metab 2002;87:4515–4521
7. Wood PJ, Barth JH, Freedman DB, Perry L, Sheridan B. Evidence for the low dose dexamethasone suppression test to screen for Cushing's syndrome—recommendations for a protocol for biochemistry laboratories. Ann Clin Biochem 1997;34(Pt 3):222–229
8. Dichek HL, Nieman LK, Oldfield EH, Pass HI, Malley JD, Cutler GB Jr. A comparison of the standard high dose dexamethasone suppression test and the overnight 8-mg dexamethasone suppression test for the differential diagnosis of adrenocorticotropin-dependent Cushing's syndrome. J Clin Endocrinol Metab 1994;78:418–422
9. Tyrrell JB, Findling JW, Aron DC, Fitzgerald PA, Forsham PH. An overnight high-dose dexamethasone suppression test for rapid differential diagnosis of Cushing's syndrome. Ann Intern Med 1986;104:180–186
10. Chrousos GP, Schulte HM, Oldfield EH, Gold PW, Cutler GB Jr, Loriaux DL. The corticotropin-releasing factor stimulation test. An aid in the evaluation of patients with Cushing's syndrome. N Engl J Med 1984;310:622–626
11. Nieman LK. Diagnostic tests for Cushing's syndrome. Ann N Y Acad Sci 2002;970:112–118
12. Nieman LK, Chrousos GP, Oldfield EH, Avgerinos PC, Cutler GB Jr, Loriaux DL. The ovine corticotropin-releasing hormone stimulation test and the dexamethasone suppression test in the differential diagnosis of Cushing's syndrome. Ann Intern Med 1986;105:862–867
13. Nieman LK, Oldfield EH, Wesley R, Chrousos GP, Loriaux DL, Cutler GB Jr. A simplified morning ovine corticotropin-releasing hormone stimulation test for the differential diagnosis of adrenocorticotropin-dependent Cushing's syndrome. J Clin Endocrinol Metab 1993;77:1308–1312
14. Jagannathan J, Sheehan JP, Jane JA Jr. Evaluation and management of Cushing syndrome in cases of negative sellar magnetic resonance imaging. Neurosurg Focus 2007;23:E3

15. Oldfield EH, Doppman JL, Nieman LK, et al. Petrosal sinus sampling with and without corticotropin-releasing hormone for the differential diagnosis of Cushing's syndrome. N Engl J Med 1991;325:897–905
16. Tyrrell JB, Findling JW, Aron DC, Fitzgerald PA, Forsham PH. An overnight high-dose dexamethasone suppression test for rapid differential diagnosis of Cushing's syndrome. Ann Intern Med 1986;104:180–186
17. Doppman JL, Chang R, Oldfield EH, Chrousos G, Stratakis CA, Nieman LK. The hypoplastic inferior petrosal sinus: a potential source of false-negative results in petrosal sampling for Cushing's disease. J Clin Endocrinol Metab 1999;84:533–540
18. Patronas N, Bulakbasi N, Stratakis CA, et al. Spoiled gradient recalled acquisition in the steady state technique is superior to conventional postcontrast spin echo technique for magnetic resonance imaging detection of adrenocorticotropin-secreting pituitary tumors. J Clin Endocrinol Metab 2003;88:1565–1569
19. Colombo N, Loli P, Vignati F, Scialfa G. MR of corticotropin-secreting pituitary microadenomas. AJNR Am J Neuroradiol 1994;15:1591–1595
20. Doppman JL, Frank JA, Dwyer AJ, et al. Gadolinium DTPA enhanced MR imaging of ACTH-secreting microadenomas of the pituitary gland. J Comput Assist Tomogr 1988;12:728–735
21. Peck WW, Dillon WP, Norman D, Newton TH, Wilson CB. High-resolution MR imaging of pituitary microadenomas at 1.5 T: experience with Cushing disease. AJR Am J Roentgenol 1989;152:145–151
22. Tabarin A, Laurent F, Catargi B, et al. Comparative evaluation of conventional and dynamic magnetic resonance imaging of the pituitary gland for the diagnosis of Cushing's disease. Clin Endocrinol (Oxf) 1998;49:293–300
23. Hall WA, Luciano MG, Doppman JL, Patronas NJ, Oldfield EH. Pituitary magnetic resonance imaging in normal human volunteers: occult adenomas in the general population. Ann Intern Med 1994;120:817–820
24. Ratliff JK, Oldfield EH. Multiple pituitary adenomas in Cushing's disease. J Neurosurg 2000;93:753–761
25. Pluta RM, Nieman L, Doppman JL, et al. Extrapituitary parasellar microadenoma in Cushing's disease. J Clin Endocrinol Metab 1999;84:2912–2923
26. Mason RB, Nieman LK, Doppman JL, Oldfield EH. Selective excision of adenomas originating in or extending into the pituitary stalk with preservation of pituitary function. J Neurosurg 1997;87:343–351
27. Hofmann BM, Hlavac M, Martinez R, Buchfelder M, Müller OA, Fahlbusch R. Long-term results after microsurgery for Cushing disease: experience with 426 primary operations over 35 years. J Neurosurg 2008;108:9–18
28. Patil CG, Prevedello DM, Lad SP, et al. Late recurrences of Cushing's disease after initial successful transsphenoidal surgery. J Clin Endocrinol Metab 2008;93:358–362
29. Dehdashti AR, Gentili F. Current state of the art in the diagnosis and surgical treatment of Cushing disease: early experience with a purely endoscopic endonasal technique. Neurosurg Focus 2007;23:E9
30. Netea-Maier RT, van Lindert EJ, den Heijer M, et al. Transsphenoidal pituitary surgery via the endoscopic technique: results in 35 consecutive patients with Cushing's disease. Eur J Endocrinol 2006;154:675–684
31. Atkinson JL, Young WF Jr, Meyer FB, et al. Sublabial transseptal vs transnasal combined endoscopic microsurgery in patients with Cushing disease and MRI-depicted microadenomas. Mayo Clin Proc 2008;83:550–553
32. Friedman RB, Oldfield EH, Nieman LK, et al. Repeat transsphenoidal surgery for Cushing's disease. J Neurosurg 1989;71:520–527
33. Ram Z, Nieman LK, Cutler GB Jr, Chrousos GP, Doppman JL, Oldfield EH. Early repeat surgery for persistent Cushing's disease. J Neurosurg 1994;80:37–45
34. Estrada J, García-Uría J, Lamas C, et al. The complete normalization of the adrenocortical function as the criterion of cure after transsphenoidal surgery for Cushing's disease. J Clin Endocrinol Metab 2001;86:5695–5699
35. Wagenmakers MA, Netea-Maier RT, van Lindert EJ, Timmers HJ, Grotenhuis JA, Hermus AR. Repeated transsphenoidal pituitary surgery (TS) via the endoscopic technique: a good therapeutic option for recurrent or persistent Cushing's disease (CD). Clin Endocrinol (Oxf) 2009;70:274–280
36. Dickerman RD, Oldfield EH. Basis of persistent and recurrent Cushing disease: an analysis of findings at repeated pituitary surgery. J Neurosurg 2002;97:1343–1349
37. Nakane T, Kuwayama A, Watanabe M, et al. Long term results of transsphenoidal adenomectomy in patients with Cushing's disease. Neurosurgery 1987;21:218–222
38. Estrada J, Boronat M, Mielgo M, et al. The long-term outcome of pituitary irradiation after unsuccessful transsphenoidal surgery in Cushing's disease. N Engl J Med 1997;336:172–177
39. Höybye C, Grenbäck E, Rähn T, Degerblad M, Thorén M, Hulting AL. Adrenocorticotropic hormone-producing pituitary tumors: 12- to 22-year follow-up after treatment with stereotactic radiosurgery. Neurosurgery 2001;49:284–291, discussion 291–292
40. Sonino N, Boscaro M, Paoletta A, Mantero F, Ziliotto D. Ketoconazole treatment in Cushing's syndrome: experience in 34 patients. Clin Endocrinol (Oxf) 1991;35:347–352
41. Nagesser SK, van Seters AP, Kievit J, Hermans J, Krans HM, van de Velde CJ. Long-term results of total adrenalectomy for Cushing's disease. World J Surg 2000;24:108–113

12 Thyroid-Stimulating Hormone Tumors

Stephen J. Monteith, Jonathan H. Sherman, John A. Jane Jr., and Edward R. Laws Jr.

Epidemiology

As early as the 1950s it was postulated that some forms of hyperthyroidism could have their origins in the pituitary gland.[1] However, it was not until the 1960s that the first cases of thyroid-stimulating hormone (TSH)–secreting tumors were reported by Jailer and Holub.[2] With the advent of newer immunostaining techniques, the incidence of TSH adenomas is reported as 2%.[3] However, the incidence varies among series and is commonly reported to be approximately 0.5 to 3%.[4,5]

It is reported that TSH adenomas are more common in females.[4,6] The female-to-male ratio varies widely in the literature from between 5:1 and 10:1[7] to 1:1.6.[8] It has been suggested that males are diagnosed earlier than females due to the rarity of Graves' disease in males, thus prompting early investigation for secondary hyperthyroidism.[6] The age of diagnosis tends to be in middle adulthood, usually in the fifth or sixth decade. Though uncommon, TSH adenomas have been reported in children as young as 15 and in adults older than 80 years.[6] Some studies have found that women tend to develop their adenomas at a younger age, have a longer history of symptoms, and have smaller tumors that are less invasive when compared with these tumors in men.[4]

Pathology

Histopathology

Thyrotrophic adenoma cells usually appear chromophobic with mild periodic acid-Schiff positivity. Immunostaining is positive for TSH-β in virtually all adenomatous cells from TSH adenomas (**Fig. 12.1**). Under electron microscopy the cells demonstrate moderate differentiation, scant rough endoplasmic reticulum (RER), and Golgi complexes. Secretory granules are small, round, evenly electron dense and are found along the cytoplasmic membrane[9] (**Fig. 12.2**). Specialized techniques have identified the presence of TSH and other pituitary hormones within the same adenomatous cell and even from within the same secretory granule. Pituitary adenomas of the growth hormone (GH), prolactin (PRL), and TSH lineage may originate from a common

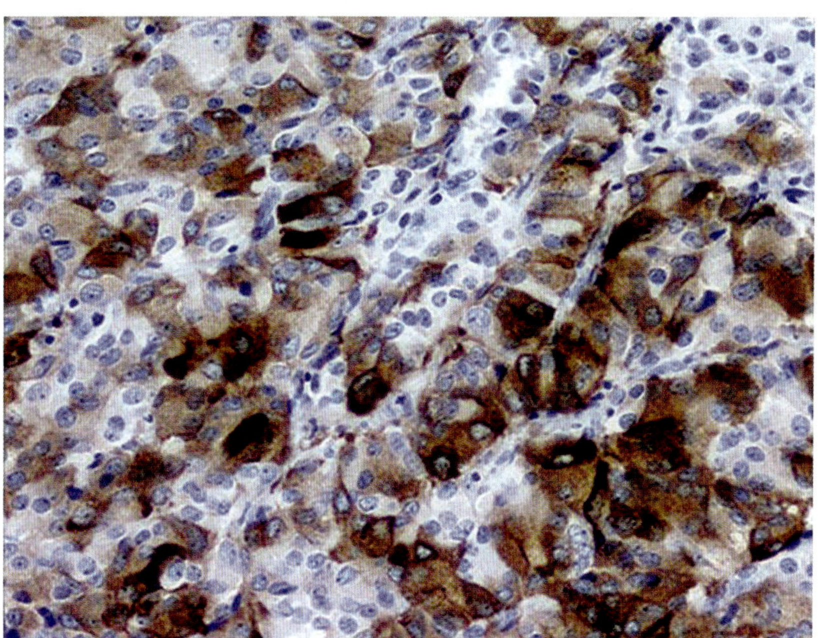

Fig. 12.1 Immunohistochemistry specimen demonstrating thyroid-stimulating hormone positivity.

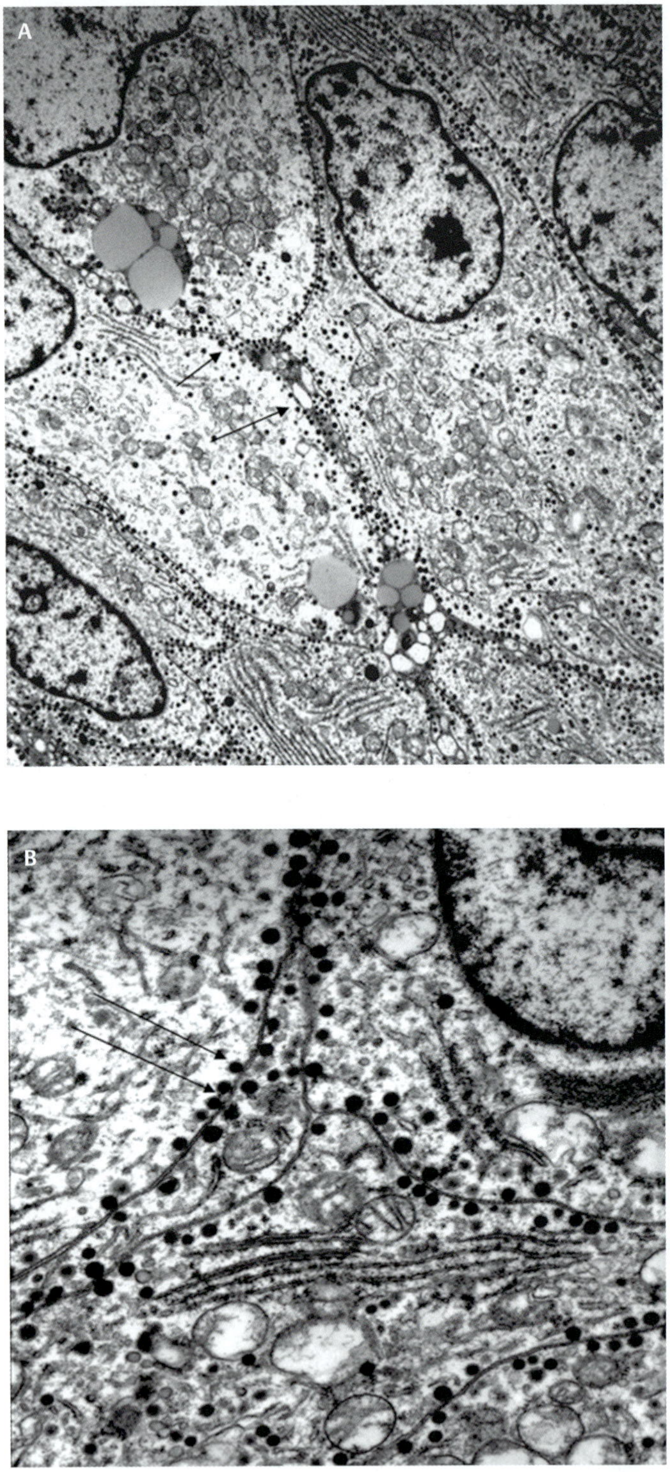

Fig. 12.2 **(A)** Low-power and **(B)** high-power electron microscopy demonstrating small, round, evenly dense secretory granules along the cytoplasmic membrane (*arrows*).

progenitor cell; however, the presence of positive immunohistochemistry does not necessarily mean that the patient will have hypersecretion of that hormone. It has been suggested that the production of two seemingly unrelated hormones by the same adenomatous cell is due to TSH adenomas developing from this common progenitor cell.

Molecular Pathology

The anterior pituitary transcription factor Pit-1 is required for the growth of somatotrophs, lactotrophs, and thyrotrophs. Mutations in Pit-1 result in the lack of expression of these three cell lineages in both humans and transgenic organisms.[10,11] Pit-1 expression and the development of pituitary tumors have been explored in both humans and in the laboratory. Although Pit-1 overexpression can result in the development of GH, PRL, and TSH adenomas, the *Pit-1* gene itself may not demonstrate any mutation.[12–15]

Several oncogenes have been investigated in relation to TSH adenomas but none has consistently been found to be abnormal. The *gsp* oncogene is expressed in approximately 40% of GH adenomas; however, in Beck-Peccoz et al's[5] review of TSH adenomas that included 11 specimens, none was found to express *gsp*. The *gsp* oncogene is responsible for production of G-protein subunits, and thus it has been suggested that disruption of guanosine triphosphatase activity is unlikely to be the underlying pathologic mechanism of TSH adenomas.[5]

Oncogenes such as c-*myc*, c-*fos*, and c-*myb* have been implicated in pituitary adenomas. The literature on such mutations in TSH adenomas is sparse, but there appears to be no overexpression of these oncogenes in TSH adenomas.[16] *Ras* oncogene and protein kinase C mutations have been found in pituitary adenomas. Nevertheless, data on mutations in p53, retinoblastoma gene, and 11q13 deletions in the context of TSH adenomas are insufficient to draw any reliable conclusion.

Presentation

The presenting signs and symptoms leading to the diagnosis of TSH adenomas usually relate to thyrotoxicosis. Patients may present with a short history, but the duration of signs and symptoms may be greater than 25 years in some cases and can range in severity from mild to the severe. Symptoms related to tumor size or mass effect include visual field abnormalities, cranial nerve palsies, and headache. One large study of 25 patients from the National Institutes of Health found that headaches were present in 39% and visual fields were impaired in 36%.[6] Thyrotoxicosis commonly presents with palpitations, arrhythmias, weight loss, tremor, sweating, and nervousness.[6,17] Up to 90% of patients may present with goiter.[17,18] TSH adenomas may also be associated with multiple endocrine neoplasia type 1 syndrome; however, the pituitary lesions may be found prior to the systemic disease.[19] Familial cases of TSH adenoma have not yet been reported in the literature.[17]

About 30% of cases have associated dysregulation of another pituitary hormone axis.[5] With dysregulation of another hormone pathway, the signs and symptoms of other pituitary disorders may also precipitate diagnosis, such as amenorrhea, galactorrhea, loss of libido, and acromegaly. Despite the presence of signs and symptoms related to dysregulation of another pituitary-hormone axis, the associated hormones may not be elevated on serum hormone evaluation. It has been postulated that in cases without elevated levels of associated hormones the mechanism of dysregulation revolves around compression of the pituitary gland or disconnection of the pituitary-hypothalamic axis.[17] Patients may also be asymptomatic and are diagnosed incidentally when undergoing neuroimaging of the brain for other reasons.

Unfortunately, because of the rarity of these lesions, many patients present to neurosurgical services after having undergone a lengthy and invasive course over many years prior to diagnosis. In some series the majority of patients have undergone thyroid surgery for excision of goiter. Some receive radioactive iodine or antithyroid drugs. Earlier studies from the 1980s were more likely to include patients who underwent additional treatment prior to diagnosis. Since the advent of commercially available laboratory assays for TSH, from the 1990s to the present these events are becoming less common.[6,17]

The consequences of misdiagnosis in the setting of a TSH adenoma can be severe. It has been suggested that a similar mechanism involved in Nelson's syndrome leading to transformation of pituitary cells after adrenalectomy may occur following thyroidectomy in a patient with a TSH adenoma. In addition, it has been postulated that patients with previous thyroid surgery had more aggressive, fibrous, firm, invasive tumors.[17,20] It has also been suggested that reactive TSH adenomas may develop as a consequence of primary hypothyroidism.[21,22]

Diagnosis

Biochemical

The diagnosis of a TSH adenoma requires the appropriate history, physical examination, and radiographic findings as well as multiple biochemical markers. A patient with weight loss, tremor, sweating, palpitations, or a goiter in combination with headaches or visual field or eye movement abnormalities should prompt the clinician to consider a TSH adenoma. A routine panel of pituitary hormone tests should be performed in all patients and includes PRL, GH, insulin-like growth factor-1 (IGF-1), luteinizing hormone (LH), follicle-stimulating hormone (FSH), and adrenocorticotropic hormone (ACTH). There is no one serum biochemical marker or test that can be used solely to diagnose TSH adenomas. In addition, the biochemical parameters used to diagnose TSH adenomas have changed over the years as more sensitive assays have become commercially available. This has undoubtedly led to an increase in the rate of diagnosis of these lesions.

A TSH adenoma can be suspected when free triiodothyronine and free thyroxine levels are elevated, TSH is inappropriately normal or elevated, and markers of thyroid hormone activity (sex hormone–binding globulin, cholesterol, angiotensin-converting enzyme, carboxyterminal cross-linked telopeptide of type 1 collagen are elevated. More specialized tests and dynamic studies are then used to further evaluate the biochemical profile. A baseline α-subunit level may be elevated and the α-subunit:TSH ratio may be elevated also. Patients with prior treatment for hyperthyroidism tend to have a lower α-subunit:TSH ratio. Other test results that favor a diagnosis of TSH adenoma include a negative thyrotropin-releasing hormone (TRH) stimulation test (less than a twofold increase of TSH after TRH administration), and a negative triiodothyronine suppression test. Nocturnal increases of TSH may also be absent. The diagnosis can usually be made in these patients when combining the α-subunit:TSH ratio and the results of a TRH test.[17]

Imaging

The use of magnetic resonance imaging (MRI) as the imaging modality of choice for the identification of pituitary tumors has been well established. High-resolution computed tomography (CT) scanning can identify macroadenomas and delineate bony anatomy or invasion. However, MRI offers higher sensitivity in identifying microadenomas and defining the relationship of the tumor to surrounding structures.

A detailed study of the radiographic findings in 21 patients with TSH adenomas demonstrated a high proportion of macroadenomas (20 of 21 cases).[23] The same authors suggest that with the advent of more sensitive biochemical techniques to allow earlier diagnosis of TSH adenomas, the proportion of macroadenomas and invasive tumors will decline in future study populations.

Thyroid-stimulating hormone (TSH)–secreting macroadenomas tend to adopt an aggressive pattern of growth. They tend to extend into the suprasellar space (**Fig. 12.3**) and may compress the optic chiasm. In addition, they may invade the cavernous sinus (**Fig. 12.4**) and sphenoid sinus. Thyrotropin-producing adenomas tend to be hypointense on MRI T1-weighted postgadolinium images compared with normal pituitary gland. However, they may also be isodense to normal pituitary on T1-weighted imaging following gadolinium.[19,23]

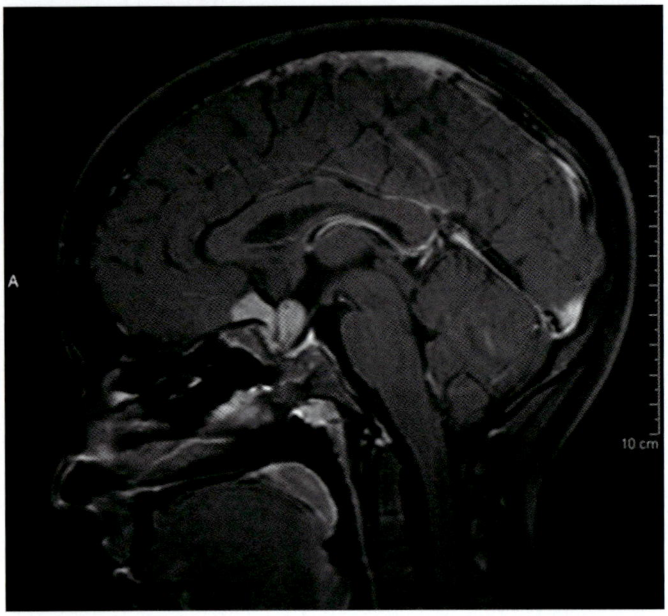

Fig. 12.3 T1-weighted postgadolinium sagittal magnetic resonance imaging demonstrating suprasellar extension of a pure TSH adenoma.

Growth Pattern

A review of 43 patients with TSH adenomas by Socin et al[19] found a preponderance (20 of 31 cases) of macroadenomas with suprasellar or sphenoidal extension as well as growth medially within the pituitary gland. It has been postulated that the medial extension of TSH adenomas is due to the medial location of thyrotrophs in the pituitary gland. This growth pattern is in contrast to GH-secreting adenomas, which tend to spread laterally, and have the associated GH-producing cells located laterally. The same study also found that there was a statistically significant ($p < .01$) correlation between the size of the tumor and nature of the hormonal secretions. In addition to the secretion of TSH, macroadenomas were more likely to secrete GH or PRL.[19]

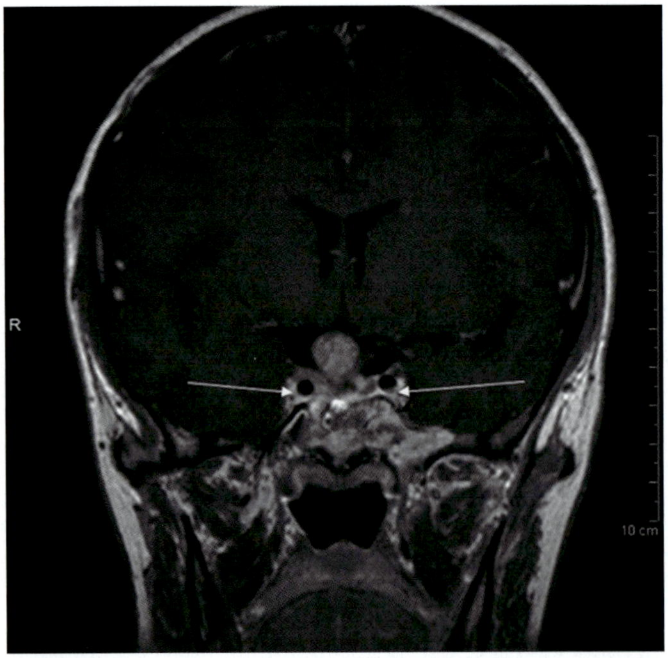

Fig. 12.4 T1-weighted postgadolinium coronal MRI of a pure TSH adenoma with suprasellar extension and invasion of the cavernous sinus bilaterally (*arrows*).

Other studies have found that TSH adenomas tend to be invasive.[4,6,18] A staging system of tumor invasion was proposed for TSH adenomas that incorporates cavernous and sphenoid sinus invasion and suprasellar extension.[23] The same authors found that a high staging score for invasion was a predictor of unfavorable response to surgery.

Additional Diagnostic Modalities

In addition to routine imaging with CT and MRI scanning, inferior petrosal sinus sampling following a hormone stimulation test can be used in an attempt to isolate the correct side of the tumor. Petrosal sinus testing has been used extensively with Cushing's disease with variable accuracy of lateralization but less frequently with TSH-secreting adenomas.[24] With a TRH stimulation test, a central to peripheral gradient of the TSH level can be expected on the side of the tumor. However, some authors describe incorrect localization by this technique, finding the tumor on the contralateral side at the time of surgery.[19]

Positron emission tomography (PET) scanning can also be combined with traditional imaging modalities. A radioactive isotope (such as fluorodeoxyglucose), which decays by emitting a positron, is injected into the patient and binds to pituitary adenoma receptors. After a suitable waiting period the decay of the particles is picked up by the PET scanner and co-registered with CT or MRI imaging. This technique demonstrates location of tumor cells and can demonstrate the metabolic demands of the tumor. The treatment can also be used before and after medical treatment as a determinant of treatment effect.[25]

Treatment

Surgical Management

The primary goals of treatment of TSH-secreting tumors are to restore euthyroidism and maintain normal pituitary function. Surgical intervention also addresses symptoms due to mass effect such as headache, visual loss, or diplopia as a result of cavernous sinus involvement or compression of the optic chiasm. Transsphenoidal surgery is usually the method of choice for resection once the diagnosis of a TSH adenoma has been made. In addition to the benefits above, microsurgical treatment has the added benefit of providing pathologic tissue for immunocytochemical analysis. This analysis can help differentiate the tumor as an isolated TSH adenoma versus a mixed tumor secreting multiple hormones. Although standard microsurgical techniques for resection of pituitary macroadenomas have been well established, the use of rigid endoscopic techniques are now becoming more common. Proponents of endoscopic transsphenoidal surgery advocate its use based on more favorable visualization of the tumor, the pituitary gland–tumor interface, and structures such as the diaphragm sellae and the medial cavernous sinus wall as compared with the microscopic approach. The increased view of the latter two structures can assist the surgeon in directly visualizing residual tumor.[26]

Macroscopic findings with TSH adenomas include suprasellar extension and invasion of the cavernous sinus, dura, and bone. These findings may make complete resection of macroadenomas difficult or impossible. However, microadenomas rarely invade the cavernous sinus, making complete surgical resection more of a reality. TSH adenomas may also be particularly fibrous, which increases the difficulty in achieving maximal tumor resection.[5,18] In addition, some authors have reported more difficultly resecting TSH adenomas following prolonged duration of hyperthyroidism, surgical ablation of the thyroid, and antithyroid therapy.[18] It is thought that the marked fibrosis of these tumors may be related to the high expression of a form of fibroblast growth factor.[5,27]

The criterion for cure varies in study populations; however, euthyroidism and a postoperative normalization of a previously elevated TSH is usually employed. Some groups have also included absence of tumor on postoperative MRI scanning, normal TRH stimulation tests, vision improvement, or improvement in neurologic symptoms.

The outcome of surgery depends on the criteria used to define remission. Surgical remission rates range from 35 to 83% depending on the duration of follow-up and the remission criteria. Not surprisingly, microadenomas tended to have improved rates of cure when compared with macroadenomas, which have usually spread into the suprasellar compartment or invaded the cavernous sinus, rendering complete resection difficult or impossible. Recurrence rates range from 8 to 10% within 10 years of surgery.[6,8,18,19,28–31]

A large case series from the National Institutes of Health found that prognosis after surgery depends largely on the size of the tumor and its invasiveness.[6] Delay in diagnosis and female gender also carried a poorer prognosis.

Complications of surgery are similar to those for other pituitary tumors. The size of TSH adenomas and their invasive nature increase the risk of damage to surrounding structures if attempts at aggressive surgical resection are made. Early complications such as cerebrospinal fluid leak, panhypopituitarism, diabetes insipidus (transient or permanent), and the syndrome of inappropriate antidiuretic hormone (SIADH) secretion have all been reported. The late complication of central hypothyroidism following remission by surgery can also occur.[6] In the large series by Brucker-Davis et al,[6] death from tumor progression to metastatic thyrotrophic carcinoma was also reported in one of 25 patients. Because adjunctive treatments are available, it is recommended that a more conservative surgical approach should be employed and any residual tumor can be treated medically or with radiation. All postoperative patients should be evaluated with a full pituitary panel to assess for hypopituitarism.

Medical Therapy

For patients who cannot tolerate surgical resection or for whom surgical intervention is contraindicated, medical therapy can be very effective. Somatostatin analogues such as octreotide can be used in the long term to effectively reduce or normalize free thyroid hormone levels in patients with TSH adenomas. Octreotide may stabilize or even reduce the size of the tumor on MRI. In addition to the reduction in tumor size, the metabolism of the tumor and effectiveness of medical treatment may be monitored using PET scanning.[5,17,19,32] Octreotide can also be used preoperatively to stabilize thyrotoxicosis and to try to shrink tumor size to improve surgical resection. Tachyphylaxis may occur and may successfully be treated by increasing the octreotide dose. Resistance to octreotide has also been reported as a cause of medical treatment failure. Patients being treated with octreotide need to be followed closely as side effects may manifest, such as carbohydrate intolerance, cholelithiasis, and gastrointestinal side effects.

Dopamine agonists have also been used to treat TSH adenomas; however, their success has been limited. Treatment may be more effective in tumors that demonstrate a mixed TSH/PRL profile with lactotroph differentiation than pure TSH adenomas.[19]

In a large proportion of patients, the degree of thyrotoxicosis can be severe. Preoperative treatment with the use of beta-blockers is recommended. Some authors advocate the use of antithyroid medications, whereas others do not, citing confusion in the interpretation of postoperative laboratory studies in trying to determine cure. Somatostatin analogues can also be useful and result in control of hyperthyroidism and may even shrink the tumor preoperatively.[18] On rare occasions TSH adenomas may respond to methimazole.[33]

Radiotherapy

Patients who are not cured or stabilized following surgical resection or medical treatment may be treated with radiation therapy. In a study by Socin et al,[19] eight of 17 patients for whom surgical resection failed underwent radiation therapy. Seven of these patients underwent fractionated external-beam radiation therapy with the total radiation dose ranging from 42 to 65 Gy in 28 treatments via at least three ports. One underwent gamma knife radiosurgery. Gamma knife radiosurgery using stereotactic focused radiation has been used to treat these lesions as well. There are limited published reports establishing the role of this treatment modality.[6,19] Of those eight patients, five had their tumors controlled by radiotherapy alone, whereas the remaining three required radiation and somatostatin analogues to obtain tumor control.[19]

Conclusion

The diagnosis of a TSH adenoma in the setting of hyperthyroidism is rare. Once the diagnosis of a TSH-producing adenoma has been made, the treatment of choice is surgical resection by the transsphenoidal approach. Surgery offers the benefits of normalization of TSH secretion while at the same time relieving the symptoms produced by mass effect. The pathologic specimen obtained at surgery confirms the diagnosis and provides immunohistochemical staining information for the other pituitary hormones. Second-line therapy such as somatostatin analogues are indicated following a subtotal resection or if surgery is contraindicated. If TSH levels remain high after medical or surgical treatment, or if there is significant residual tumor burden or mass effect, then radiation therapy or radiosurgery should be considered.

References

1. Werner SC, Stewart WB. Hyperthyroidism in a patient with a pituitary chromophobe adenoma and a fragment of normal pituitary. J Clin Endocrinol Metab 1958;18:266–270
2. Jailer JW, Holub DA. Remission of Graves' disease following radiotherapy of a pituitary neoplasm. Am J Med 1960;28:497–500
3. Samuels MH, Ridgway EC. Glycoprotein-secreting pituitary adenomas. Baillieres Clin Endocrinol Metab 1995;9:337–358
4. Mindermann T, Wilson CB. Thyrotropin-producing pituitary adenomas. J Neurosurg 1993;79:521–527
5. Beck-Peccoz P, Brucker-Davis F, Persani L, Smallridge RC, Weintraub BD. Thyrotropin-secreting pituitary tumors. Endocr Rev 1996;17:610–638
6. Brucker-Davis F, Oldfield EH, Skarulis MC, Doppman JL, Weintraub BD. Thyrotropin-secreting pituitary tumors: diagnostic criteria, thyroid hormone sensitivity, and treatment outcome in 25 patients followed at the National Institutes of Health. J Clin Endocrinol Metab 1999;84:476–486
7. Smallridge RC. Thyrotropin-secreting pituitary tumors. Endocrinol Metab Clin North Am 1987;16:765–792
8. Wynne AG, Gharib H, Scheithauer BW, Davis DH, Freeman SL, Horvath E. Hyperthyroidism due to inappropriate secretion of thyrotropin in 10 patients. Am J Med 1992;92:15–24
9. Fletcher CDM. Diagnostic Histopathology of Tumors, Vol 2, 2nd ed. London, New York: Churchill Livingstone; 2000
10. Pellegrini-Bouiller I, Morange-Ramos I, Barlier A, Gunz G, Enjalbert A, Jaquet P. Pit-1 gene expression in human pituitary adenomas. Horm Res 1997;47:251–258
11. Asa SL, Puy LA, Lew AM, Sundmark VC, Elsholtz HP. Cell type-specific expression of the pituitary transcription activator pit-1 in the human pituitary and pituitary adenomas. J Clin Endocrinol Metab 1993;77:1275–1280
12. Sanno N, Teramoto A, Matsuno A, Takekoshi S, Osamura RY. GH and PRL gene expression by nonradioisotopic in situ hybridization in TSH-secreting pituitary adenomas. J Clin Endocrinol Metab 1995;80:2518–2522
13. Sanno N, Teramoto A, Matsuno A, Inada K, Itoh J, Osamura RY. Clinical and immunohistochemical studies on TSH-secreting pituitary adenoma: its multihormonality and expression of Pit-1. Mod Pathol 1994;7:893–899
14. Pellegrini I, Barlier A, Gunz G, et al. Pit-1 gene expression in the human pituitary and pituitary adenomas. J Clin Endocrinol Metab 1994;79:189–196
15. Delhase M, Vergani P, Malur A, et al. Pit-1/GHF-1 expression in pituitary adenomas: further analogy between human adenomas and rat SMtTW tumours. J Mol Endocrinol 1993;11:129–139
16. Woloschak M, Roberts JL, Post K. c-myc, c-fos, and c-myb gene expression in human pituitary adenomas. J Clin Endocrinol Metab 1994;79:253–257
17. Kienitz T, Quinkler M, Strasburger CJ, Ventz M. Long-term management in five cases of TSH-secreting pituitary adenomas: a single center study and review of the literature. Eur J Endocrinol 2007;157:39–46
18. Sanno N, Teramoto A, Osamura RY. Long-term surgical outcome in 16 patients with thyrotropin pituitary adenoma. J Neurosurg 2000;93:194–200
19. Socin HV, Chanson P, Delemer B, et al. The changing spectrum of TSH-secreting pituitary adenomas: diagnosis and management in 43 patients. Eur J Endocrinol 2003;148:433–442
20. Sanno N, Teramoto A, Osamura RY. Thyrotropin-secreting pituitary adenomas. Clinical and biological heterogeneity and current treatment. J Neurooncol 2001;54:179–186
21. Caughey JE. The aetiology of pituitary tumours: the role of hypogonadism and hypothyroidism. Australas Ann Med 1957;6:93–97
22. Samaan NA, Osborne BM, Mackay B, Leavens ME, Duello TM, Halmi NS. Endocrine and morphologic studies of pituitary adenomas secondary to primary hypothyroidism. J Clin Endocrinol Metab 1977;45:903–911
23. Sarlis NJ, Gourgiotis L, Koch CA, et al. MR imaging features of thyrotropin-secreting pituitary adenomas at initial presentation. AJR Am J Roentgenol 2003;181:577–582
24. Batista D, Gennari M, Riar J, et al. An assessment of petrosal sinus sampling for localization of pituitary microadenomas in children with Cushing disease. J Clin Endocrinol Metab 2006;91:221–224
25. Francavilla TL, Miletich RS, DeMichele D, et al. Positron emission tomography of pituitary macroadenomas: hormone production and effects of therapies. Neurosurgery 1991;28:826–833
26. Jane JA Jr, Han J, Prevedello DM, Jagannathan J, Dumont AS, Laws ER Jr. Perspectives on endoscopic transsphenoidal surgery. Neurosurg Focus 2005;19:E2
27. Ezzat S, Horvath E, Kovacs K, Smyth HS, Singer W, Asa SL. Basic fibroblast growth factor expression by two prolactin and thyrotropin-producing pituitary adenomas. Endocr Pathol 1995;6:125–134
28. Losa M, Giovanelli M, Persani L, Mortini P, Faglia G, Beck-Peccoz P. Criteria of cure and follow-up of central hyperthyroidism due to

thyrotropin-secreting pituitary adenomas. J Clin Endocrinol Metab 1996;81:3084–3090
29. Grisoli F, Leclercq T, Winteler JP, et al. Thyroid-stimulating hormone pituitary adenomas and hyperthyroidism. Surg Neurol 1986;25: 361–368
30. Beckers A, Abs R, Mahler C, et al. Thyrotropin-secreting pituitary adenomas: report of seven cases. J Clin Endocrinol Metab 1991;72:477–483
31. Laws ER, Vance ML, Jane JA Jr. TSH adenomas. Pituitary 2006;9: 313–315
32. Mannavola D, Persani L, Vannucchi G, et al. Different responses to chronic somatostatin analogues in patients with central hyperthyroidism. Clin Endocrinol (Oxf) 2005;62:176–181
33. Inukai T, Fujiwara Y, Aso Y, Yamamoto A, Takemura Y. A rare case of a thyrotropin-secreting pituitary tumor which responded to methimazole. J Med 1998;29:185–198

13 Clinical Management of Nonfunctioning Pituitary Adenomas

Gabriel Zada, Jeroen R. Coppens, William T. Couldwell, and Martin H. Weiss

In the past, nonfunctioning pituitary adenomas were known as chromophobe adenomas based on characteristic results observed with standard hematoxylin and eosin staining. Subsequent refinements in immunohistochemical methods have demonstrated their relative heterogeneity. Clinically nonfunctioning adenomas (NFAs) include null-cell adenomas as well as silent adenomas with positive immunochemical staining. The clinical management of these tumors is discussed in this chapter.

Epidemiology of Nonfunctioning Adenomas

Pituitary adenomas have been reported to occur incidentally in up to 25% of the population, according to autopsy studies of the sellar region.[1] One study of more than 12,000 pituitary specimens demonstrated an 11.3% incidence of adenomas, with the vast majority being microadenomas.[2] A recent meta-analysis reported an estimated prevalence of pituitary adenomas in 16.4% of the population.[3] NFAs are the most commonly encountered form of pituitary adenomas. According to previous reports, NFAs constitute 25 to 33% of surgically resected pituitary adenomas, making them the most common subtype requiring surgical intervention.[4–6]

Although NFAs have been labeled nonsecreting tumors (i.e., characterized by no functional oversecretion) in the past, they frequently do produce various hormonal glycoprotein subunits that have little known independent functional endocrine activity.[7] On routine immunohistochemical testing, the majority of NFAs stain positive for at least one type of hormone, with gonadotropins being the most commonly produced.[7,8] Other immunopositive subtypes of NFAs that are clinically "silent" include corticotroph and somatotroph adenomas.[9] True null-cell adenomas are much rarer, representing approximately 6% of all NFAs.[1–9] Furthermore, immunohistochemical staining for subunits, such as the α- and β-subunits, is positive in almost 70% of cases.[7] Despite the ability to produce glycoprotein hormones and subunits in a majority of NFAs, the ability to secrete these proteins is significantly impaired, occurring in a minority of NFAs.[10,11]

Clinical Manifestations of Nonfunctioning Adenomas

Rather than causing symptoms related to hormone oversecretion, as occurs with functional pituitary adenomas, NFAs typically present secondary to mass effect on surrounding structures. Although patients with NFAs frequently present with headaches and visual deficits, serum laboratory studies reveal hypopituitarism in a significant proportion of patients.[12,13] In many cases, visual loss occurs secondary to mass effect on the optic chiasm from below, resulting initially in a superior bitemporal quadrantanopsia that frequently progresses to a classic bitemporal hemianopsia.[14] The most frequent hormonal abnormalities associated with NFAs are hypogonadism and hyperprolactinemia, followed by growth hormone (GH) deficiency.[12] The serum prolactin level is often elevated in patients with NFAs secondary to a "stalk effect," which prevents the tonic inhibition of prolactin-secreting cells in the anterior pituitary gland via dopamine secretion from hypothalamic cells. Serum prolactin levels in patients with nonfunctioning macroadenomas are typically less than 150 ng/mL, as compared with a maximum value in the several hundred or even thousand range for equally sized prolactinomas.[15,16]

There is typically a gradual progression in symptoms in patients with NFAs, except in cases of pituitary apoplexy, where acute progression of symptoms is observed in many cases. The diagnosis of pituitary apoplexy is primarily a clinical diagnosis and has been reported in 1 to 21% of patients with NFAs, although the majority of series report an incidence of less than 5%.[15,17,18] The clinical presentation of pituitary apoplexy frequently includes rapidly progressing headache, meningismus, visual field deficits, cranial nerve deficits, and symptoms related to hypopituitarism.[15]

Preoperative Evaluation of Patients with Nonfunctioning Pituitary Adenomas

A complete endocrine evaluation is indicated in all patients presenting with symptoms of mass effect from an NFA. This typically includes measurement of serum GH and insulin-like growth factor-1 (IGF-1), morning cortisol, free thyroxine (FT_4) and prolactin levels in all patients, luteinizing hormone/follicle-stimulating hormone (LH/FSH) levels in women, and testosterone levels in men. Furthermore, a standard Humphrey visual field examination should be performed by an ophthalmologist, as many visual field deficits are subtle on clinical examination. Standard radiographic workup includes magnetic resonance imaging (MRI) with and without contrast administration in axial, sagittal, and coronal sellar views. Key factors to consider on MRI when evaluating nonsecreting macroadenomas include the degree of extension into the infrasellar region and the thickness of the sellar floor, any evidence of cavernous sinus invasion and relationship to the internal carotid arteries and cranial nerves, the extent of suprasellar and subfrontal extension and relationship to the optic apparatus, the position of the normal pituitary gland relative to the lesion, and finally the degree of retrosellar extension and relationship to the clivus and brainstem (**Fig. 13.1**).

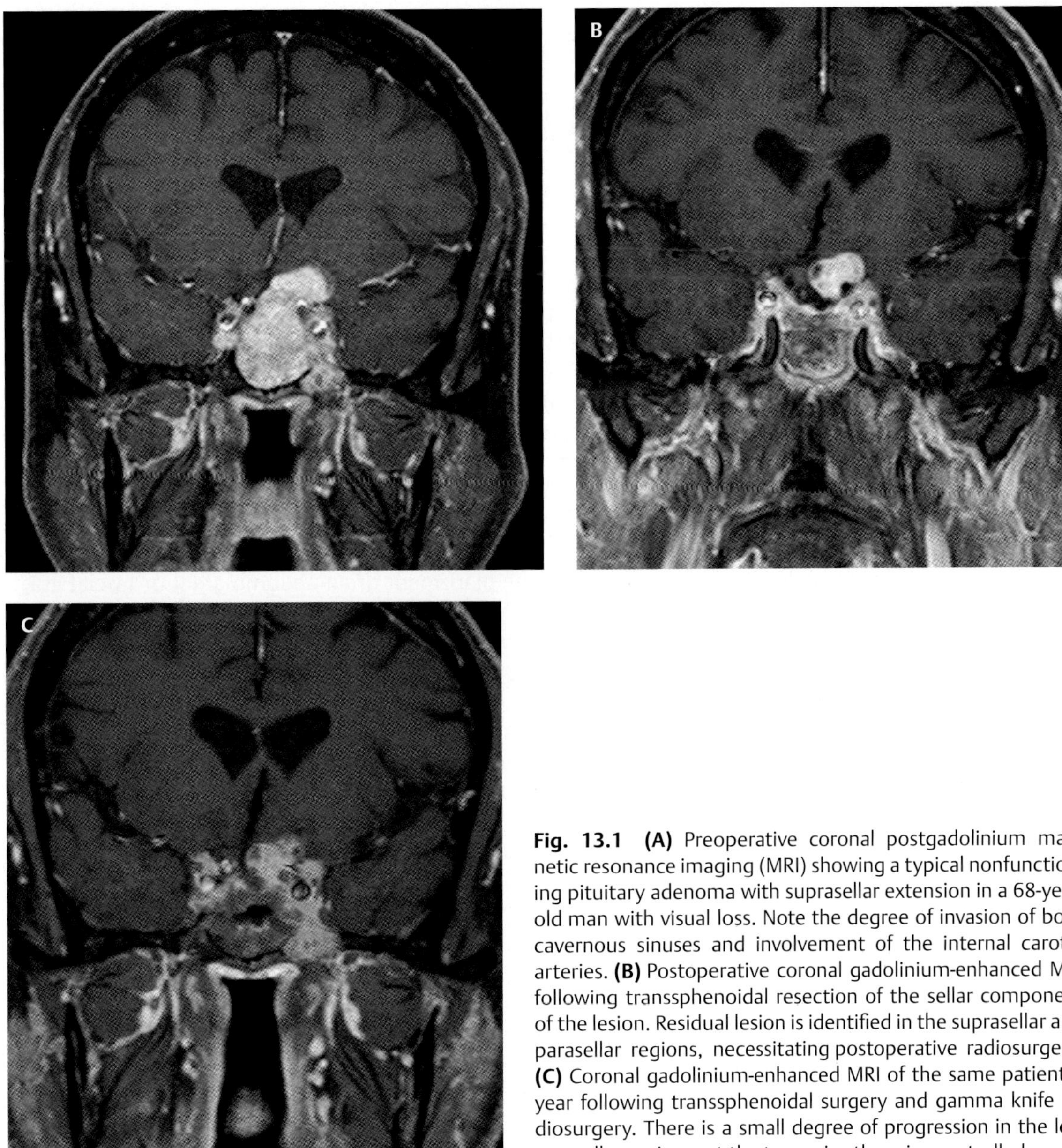

Fig. 13.1 **(A)** Preoperative coronal postgadolinium magnetic resonance imaging (MRI) showing a typical nonfunctioning pituitary adenoma with suprasellar extension in a 68-year-old man with visual loss. Note the degree of invasion of both cavernous sinuses and involvement of the internal carotid arteries. **(B)** Postoperative coronal gadolinium-enhanced MRI following transsphenoidal resection of the sellar component of the lesion. Residual lesion is identified in the suprasellar and parasellar regions, necessitating postoperative radiosurgery. **(C)** Coronal gadolinium-enhanced MRI of the same patient 1 year following transsphenoidal surgery and gamma knife radiosurgery. There is a small degree of progression in the left parasellar region, yet the tumor is otherwise controlled.

The Natural History of Nonfunctioning Adenomas

The natural history of unresected pituitary adenomas has been reported in few studies. As expected, the major factor that determines patient outcome in these cases is tumor size. The authors of one study reviewed 40 patients with NFAs who did not undergo surgery for a variety of reasons.[19] They determined that 19% of microadenomas and 44% of macroadenomas demonstrated interval growth on follow-up imaging at a 4-year follow-up. New or worsening visual deficits were observed in 67% of macroadenomas and were absent in all microadenomas. The authors recommended that a watchful waiting policy for nonfunctioning pituitary microadenomas is reasonable in the absence of significant symptoms, whereas macroadenomas should be evaluated for resection. In a separate study, the authors reviewed their experience with 28 patients with unresected nonfunctioning macroadenomas.[20] Fifty percent of these patients had an increase in tumor size in a mean follow-up time of 85 months. In turn, 50% of the patients with enlargement in tumor size had progression of visual field deficits requiring surgery.

Our institutional preference has been to offer resection of nonfunctioning pituitary macroadenomas to patients who are acceptable surgical candidates, regardless of visual status. This avoids the potential for developing irreversible symptoms and provides for safer tumor resection, as well as decreases the risk of postoperative visual deterioration. Furthermore, the risk of developing pituitary apoplexy, which has been reported to be higher in patients harboring NFAs than in those with other adenomas, is reduced.[15] In the absence of symptoms, nonfunctioning microadenomas can be observed with interval imaging, based on clinical status and patient preference. A possible exception to this rule is the category of primarily suprasellar NFAs. In this location, resection may be indicated in smaller lesions, based on the propensity of patients with these lesions for developing significant visual or hormonal deficits.[9]

Medical Management of Nonfunctional Pituitary Adenomas

In general, the medical management of NFAs has been anecdotal and unsubstantiated. Dopamine agonists may decrease gonadotropin and α-subunit production, but their clinical efficacy in patients with NFAs has been marginal. Despite occasional declines in elevated serum prolactin levels caused by tumor stalk effect, tumor shrinkage has been the exception rather than the rule.[3] Somatostatin analogues have also been used, with reports of mild visual improvement in 20 to 40% of cases, yet there is only anecdotal evidence of tumor regression.[8]

Surgical Management of Nonfunctional Pituitary Adenomas

The decision to offer resection of an NFA is based on careful evaluation of a patient's clinical presentation, MRI, serum hormonal assessment, and formal visual field testing. This decision must be individualized to each patient's particular situation and preferences. As in all cases, medical comorbidities and the patient's overall clinical status must be carefully considered. Regarding age limitations for surgery, one study demonstrated that transsphenoidal surgery for NFAs in elderly patients (older than 70 years of age) is both safe and effective, with the only significant variation in outcome being a lower rate of hormonal axis recovery.[21]

In most cases, resection of NFAs can be safely accomplished via a transsphenoidal approach. Some tumors with primarily suprasellar, parasellar, or subfrontal extension require resection via a standard transcranial approach.[9] In recent years, extended transsphenoidal techniques have been used to resect lesions with subfrontal and clival extension.[22,23] The relationship of the tumor to the optic complex and the ability to resect tumor while working around the optic apparatus will partially dictate the selection of the surgical approach.

The risk of cerebrospinal fluid (CSF) leak after transsphenoidal surgery for NFAs has been reported as 3 to 53%.[21,24–27] As expected, the incidence of CSF leaks is higher after resection of macroadenomas and lesions with suprasellar extension. Smaller CSF leaks can frequently be controlled intraoperatively using dural replacement grafts, cellulose sponge, and fibrin glue. Larger CSF leaks frequently require at times the placement of an abdominal fat or fascial graft. Adjunct lumbar drainage may be required if leaking is noted postoperatively but is not routinely performed when an intraoperative leak is observed.

Rates of total resection of NFAs have been reported as 35 to 90% in major surgical series and are limited primarily by the degree of cavernous sinus invasion and encasement of the internal carotid artery.[12,27–30] The use of the angled endoscope as a primary or adjunct modality has permitted the evaluation of residual tumor in the cavernous sinuses, although resection in this region may still be limited by proximity to or encasement of the internal carotid artery and cranial nerves. Many patients, therefore, require adjuvant radiation therapy or radiosurgery for residual or recurrent disease. Giant pituitary macroadenomas may require a staged or combined procedure using both transcranial and transsphenoidal approaches. The rates of recurrence of NFAs after gross total resection have been reported to be between 5 to 27% in previous series, depending primarily on the follow-up time of the particular study.[9,12,31–36]

Postoperative Management of Nonfunctioning Adenomas

Routine follow-up MRI is recommended 3 months after resection of NFAs and on a yearly basis thereafter. Postoperative radiosurgery may be employed, when necessary, after the 3-month postoperative time point.

From an endocrinological perspective, the major goal after resection is to ensure that panhypopituitarism has not developed. The incidence of postoperative panhypopituitarism after transsphenoidal resection of NFAs has been reported as 12 to 44%.[36,37] Endocrine evaluation is recommended between 6 and 12 weeks after resection.[38] This includes a serum-free T_4 level, a fasting serum cortisol level, a GH level, a testosterone level in men, and an FSH level in postmenopausal women.[38] Improvement in endocrine function has been reported in approximately 30% of patients after resection of NFAs, especially in cases of macroadenomas.[39–42] Improvement of visual function has been reported to occur in the vast majority of cases after resection of NFAs.[21,24,32]

Postoperative Radiation Therapy and Radiosurgery

After surgical debulking of NFAs, radiation therapy has been shown to significantly improve progression-free survival rates.[30,40,41] One study compared patients undergoing postoperative radiotherapy after surgery with patients undergoing only resection. The progression-free survival rates in the radiation group at 5 and 15 years were each 93%, compared with rates of 68% and 33%, respectively, in the unirradiated group.[41] Another study reported 10- and 20-year tumor recurrence rates of 6% and 12%, respectively, after resection and subsequent conventional radiation for NFAs.[40]

Despite these survival rates, conventional radiation therapy after transsphenoidal resection incurs its own set of risks. Panhypopituitarism, independent of tumor regrowth, has been reported in 50 to 100% of patients undergoing postoperative radiation.[42–45] In turn, panhypopituitarism has been associated with decreased survival and quality of life for affected patients compared with age-matched controls.[46–49] Furthermore, radiation therapy after resection of NFAs has been associated with some less frequent complications such as optic nerve atrophy,[45,50] secondary brain tumors,[40,51] and cerebrovascular accidents (CVAs).[40,52] Finally, conventional radiotherapy must be given in 20 to 25 daily fractions, as compared with radiosurgical methods that frequently require one treatment.[53] For these reasons, some authors have advocated observation alone after resection of NFAs.[33] The authors of one study retrospectively analyzed a series of 97 patients after transsphenoidal resection of NFAs, with a mean follow-up time of 6 years.[33] For patients with residual disease shown on postoperative MRI (72% of all cases), the 5- and 10-year tumor growth-free survival rates were 94% and 81%, respectively. For patients with no evidence of residual disease on postoperative imaging, the 5- and 10-year tumor growth-free survival rates were both 100%.

In recent years, radiosurgical treatment has essentially replaced conventional radiotherapy for residual or recurrent NFAs in most major centers. Gamma knife surgery (GKS) has demonstrated tumor growth control rates in the 88 to 97% range, with acceptable risk profiles.[28,53–57] Radiosurgery can typically be used for residual or recurrent lesions with tumor volumes of 12 to 15 cm^3 and with sufficient distance between the lesion and the optic nerve.[28] The optimal prescription dosage for NFAs using GKS has been reported to be between 14 and 20 Gy delivered to the tumor margin.[54] The typical dose used at our institution for residual or recurrent NFAs in the parasellar region is 15 to 16 Gy delivered to the 50% isodose line.[53,58] In a previous study from our institution reporting 56 patients with NFAs undergoing postoperative GKS, there were no tumor recurrences during the median follow-up period of 36 months.[59] The same study further demonstrated that a minimum distance of 3 mm between the optic complex and tumor was required to safely achieve tumor control with GKS. In cases of close tumor proximity to the optic apparatus, we rely on fractionated radiosurgical treatments, which have been shown to have excellent tumor control rates, with a reported accuracy of less than 1 mm.[60]

Complications of radiosurgery for recurrent or residual NFAs have certainly been less frequent than those encountered with the previous era of conventional radiation. The rate of GKS-induced optic neuropathy with visual loss has been quite low, with primarily individual cases reported among several large series.[53,61] Rates of GKS-induced hypopituitarism have been reported as 14 to 19%.[55,57] Transient expansion of tumor has been reported in 3 to 13% of cases after GKS, whereas cystic enlargement of tumors has been observed in only a minority of patients.[54,57,62]

There has been a paradigm shift in the surgical management of invasive pituitary adenomas since the advent of radiosurgery. Aggressive tumor resection in the cavernous sinus region carries a high risk of vascular and cranial nerve injury, making gross total resection an impractical and unsafe goal in many instances. Tumor debulking of the sellar and suprasellar region, followed by radiosurgery of the residual cavernous sinus component, has been advocated by many authors and is gradually becoming the standard of care for these lesions.[28,63]

Conclusion

Nonfunctioning adenomas are the most commonly encountered subtype of pituitary adenomas. They can be classified according to their size as well as their immunohistochemical staining characteristics. Nonfunctioning microadenomas are frequently incidental findings and can be managed with a watchful waiting approach until documented growth is demonstrated or clinical symptoms develop. Macroadenomas commonly present with symptoms related to mass effect on surrounding structures, yet hypopituitarism is frequently diagnosed as well. The natural history of these lesions suggests a high propensity for growth, making their treatment primarily surgical. Medical treatment of NFAs remains anecdotal. Resection rates of 90% have been reported in cases without invasion of the cavernous sinus. The transsphenoidal route is preferred in most cases and has demonstrated excellent rates of tumor resection with acceptable risk profiles. Complete resection may not be a practical goal in cases of NFAs with cavernous sinus involvement, and multimodal treatment including surgery and radiation is often necessary. Recurrence rates in long-term surgical series mandate close follow-up and high likelihood for subsequent radiosurgery for recurrent or residual tumors.

References

1. Asa SL, Ezzat S. The pathogenesis of pituitary tumours. Nat Rev Cancer 2002;2:836–849
2. Molitch ME. Pituitary incidentalomas. Endocrinol Metab Clin North Am 1997;26:725–740
3. Ezzat S, Asa SL, Couldwell WT, et al. The prevalence of pituitary adenomas: a systematic review. Cancer 2004;101:613–619
4. Milker-Zabel S, Debus J, Thilmann C, Schlegel W, Wannenmacher M. Fractionated stereotactically guided radiotherapy and radiosurgery in the treatment of functional and nonfunctional adenomas of the pituitary gland. Int J Radiat Oncol Biol Phys 2001;50:1279–1286
5. Sanno N, Teramoto A, Osamura RY, et al. Pathology of pituitary tumors. Neurosurg Clin N Am 2003;14:25–39, vi
6. Zada G, Liu CY, Fishback D, Singer PA, Weiss MH. Recognition and management of delayed hyponatremia following transsphenoidal pituitary surgery. J Neurosurg 2007;106:66–71
7. Black PM, Hsu DW, Klibanski A, et al. Hormone production in clinically nonfunctioning pituitary adenomas. J Neurosurg 1987;66:244–250
8. Shomali ME, Katznelson L. Medical therapy of gonadotropin-producing and nonfunctioning pituitary adenomas. Pituitary 2002;5:89–98
9. Fahlbusch R, Buchfelder M, Honegger J, Nomikos P. Nonfunctional pituitary adenomas. In: Krisht A, Tindall GT, ed. Pituitary Disorders: Comprehensive Management. Baltimore: Lippincott Williams & Wilkins; 1999:281–285
10. Saccomanno K, Gil del Alamo P, Bassetti M, Reza-Elahi F, Spada A. In vitro detection of glycoprotein production and secretion by human nonfunctioning pituitary adenomas. J Endocrinol Invest 1993;16:109–115
11. Yamada S, Asa SL, Kovacs K, Muller P, Smyth HS. Analysis of hormone secretion by clinically nonfunctioning human pituitary adenomas using the reverse hemolytic plaque assay. J Clin Endocrinol Metab 1989;68:73–80
12. Ferrante E, Ferraroni M, Castrignanò T, et al. Non-functioning pituitary adenoma database: a useful resource to improve the clinical management of pituitary tumors. Eur J Endocrinol 2006;155: 823–829
13. Tindall G, Barrow D. Disorders of the Pituitary. St. Louis: CV Mosby; 1986
14. Patten J. Neurological Differential Diagnosis, 2nd ed. London: Springer; 1996
15. Nielsen EH, Lindholm J, Bjerre P, et al. Frequent occurrence of pituitary apoplexy in patients with non-functioning pituitary adenoma. Clin Endocrinol (Oxf) 2006;64:319–322
16. Simard MF. Pituitary tumor endocrinopathies and their endocrine evaluation. Neurosurg Clin N Am 2003;14:41–54, vi
17. Bonicki W, Kasperlik-Załuska A, Koszewski W, Zgliczyński W, Wisławski J. Pituitary apoplexy: endocrine, surgical and oncological emergency. Incidence, clinical course and treatment with reference to 799 cases of pituitary adenomas. Acta Neurochir (Wien) 1993;120:118–122
18. Dubuisson AS, Beckers A, Stevenaert A. Classical pituitary tumour apoplexy: clinical features, management and outcomes in a series of 24 patients. Clin Neurol Neurosurg 2007;109:63–70
19. Karavitaki N, Collison K, Halliday J, et al. What is the natural history of nonoperated nonfunctioning pituitary adenomas? Clin Endocrinol (Oxf) 2007;67:938–943
20. Dekkers OM, Hammer S, de Keizer RJ, et al. The natural course of non-functioning pituitary macroadenomas. Eur J Endocrinol 2007;156:217–224
21. Kurosaki M, Lüdecke DK, Flitsch J, Saeger W. Surgical treatment of clinically nonsecreting pituitary adenomas in elderly patients. Neurosurgery 2000;47:843–848, discussion 848–849
22. Couldwell WT, Weiss MH, Rabb C, Liu JK, Apfelbaum RI, Fukushima T. Variations on the standard transsphenoidal approach to the sellar region, with emphasis on the extended approaches and parasellar approaches: surgical experience in 105 cases. Neurosurgery 2004;55:539–547, discussion 547–550
23. Kitano M, Taneda M, Shimono T, Nakao Y. Extended transsphenoidal approach for surgical management of pituitary adenomas invading the cavernous sinus. J Neurosurg 2008;108:26–36
24. Black PM, Zervas NT, Candia G. Management of large pituitary adenomas by transsphenoidal surgery. Surg Neurol 1988;29: 443–447
25. Neal JG, Patel SJ, Kulbersh JS, Osguthorpe JD, Schlosser RJ. Comparison of techniques for transsphenoidal pituitary surgery. Am J Rhinol 2007;21:203–206
26. Nishioka H, Haraoka J, Ikeda Y. Risk factors of cerebrospinal fluid rhinorrhea following transsphenoidal surgery. Acta Neurochir (Wien) 2005;147:1163–1166, discussion 1166
27. Zada G, Kelly DF, Cohan P, Wang C, Swerdloff R. Endonasal transsphenoidal approach for pituitary adenomas and other sellar lesions: an assessment of efficacy, safety, and patient impressions. J Neurosurg 2003;98:350–358
28. Losa M, Valle M, Mortini P, et al. Gamma knife surgery for treatment of residual nonfunctioning pituitary adenomas after surgical debulking. J Neurosurg 2004;100:438–444
29. Saito K, Kuwayama A, Yamamoto N, Sugita K. The transsphenoidal removal of nonfunctioning pituitary adenomas with suprasellar extensions: the open sella method and intentionally staged operation. Neurosurgery 1995;36:668–675, discussion 675–676

30. Woollons AC, Hunn MK, Rajapakse YR, et al. Non-functioning pituitary adenomas: indications for postoperative radiotherapy. Clin Endocrinol (Oxf) 2000;53:713–717
31. Bradley KM, Adams CB, Potter CP, Wheeler DW, Anslow PJ, Burke CW. An audit of selected patients with non-functioning pituitary adenoma treated by transsphenoidal surgery without irradiation. Clin Endocrinol (Oxf) 1994;41:655–659
32. Ciric I, Mikhael M, Stafford T, Lawson L, Garces R. Transsphenoidal microsurgery of pituitary macroadenomas with long-term follow-up results. J Neurosurg 1983;59:395–401
33. Dekkers OM, Pereira AM, Roelfsema F, et al. Observation alone after transsphenoidal surgery for nonfunctioning pituitary macroadenoma. J Clin Endocrinol Metab 2006;91:1796–1801
34. Ebersold MJ, Quast LM, Laws ER Jr, Scheithauer B, Randall RV. Long-term results in transsphenoidal removal of nonfunctioning pituitary adenomas. J Neurosurg 1986;64:713–719
35. Jaffrain-Rea ML, Derome P, Bataini JP, Thomopoulos P, Bertagna X, Luton JP. Influence of radiotherapy on long-term relapse in clinically non-secreting pituitary adenomas. A retrospective study (1970-1988). Eur J Med 1993;2:398–403
36. Petruson B, Jakobsson KE, Elfverson J, Bengtsson BA. Five-year follow-up of nonsecreting pituitary adenomas. Arch Otolaryngol Head Neck Surg 1995;121:317–322
37. Nielsen EH, Lindholm J, Laurberg P, et al. Nonfunctioning pituitary adenoma: incidence, causes of death and quality of life in relation to pituitary function. Pituitary 2007;10:67–73
38. Singer PA, Sevilla LJ. Postoperative endocrine management of pituitary tumors. Neurosurg Clin N Am 2003;14:123–138
39. Nomikos P, Ladar C, Fahlbusch R, Buchfelder M. Impact of primary surgery on pituitary function in patients with non-functioning pituitary adenomas—a study on 721 patients. Acta Neurochir (Wien) 2004;146:27–35
40. Breen P, Flickinger JC, Kondziolka D, Martinez AJ. Radiotherapy for nonfunctional pituitary adenoma: analysis of long-term tumor control. J Neurosurg 1998;89:933–938
41. Gittoes NJ, Bates AS, Tse W, et al. Radiotherapy for non-function pituitary tumours. Clin Endocrinol (Oxf) 1998;48:331–337
42. Littley MD, Shalet SM, Beardwell CG, Ahmed SR, Applegate G, Sutton ML. Hypopituitarism following external radiotherapy for pituitary tumours in adults. QJM 1989;70:145–160
43. McCord MW, Buatti JM, Fennell EM, et al. Radiotherapy for pituitary adenoma: long-term outcome and sequelae. Int J Radiat Oncol Biol Phys 1997;39:437–444
44. Nelson PB, Goodman ML, Flickenger JC, Richardson DW, Robinson AG. Endocrine function in patients with large pituitary tumors treated with operative decompression and radiation therapy. Neurosurgery 1989;24:398–400
45. Tsang RW, Brierley JD, Panzarella T, Gospodarowicz MK, Sutcliffe SB, Simpson WJ. Radiation therapy for pituitary adenoma: treatment outcome and prognostic factors. Int J Radiat Oncol Biol Phys 1994;30:557–565
46. Bates AS, Bullivant B, Sheppard MC, Stewart PM. Life expectancy following surgery for pituitary tumours. Clin Endocrinol (Oxf) 1999;50:315–319
47. Bülow B, Hagmar L, Mikoczy Z, Nordström CH, Erfurth EM. Increased cerebrovascular mortality in patients with hypopituitarism. Clin Endocrinol (Oxf) 1997;46:75–81
48. Clayton RN. Mortality, cardiovascular events and risk factors in hypopituitarism. Growth Horm IGF Res 1998;8(Suppl A):69–76
49. Rosén T, Bengtsson BA. Premature mortality due to cardiovascular disease in hypopituitarism. Lancet 1990;336:285–288
50. Brada M, Rajan B, Traish D, et al. The long-term efficacy of conservative surgery and radiotherapy in the control of pituitary adenomas. Clin Endocrinol (Oxf) 1993;38:571–578
51. Minniti G, Traish D, Ashley S, Gonsalves A, Brada M. Risk of second brain tumor after conservative surgery and radiotherapy for pituitary adenoma: update after an additional 10 years. J Clin Endocrinol Metab 2005;90:800–804
52. Flickinger JC, Nelson PB, Taylor FH, Robinson A. Incidence of cerebral infarction after radiotherapy for pituitary adenoma. Cancer 1989;63:2404–2408
53. Sheehan JP, Kondziolka D, Flickinger J, Lunsford LD. Radiosurgery for residual or recurrent nonfunctioning pituitary adenoma. J Neurosurg 2002;97(5, Suppl):408–414
54. Iwai Y, Yamanaka K, Yoshioka K. Radiosurgery for nonfunctioning pituitary adenomas. Neurosurgery 2005;56:699–705, discussion 699–705
55. Mokry M, Ramschak-Schwarzer S, Simbrunner J, Ganz JC, Pendl G. A six year experience with the postoperative radiosurgical management of pituitary adenomas. Stereotact Funct Neurosurg 1999;72(Suppl 1):88–100
56. Pollock BE, Carpenter PC. Stereotactic radiosurgery as an alternative to fractionated radiotherapy for patients with recurrent or residual nonfunctioning pituitary adenomas. Neurosurgery 2003;53:1086–1091, discussion 1091–1094
57. Wowra B, Stummer W. Efficacy of gamma knife radiosurgery for nonfunctioning pituitary adenomas: a quantitative follow up with magnetic resonance imaging-based volumetric analysis. J Neurosurg 2002;97(5, Suppl):429–432
58. Sheehan JP, Kondziolka D, Flickinger J, Lunsford LD. Radiosurgery for nonfunctioning pituitary adenoma. Neurosurg Focus 2003;14: e9
59. Petrovich Z, Yu C, Giannotta SL, Zee CS, Apuzzo ML. Gamma knife radiosurgery for pituitary adenoma: early results. Neurosurgery 2003;53:51–59, discussion 59–61
60. Pham CJ, Chang SD, Gibbs IC, Jones P, Heilbrun MP, Adler JR Jr. Preliminary visual field preservation after staged CyberKnife radiosurgery for perioptic lesions. Neurosurgery 2004;54:799–810, discussion 810–812
61. Izawa M, Hayashi M, Nakaya K, et al. Gamma knife radiosurgery for pituitary adenomas. J Neurosurg 2000;93(Suppl 3):19–22
62. Hayashi M, Izawa M, Hiyama H, et al. Gamma knife radiosurgery for pituitary adenomas. Stereotact Funct Neurosurg 1999;72(Suppl 1): 111–118
63. Kuo JS, Chen JC, Yu C, et al. Gamma knife radiosurgery for benign cavernous sinus tumors: quantitative analysis of treatment outcomes. Neurosurgery 2004;54:1385–1393, discussion 1393–1394

14 Neuro-Ophthalmologic Considerations

Jacqueline M.S. Winterkorn, Richard L. Levy, and Marc J. Dinkin

A neuro-ophthalmologist is an essential member of the team of physicians caring for patients with pituitary lesions, along with a neurosurgeon, a neurologist, a radiologist, and an endocrinologist. The neuro-ophthalmologist quantifies and evaluates the impact of sellar lesions on the afferent and efferent visual pathways, helps to determine the tempo of tumor growth, and monitors the success and possible complications of treatment. In cases where vision loss or blurred or double vision is the presenting symptom, the neuro-ophthalmologist may be the first to recognize a pituitary lesion. In previously diagnosed cases, the neuro-ophthalmologist's role is to follow sequential visual fields and determine progression or stability of defects. By supplying information about functioning in the visual pathway, the neuro-ophthalmologist influences decisions about the modality and timing of treatment.

Pituitary adenomas are among the most common lesions in the head, with small ones found at autopsy in a quarter of otherwise normal individuals. Therefore, most pituitary adenomas do not have neuro-ophthalmologic symptoms. Pituitary adenomas greater than 1 cm in height are likely to cause symptoms by compressing the anterior visual pathway or the nerves controlling ocular motility. A similar syndrome of visual loss can be caused by craniopharyngiomas, meningiomas, or gliomas. Information supplied by the neuro-ophthalmologist may move the team toward a therapeutic decision.

This chapter begins with a description of the structures surrounding the pituitary, including the afferent visual pathways and the cavernous sinus, and how their anatomy is affected by pituitary lesions. It goes on to consider various neuro-ophthalmologic presentations of pituitary lesions, especially visual field loss. It outlines indications for treatment, with special attention to pituitary apoplexy, hypophysitis, and pregnancy. After discussing visual recovery, complications of treatment, and follow-up, the chapter concludes with a note on the place of neuro-ophthalmology in the care of patients with pituitary adenomas.

Anatomical Considerations

The Afferent Visual Pathway

The pituitary sets in the sella turcica just above the sphenoid sinus and between the paired cavernous sinuses. The proximity of the pituitary to the anterior visual pathway and to the cavernous sinuses makes knowledge of their anatomy critical. Axons of the retinal ganglion cells destined to synapse in the dorsal lateral geniculate nuclei pass through the optic nerves, optic chiasm, and optic tracts to reach their termination. Each eye provides information about both hemifields, that is, both the right and left halves of visual space, which are distributed at the optic chiasm. Within the optic nerve, axons originating in the temporal retina remain temporal and subserve the contralateral visual hemifield. Axons from the nasal retina subserve the temporal visual field. Axons from retinal ganglion cells in the superior retina are located superiorly in the optic nerve, optic tract, and cerebral cortex, and subserve vision in the inferior hemifield. More than half of the 1.1 to 1.3 million axons in each human optic nerve decussate in the optic chiasm. Axons from the nasal half of the right eye carry information about the right half of visual space and decussate in the optic chiasm to join the left optic tract, and axons from the temporal half of the right eye that carry information about the left half of space remain on the right, to be joined by the nasal axons crossing from the left eye. Hemidecussation allows a neat topographical map of visual space to be projected on the various visual brain centers and allows precise localization of lesions along the pathway from the retina to the occipital cortex. **Figure 14.1** shows a retinotopic map of the visual system.

The optic nerves are considered "cranial nerve II," even though they are embryologically and histologically white matter tracts of the brain and their axons are myelinated by oligodendrocytes like other central fibers. In each eye, axons of retinal ganglion cells run in the nerve fiber layer to reach the optic disk and then pass through the lamina cribrosa, a collection of windows through the posterior sclera of the eye, which is continuous with the dura mater of the brain. Just behind the eye, the axons become myelinated and the optic nerve reaches its greatest diameter of 4 mm, which declines to 3.5 mm posteriorly. After traversing the orbit, the optic nerve passes through the optic canal, where its dural sheath is fused to the wall of the canal, rendering it particularly susceptible to traumatic injury. In 4% of patients, a defect in the wall of the canal exposes the optic nerve to the sphenoid sinus.[1] The intracranial portion of the optic nerve passes beneath the falciform ligament, along the planum sphenoidale, and turns superiorly and medially to form the

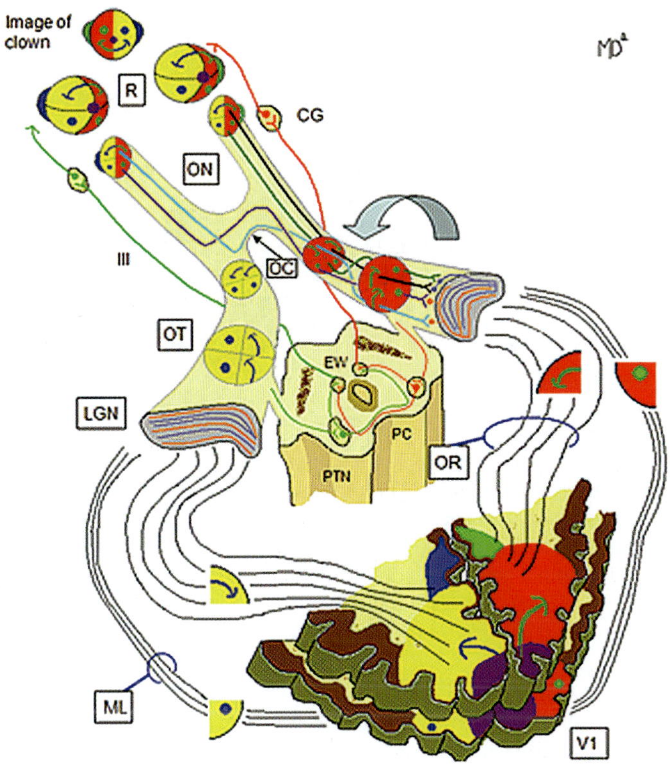

Fig. 14.1 A simplified representation of a clown throughout the visual pathways. First, retinotopic representation (R) is inverted and reversed as light rays cross through the lens. Second, in the optic nerves (ON), reversed and inverted representation is maintained. Third, in the optic chiasm (OC), fibers carrying temporal information cross, whereas fibers carrying nasal information remain ipsilateral. Fibers carrying superior temporal information cross anteriorly in the chiasm (purple path), while those carrying inferior temporal information cross posteriorly (aqua path). Fourth, the optic tracts (OT) carry information from the contralateral visual field. Note that orientation changes as superior fibers (inferior field) move medially and inferior fibers (superior field) move laterally. Fifth, in the lateral geniculate nucleus (LGN), fibers synapse within six layers. Fibers originating in the contralateral eye synapse in layers 1, 4, and 6 (orange), whereas fibers from ipsilateral eye synapse in layers 2, 3, and 5 (lavender). Sixth, optic radiation (OR) carries the inferior half of the contralateral field through the parietal lobe. Seventh, Meyer's loop (ML) carries the superior contralateral field through the temporal lobe. Eighth, in the occipital (striate) cortex (V1), each side receives the contralateral field. Representation of the clown's face is shown overlying the two halves of the cortex, which is shown in two axial slices, one superior and one inferior to the calcarine fissure. Macular information (the purple nose) is disproportionately represented at the occipital tip. Ninth, the clown's ears are contained within the temporal crescent, which is only seen by the ipsilateral eye. Its representation is in the contralateral occipital cortex, anteriorly and medially. Finally, consensual pupillary reactions are shown. Some fibers (light green on the left, red on the right) peel off the optic tracts and synapse in the pretectal nuclei (PTN). From each PTN, fibers reach the ipsilateral Edinger Westphal (EW) nucleus, a subnucleus of the oculomotor nuclear complex where they synapse with parasympathetic fibers of the oculomotor nerve (III). These fibers then synapse in the ciliary ganglion (CG) with postganglionic fibers that travel to the iris sphincter muscle, which constricts the pupil. From each PTN, fibers also travel to the contralateral EW, thereby ensuring consensual constriction of the contralateral pupil.

optic chiasm. This intracranial segment is the most variable portion of the nerve, with an average length of 10 mm but commonly ranging from 5 to 15 mm, depending on the position of the optic chiasm. In 25% of patients the optic nerves follow such an upturned course that the incident angle with the chiasm is acute.[2]

The optic chiasm is named for the Greek letter Chi (τττ), but its shape more closely resembles the letter H. The dimensions of the chiasm are roughly 12 to 13 mm wide, 3 to 4 mm high, and 8 mm long, varying in size depending on the individual and the method of measurement. In the human brain, slightly more than half (53%) of the axons decussate in the optic chiasm. Nondecussating axons travel in a lateral position through the chiasm. Decussating axons cross left to right or right to left, arranged in parallel bundles across the cross-bar of the "H."

The location of the chiasm relative to the pituitary and pituitary stalk can vary. In approximately 80% of patients the optic chiasm is located directly above the pituitary. However, in 5 to 10% of the population, the chiasm is pre-fixed, meaning that it lies anterior to the pituitary adjacent to the posterior optic nerves, and in 11 to 15% it is post-fixed, lying above the dorsum sella, not far from the optic tracts. This is diagrammed in **Fig. 14.2**.

The optic chiasm lies an average of 10 mm above the pituitary, but in 14% of patients this distance may be as little as 2 mm.[2] Axons from the macula, the central region of the retina, cross in the posterior portion of the chiasm, whereas axons from the periphery cross more anteriorly.

From the optic chiasm, the optic tracts run posteriorly, superiorly, and laterally, passing between the anterior perforated substance and the tuber cinereum. After curving around the cerebral peduncle, each optic tract gives off the retinal ganglion cell axons that subserve the pupillary light reflex. These axons leave the optic tract and pass medially in the brachium of the superior colliculus to synapse in the pretectum. Other populations of retinal ganglion cells project to the superior colliculus and to the accessory optic system. Nerve fibers responsible for entrainment of circadian rhythms to ambient light come off the dorsal optic chiasm and project into the hypothalamus. The remaining 90% of retinal ganglion cell axons carry visual information to the lateral geniculate nucleus (LGN). The retinotopic organization of axons is maintained in the optic tracts but is rotated in the lateral geniculate such that superior ganglion cell fibers are found more medially and inferior fibers more laterally. The LGN has six cellular layers, with contralateral fibers synapsing in layers 1, 4, and 6, and ipsilateral fibers synapsing in layers 2, 3, and 5 (**Fig. 14.1**).

Neurons of the LGN give off axons that ultimately synapse in the primary visual cortex (V1) of the occipital lobe. Fibers transferring inferior visual field information from the superior retinal ganglion cells travel through the parietal lobe and synapse superior to the calcarine fissure that divides the occipital cortex in two. In contrast, fibers

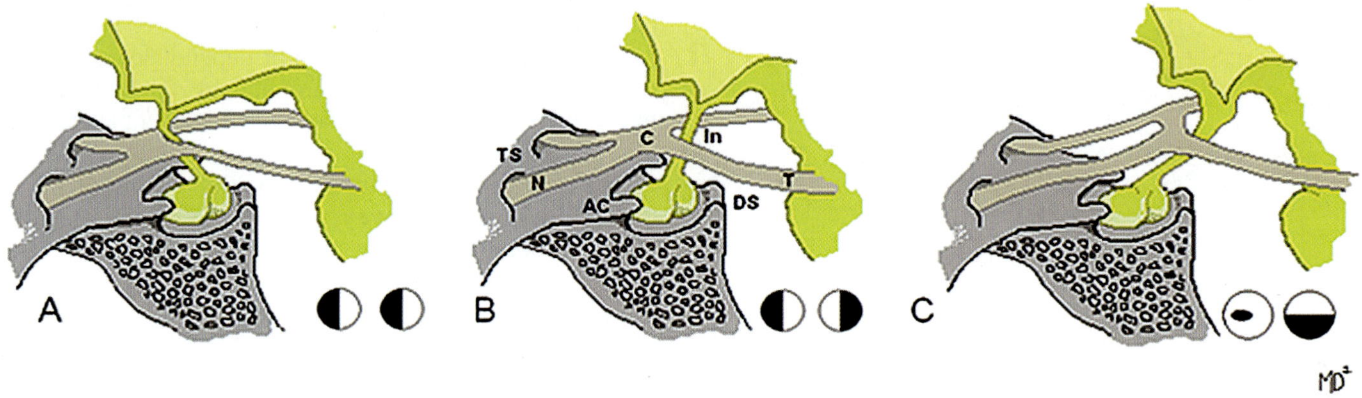

Fig. 14.2 Variable anatomy of the chiasm determines type of visual loss from pituitary tumors. **(A)** The chiasm is pre-fixed, above the tuberculum sellae, placing the optic tracts in the line of an expanding pituitary tumor. Field loss may include a homonymous hemianopia. **(B)** The optic chiasm is normal, lying above the diaphragma sella and the pituitary gland. Typical field loss from an expanding pituitary tumor would be bitemporal hemianopia. **(C)** The chiasm is post-fixed above the dorsum sellae. The pituitary lies below the optic nerves, so that monocular field defects (cecocentral, arcuate, and altitudinal) result. Note that the angle of the infundibulum varies accordingly. AC, anterior clinoid process; C, optic chiasm; DS, dorsum sellae; In, infundibulum; N, optic nerves; T, optic tracts; TS, tuberculum sellae.

subserving the superior field travel anteriorly in the temporal lobe and then posteriorly back to the inferior occipital cortex through a bundle of fibers called Meyer's loop. From the primary visual cortex, information is passed to visual processing areas that are concerned with object recognition (the temporal stream) and visuospatial mapping (the parietal stream).

Blood Supply

The blood supply to the anterior visual system is provided by an extensive pial network on its surface, derived from the carotid artery and its branches. The intracanalicular optic nerve receives blood from the ophthalmic artery, with some of its short branches, the posterior ciliary arteries, meeting to form an anastomosis around the anterior optic nerve called the circle of Zinn-Haller. The intracranial portion of the nerve is fed from the internal carotid, anterior cerebral, and anterior communicating arteries, with some recurrent branches from the ophthalmic artery. Some authors have found major input from the anterior superior hypophyseal artery.[3,4]

The blood supply to the optic chiasm is complex.[1,3–5] The inferior aspect is fed by the anterior superior hypophyseal and posterior communicating arteries. The lateral aspect receives blood directly from the ophthalmic (C6) segment of the internal carotid. The superior aspect is fed mainly from the anterior cerebral and anterior communicating arteries. The rich anastomoses among these arteries account for the rarity of ischemic lesions of the optic chiasm. The crossing macular fibers in the central chiasm are susceptible to compression because once the pituitary expands more than about a centimeter, the chiasm begins to be compressed.

The anterior optic tract is fed by a continuation of the chiasmal pial plexus. Posterior to that, its main contributor is the anterior choroidal artery. The lateral geniculate nucleus has a dual blood supply; the anterior aspect is fed by the anterior choroidal artery (arising from the internal carotid), whereas the posterior aspect is fed by the lateral choroidal artery, a tributary of the posterior cerebral artery. Ischemia to the anterior choroidal artery leads to contralateral sectoral defects superiorly and inferiorly, sparing a central zone, whereas the converse is true for lateral choroidal artery infarcts.

Efferent Pathways: Cavernous Sinus

The cavernous sinus is a rete or plexus of blood vessels surrounding the carotid artery on either side of the pituitary fossa. A diagram of its structures is shown in **Fig. 14.3**.

Cranial nerves responsible for eye movements and pupillary responses to light pass through the cavernous sinuses on their way to the orbit. Expanding pituitary lesions can lead to compression or hemorrhage into the cavernous sinus on either side, resulting in ophthalmoplegia.

The oculomotor nerve (cranial nerve III) is the motor nerve most frequently involved by pituitary adenomas. It exits the midbrain ventrally in the interpeduncular fossa, passing between the posterior cerebral and superior cerebellar arteries, and runs parallel and just lateral to the posterior communicating artery, to reach the cavernous sinus. Fibers controlling pupillary constriction to light are situated together in a bundle on the medial surface of the nerve, in a position where they are vulnerable to compression by a posterior communicating artery aneurysm. In contrast, ischemic third nerve palsies tend to spare this bundle. Just

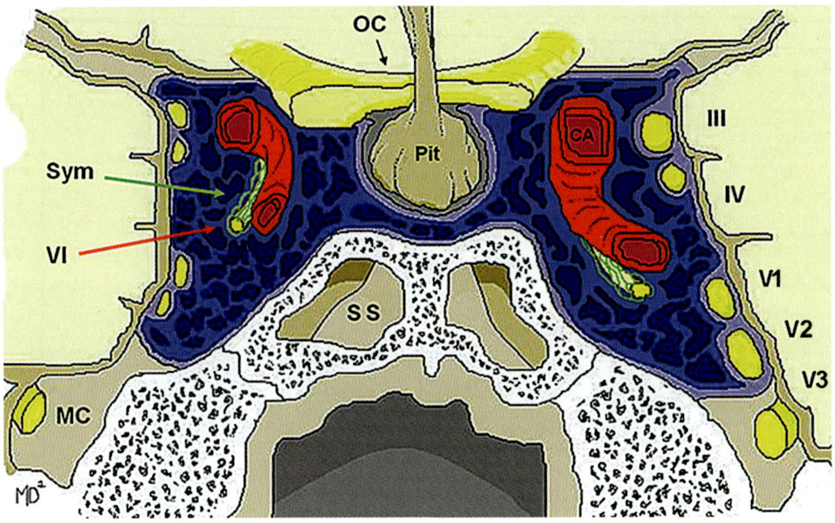

Fig. 14.3 The cavernous sinus (blue) is collection of venous pockets that drain blood from the sphenoparietal veins, superficial middle cerebral veins, and the superior and inferior ophthalmic veins. Blood exits to the petrosal sinus and emissary veins. It is the only location in the body where an artery, in this case the carotid artery (CA), is completely surrounded by a vein. It is also traversed by cranial nerves III, IV, V1, V2, and VI, the latter of which can be seen adjacent to the CA. The sympathetic fibers traveling toward the eye are near the abducens nerve and, in some studies, form a plexus around it. V3 travels through Meckel's cave (MC), which lies inferior to the sinus. The pituitary gland sits in between the two halves of the sinus, whereas the chiasm sits above. OC, optic chiasm; MC, Meckel's cave; Pit, pituitary gland; SS, sphenoid sinus; Sym, sympathetic nerves in plexus around VI; III, oculomotor nerve; IV, trochlear nerve; V1, ophthalmic branch of trigeminal nerve; V2, maxillary branch of trigeminal nerve; V3, mandibular branch of trigeminal nerve; VI, abducens nerve.

behind the cavernous sinus, the oculomotor nerve travels through the triangle of dura composed of the interclinoid ligament and the anterior and posterior petroclinoidal folds. It pierces the dura anterior and lateral to the posterior clinoid process and then passes within the lateral wall of the cavernous sinus. The oculomotor nerve is organized into two divisions: the superior division controls the levator palpebrae and superior rectus muscles, whereas the inferior division controls the medial rectus, inferior rectus, inferior oblique, and iris sphincter muscles. At the anterior end of the cavernous sinus, the two divisions pass just inferior to the anterior clinoid process before exiting the skull through the superior orbital fissure.

The trochlear nerve (cranial nerve IV) exits the midbrain dorsally just behind the inferior colliculus. The paired nerves cross in the anterior medullary velum, and each passes around the brainstem within the subarachnoid space. After piercing the dura to enter the cavernous sinus just inferior to the oculomotor nerve, each trochlear nerve runs in the wall of the cavernous sinus parallel to and just below the third nerve.

The abducens nerve (cranial nerve VI) is the only ocular motor nerve to run through the substance of the cavernous sinus rather than in its wall and is located between the trigeminal nerve and the intracavernous carotid. Theoretically, this makes it more susceptible to compression from the lateral wall of the sella turcica. The sympathetic fibers responsible for dilation of the pupil and widening of the palpebral fissure also pass through the cavernous sinus. They enter around the internal carotid artery, "hitchhike" briefly on the abducens nerve, and exit the cavernous sinus with the ophthalmic nerve. This accounts for the co-occurrence of abducens paresis and oculosympathetic defects with lesions in the cavernous sinus. Behind and inferior to the cavernous sinus, in Meckel's cave, the trigeminal ganglion gives off its third (mandibular) branch into the foramen ovale, leaving only the first and second divisions of the trigeminal (ophthalmic and maxillary branches) to pass through the cavernous sinus. Both divisions lie in the wall of the cavernous sinus, inferior to the trochlear nerve. The maxillary branch leaves the skull through the foramen rotundum, and the ophthalmic branch continues on in the wall of the cavernous sinus and exits through the superior orbital fissure.

■ Neuro-Ophthalmologic Presentations of Pituitary Lesions

Presenting Signs and Symptoms

Pituitary lesions can present with specific symptoms or can be discovered incidentally, for example, when neuroimaging is performed after unrelated trauma or head pain as in the case presented in **Fig. 14.4A**. Although magnetic resonance imaging (MRI) or computed tomography (CT) can indicate that a pituitary mass is of sufficient size to be in contact with the optic chiasm or the cavernous sinuses, only careful clinical examination can determine the compressive effect of the mass on the visual system. A full neuro-ophthalmologic exam should be performed, including visual acuity, color vision, stereoacuity, visual fields, pupil response, evaluation of eye movements (especially for subtle motility disturbances or nystagmus), and assessment of the optic disk for pallor and patterns of nerve fiber layer dropout.

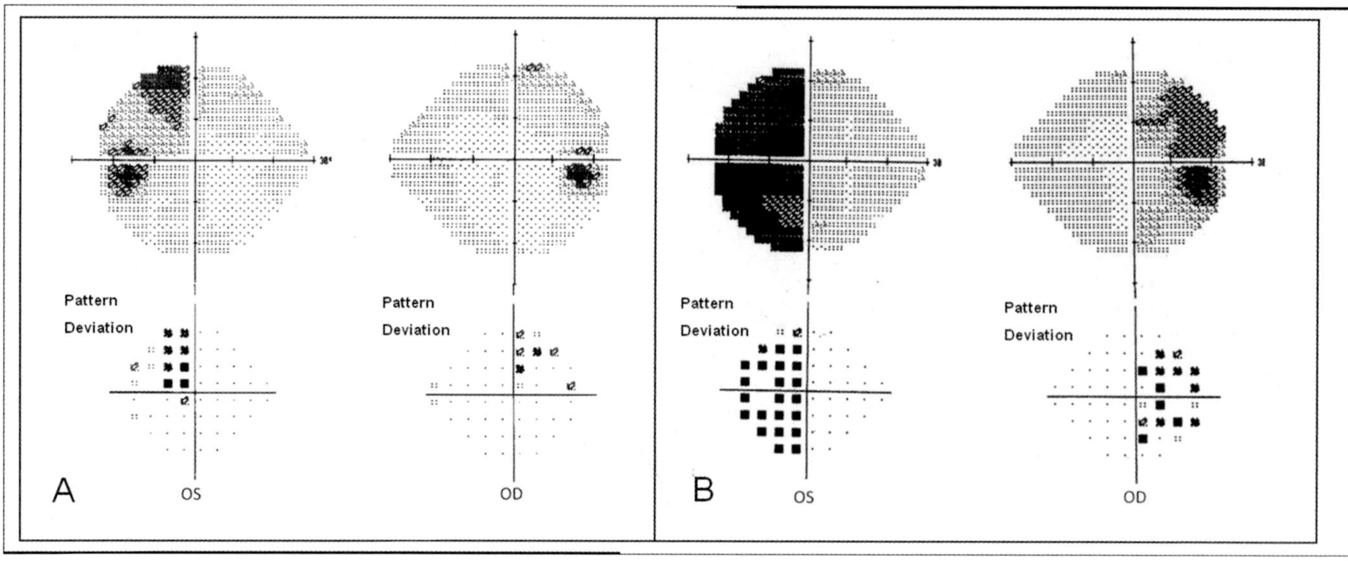

Fig. 14.4 Bitemporal defects due to chiasmal compression. **(A)** In early compression from below, superior bitemporal defects may be seen. Note that the defects hug the vertical meridian. **(B)** In more advanced compression, the superior fibers have been affected as well, and a bitemporal hemianopia has evolved.

Bitemporal Hemianopia

The classic ophthalmologic presentation of a pituitary tumor is a bitemporal hemianopia caused by compression of the crossing axons in the optic chiasm. The superior quadrants of the temporal visual field typically are affected first, corresponding to compression of the optic chiasm from below. However, depending on the patient's underlying anatomy and the growth pattern of the lesion, other loci of visual field loss are possible. A post-fixed optic chiasm is likely to produce monocular retinal nerve fiber layer defects from optic nerve compression, and an ipsilateral relative afferent pupillary defect (RAPD). A pre-fixed chiasm is likely to produce a homonymous hemianopia resulting from compression of the optic tract along with a contralateral RAPD.

The visual field has been described as an "island of vision surrounded by a sea of darkness"[6] because sensitivity to stimuli is greatest in the center at fixation and then declines toward the periphery until complete darkness is reached. Therefore, an object must be larger or brighter to be seen in the periphery than at fixation. A defect in the visual field can be thought of as part of this island sinking into darkness. Two approaches can be taken to map out a visual field defect: kinetic, in which a test object of specified size and luminance is moved from the periphery to the center until it is perceived; and static, in which a stationary stimulus is presented with increasing brightness until it reaches the threshold of perception. Formal kinetic perimetry is performed using either a tangent screen, which is a wall-mounted flat screen against which the examiner moves standardized test objects from the periphery to the center, or a Goldmann perimeter, which is a bowl-shaped background of uniform luminance against which a pantograph projects spots of different size, luminance, and color. In Goldmann perimetry, a peephole in the center of the bowl allows the examiner to monitor the patient's fixation while controlling the presentation of stimuli. For both Goldmann and tangent screen methods, the result is a series of isopters or concentric topographical curves, representing the distance from fixation at which the patient became aware of test objects.

Static perimetry has largely replaced kinetic perimetry as the standard method for obtaining visual fields, and usually is performed on a Humphrey visual field analyzer. The Humphrey analyzer consists of a similar bowl-shaped background of set luminance, and tests vision by having the patient fixate on a central target and press a button when a stimulus is perceived. The Humphrey machine offers a variety of standardized strategies that differ in the extent of grid tested, and the color, size, and luminance of the test object or background. The most common test, the 24–2 threshold test, obtains sensitivity at points within 24 degrees of fixation; the "dash 2" signifies that the grid is arranged with test points not on the axes but rather straddling the vertical and horizontal meridians, providing more value in localizing pathology. A "full-threshold" test, where sensitivity is determined at numerous points within the test grid, can be a grueling ordeal, requiring up to 30 minutes per eye. The Swedish Interactive Threshold Algorithm (SITA) was developed to shorten the testing time by eliminating empirically redundant tests. SITA Standard testing takes up to 15 minutes per eye for a 24–2 field. The more recently developed SITA Fast strategy is even more efficient, taking 3 to

5 minutes per eye. All Humphrey threshold strategies include internal controls for fixation and for false-positive and false-negative errors. The machine is automated, so that while a human operator is required to set up the test, monitoring of the patient, presentation of stimuli, and data processing are performed by the machine.

The typical visual field heralding a pituitary tumor—the bitemporal hemianopia—may be demonstrated by either static perimetry (**Fig. 14.4**) or by kinetic perimetry (**Fig. 14.5**).

Each method has a characteristic appearance. With kinetic perimetry, such as a Goldmann, early bitemporal lesions appear as a constriction of each isopter as it courses through the temporal field, often beginning in the superior quadrant, and resulting in sharp step-off of the isopter as it crosses the midline into the seeing nasal hemifield. In static perimetry, such as a Humphrey test, there is loss of sensitivity to stimuli at points temporal to the vertical midline, where the threshold stimulus is brighter than its nasal counterpart. The defect is often more pronounced in the superior quadrants. In either method, the defects strictly obey the vertical midline, which can help to differentiate pituitary lesions from masquerade syndromes such as tilted optic disks or ceco-central scotomas from hereditary dystrophies or toxicities that can create similar bitemporal defects, but which cross the midline.

The chiasmal visual field defect does not begin in the far periphery and migrate inward. Indeed, if the defect is sought in the periphery, it may be missed. Instead, the macular fibers that cross in the inferior optic chiasm are the first affected with the earliest defects near fixation. This principle is corroborated by studies with Goldmann, Humphrey, and bedside testing. Trobe et al[7] showed that to obtain a valid visual field screening for chiasmal injury using Goldmann perimetry, the tester need only explore points along the vertical midline to screen for a defect; information from the far periphery was superfluous. Similarly, confrontational testing with a red object can disclose a bitemporal desaturation missed by formal perimetry and has the additional advantage that it can be done at bedside. Most importantly for the choice of testing methods, although Humphrey perimetry does not test points as far in the periphery as Goldmann perimetry, the Humphrey is much more sensitive than the Goldmann in detecting temporal defects[8] because it compares loci across the midline quantitatively.

For multiple reasons, Humphrey perimetry has become the test of choice for patients with pituitary lesions. As stated above, it is very sensitive to hemianopic field defects. The results are quantitative and minimally dependent on the technician. Specifically, the Humphrey 24–2 testing strategy is preferred for most neuro-ophthalmologic indications, whether ocular or neurologic pathology is being evaluated. Testing the central 24 degrees around fixation accounts for more than 90% of cells in the visual cortex.[9] Indeed, cortical magnification of the macula, by which 60% of cortical cells are devoted to the central 10 degrees, makes the central 10 degrees more important than the periphery. Conversely, a Humphrey 30–2 (a 30-degree field) study may provide less reliable visual field data because peripheral loci are more likely to be influenced by eyelid position, lens artifacts, loss of patient interest, and fatigue. SITA-Standard and SITA-Fast strategies, as opposed to the more tedious full-threshold strategies, are widely preferred for detecting

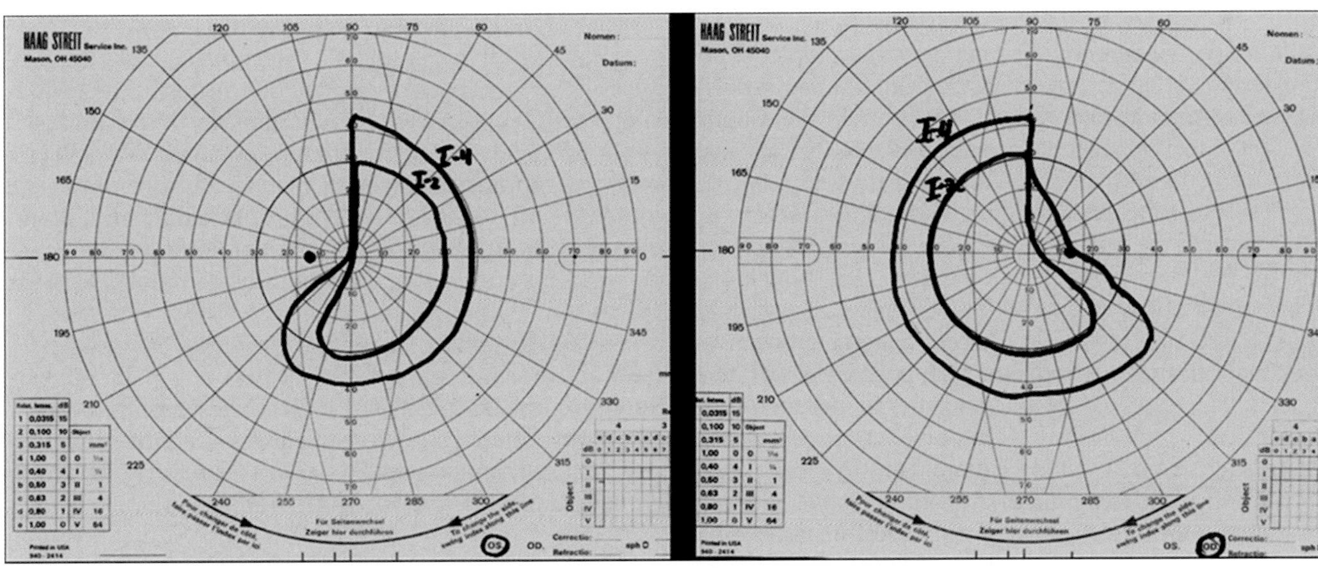

Fig. 14.5 Goldmann visual fields revealing bitemporal hemianopia with a superior predominance. This type of perimetry has the advantage of a full 180 degrees' worth of horizontal field and the ability of the physician to retest points as needed to confirm reliability. I-4e and I-2e describe light stimuli. The Roman numeral describes size, whereas the arabic numeral and letter are a function of luminosity.

and following visual field defects resulting from pituitary lesions.[10] The SITA strategy is recognized to be as sensitive as full-threshold testing for neurologic defects.[11] In addition, for patients who require shorter testing times, such as elderly, very young, or neurologically impaired patients, SITA-Fast testing may be the only way to acquire reliable data.

The use of high-pass resolution perimetry, a technique correlating neuroimaging with visual field data, has suggested that an elevation of the chiasm by 6.3 mm will create a detectable visual field defect in 50% of patients, and an elevation of 11 mm will raise this incidence to 90%. To create a complete bitemporal hemianopia, therefore, requires much more deformation of the visual structures.[12] However, the extent to which the MRI finding is correlated with the visual field is dependent on myriad other factors such as tempo of growth, the visual field test used, and individual variability. Indeed, tumors that are apparently compressing and distorting the chiasm may not necessarily be associated with any field loss.

For larger tumors, in which visual structures are extremely deformed, the visual field may offer clues to the tumor's origin. Specifically, a bitemporal defect that is denser in the inferior quadrants strongly suggests a mass originating above the chiasm, such as a craniopharyngioma. Other clinical features suggesting a nonpituitary origin include absolute field defects (blindness), asymmetric optic disk pallor, and a relative afferent pupillary defect.[13] Such clinical clues may provide a warning as to what might be encountered at the time of surgery and even influence the choice of surgical approach.

Anterior Chiasmal and Optic Tract Syndromes

Despite the preponderance of bitemporal hemianopias in pituitary lesions, other patterns of visual field loss may be present. When a tumor involves the posterior portion of one optic nerve at its junction with the chiasm, an "anterior chiasmal syndrome" is created, and the characteristic field defect is referred to as a junctional scotoma: an optic neuropathy or central defect in the ipsilateral eye, with a wedge-shaped defect in the superotemporal field of the other eye. At one time, this defect was attributed to Wilbrand's knee, an invagination of the crossing fibers into the contralateral optic nerve, but anatomical studies have shown that the inferonasal fibers take no such detour.[14] However, the anterior chiasmal syndrome remains a robust clinical phenomenon. The finding of a wedge-shaped defect, often asymptomatic, in the eye contralateral to an optic neuropathy should point the clinician toward the anterior chiasm. In these cases, neuroimaging usually finds a lesion at the junction of the anterior chiasm and the optic nerve. In some cases, chiasmal compression is associated with a temporal defect in only one eye, ostensibly because only its crossing nasal fibers have been affected.

A lesion located posterior to the chiasm produces an optic tract syndrome, characterized by an incongruent homonymous hemianopia and a contralateral afferent pupillary defect. Posterior to the chiasm, the fibers originating in the nasal retina of one eye come together with those from the contralateral temporal retina, and therefore visual field defects take on a homonymous hemianopic pattern. However, in contrast to the congruent homonymous hemianopias owing to lesions in the occipital cortex, optic tract lesions are said to produce incongruent loss, because the corresponding fibers from each side have not yet fully intermingled, although Kedar et al's[15] review of this subject showed that over 50% of optic tract lesions produce congruent defects as well.

An optic tract lesion, unique among postchiasmal syndromes, is associated with an afferent pupillary defect. Because 53% of axons originating in the retina decussate in the chiasm,[16] and of these 53% a disproportionate number may project to the pupillary centers in the pretectum, each optic tract carries more of the stimulus for pupil constriction from the contralateral eye than from the ipsilateral eye. Therefore, a light shone in the eye contralateral to a tract lesion will elicit a smaller bilateral pupillary response. The size of this relative afferent pupillary defect can be quantified by balancing it with a neutral density filter held over the other eye; this is an excellent way to follow progression or resolution of the lesion postoperatively and in years to come. Behr,[17] in 1924, described dilation of the contralateral pupil in patients with optic tract lesions, but later studies have not confirmed this finding.[18] Interestingly, careful stimulation of the nonseeing half of either eye may produce decreased or no pupillary reaction, but this phenomenon, known as pupillary hemiakinesia or Wernicke's sign,[19] has limited utility because of the scatter of light. The complete optic tract syndrome, in which one optic tract is completely disabled, produces a "bowtie" pattern of optic disk pallor in the contralateral eye (**Fig. 14.6**), temporal disk pallor in the ipsilateral eye, a contralateral relative afferent pupillary defect, and a complete contralateral homonymous hemianopia. Although complete and isolated lesions of the optic tract are uncommon with pituitary adenomas, any homonymous hemianopic visual field defect suggests extension of tumor behind the chiasm.

With larger tumors, combinations of the above field defects are possible, and all clinical data and neuroimaging findings must be considered together. For example, a relative afferent pupillary defect might suggest either an anterior chiasmal syndrome or else a tract lesion, and the details of the visual fields will help to differentiate them.

Ocular Motor Signs and Symptoms

Although pituitary lesions tend to expand upward, compressing the afferent visual system, they may grow so large

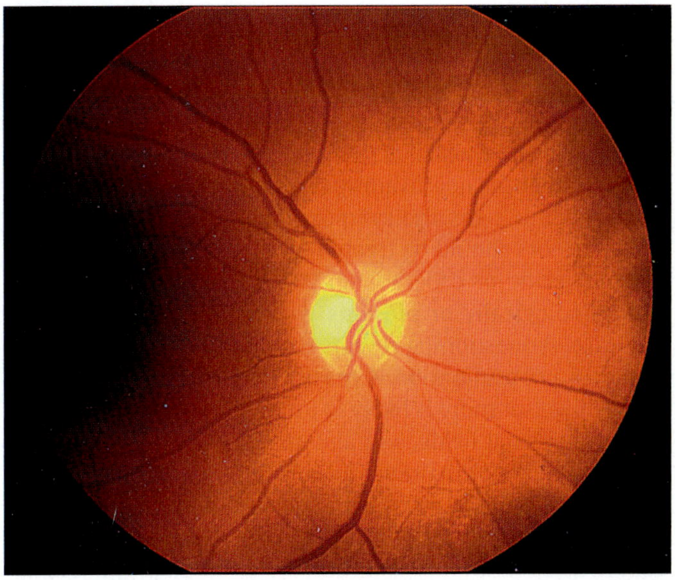

Fig. 14.6 Bowtie atrophy of the right optic disk. This is a band of pallor reflecting loss of the peripheral nasal retina and the nasal half of the macula. It is commonly seen when an enlarged pituitary compresses the nasal fibers that cross in the optic chiasm. It indicates a poor prognosis for recovery from the associated temporal visual field deficit.

that they invade or compress the adjacent cavernous sinuses. Lateral growth may even preferentially compress the cavernous sinuses without causing visual field defects. Any combination of defects can be seen involving palsies of cranial nerves III, IV, or VI, Horner syndrome from disruption of the sympathetic fibers, and facial and ocular hypesthesia from trigeminal involvement. One series[20] described five patients with pituitary adenomas who presented with cranial nerve III palsies, four of whom had no additional visual signs or symptoms. The authors concluded that oculomotor involvement is usually a late sign of an adenoma and carries a poor prognosis, but when it is the only presenting sign it may be compatible with a good outcome. Another patient had elevation of the eyelid on downgaze due to aberrant regeneration of the cranial nerve III[21] in a pituitary adenoma invading the cavernous sinus. Third nerve palsies with aberrant regeneration may be subtle, requiring careful sensorimotor evaluation. Other patterns of aberrant innervation involving the pupil, the eyelid, and the extraocular muscles occur and can be overlooked if not specifically sought.

Seesaw nystagmus, a rare presentation of pituitary adenoma, is a cyclical movement of the eyes in which one eye moves upward and rotates inward while the other eye moves downward and rotates outward, as if the two eyes were playing on a seesaw across the midline. The nystagmus is typically pendular, in which case it is thought to localize to the chiasm or midline diencephalon. However, occasionally the nystagmus has a jerk waveform, resulting in a hemi-seesaw nystagmus. This subtype has been associated with mesodiencephalic lesions and is thought to result from injury to the interstitial nucleus of Cajal (INC),[22] which integrates velocity commands for torsional and vertical eye movements.

Although the majority of cases of seesaw nystagmus have been described with sellar tumors, seesaw nystagmus may also result from a variety of other causes including neurodegenerative disease, congenital anomalies of the chiasm, and after radiation.

When seesaw nystagmus is the presenting sign of a pituitary lesion, it is rarely an isolated finding, because such significant compression of the chiasm results in other signs or symptoms.

Other Visual Disturbances

Although bitemporal hemianopia is by far the most frequent defect associated with a pituitary mass, patients with pituitary lesions often present first with poorly localizing visual complaints, such as photophobia, amaurosis fugax, and frontal headache.

A series of five patients with photophobia had lesions compressing the chiasm. Three of the patients had pituitary adenomas.[23] Photophobia can be a confusing presenting sign because it is poorly localizing and is seen with pathology anywhere in the visual system, including corneal opacities, inflammation within the eye, cataracts, retinal dystrophy, albinism, and thalamic infarcts. When photophobia is due to compression of the anterior visual pathways by tumor, it is frequently accompanied by headache and may produce positive visual phenomena such as glare and twinkling lights.

Pituitary patients who experience transient vision loss represent a diagnostic challenge, as amaurosis fugax is also seen with retinal emboli, vertebrobasilar ischemia, papilledema, vasospasm, and optic disk drusen. Workup of a patient complaining of amaurosis fugax may have delayed the diagnosis of a pituitary adenoma until visual field loss and optic atrophy became apparent, at which time a large pituitary adenoma was discovered.[24]

Bitemporal visual field defects are often asymptomatic, and a patient with preserved central acuity who has no difficulty ambulating or participating in daily activities may not be aware of his impairment even when it is profound, especially if it is progressing slowly. Even with near-complete bitemporal hemianopia, the eyes send complementary information to the brain, and both central acuity and a good deal of binocular field are preserved. In these patients, other disturbances of binocular visual function, rather than visual field loss, may first bring a pituitary lesion to awareness. Stereopsis is true binocular vision, produced by comparison of images from the two eyes of an object projected onto the two retinas. Whereas much of human depth perception relies on monocular cues, such as object size, brightness, and parallax, stereopsis is exclusively a binocular product, and in those who have stereopsis it is invaluable in perceiving the depth and contour of objects within our reach. Stereopsis can be quantified as "stereoacuity," and many different clinical tests for it are available. When the temporal field of each eye is selectively impaired, then the amount of overlapping visual field from which the brain can extract comparative information is reduced, and therefore a flattened world is perceived. Reduced stereo acuity was found in 85% of patients with lesions of the optic chiasm, but half of those patients had no scotoma on monocular visual field testing. In those patients, loss of the temporal field was so subtle and so close to central fixation that the loss of stereopsis was more sensitive than any monocular test.[25] Loss of stereopsis may be an underreported phenomenon in pituitary patients because it is not as routinely tested as acuity or visual fields.

The patient with complete bitemporal hemianopia who sees nothing temporal to fixation in either eye may experience two additional binocular impairments: post-fixation blindness and the hemifield-slide phenomenon.[26] In post-fixation blindness, when the eyes converge onto a near target, the nasal fields overlap to create a cone of sight with its apex at the fixation target. Any stimulus present beyond the fixation target falls onto the temporal fields of both eyes and is therefore not visible. Post-fixation blindness may be reported spontaneously by a patient, or it may be specifically tested for on confrontation by asking the patient to count fingers behind a target under binocular conditions.

In the hemifield-slide phenomenon, the two nonoverlapping nasal fields slide along each other, creating intermittent double vision. In many normal patients, the eyes have a latent tendency to drift with respect to each other, either horizontally or vertically, and only the active fusion of the two retinal images keeps the eyes straight. Such patients may never experience diplopia, except when very tired or inebriated. However, if all overlapping information is removed (for example, intermittent convergence produces a central strip that is not seen) the patient cannot "line up" the two fields, and the latent deviation becomes manifest. Almost always, if some temporal field can be restored in at least one eye, the double vision resolves.

Funduscopic Findings

The fibers that originate nasal to the fovea (and subserve temporal vision) enter the disk nasally and temporally. Compression of these fibers produces atrophy of the optic disk in a characteristic "butterfly," "bowtie," or "band" pattern (**Fig. 14.6**). This is similar to the atrophy seen in the contralateral eye in the optic tract syndrome, except in chiasmal injury it is bilateral. The earliest appearance of this pattern of atrophy can be quite subtle and if noted can be a valuable indicator for intervention. Moderate to severe or generalized atrophy, on the other hand, is a poor prognostic indicator.

Indications for Treatment

Medical management for prolactinomas has been reviewed by Schlechte.[27] A microadenoma confined to the sella is unlikely to produce visual disturbance even during pregnancy. A microadenoma not invading the suprasellar space can produce systemic signs and symptoms before vision is affected. These tumors should be treated by the endocrinologist with bromocriptine or cabergoline. When an adenoma is silent endocrinologically or presents with visual impairment before careful questioning reveals the endocrinopathy, surgery becomes a consideration. A macroadenoma with a height of a centimeter or more is likely to impinge on the optic chiasm, impairing visual fields, and also to compress the cavernous sinus, causing ophthalmoparesis. The patient is an immediate surgical candidate unless the adenoma secretes prolactin. Prolactinomas, producing menstrual cycle irregularity and galactorrhea in women and decreased libido and infertility in men, usually can be managed medically by administration of a dopamine agonist, such as cabergoline, or bromocriptine. Visual parameters must be monitored, including acuity, color vision, visual fields, afferent pupillary defect, and ocular motility. The patient can be treated medically as long as these parameters have normalized. If the patient cannot tolerate the dopamine agonist or if the suprasellar lesion continues to enlarge, compromising visual fields and producing optic atrophy, surgical intervention is necessary. Patients with macroadenomas that persist in filling the suprasellar space and compressing the optic chiasm or cavernous sinus require surgery. Most of these patients complain of neuro-ophthalmologic symptoms. A growth hormone secreting adenoma may go undetected even after disfiguring acromegaly because the patient and family attribute the patient's coarsening features to aging. The patient may eventually present with skull and joint pain, prompting a workup.

Pituitary Apoplexy

Pituitary apoplexy is a life-threatening condition that occurs when the rapidly expanding pituitary suddenly infarcts or hemorrhages into the cavernous sinus and the subarachnoid space. It is characterized by severe headache accompanied by visual loss and ophthalmoplegia. The patient may be too obtunded to provide a history or cooperate with the examination. Any combination of afferent and efferent disturbances may occur. This must be considered in any patient in whom such signs or symptoms rapidly evolve.[28] Acute addisonianism may be associated with severe hypotension. In a series of 560 pituitary adenomas, 6.8% had a history of an acute process involving altered consciousness and loss of vision or an oculomotor palsy. In another series of 24 patients with apoplexy,[29] half had visual field loss and half had oculomotor palsies. Among oculomotor palsies, presumably because of its location in the superior portion of the cavernous sinus, the third nerve seems the most commonly affected. The patient most often does not know of a preexisting pituitary adenoma. Patients with pituitary adenomas undergoing coronary bypass grafting are particularly susceptible to pituitary apoplexy,[30] which occurs in 10%. Pituitary apoplexy requires steroid replacement therapy and immediate transsphenoidal decompression.

Hypophysitis

Although enlargement of the pituitary sufficient to compress the optic chiasm is usually the result of a pituitary macroadenoma, and less often meningioma, glioma, or lymphoma, the diagnosis of inflammatory or lymphocytic hypophysitis must be considered in certain cases. Hypophysitis occurs mostly in women, especially during pregnancy or in the peripartum period. The patient presents with headache, resulting from the rapid enlargement of both the pituitary and the stalk, infiltrated by inflammatory cells and fibrosis. The patient may suffer oversecretion of prolactin or growth hormone, mimicking a pituitary adenoma, but accompanied by progressive panhypopituitarism and rheumatologic diatheses. The patient's autoimmunity may manifest as systemic lupus erythematosus, thyroiditis, diabetes insipidus, or adrenal insufficiency heralding death.[31] Typical of autoimmune disorders, hypophysitis responds to steroid therapy. Complications occur with aggressive surgery. A diagnostic biopsy should be taken before aggressive removal of the pituitary in such cases.

The Pituitary in Pregnancy

A small percentage of pregnant women with macroadenoma may be at unique risk of visual loss resulting from enlargement of the pituitary during pregnancy. The risk is greater for macroadenomas than for microadenomas.[32] Sheehan's syndrome, a delayed infarct of the pituitary following peripartum hemorrhage, may lead to severe hypopituitarism but usually has no neuro-ophthalmologic consequences.

Visual Recovery After Treatment of Pituitary Tumors

All large series of transsphenoidal pituitary surgery report visual improvement in the majority of patients, with full recovery in many. Gradual improvement continued for months to years postoperatively. The prognosis for recovery was decreased in cases with poor preoperative acuity and visual fields or a long duration of preoperative deficits, resulting in optic atrophy. In Wilson and Dempsey's[33] 1978 series of 250 adenomas, one fourth presented with visual impairment, and of these patients 66.7% had postoperative improvement or complete resolution of field defects. Cohen et al[34] reported on 100 consecutive patients with pituitary adenomas, all of whom had preoperative visual impairment. Acuity improved or normalized in 79% of eyes, and the visual field improved or normalized in 74%. Patients with severely reduced preoperative acuity had less recovery of acuity; in contrast, visual field improvement was impressive regardless of the degree of preoperative field loss. Powell[35] reported on 67 patients who underwent resection of adenomas that were compressing the visual pathway. He found that 88% showed improved visual function, measured by visual field, acuity, or both. Even among patients with optic atrophy, half showed some improvement in acuity and visual fields. Overall, 13.4% of patients had complete recovery of acuity, and 34.3% had complete normalization of fields. In 2005, Gnanalingham et al[36] described 41 patients who underwent transsphenoidal resection of pituitary adenomas, 88% of whom had preoperative visual disturbance. The visual field normalized in 35% of these patients' eyes, and improved in 60%. As in previous reports, poor prognostic indicators included longer duration of preoperative deficits, worse preoperative acuity, and worse impairment of visual fields.

Three stages of improvement in visual fields following tumor resection have been recognized. The earliest is recovery immediately after surgery, which can be demonstrated by visual evoked potentials within 10 minutes.[37] This is attributed to the return of normal nerve conduction by fully functional axons that had been compressed but not otherwise compromised. Further improvement in visual fields or acuity occurring weeks to months after treatment is attributed to restoration of axonal transport or remyelination. Late improvement, a year or more after treatment, is described but less well understood. Serial postoperative visual fields of 62 patients were analyzed to study the course of recovery after pituitary surgery.[38] Some patients exhibited significant improvement during the first postoperative week, and even severely impaired visual fields could normalize during this early period. Additional improvement took place in 1 to 4 months, which suggested a separate, slow phase of recovery, and this improvement was more consistently achieved than the immediate postoperative recovery. Many patients continued to improve at the 1-year visit and beyond, implying a possible additional phase of recovery and even an additional biologic mechanism, such as remodeling of the visual system. Interestingly, despite the potential for continuing recovery, no eye with severe visual field loss normalized if it had not normalized by the first postoperative week; therefore, if one is to speak of a "delayed" recovery in pituitary tumors, the capacity for continued recovery should not be overemphasized. Serial visual fields showing prolonged postoperative improvement are depicted in **Fig. 14.7**.

Visual recovery also occurs in the majority of patients with endocrinologically active tumors treated medically and then with radiation. In prolactinomas treated with bromocriptine, restoration of vision is not as dramatic as in

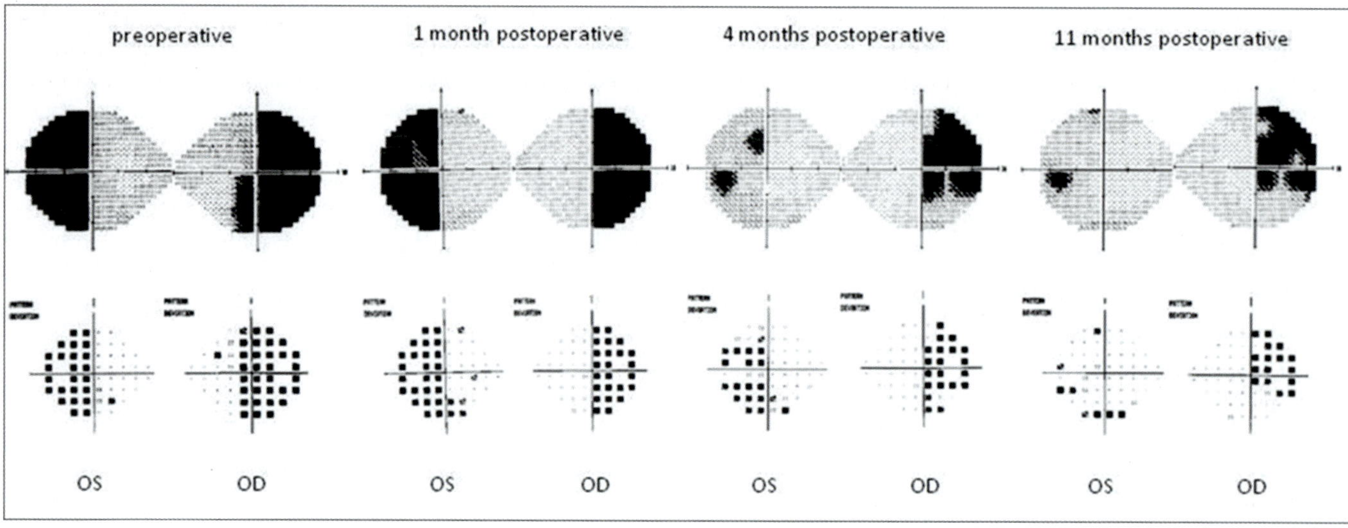

Fig. 14.7 Delayed recovery of temporal visual fields following resection of a pituitary adenoma. The bulk of visual field recovery typically occurs within the first few weeks after surgery.

surgical decompression, but can begin within days of initiating therapy, and thereafter may follow a similar time course.[39] Therefore, even with severely impaired visual function, medical management should be tried before surgical decompression of a prolactinoma.[5]

Optical coherence tomography (OCT) produces high-resolution two-dimensional images of the posterior ocular structures by examining the time of reflection of low-coherent light from the various layers of the retina. It is now routinely used to quantify retinal structural lesions and may also be used to measure the thickness of the retinal nerve fiber layer (RNFL). Because the axons of retinal ganglion cells that make up the RNFL are unmyelinated, thinning should occur only as a consequence of axonal degeneration, not from reversible demyelination related to downstream compression.

Preserved thickness of the nerve fiber layer, even in the face of significant visual field loss, suggests a good prognosis in patients with chiasmal compression, though swelling also should be considered. Kanamori et al[45] were the first to use OCT to show RNFL thinning corresponding to the band atrophy seen with chiasmal compression. OCT-determined RNFL thickness has been found to correlate well with visual field defects in patients with chiasmal compression, and the correlation improved as time from the surgery increased.[46] Patients with severe visual defects with normal preoperative RNFL measurements showed a greater degree of postoperative improvement in visual fields and acuity when retested at 6 weeks following resection.[47] A similar outcome was observed when patients were reexamined 3 months postoperatively.[48] In both of these studies, inferior RNFL thinning appeared to be a particularly strong prognostic factor. However, because visual recovery may occur later than 3 months following resection, longer-term studies are needed to better understand the utility of OCT in predicting final visual outcome. Newer OCT technology uses a Fourier-domain analysis (as opposed to time-domain) but has not been found to enhance the ability to detect band atrophy in 36 patients with chiasmal compression.[49]

A decrement in the pattern electroretinogram (PERG) signal has been observed in three patients with pituitary adenomas, two of which were abutting the chiasm. Signal recovery in all six eyes followed tumor resection.[50] The suggestion that chiasmal compression may lead to retrograde dysfunction of retinal ganglion cells remains controversial. A more recent study showed a correlation of visual field loss with nasal or full-field PERG signal.[51]

Preoperative diplopia from cavernous sinus involvement is likely to improve or resolve after surgery. New diplopia is less common than visual loss after transsphenoidal surgery. In two large series[43,52] there were no incidents of new-onset diplopia. In a national survey, only 86 of 1162 neurosurgeons had encountered diplopia as a complication of transsphenoidal surgery.[44] In one unusual case, a transient third nerve palsy developed and resolved within a week after resection of a pituitary adenoma, without any evidence of cavernous sinus compression.[53]

Neuro-Ophthalmologic Complications of Treatment

Although the majority of patients experience an improvement in, or even complete restoration of, visual function following treatment of pituitary tumors, there are potential neuro-ophthalmologic complications in every form of therapy. Vision loss, double vision, and other complaints may occur immediately following treatment or may be delayed by months to years. The task of the treating physician is to recognize these complications early and to differentiate them from recurrence of the original pathology.

The empty sella syndrome is a complication common to all treatment modalities and may be delayed in onset or slowly progressive, mimicking tumor recurrence. In primary empty sella syndrome, a defect in the diaphragma sella, possibly combined with an increase in cerebrospinal fluid pressure or pulse pressure, creates a gradual enlargement of the bony sella and pushes the pituitary flat against its expanding floor. Although primary empty sella may be an incidental radiographic finding, especially in a multipara, it may also be associated with clinical signs and symptoms, including endocrinologic derangement and vision loss. The same pulsations that enlarge the sella put pressure on the optic structures and may force the chiasm and optic nerves down into the empty space, putting traction on the axons, and causing transient visual obscurations or chronic central or peripheral vision loss. Even if the chiasm is in its normal position radiographically, vision may be compromised. Secondary empty sella syndrome has a similar etiology, except that the defect in the sella follows shrinkage or removal of a tumor. It has been described after endocrine therapy for prolactinomas[40] and surgical resection.[41] It may be an underrecognized phenomenon, and delayed vision loss in the absence of tumor recurrence may be empty sella syndrome with or without the characteristic MRI findings.[41] Buttressing the chiasm and nerves with exogenous fat at the time of surgery may help to reduce this complication, but this practice carries its own risk of compression.

The visual system or its blood supply can be damaged directly at the time of surgery. Manipulations of the nerves, chiasm, or tracts can cause postoperative vision loss even in the absence of surgical complications and has been reported to occur in 0.6 to 1.6% of patients, depending on the series.[33,42,43] In a nationwide survey, the incidence of vision loss was 1.8%, ranging from 0.4 to 2.4% depending on the experience of the surgeon.[44] Occult vision loss may be attributable to traction, contusion, or ischemia, and therefore prognosis is often uncertain. Sudden decompression of the chiasm may lead to visual loss from ischemia. In some cases, swelling or hemorrhage may temporarily impair vision, and neuroimaging will offer some prognostic information.[42] Factors associated with increased risk of vision loss include larger tumors and dumbbell-shaped tumors. Recurrent tumors in particular incur a higher incidence of postoperative vision loss when approached transsphenoidally, perhaps owing to adhesions with the meninges and a delicate blood supply.[44]

Because endoscopic surgery minimizes manipulation of intracranial structures, it potentially minimizes complications as well. However, transsphenoidal surgery may impair vision in a variety of ways. Orbital fractures can occur especially in elderly patients when the surgical approach is misdirected laterally and can even cause blindness in one eye.[42,54] The chiasm can be compressed by the fat used to pack the surgical void, with variable visual recovery after the fat is removed.[55] Following transsphenoidal resection, a pneumatocele can form in the sella as a result of air transfer and trapping, and can compress the chiasm, resulting in visual loss. This rare complication may reflect poor packing of the sinus, but excellent recovery has been reported with removal of packing.[56] One of the authors has seen quadrantic visual field loss and cerebrospinal fluid leak resulting from an endoscope inadvertently entering the temporal lobe and damaging the inferior optic radiations, but no such cases were found in the literature. Prevedello et al[57] advocate a team approach to endoscopic procedures to minimize morbidity, with a second experienced endoscopist assisting the cutting surgeon.

Whenever radiation is employed as a primary or adjunctive therapy, there is a risk of radiation necrosis affecting the optic nerves, chiasm, or tracts. Radiation necrosis is an ischemic response owing to radiation damage to small blood vessels. It may follow treatment by weeks, months, or even years. It may be associated with enhancement of the intracranial optic nerves or chiasm and sometimes optic disk swelling or pallor.[58] It tends to be fulminant and to respond poorly to treatment with steroids, anticoagulants, and hyperbaric oxygen.

Ocular neuromyotonia also has been reported as a result of radiation therapy to the chiasm, occurring many years after treatment.[59] This rare phenomenon consists of an episodic strabismus brought on by sustained eccentric gaze. It is attributed to the inappropriate firing of unstable axonal membranes and ephaptic transmission in affected ocular motor nerves. For example, a patient with right third nerve neuromyotonia might develop a transient right hypertropia in primary gaze following sustained upgaze but then might display a right hypotropia and ptosis after returning to primary gaze following sustained downgaze. It is typically controlled with membrane stabilizing agents such as carbamazepine.

Limiting the dose and selecting the form of radiation can avert damage to the visual system. Technologic advances in the delivery of radiation to the tumor bed have progressively reduced the incidence of damage to the visual system. Nevertheless, any acute or subacute loss of vision in a patient who has received intracranial radiation should raise suspicion of radiation necrosis and prompt an immediate ophthalmologic examination and contrast-enhanced MRI.

■ Follow-Up

Every patient who has been treated for a pituitary adenoma requires periodic follow-up forever. Visual fields should be followed up monthly at first in the perioperative period, then annually for 5 years, after which every other year should be adequate unless the patient reports new symptoms.

This visual field schedule approximating the schedule for MRI should help the surgeon determine whether a lesion or recrudescence that appears to be touching the chiasm is in fact causing neurologic damage requiring intervention.

Conclusion

Because structures vital to vision and eye movement surround the pituitary, neuro-ophthalmologic implications are present at every stage of managing patients with pituitary lesions, including diagnosis, neuroimaging, decisions to treat, monitoring for complications and tumor recurrence, and postoperative follow-up. The primary contributions of the neuro-ophthalmologist are (1) performing and interpreting the visual field exam, which is generally more sensitive than MRI in revealing and localizing compression of the anterior visual pathways; and (2) the early detection of cavernous sinus involvement by uncovering subtle eye movement defects. The majority of patients experience improvement in visual function following treatment of a pituitary lesion, but care must be taken in patient selection and operative technique to avoid neuro-ophthalmologic complications.

References

1. Perlmutter D, Rhoton AL Jr. Microsurgical anatomy of the anterior cerebral-anterior communicating-recurrent artery complex. J Neurosurg 1976;45:259–272
2. Renn WH, Rhoton AL Jr. Microsurgical anatomy of the sellar region. J Neurosurg 1975;43:288–298
3. Bergland R. The arterial supply of the human optic chiasm. J Neurosurg 1969;31:327–334
4. Blunt MJ, Steele EJ. The blood supply of the optic nerve and chiasma in man. J Anat 1956;90:486–493
5. Gittinger JW Jr. Pituitary tumors. In: Miller NR, Newman NJ, eds. Walsh and Hoyt's Clinical Neuro-Ophthalmology, Vol 2, 6th ed. Philadelphia: Lippincott Williams & Wilkins; 2005
6. Traquair HM. An Introduction to Clinical Perimetry. St. Louis: CV Mosby; 1948
7. Trobe JD, Acosta PC, Krischer JP. A screening method for chiasmal visual-field defects. Arch Ophthalmol 1981;99:264–271
8. Fujimoto N, Saeki N, Miyauchi O, Adachi-Usami E. Criteria for early detection of temporal hemianopia in asymptomatic pituitary tumor. Eye (Lond) 2002;16:731–738
9. Khoury JM, Donahue SP, Lavin PJ, Tsai JC. Comparison of 24-2 and 30-2 perimetry in glaucomatous and nonglaucomatous optic neuropathies. J Neuroophthalmol 1999;19:100–108
10. Szatmáry G, Biousse V, Newman NJ. Can Swedish interactive thresholding algorithm fast perimetry be used as an alternative to Goldmann perimetry in neuro-ophthalmic practice? Arch Ophthalmol 2002;120:1162–1173
11. Wall M, Punke SG, Stickney TL, Brito CF, Withrow KR, Kardon RH. SITA standard in optic neuropathies and hemianopias: a comparison with full threshold testing. Invest Ophthalmol Vis Sci 2001;42:528–537
12. Frisén L, Jensen C. How robust is the optic chiasm? Perimetric and neuro-imaging correlations. Acta Neurol Scand 2008;117:198–204
13. Mejico LJ, Miller NR, Dong LM. Clinical features associated with lesions other than pituitary adenoma in patients with an optic chiasmal syndrome. Am J Ophthalmol 2004;137:908–913
14. Horton JC. Wilbrand's knee of the primate optic chiasm is an artefact of monocular enucleation. Trans Am Ophthalmol Soc 1997;95:579–609
15. Kedar S, Zhang X, Lynn MJ, Newman NJ, Biousse V. Congruency in homonymous hemianopia. Am J Ophthalmol 2007;143:772–780
16. Kupfer C, Chumbley L, Downer JC. Quantitative histology of optic nerve, optic tract and lateral geniculate nucleus of man. J Anat 1967;101(Pt 3):393–401
17. Behr C. Die Lehre von den Pupillen Bewegungen, Vol 6. Berlin: Springer; 1924:224
18. Herman P. The Behr pupil revisited. Anisocoria following cerebrovascular accidents. Stroke 1975;6:697–702
19. Wernicke G. Uberhemiopische Pupillenreaction. Fortschr Med 1883;1:49–53
20. Saul RF, Hilliker JK. Third nerve palsy: the presenting sign of a pituitary adenoma in five patients and the only neurological sign in four patients. J Clin Neuroophthalmol 1985;5:185–193
21. Landau K. Discovering a dys-covering lid. Surv Ophthalmol 1997; 42:87–91
22. Kanter DS, Ruff RL, Leigh RJ, Modic M. See-saw nystagmus and brainstem infarction: MRI findings. Neuroophthalmology 1987;7:279–283
23. Kawasaki A, Purvin VA. Photophobia as the presenting visual symptom of chiasmal compression. J Neuroophthalmol 2002;22:3–8
24. Dirr LY, Troost BT, Elster AD, Fiedler AJ. Amaurosis fugax due to pituitary tumor. J Clin Neuroophthalmol 1991;11:254–258
25. Hirai T, Ito Y, Arai M, et al. Loss of stereopsis with optic chiasmal lesions and stereoscopic tests as a differential test. Ophthalmology 2002;109:1692–1702
26. Kirkham TH. The ocular symptomatology of pituitary tumours. Proc R Soc Med 1972;65:517–518
27. Schlechte JA. Clinical practice. Prolactinoma. N Engl J Med 2003; 349:2035–2041
28. Wakai S, Fukushima T, Teramoto A, Sano K. Pituitary apoplexy: its incidence and clinical significance. J Neurosurg 1981;55:187–193
29. Dubuisson AS, Beckers A, Stevenaert A. Classical pituitary tumour apoplexy: clinical features, management and outcomes in a series of 24 patients. Clin Neurol Neurosurg 2007;109:63–70
30. Levy E, Korach A, Merin G, Feinsod M, Glenville B. Pituitary apoplexy and CABG: should we change our strategy? Ann Thorac Surg 2007;84:1388–1390
31. Winterkorn JMS, Gabbay M, Klein I, Farmer P, and Carras R. 4-H Club: Headache, Hemianopia, Hypopituitarism, Hypophysitis. 24th annual Frank B. Walsh Society; Los Angeles:1992. http://content.lib.Utah.edu/cdm4/item_viewer.php?CISROOT=/EHSL-FBWNOC8.CISOPTR=739.
32. Kupersmith MJ, Rosenberg C, Kleinberg D. Visual loss in pregnant women with pituitary adenomas. Ann Intern Med 1994;121:473–477
33. Wilson CB, Dempsey LC. Transsphenoidal microsurgical removal of 250 pituitary adenomas. J Neurosurg 1978;48:13–22
34. Cohen AR, Cooper PR, Kupersmith MJ, Flamm ES, Ransohoff J. Visual recovery after transsphenoidal removal of pituitary adenomas. Neurosurgery 1985;17:446–452

35. Powell M. Recovery of vision following transsphenoidal surgery for pituitary adenomas. Br J Neurosurg 1995;9:367–373
36. Gnanalingham KK, Bhattacharjee S, Pennington R, Ng J, Mendoza N. The time course of visual field recovery following transsphenoidal surgery for pituitary adenomas: predictive factors for a good outcome. J Neurol Neurosurg Psychiatry 2005;76:415–419
37. Feinsod M, Selhorst JB, Hoyt WF, Wilson CB. Monitoring optic nerve function during craniotomy. J Neurosurg 1976;44:29–31
38. Kerrison JB, Lynn MJ, Baer CA, Newman SA, Biousse V, Newman NJ. Stages of improvement in visual fields after pituitary tumor resection. Am J Ophthalmol 2000;130:813–820
39. Lesser RL, Zheutlin JD, Boghen D, Odel JG, Robbins RJ. Visual function improvement in patients with macroprolactinomas treated with bromocriptine. Am J Ophthalmol 1990;109:535–543
40. Dorotheo EU, Tang RA, Bahrani HM, Schiffman JS, Bhatti MT, Lewis SB. Her vision was tied down. Surv Ophthalmol 2005;50:588–597
41. Czech T, Wolfsberger S, Reitner A, Görzer H. Delayed visual deterioration after surgery for pituitary adenoma. Acta Neurochir (Wien) 1999;141:45–51
42. Barrow DL, Tindall GT. Loss of vision after transsphenoidal surgery. Neurosurgery 1990;27:60–68
43. Mampalam TJ, Tyrrell JB, Wilson CB. Transsphenoidal microsurgery for Cushing disease. A report of 216 cases. Ann Intern Med 1988;109:487–493
44. Ciric I, Ragin A, Baumgartner C, Pierce D. Complications of transsphenoidal surgery: results of a national survey, review of the literature, and personal experience. Neurosurgery 1997;40:225–236, discussion 236–237
45. Kanamori A, Nakamura M, Matsui N, et al. Optical coherence tomography detects characteristic retinal nerve fiber layer thickness corresponding to band atrophy of the optic discs. Ophthalmology 2004;111:2278–2283
46. Danesh-Meyer HV, Carroll SC, Foroozan R, et al. Relationship between retinal nerve fiber layer and visual field sensitivity as measured by optical coherence tomography in chiasmal compression. Invest Ophthalmol Vis Sci 2006;47:4827–4835
47. Danesh-Meyer HV, Papchenko T, Savino PJ, Law A, Evans J, Gamble GD. In vivo retinal nerve fiber layer thickness measured by optical coherence tomography predicts visual recovery after surgery for parachiasmal tumors. Invest Ophthalmol Vis Sci 2008;49:1879–1885
48. Jacob M, Raverot G, Jouanneau E, et al. Predicting visual outcome after treatment of pituitary adenomas with optical coherence tomography. Am J Ophthalmol 2009;147:64–70, e2
49. Costa-Cunha LV, Cunha LP, Malta RF, Monteiro ML. Comparison of Fourier-domain and time-domain optical coherence tomography in the detection of band atrophy of the optic nerve. Am J Ophthalmol 2009;147:56–63, e2
50. Ventura LM, Venzara FX III, Porciatti V. Reversible dysfunction of retinal ganglion cells in non-secreting pituitary tumors. Doc Ophthalmol 2009;118:155–162
51. Monteiro ML, Cunha LP, Costa-Cunha LV, Maia OO Jr, Oyamada MK. Relationship between optical coherence tomography, pattern electroretinogram and automated perimetry in eyes with temporal hemianopia from chiasmal compression. Invest Ophthalmol Vis Sci 2009;50:3535–3541
52. Black PM, Zervas NT, Candia GL. Incidence and management of complications of transsphenoidal operation for pituitary adenomas. Neurosurgery 1987;20:920–924
53. Foroozan R, Bhatti MT, Rhoton AL. Transsphenoidal diplopia. Surv Ophthalmol 2004;49:349–358
54. Newmark H III, Kant N, Duerksen R, Pribram HW. Orbital floor fracture: an unusual complication of trans-septal trans-sphenoidal hypophysectomy. Neurosurgery 1983;12:555–556
55. Slavin ML, Lam BL, Decker RE, Schatz NJ, Glaser JS, Reynolds MG. Chiasmal compression from fat packing after transsphenoidal resection of intrasellar tumor in two patients. Am J Ophthalmol 1993;115:368–371
56. Lee AG, Van Gilder JC, White ML. Progressive visual loss because of a suprasellar pneumatocele after trans-sphenoidal resection of a pituitary adenoma. J Neuroophthalmol 2003;23:142–144
57. Prevedello DM, Kassam AB, Snyderman C, et al. Endoscopic cranial base surgery: ready for prime time? Clin Neurosurg 2007;54:48–57
58. Lessell S. Friendly fire: neurogenic visual loss from radiation therapy. J Neuroophthalmol 2004;24:243–250
59. Shults WT, Hoyt WF, Behrens M, MacLean J, Saul RF, Corbett JJ. Ocular neuromyotonia. A clinical description of six patients. Arch Ophthalmol 1986;104:1028–1034

15 Endoscopic Transsphenoidal Approach to the Sella

Lewis Z. Leng, Vijay K. Anand, and Theodore H. Schwartz

First performed by Schloffer over a hundred years ago, the transsphenoidal approach has become the standard approach for the removal of sellar lesions.[1] In the early 1990s, Cushing[2] and Hirsch[3] went on to develop and refine the transsphenoidal approach. However, the approach fell out of favor after Cushing abandoned it for the transcranial approach. It was not until the 1950s and 1960s, with the addition of intraoperative fluoroscopy and the operating microscope, that Guiot[4] and Hardy[5] revitalized the transsphenoidal approach. The next major stage in the evolution of pituitary surgery began when Guiot et al[6] introduced the use of endoscopy into transsphenoidal surgery in 1963. The endoscope was later reintroduced into clinical practice in the early 1990s.[7] Since that time larger contemporary endoscopic series by Jho and Carrau[8,9] and by Cappabianca et al[10–13] have established the endoscopic, endonasal, transsphenoidal approach as an accepted technique and arguably new standard of care in pituitary surgery[14] (**Fig. 15.1**).

For surgery within the sella, the endoscope has numerous advantages over the microscope. The endoscope produces a more panoramic view of the operative field.[15] The endoscopic, endonasal approach may be associated with less postoperative swelling, avoidance of nasal packing, improved patient comfort, decreased length of stay, and less postoperative complications.[16,17] With this approach, normal mucociliary transport is preserved because the nasal passage is not disrupted and the mucosa of the sphenoid sinus remains intact. Most importantly, the endoscope dramatically improves intra- and suprasellar visualization, especially with the use of angled scopes.[18–20] Angled scopes can be advanced into the sphenoid sinus and sella to explore around corners to look for residual tumor, particularly laterally, against the medial wall of the cavernous sinus (**Fig. 15.2**). Similarly, extended approaches can be used to remove tumor in the suprasellar cistern and cavernous sinus.[21–25] As a result the endoscopic approach has a lower incidence of

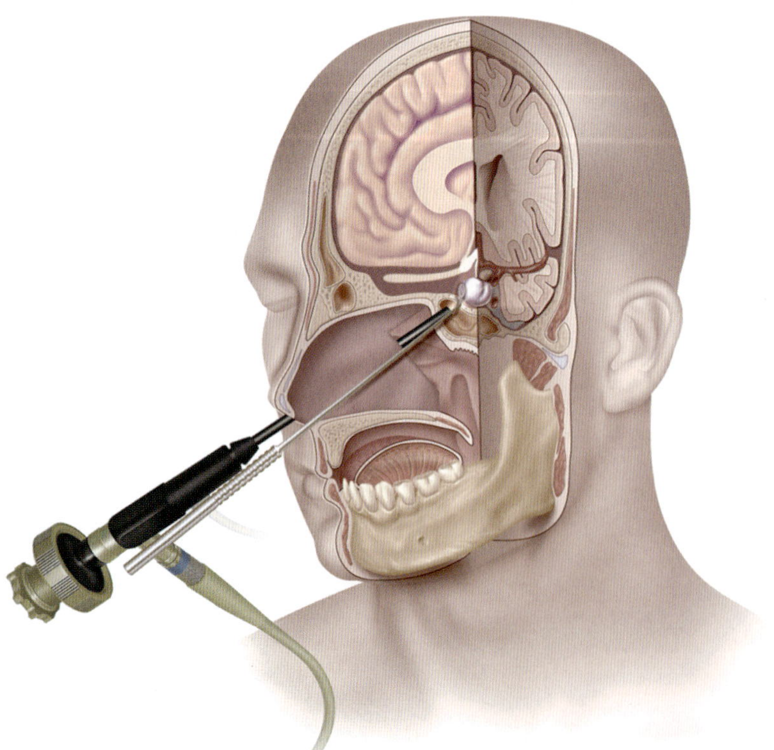

Fig. 15.1 The endonasal endoscopic approach to the sella is the most direct, minimally invasive approach to intrasellar lesions.

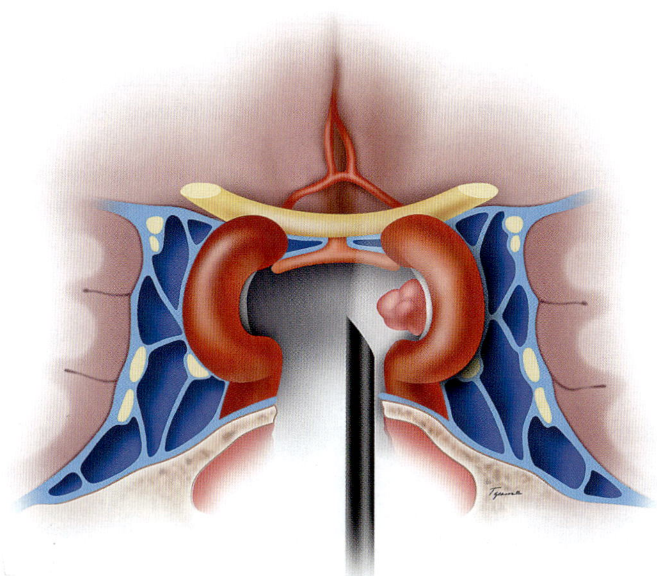

Fig. 15.2 Angled endoscopes can be used to visualize residual tumor in the lateral recesses of the sella, adjacent to the cavernous sinus, which would not be visualized with the microscope. (From Anand VK, Schwartz TH. Practical Endoscopic Skull Base Surgery. San Diego: Plural Publishing; 2007. Reprinted with permission.)

residual tumor on postoperative magnetic resonance imaging (MRI) scans.[26] The main disadvantage of the endoscope compared with the microscope is the lack of stereoscopic vision. However, this is not a significant limitation once the surgeon gains sufficient experience.[18,27,28] In addition, three-dimensional stereoendoscopes are now available that provide stereoscopic vision.[29–31]

Indications

The endoscopic, endonasal, transsphenoidal approach is suitable for pituitary tumors, both microadenomas and macroadenomas. Other lesions that are confined to the sella or that enlarge the sella and extend into the suprasellar cistern, such as some craniopharyngiomas and Rathke cleft cysts, are also suitable candidates for this approach (**Fig. 15.3**).

Surgery continues to be the standard of care for hormone-producing pituitary tumors, such as ones that cause Cushing's disease or acromegaly, and for nonsecreting pituitary macroadenomas that cause either optic nerve compression or have documented growth.[28,32] For asymptomatic nonsecreting pituitary tumors that are stable in size and not compressing the optic chiasm, either conservative management with expectant observation or surgical resection should be considered, depending on the situation. Prolactinomas are not routinely removed as a first-line therapy. However, when

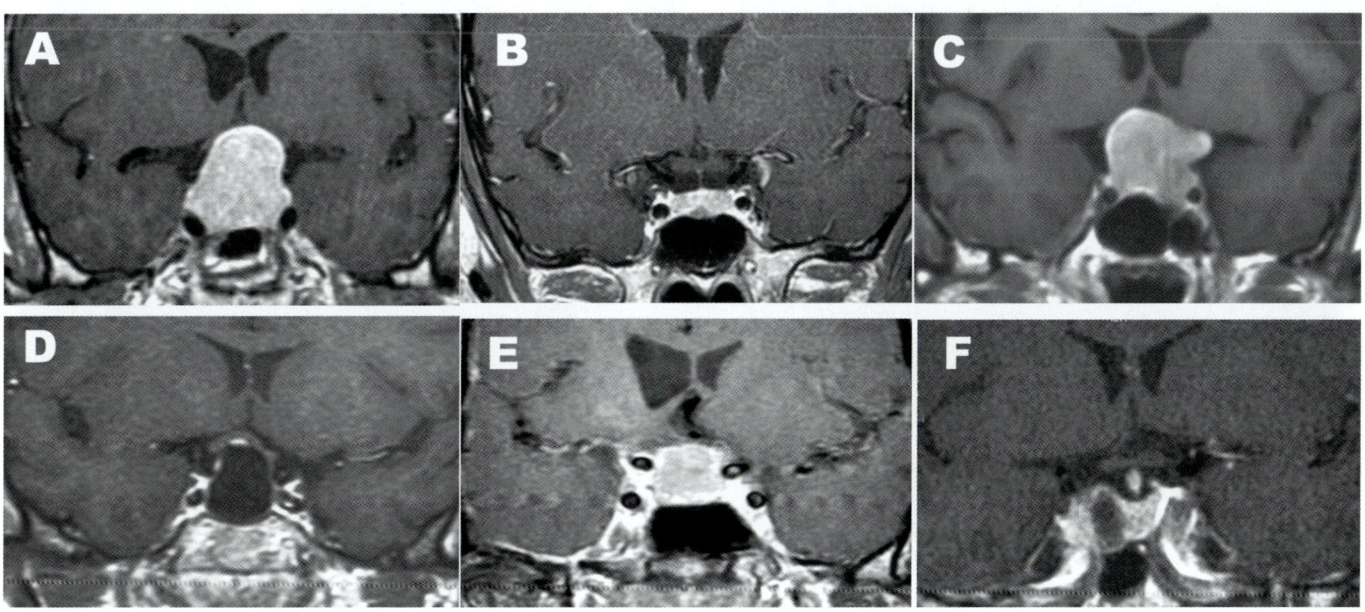

Fig. 15.3 Multiple types of intrasellar and intra- and suprasellar lesions are suitable for the endonasal, endoscopic transsphenoidal, transsellar approach: **(A)** pituitary macroadenomas with suprasellar extensions, **(B)** pituitary microadenomas, **(C)** macroadenomas with moderate lateral extension, **(D)** Rathke cleft cysts, and **(E)** intrasellar craniopharyngiomas. A unilateral approach can be used for small tumors such as that shown in B. Note that in this case, a right-sided approach can be used, and only half of the sphenoid sinus needs to be opened because there is a septum that marks the lateral extent of the tumor. A unilateral left-sided approach can be used for tumors that are on the right side of the sella, such as the adenoma shown in **F**. (From Anand VK, Schwartz TH. Practical Endoscopic Skull Base Surgery. San Diego: Plural Publishing; 2007. Reprinted with permission.)

surgical resection is considered, a preoperative prolactin level >250 μg/L has been shown to predict a lower probability of cure from surgery than is obtained with medical management. If the prolactin level is <250 μg/L, and the tumor is a microadenoma with no cavernous sinus involvement, then the chance of surgical cure is almost 90%.[33] Other factors that support surgical debulking include significant visual loss, apoplexy, and resistance to medical treatment.

The role of surgical intervention for Rathke cleft cysts is somewhat controversial. Hypopituitarism is improved in only approximately 20 to 30% of patients, but symptoms of optic chiasm compression improve in 98%.[34,35] In addition, headaches are relieved in approximately 90% of patients and can be an indication for surgery.[36] Although some authors recommend aggressive removal of the cyst wall to prevent recurrence, this strategy increases the risk of postoperative hypopituitarism.[37] Drainage and subtotal cyst wall removal is a less risky procedure and prevents recurrence in up to 84% of cases.[13,34–36] Endoscopic, endonasal resection of Rathke cleft cysts is an effective minimally invasive approach.[13,35] Evidence of squamous metaplasia in the cyst wall predicts recurrence, as does residual cyst on postoperative imaging.[34,36]

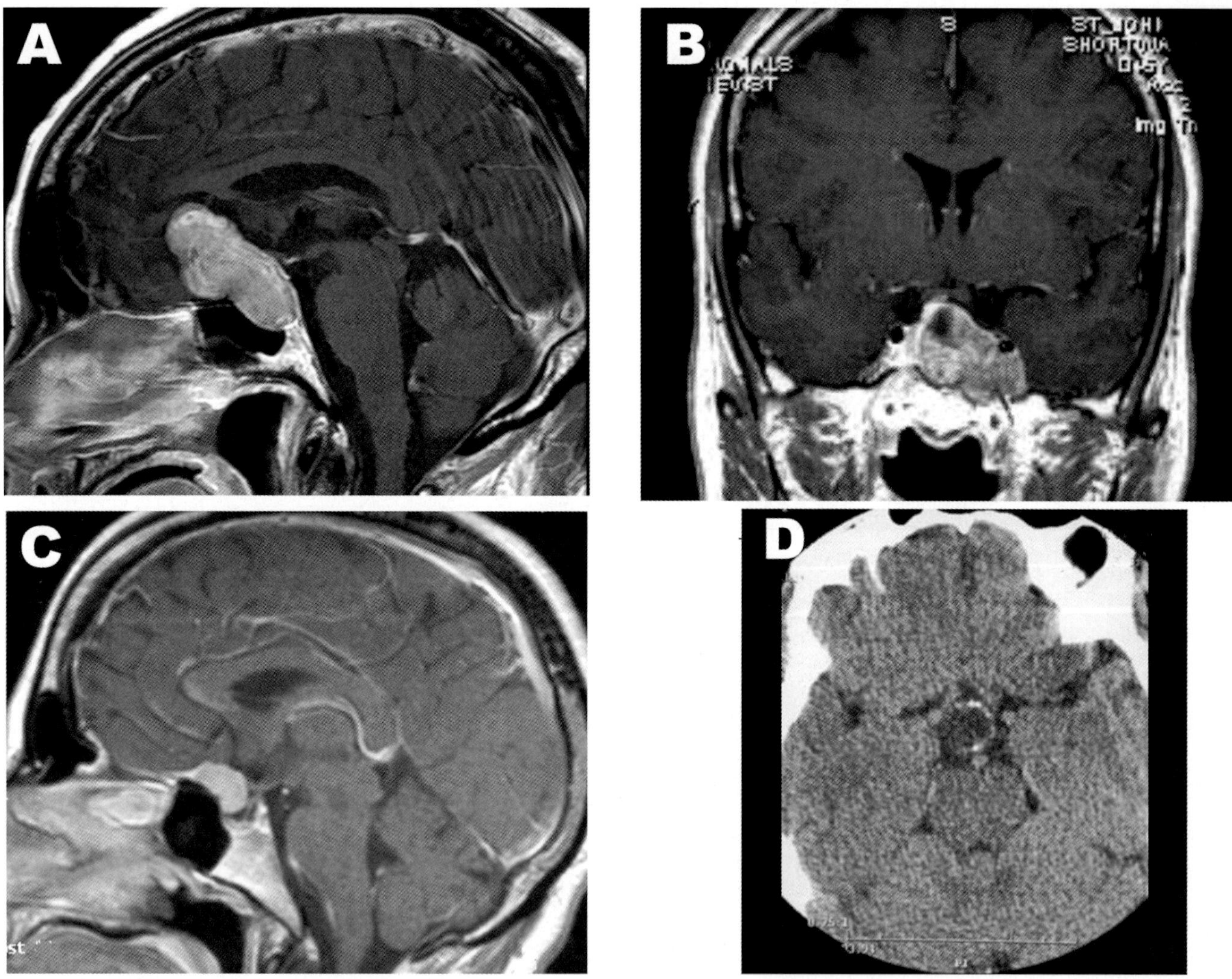

Fig. 15.4 Considerations in choosing the transsellar approach. **(A)** A pituitary macroadenoma with significant suprasellar extension that extends anteriorly. This tumor cannot reliably be completely removed with a sellar approach but requires a more extensive approach such as the endonasal, endoscopic, transplanum, transtuberculum approach. In some cases removal of the posterior ethmoids is required. **(B)** A tumor with significant cavernous sinus extension cannot be completely removed through a transsellar approach. If the goal is to remove the entire tumor, a transcavernous approach is required. However, a limited resection followed by radiosurgery to the cavernous sinus remnant may be more prudent in this situation. **(C)** Meningiomas of the tuberculum sellae can extend into the sella and mimic pituitary adenomas. These tumors require a larger transtuberculum opening for removal. **(D)** Calcification is the hallmark of the craniopharyngiomas, which can be removed only through a transsellar approach if there is significant involvement of the sella. (From Anand VK, Schwartz TH. Practical Endoscopic Skull Base Surgery. San Diego: Plural Publishing; 2007. Reprinted with permission.)

The standard treatment for craniopharyngiomas has been surgery for many years. The transsphenoidal approach is appropriate when an enlarged sella is present. Purely intrasellar craniopharyngiomas are rare and occur only 4% of the time. Intra- or suprasellar lesions occur 21% of the time, and primarily suprasellar lesions are observed 75% of the time.[38] Controversy remains regarding conservative versus aggressive resection.[39] Aggressive surgery is associated with better control but also greater morbidity secondary to hypothalamic and pituitary injury. The transsphenoidal approach has been broadened to lesions other than purely intrasellar craniopharyngiomas.[40] Application of the endoscope to the transsphenoidal approach for craniopharyngiomas takes advantage of the less invasive nature of the approach with improved intra- and suprasellar visualization.[41]

Contraindications and Considerations

The endonasal, endoscopic, transsphenoidal approach to the sella can be used to resect the majority of suprasellar tumors that arise within and enlarge the sella by using straight and angled endoscopes. However, for exceptionally large tumors with a considerable amount of anterior suprasellar extension, we do not advise a direct transsellar method (**Fig. 15.4A**). In such cases, a transplanum, transtuberculum approach to enlarge the bony and dural opening can be applied, which provides a direct view of the suprasellar component of the tumor to allow a safe and maximal resection.

Another major consideration is the lateral extent of the lesion, into the cavernous sinus (**Fig. 15.4B**). Only when the tumor completely encircles the carotid artery can cavernous sinus involvement be guaranteed (**Fig. 15.5B**). Often, compression of the medial wall can mimic invasion (**Fig. 15.5C,D**), and in these cases the entire tumor can be removed through an endonasal, transsellar approach. Lateral extension into the cavernous sinus is not an absolute contraindication, but the decision should be made preoperatively whether the goal of surgery is to decompress the optic apparatus by resecting sellar and suprasellar components of tumor or to remove intracavernous tumor by opening the cavernous sinus. If the goal is to remove tumor from the cavernous sinus, there are two options. In some circumstances, the tumor passes through a fenestration in the medial wall of the cavernous sinus. By using angled endoscopes and instruments, this opening can be followed from within the sella into the cavernous sinus to remove intracavernous tumor. The alternative method is a transethmoidal or

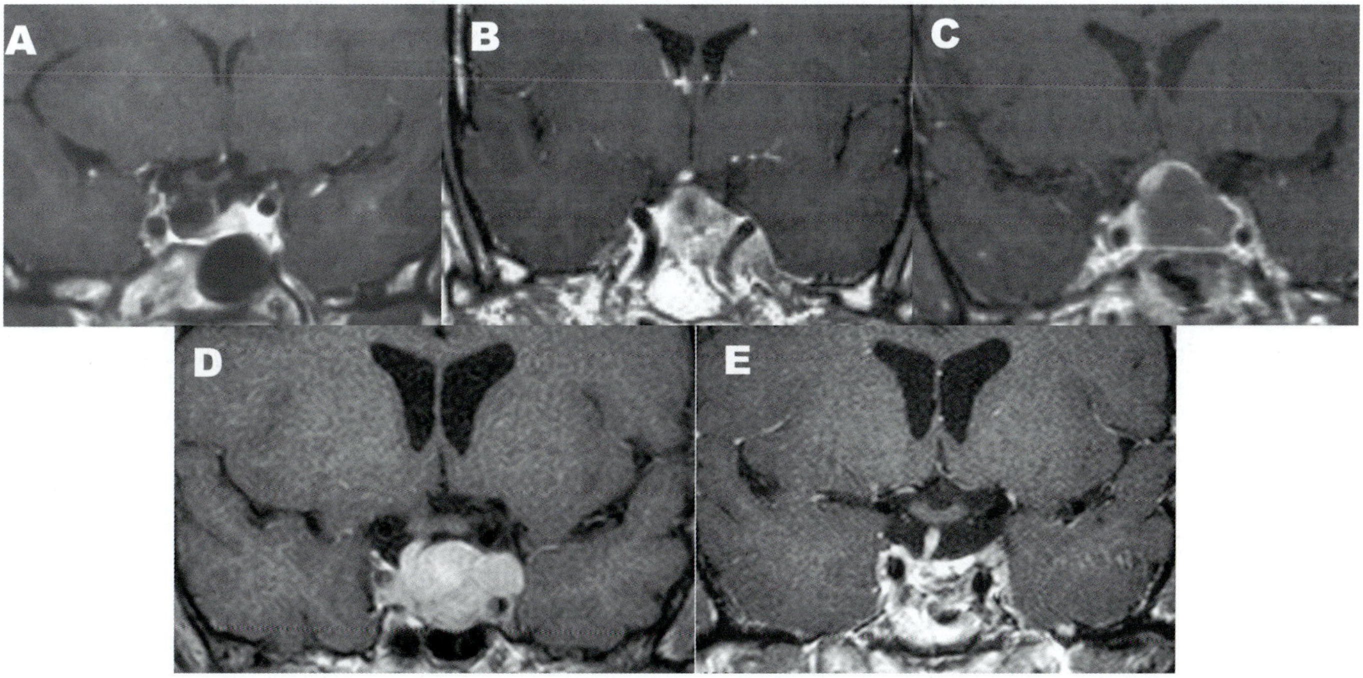

Fig. 15.5 Anatomic considerations as demonstrated by preoperative magnetic resonance imaging (MRI). **(A)** Empty sella syndrome can mimic a Rathke cleft cyst or cystic pituitary adenoma. **(B)** True cavernous sinus invasion, in which the tumor encircles the cavernous sinus. **(C)** This macroadenoma compresses the cavernous sinus but does not actually invade. Note the normal pituitary gland compressed superiorly. **(D)** Recurrent tumor following radiosurgery shows the possibility of cavernous sinus invasion on the left. **(E)** Postoperative films reveal that the entire tumor was removed via an endonasal, endoscopic transsellar approach. (From Anand VK, Schwartz TH. Practical Endoscopic Skull Base Surgery. San Diego: Plural Publishing; 2007. Reprinted with permission.)

transpterygoidal approach, which provides a more direct exposure of the parasellar region.[42] In cases when intracavernous tumor is intentionally left, stereotactic radiation therapy can be used to control growth as long as the tumor mass is at least 4 to 5 mm from the optic apparatus.[43]

Preoperative Considerations

Other lesions such as meningiomas, germinomas, hypothalamic hamartomas, and basilar tip aneurysms can be mistaken for pituitary macroadenomas. Such lesions must be ruled out preoperatively. In comparison to meningiomas, pituitary tumors typically enlarge the sella and lack a dural tail. Furthermore, meningiomas with cavernous sinus extension tend to constrict the carotid artery, whereas pituitary tumors do not. Calcifications that are more commonly present in either craniopharyngiomas or meningiomas can be identified with computed tomography (CT) scanning (**Fig. 15.4D**). If an aneurysm is suspected, an angiogram should be performed.

All patients with pituitary adenomas should be evaluated for endocrine abnormalities. Patients should be questioned about symptoms of endocrine abnormalities, which include amenorrhea; galactorrhea; impotence or decreased libido; arthropathy; hyperhidrosis; changes in facial features; changes in foot, hand, and hat size; weight gain or loss; hypertension; polyuria; polydipsia; hypotension; hirsutism; bruising; stretch marks; and development of adipose deposits. A comprehensive endocrinologic evaluation of the hypothalamic-pituitary axis should be undertaken with each patient. Patients with chiasmal compression are evaluated with formal visual field testing. Previously instituted medical therapy such as dopaminergic or somatostatin analogues do not need to be stopped before surgery, as these agents do not appear to decrease the efficacy of surgery.[44] In the case of stereotactic radiosurgery, medical therapy should be stopped before treatment as it appears to be more effective if the tumor is more metabolically active.[45,46] Identification of the pituitary microadenoma on preoperative imaging is critical. One clue is that the stalk is generally shifted away from the tumor, although this is neither 100% sensitive nor specific.[47] Pituitary adenomas are typically hypointense on T1-weighted MRI (**Fig. 15.3**) and variable in appearance on T2-weighted imaging. Because the normal pituitary gland takes up gadolinium rapidly, microadenomas appear nonenhancing on early postcontrast images and isointense at later time points. If imaging does not demonstrate a tumor in a patient with possible Cushing's disease, bilateral petrosal sinus sampling after administration of corticotropin-releasing hormone can be performed to measure adrenocorticotropic hormone (ACTH) levels to confirm the diagnosis. However, the reliability of this test in lateralizing the tumor is questionable.

Rathke cleft cysts are benign epithelium-lined cysts, probably arising from the remnants of a Rathke pouch (**Fig. 15.3D**). Preoperatively, mucoid Rathke cleft cysts are hyperintense on T1- and hypointense on T2-weighted MRI. Serous cysts are isointense to cerebrospinal fluid (CSF), as compared with cysts that contain cellular remnants, which can resemble more solid tumors.[47] Craniopharyngiomas arise from squamous epithelial remnants of a Rathke pouch in the region of the pars tuberalis. These tumors commonly extend into the sella. Adamantinomatous craniopharyngiomas, often found in children, generally contain cysts that are hypointense on T1- and hyperintense on T2-weighted MRI with rim enhancement (**Fig. 15.3E**). Characteristically, these lesions have a calcified ring and a hyperintense nodular component (**Fig. 15.4D**). Squamopapillary craniopharyngiomas, more common in adolescents and young adults, can extend further into the third ventricle and are both cystic and solid.

One important diagnosis to rule out preoperatively is empty sella syndrome, as these patients are likely to have previously unrecognized increased intracranial pressure and subsequently a high likelihood of postoperative CSF leak. Empty sella can be caused by a dehiscent sellar diaphragm, increased intracranial pressure, or prior pituitary surgery. It can mimic a Rathke cleft cyst (**Fig. 15.5A**). The sella may even be enlarged. One distinction is the absence of optic nerve compression in empty sella syndrome. In fact, the chiasm can even herniate into the sella.

Careful preoperative evaluation of the nasal and paranasal sinuses, in particular the sphenoid sinus anatomy, is critical (**Fig. 15.6**). We generally obtain a fine-cut CT preoperatively, which is then used for intraoperative navigation because MRI scanning alone is usually not adequate. We take note of the curvature of the middle turbinate and deviations of the septum. The endoscopic view may be obstructed by a deviated or bowed septum, precipitating a change to the side of the approach. Alternatively, a deviated septum can be repaired during the approach. Concha bullosa, or a pneumatized middle turbinate, may occur in as many as 80% of patients, depending on the definition of the term.[48] The pattern of sphenoid sinus pneumatization is critically important. Three patterns of pneumatization have been described (**Fig. 15.6A–C**). In the most common "sellar" variant (75%), the sinus is aerated in front of and below the sella. This variation is the most amenable to the transsphenoidal approach, as the anterior and inferior walls of the sella are easily accessed. In the "presellar" variant (24%), aeration permits access only to the front of the sella. To provide adequate visualization, the clivus is drilled down below the sella. In the last "conchal" variant (<1%), there is minimal or no aeration of the sphenoid. The transsphenoidal approach requires extensive drilling of the clivus and is significantly aided by stereotactic navigation in this situation. Finally, detailed analysis of the intrasphenoidal anatomy preoperatively is important. Intra-

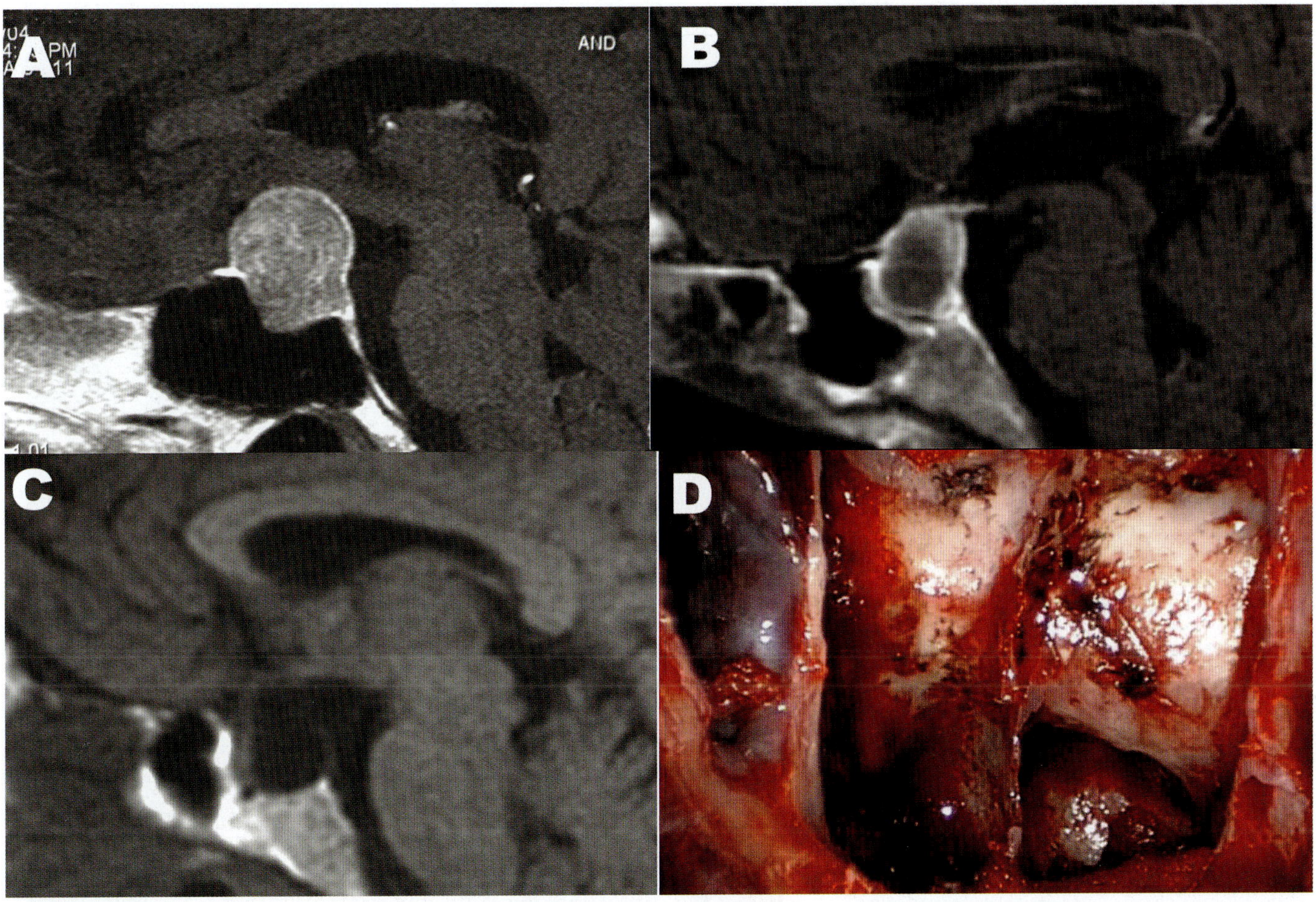

Fig. 15.6 Sphenoid sinus anatomy. **(A)** "Sellar" aeration of the sphenoid sinus. **(B)** "Presellar" aeration of the sphenoid sinus. **(C)** "Conchal" aeration of the sphenoid sinus. **(D)** Sphenoid septations can be useful landmarks in mapping out the location of the pituitary tumor, the carotid arteries, and the cavernous sinuses when compared with a preoperative MRI or computed tomography scan. (From Anand VK, Schwartz TH. Practical Endoscopic Skull Base Surgery. San Diego: Plural Publishing; 2007. Reprinted with permission.)

sphenoidal septa are helpful landmarks for confirming the locations of the carotid arteries and small microadenomas intraoperatively (**Fig. 15.6D**). Midline septa are often drilled away on the approach. However, more laterally located septa can occasionally be left in place if they do not interfere with the operative approach.

Patient Positioning and Preparation

The patient is placed under general anesthesia and given antibiotics, glucocorticoids, and antihistamines. We routinely use cefazolin (2 g, intravenous), dexamethasone (10 mg, intravenous), and diphenhydramine (50 mg, intravenous). Corticosteroids are not given to patients with Cushing's disease.[49] Both a Foley catheter and arterial line are placed. A lumbar puncture can be performed and 0.2 mL of 10% fluorescein (AK Fluor; Akorn Pharmaceutical, Buffalo Grove, IL) injected in 10 mL of CSF to help visualize CSF leakage and determine the method of closure. Although there have been reports of this maneuver causing seizures or radiculopathy, at low doses with glucocorticoids and antihistamine pretreatment, the procedure has been shown to be safe.[50,51] Cottonoids soaked in 4 mL of 4% cocaine (topical) are used to vasoconstrict the nasal mucosa. The patient's head can be placed either on a horseshoe or in rigid fixation, slightly extended, and turned slightly to the right. To facilitate venous drainage, the head is elevated above the heart. One advantage of avoiding rigid fixation is that the head can be moved during the case to improve exposure and to avoid the postoperative discomfort of the pin sites. In this case a skull clamp or headset should be used for navigation. The otolaryngologist and neurosurgeon stand on either side of the patient during the majority of the procedure. A scope holder can be used at certain times when the field of view is static (**Fig. 15.7**).

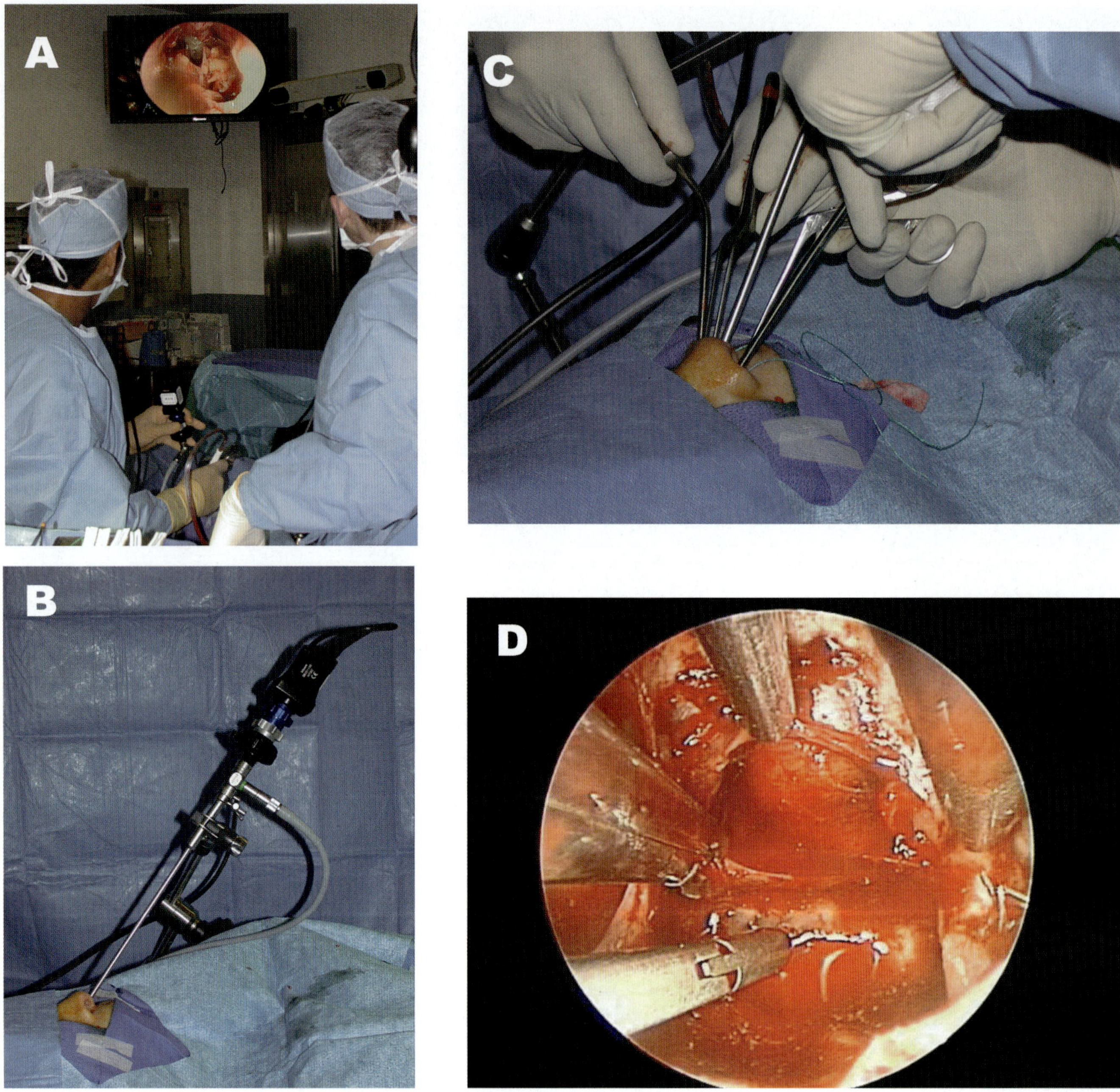

Fig. 15.7 Two surgeons **(A)** facing a plasma screen can use a scope holder **(B)** to maintain a steady view of the sella. This permits the use of four separate hands **(C)** to manipulate four instruments **(D)** within the operative field. (From Anand VK, Schwartz TH. Practical Endoscopic Skull Base Surgery. San Diego: Plural Publishing; 2007. Reprinted with permission.)

Nasal and Sinus Portion

The sphenopalatine arteries and middle turbinates are injected with a mixture of lidocaine 1% and epinephrine (1:100,000) using a rigid 0-degree, 18-cm-long, 4-mm-diameter endoscope (Karl Storz, Tuttlingen, Germany) (**Fig. 15.8A–C**). In the case of a microadenoma, the approach can be unilateral, through one nostril (**Fig. 15.9**), although we currently use both nostrils in all cases to increase our working room. For a right-handed surgeon, the approach is easiest through the right nostril. However, if a small adenoma is located eccentrically on the right of the gland, a unilateral left-sided approach provides the best trajectory. Under endoscopic view, the inferior, middle, and superior turbinates are identified. The endoscope is advanced into the choana, which is bordered by the tail of the inferior

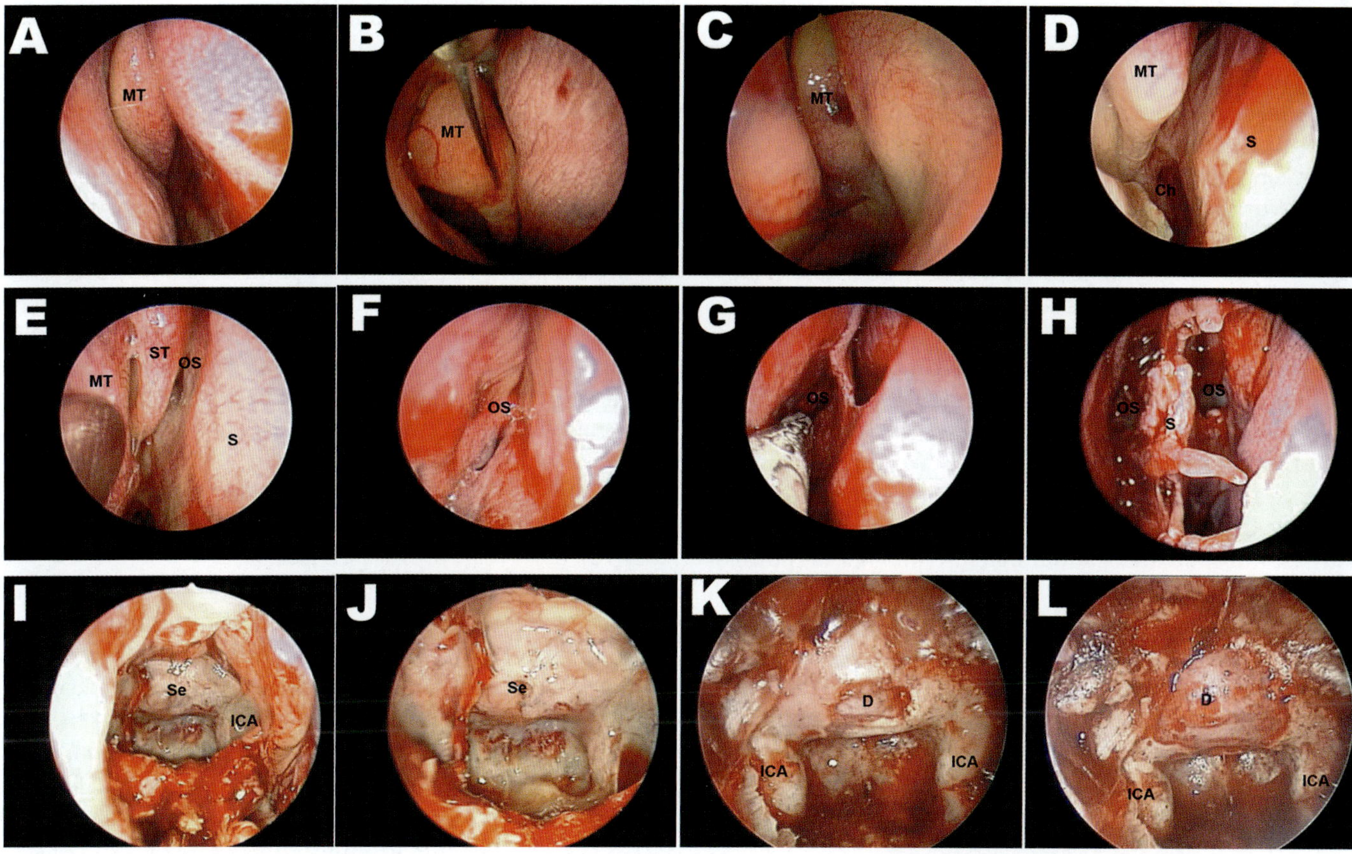

Fig. 15.8 Endoscopic, endonasal approach to the sella. **(A)** The middle turbinate (MT) is usually the first anatomical landmark seen when the endoscope is advanced into the nostril. **(B)** The middle turbinate is injected with lidocaine and epinephrine, as is **(C)** the sphenopalatine artery. **(D)** The choana (Ch) is below and medial to the middle turbinate, and it can be followed superiorly along the sphenoethmoid recess to find the **(E)** ostium of the sphenoid sinus (OS), which is generally tucked behind the superior turbinate (ST). Once the superior turbinate is retracted, the **(F)** ostium comes into better view. The ostium is enlarged with a mushroom punch, and for the bilateral approach the posterior 1 cm of the septum (S) is opened **(G)** to expose the contralateral ostium **(H)**. The septum between the ostia is removed to reveal **(I)** a panoramic view of the sphenoid sinus and the internal carotid artery (ICA) protuberances. **(J)** The floor of the sella (Se) is visualized and the mucosa is stripped. **(K)** A small bone opening can be made with a high-speed drill to reveal the dura (D), which is **(L)** enlarged to fully visualize the adenoma before removal.

turbinate laterally, the vomer medially, and the floor of the sphenoid sinus superiorly (**Fig. 15.8D**). After the middle and superior turbinates are retracted laterally, the sphenoid ostium is identified (**Fig. 15.8E,F**). The ostia lie just above the sphenoethmoid recess, approximately 1.5 cm above the choana.[52] Occasionally, the ostium is obstructed by a supreme turbinate, which can be gently retracted laterally or removed if necessary. The mucosa around the ostium is first

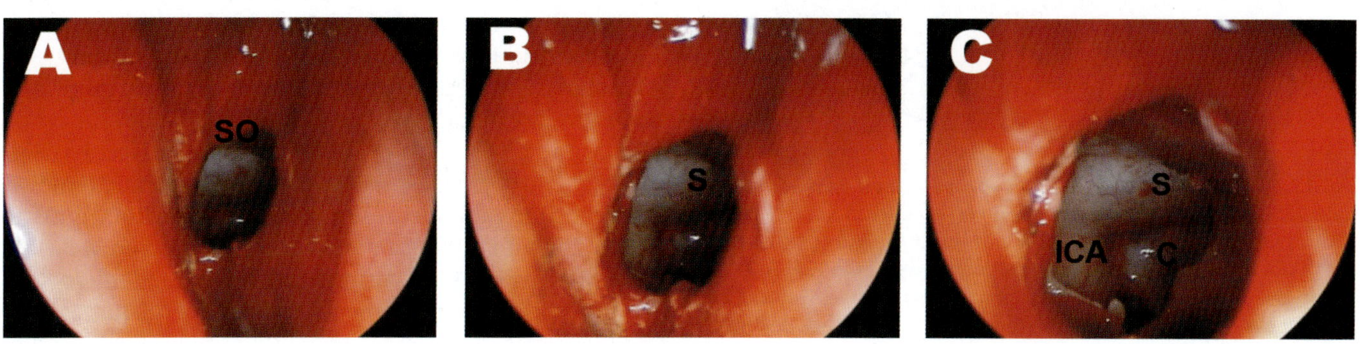

Fig. 15.9 **(A)** A unilateral approach though one sphenoid ostium (SO). **(B)** As the scope is advanced into the sphenoid sinus **(C)**, the floor of the sella (S), internal carotid artery (ICA), carotid protuberances, and clivus (C) come into view.

cauterized and then enlarged with a mushroom punch and Kerrison rongeur. The territory of the sphenopalatine artery, which is located inferolaterally from the ostia, should be avoided. For macroadenomas, we perform a complete submucosal resection of the nasal septum using a hemitransfixion incision including vomeric bone. The hemitransfixion is closed with a 4–0 chromic suture. After completion of the submucous resection of the septum, the posterior third of the nasal septum adjacent to the vomeric bone and maxillary crest is removed with a tissue shaver (**Fig. 15.8G**). In the case of large macroadenomas, removal of the nasal septum allows for the two-nostril, four-handed approach. The bilateral approach provides greater flexibility and facilitates the use of two or even four instruments during the tumor resection when a flexible scope holder (Karl Storz, Tuttlingen, Germany) is employed (**Fig. 15.7**). Moreover, the endoscope can be maneuvered closer to the lesion without interfering with the introduction of additional instruments. Removal of the nasal septum is not necessary in the unilateral approach for microadenomas. The unilateral approach is less traumatic to the patient, and there is less postoperative discomfort and drainage than with a bilateral approach. Furthermore, some surgeons advocate removal of a single middle turbinate to increase maneuverability when resecting large tumors.

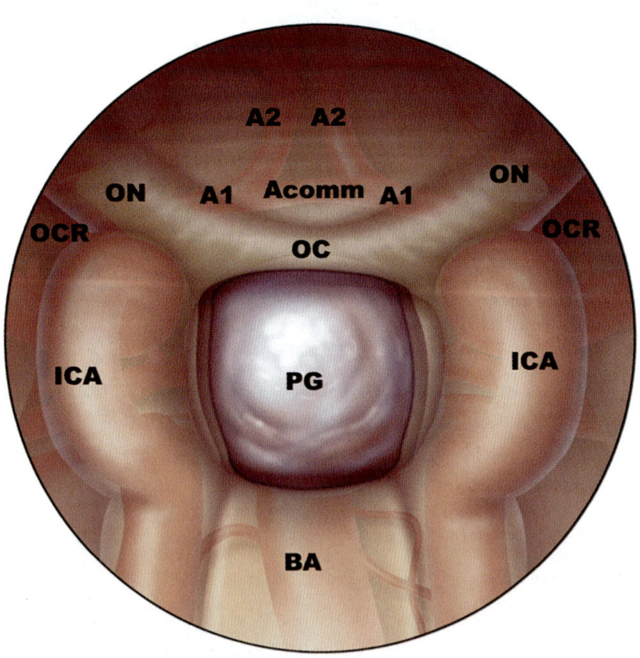

Fig. 15.10 Illustration of the endoscopic panoramic view within the sphenoid sinus. One can see the optic nerves (ON) and optic chiasm (OC) as well as the internal carotid arteries (ICA). The opticocarotid recess (OCR) demarcates the intersection between the ICA and ON. Above the OC lies the anterior communicating artery (Acomm) between the A1 and A2 branches of the anterior cerebral artery. Below the sella and pituitary gland (PG) lies the basilar artery (BA). Most of these structures are hidden by bone, but the neurosurgeon must be aware of their locations based on the bony prominences and landmarks.

In our experience, this is usually not necessary. The mucosa of the sphenoid sinus rostrum is retracted laterally, and the intrasinus sphenoid septum is removed with a rongeur forceps, which brings the posterior wall of the sphenoid sinus into full view. The carotid prominences overlying the internal carotid arteries (ICAs), optic nerve prominences overlying the optic nerves, and opticocarotid recesses are identified (**Fig. 15.10**). Localization is confirmed with stereotactic image guidance. At this point a rigid 0-degree, 30-cm-long, 4-mm-diameter endoscope (Karl Storz, Tuttlingen, Germany) is introduced through the left nostril (right nostril for unilateral approach) and held in place with a scope holder (**Fig. 15.7**). Additional intrasinus septa are removed as needed.

Intrasellar Portion

Through the right nostril, the floor of the sella is accessed with an osteotome or high-speed drill, curette, and Kerrison rongeur (**Fig. 15.11**). The bone opening generally extends from one cavernous sinus to the other and from the tuberculum sellae to the floor of the sella (**Figs. 15.8L, 15.11B,** and **15.12B**). The attachments of the sphenoid septa can help determine the location of the carotid arteries and lesion. Doppler ultrasound is valuable in identifying the carotid arteries. A wider opening facilitates maximal resection of the tumor and advancement of the endoscope into the sella for inspection at the end of the procedure. The dura is opened in a cruciate fashion below the intercavernous sinus to avoid unnecessary dural bleeding (**Fig. 15.11C,D**). Monopolar cautery of the dura is avoided, particularly with microadenomas, because of the thermal injury to the pituitary and optic chiasm. Dural bleeding is controlled with gentle pressure and hemostatic agents. The dural leaflets can be cauterized back with a bipolar or removed with microscissors. It is important to try to open the dura without cutting into the gland to find the pseudocapsule around the adenoma (**Fig. 15.11D**). To search for invasion, dural specimens can be sent to the laboratory. Occasionally, intrasellar cystic contents can be released at this time to decompress the gland and facilitate dissection around the capsule of the tumor.

At this stage of the operation we carefully probe the gland with a straight dissector to determine whether there is a plane around the adenoma (**Fig. 15.11D**). Some microadenomas can be removed en bloc with gentle dissection (**Fig. 15.12**).[53] For hormone-producing tumors, en-bloc removal is useful if possible because a complete resection is critical. For adenomas that cannot be removed en bloc, we use a variety of ring curettes, coring instruments, and micropituitary rongeurs to gently remove the center of the tumor (**Fig. 15.11E,F**). Once the sella is slightly decompressed, venous bleeding from the dural leaflets can be brisk, which is best controlled with gentle pressure and hemostatic agents. The

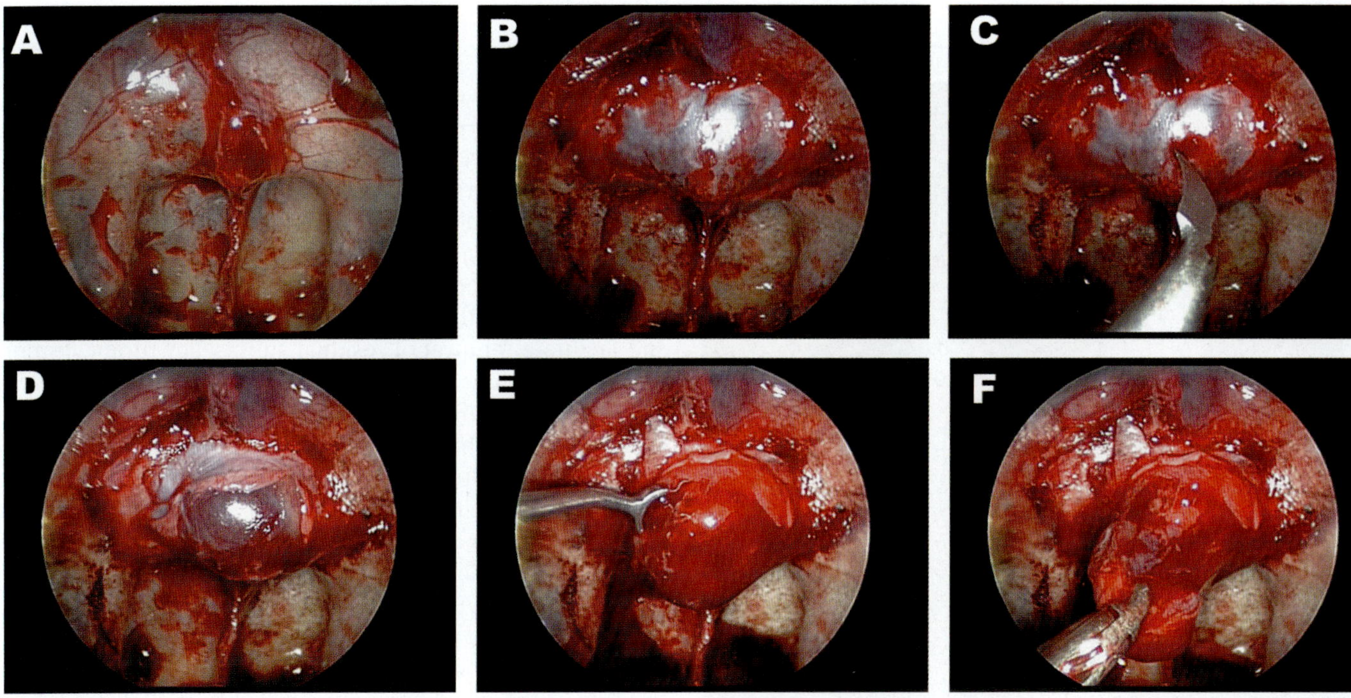

Fig. 15.11 Intrasellar surgery. **(A)** The endoscopic view of the sella. **(B)** The anterior wall of the sella has been opened from the tuberculum to the floor of the sella and from one cavernous sinus to the other. The dura is exposed. **(C)** A sickle knife is used to open the dura and expose the pituitary tumor. **(D)** The dura has been opened, and the pituitary tumor is bulging forward. **(E)** A ring curette is helpful in removing the central portion of the tumor. **(F)** A small pituitary rongeur is used to pull out a specimen.

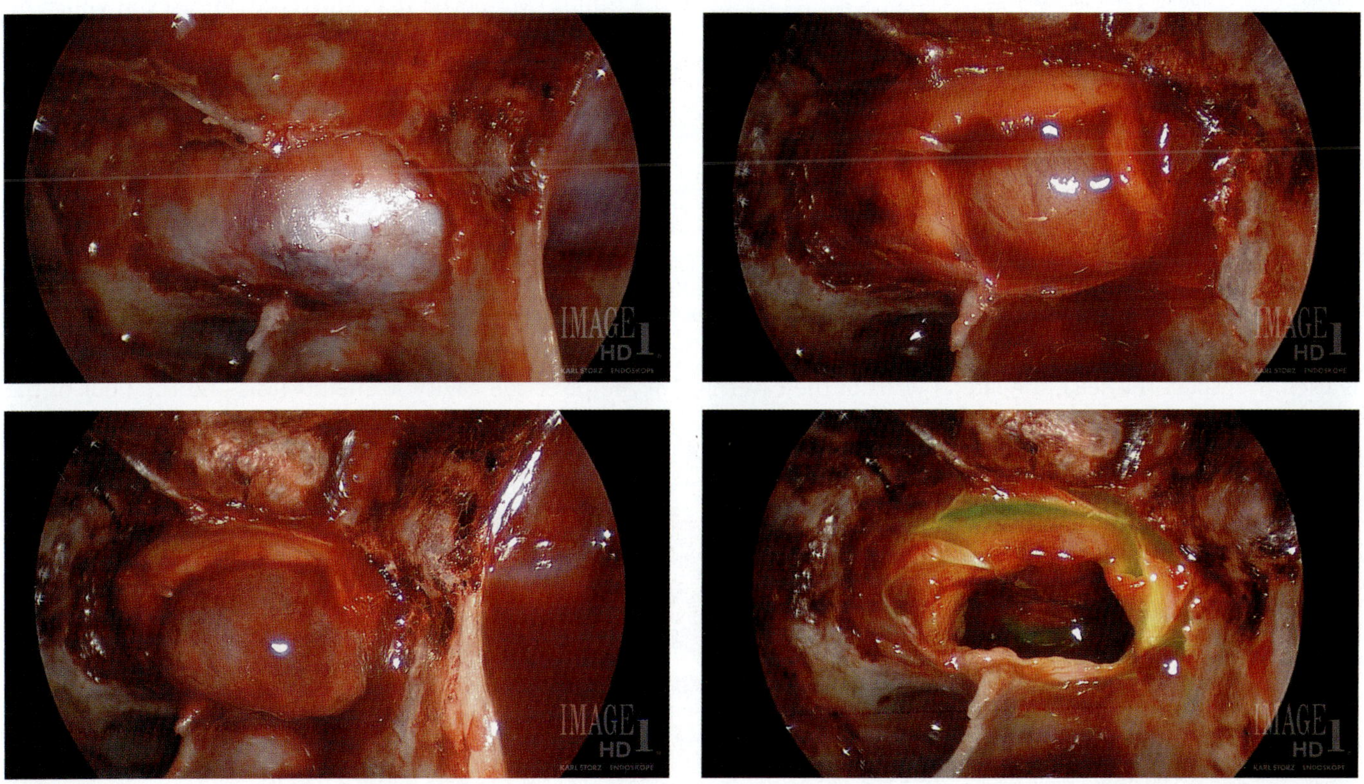

A B C D

Fig. 15.12 Removal of microadenoma en bloc using the pseudocapsule. **(A)** A wide opening is made in the floor of the sella. The tumor bulge on the dura can be seen on the patient's left (right of photo). **(B)** The pituitary gland is opened to reveal the tumor, and the pseudocapsule is carefully dissected away from the gland. **(C)** The tumor is almost completely removed, and the posterior margin is dissected free from the gland. **(D)** Once the tumor is removed, the normal gland is visualized as well as a small cerebrospinal fluid leak dyed with green fluorescein.

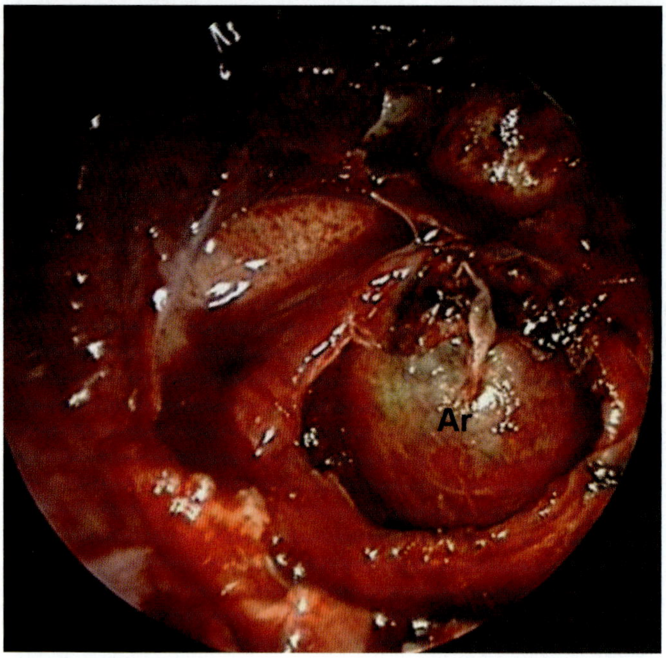

Fig. 15.13 Removal of a macroadenoma causes the arachnoid (Ar) to herniate into the sella. If the lateral component of the tumor is not completely removed, it can obscure the field of view, rendering removal of the residual tumor difficult.

order of tumor removal is first the inferior portion, followed by the lateral components, and lastly the superior portion. Premature removal of the superior component of the tumor can precipitate descent of the arachnoid, which can herniate down and obscure the field of view (**Fig. 15.13**). Firm tumors can be resected with a Cavitron ultrasonic surgical aspirator (Valleylab, Boulder, CO). After the superior aspect of the tumor is removed, the arachnoid and normal pituitary fall into view. The arachnoid can be retracted superiorly, and a rigid 45-degree, 30-cm-long, 4-mm-diameter endoscope is used to inspect the sella, the lateral walls of the cavernous sinus, and the suprasellar cistern for residual tumor. To facilitate visualization, continuous irrigation through a sheath can be used. Although some surgeons use an intrathecal injection of air to induce the descent of large suprasellar tumors, we prefer to use an extended transtuberculum, transplanum approach for tumors with a large suprasellar extension to obtain direct visualization of the suprasellar tumor. Conversely, a rigid 30-degree, 30 cm in length, 4-mm diameter endoscope (Karl Storz, Tuttlingen, Germany) can be advanced into the sella to visualize the suprasellar cistern and facilitate removal of residual suprasellar tumor. Tumor extension into the cavernous sinus through the medial wall can be removed through a transsellar approach (**Fig. 15.14**). Working behind the carotid artery, the cranial nerves are lateral, which permits removal of soft tumors in this area. This is indicated either to try to cure hormone-producing tumors or to create room between residual cavernous sinus tumor and the normal gland in preparation for radiosurgery.

For patients with Cushing's disease and a normal MRI scan but positive petrosal sinus sampling, exploration of the pituitary gland is required. One method is to start on the side of the gland corresponding with the lateralization of the petrosal sinus sampling, but the accuracy of this test is unreliable. In our practice, we place several vertical incisions every few millimeters until the tumor is found. After localization of the tumor, the half of the gland containing the tumor is removed to ensure cure. In cases in which no tumor is identified, one can perform a hypophysectomy or bilateral adrenalectomy.

Closure

After tumor removal, a careful examination for CSF leakage is undertaken, aided by the visualization of intrathecal fluorescein (**Fig. 15.12D**). We generally close the sella in one of three ways.[54] If there is no evidence of CSF leak, a small piece of thrombin-soaked Gelfoam (Pfizer, Brooklyn, NY) is placed in the resection cavity for hemostasis and the floor of the sella is reconstructed with vomeric bone harvested during the approach. If no bone is available then we use Medpor

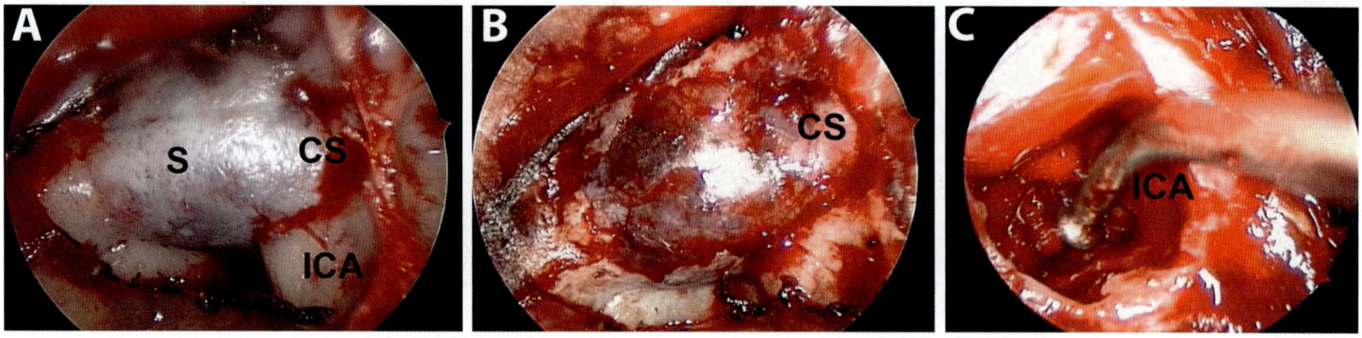

Fig. 15.14 **(A)** Tumors in the cavernous sinus (CS) can also be removed through the sella if they invade though the medial wall. ICA, internal carotid artery; S, sella. **(B)** Bone over the CS is removed to facilitate visualization. **(C)** Using angled instruments it is possible to work behind the ICA to evacuate soft tumors extending into the CS.

(Porex, Newnan, GA). If CSF leakage is observed and the approach has been transsellar only, then we harvest abdominal fat and fill but do not overpack the sella. The floor of the sella is then reconstructed with vomeric bone or Medpor (**Fig. 15.15**). If the mucosa over the sphenoid has been preserved, this can be reapproximated over the floor of the sella (**Fig. 15.15**). If there has been a large opening in the skull base, such as a transplanum, transtuberculum approach, then we use either a "gasket seal" method or pack the sella with fat followed by a nsaseoptal flap.[55] Briefly, a piece of fascia lata, larger than the defect, is first centered over the opening in the skull base. Then a piece of vomeric bone, the same size as the defect, is centered over the tissue graft and countersunk into the bony defect. This draws the tissue graft into the bony defect to form a gasket seal around the rigid graft. Recently we have begun also placing an additional nasoseptal flap[56] on top of the gasket seal, although the necessity of this last step is unknown. Finally, a thin layer of fibrin matrix (Tisseel; Baxter, Deerfield, IL) or polymerized hydrogel (Duraseal; Confluent Surgical, Waltham, MA) can be placed over the closure to obtain a watertight closure. The latter substance is preferred. Thrombin-infused gelatin matrix (FloSeal; Baxter, Deerfield, IL) is used to fill the sphenoid sinus, to aid in hemostasis. Lumbar drainage is not routinely used during transsellar surgery because the risk of CSF leak is so small and patients often go home soon after surgery. However, if a large defect in the skull base is anticipated, or if the patient has poor wound healing from diabetes, smoking, steroid use, prior radiation therapy, or renal failure, then a drain is often placed at the beginning of the operation. This is left open for only approximately 24 hours, and drainage is kept at a minimum (approximately 5 mL/h). It is best to place the drain prior to the start of resection, as the loss of CSF during the procedure makes placement more difficult at the end of the procedure. Lumbar drainage carries its own potential complications such as significant back pain, risk of spinal CSF leakage after removal, and increased length of stay. A small piece of Telfa (Kendall, Mansfield, MA) is placed in each nostril overnight to absorb any drainage and is removed in the morning. The middle turbinates are medially displaced before removal of the endoscope.

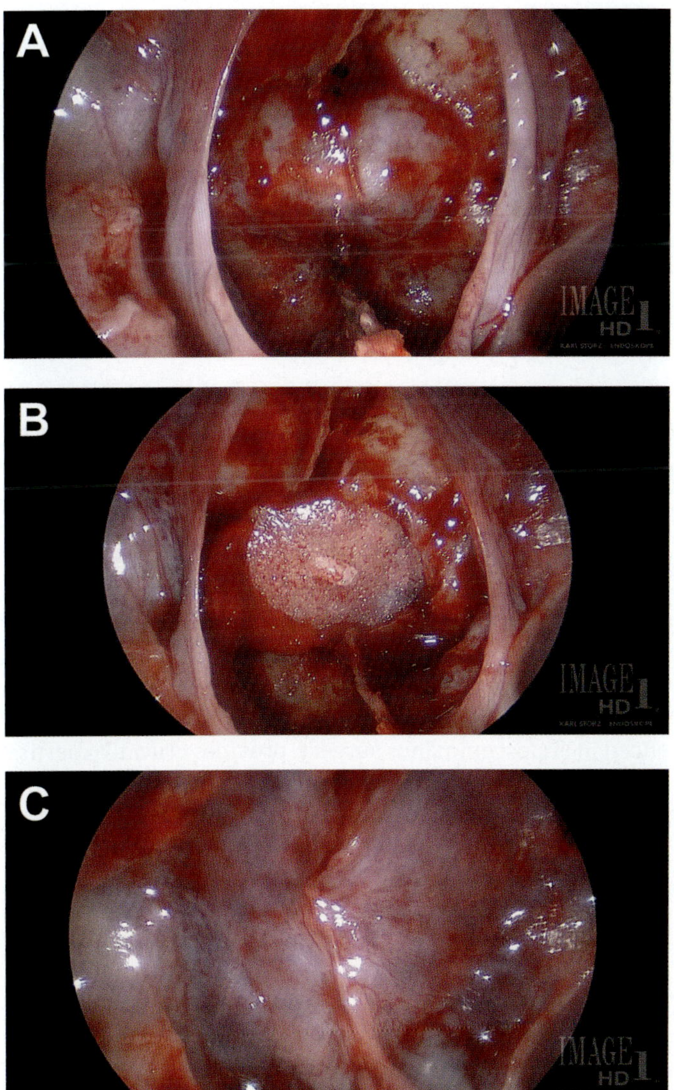

Fig. 15.15 **(A)** In some situations the mucosa over the sella can be preserved. **(B)** The sella is packed with fat, and a piece of Medpor is used to reconstruct the floor. **(C)** The mucosa can be reapproximated to allow normal mucosal transport.

Postoperative Care

All patients except those without Cushing's disease are given a single dose of dexamethasone (2 mg) the night after surgery and the following morning. A fasting morning cortisol level is obtained on the second postoperative day. Most patients after pituitary adenoma surgery have normal cortisol levels.[57] Postoperatively, patients stay in the intensive care unit (ICU) overnight. Urine output and urine specific gravity are monitored closely for signs of diabetes insipidus (DI). If there is evidence of DI and the patient is able to keep up with oral fluid intake, medical therapy is avoided. The serum sodium level is also closely monitored. Medical treatment is initiated only if there is a notable rise in the serum sodium level, the patient is unable to keep up with the urine output, or the DI lasts for more than 1 to 2 days.

In patients with hormone-producing tumors, postoperative fasting morning measurements of cortisol, ACTH, growth hormone, and prolactin are obtained to help determine endocrinologic cure after surgery. For patients with Cushing's disease, the mean ACTH level is decreased 8 to 12 hours postoperatively in those who are cured, compared with those who are not.[49] Furthermore, cortisol levels <170 nmol/L are a good indicator of cure. Until there is clinical or laboratory evidence of adrenal insufficiency, postoperative glucocorticoids are held as long as close monitoring is available.[49] In addition, patients with a cortisol level <83 mmol/L on a dexamethasone suppression test on postoperative day 3 had a 93% rate of remission at 5 years.[58] In some centers, rapid reoperation for patients with persistently elevated cortisol levels has been recommended.[59] For patients cured of Cushing's disease, glucocorticoid replacement therapy is needed for several months until the hypothalamic-pituitary-adrenal axis can make sufficient endogenous glucocorticoids. Tapering should be done judiciously under close observation. In patients with acromegaly, a fasting morning growth hormone level is obtained on the first postoperative day to assess biochemical cure. Levels less than 2 ng/mL correlate with a high likelihood of long-term remission.[60] Early measurement of insulin-like growth factor-1 (IGF-1) levels is less reliable, though free IGF-1 levels may be a better measure.[61] A fasting morning prolactin level <10 ng/mL is predictive of long-term remission in patients with prolactinomas.[62] Patients with no evidence of DI are transferred out of the ICU and usually discharged on the second postoperative day once they are ambulating and eating well.

Early MRI is obtained on the first or second postoperative day to assess the extent of resection, the location of the fat graft if one is present, and the presence of an intrasellar hematoma. Early postoperative imaging is often misleading at distinguishing residual tumor from postoperative changes. However, after normal postoperative changes are accounted for, nodular enhancement within the sella can be an indication of residual tumor.[63] After resection of macroadenomas, a large mass is often seen postoperatively with peripheral enhancement that can represent secretions, blood, packing, or residual tumor adherent to the surrounding arachnoid or brain that prevents collapse of the cavity.[47] To more definitively rule out residual tumor, an MRI scan with and without contrast at 3 months is obtained. At this point, postoperative blood and secretions should have resolved. Management options regarding residual disease include observation, repeat surgery, radiosurgery, or fractionated radiotherapy. If a complete resection is observed, radiographic follow-up is recommended with repeat imaging at 6 months postoperatively and then annually. For patients with hormone-secreting tumors, biochemical follow-up should be conducted for recurrence.

Endoscope Versus Microscope

Several studies have attempted to directly compare the endonasal, endoscopic approach with the traditional, microscope-based, transsphenoidal approach. When investigators compared a cohort of endonasal, endoscopically treated patients with a control group of patients treated with the traditional approach, it was shown that the endonasal, endoscopic approach is associated with reduced length of hospital stay and lower incidence of postoperative complications.[16,64,65] Casler et al[64] demonstrated that patients undergoing an endoscopic procedure had less postoperative discomfort, as measured by days until resolution of postoperative pain, and level of pain on postoperative day 1.[64] Some reports suggest that the endoscopic, endonasal approach only affects complications related to the nasal portion of the approach and not the resection of the tumor.[66,67] However, in a retrospective series of 50 patients, Neal et al[16] demonstrated a decreased rate of CSF leaks and lower incidence of DI as compared with the sublabial transsphenoidal and open transnasal groups. In addition to the smaller controlled studies, several larger series of endonasal, endoscopically treated pituitary lesions and a recent meta-analysis by Tabaee et al[68] report gross-total tumor removal rates, remission rates, and complication rates that are on a par with or even better than benchmarks in the medical literature for open microscope-based transsphenoidal approaches.[67–71] Frank et al[67] suggested the trend for better tumor removal appears related to the amount of extrasellar extension of the pituitary tumor, which is compatible with the acknowledged improved suprasellar and parasellar visualization of the endoscope.

Conclusion

The continued development of pituitary surgery has relied on the application and at times reapplication of new technologies and devices. The endoscope and the endonasal, endoscopic, transsphenoidal approach is one such advance that has brought about a minimally invasive technique to remove intrasellar and combined intra- and suprasellar lesions. The approach is suitable not only for pituitary adenomas but also for other lesions, depending on the exact anatomical location, such as craniopharyngiomas and Rathke cleft cysts. We advocate a team approach that comprises both an otolaryngologist and a neurosurgeon. The otolaryngologist, experienced in endoscopic sinus surgery, provides crucial expertise in navigating normal and abnormal sinus anatomy during the procedure, whereas the neurosurgeon trained in pituitary surgery brings the know-how to safely resect pituitary tumors in the setting of the intimate and complex "invisible" anatomy surrounding the sella. We continue to use intraoperative navigation but have shifted away from simple fluoroscopy to more detailed frameless stereotactic navigation. Lastly, a thorough knowledge of the hypothalamic-pituitary axis is necessary to manage these patients successfully in the perioperative period. Though the assistance of a knowledgeable endocrinologist is helpful, the operating surgeon must acquire the independent comprehension of perioperative endocrinologic issues to care for patients appropriately in situations when specialized assistance is not available.

References

1. Liu JK, Das K, Weiss MH, Laws ER Jr, Couldwell WT. The history and evolution of transsphenoidal surgery. J Neurosurg 2001;95:1083–1096
2. Cushing H, The Weir Mitchell Lecture. Surgical experiences with pituitary disorders. JAMA 1914;63:1515–1525
3. Hirsch O. Endonasal method of removal of hypophyseal tumors. With a report of two successful cases. JAMA 1910;55:772–774
4. Guiot G. Transsphenoidal approach in the surgical treatment of pituitary adenomas: general principles and indications in nonfunctioning adenomas. In: Kohler PO, Ross GT, eds. Diagnosis and Treatment of Pituitary Tumors. New York: American Elsevier; 1973:159–178
5. Hardy J, Wigser SM. Trans-sphenoidal surgery of pituitary fossa tumors with televised radiofluoroscopic control. J Neurosurg 1965;23:612–619
6. Guiot J, Rougerie J, Fourestier M, et al. [Intracranial endoscopic explorations.]. Presse Med 1963;71:1225–1228
7. Jankowski R, Auque J, Simon C, Marchal JC, Hepner H, Wayoff M. Endoscopic pituitary tumor surgery. Laryngoscope 1992;102:198–202
8. Jho HD. Endoscopic transsphenoidal surgery. J Neurooncol 2001;54:187–195
9. Jho HD, Carrau RL. Endoscopic endonasal transsphenoidal surgery: experience with 50 patients. J Neurosurg 1997;87:44–51
10. Cappabianca P, Alfieri A, de Divitiis E. Endoscopic endonasal transsphenoidal approach to the sella: towards functional endoscopic pituitary surgery (FEPS). Minim Invasive Neurosurg 1998;41:66–73
11. Cappabianca P, Cavallo LM, Colao A, et al. Endoscopic endonasal transsphenoidal approach: outcome analysis of 100 consecutive procedures. Minim Invasive Neurosurg 2002;45:193–200
12. Cappabianca P, Cavallo LM, de Divitiis E. Endoscopic endonasal transsphenoidal surgery. Neurosurgery 2004;55:933–940, discussion 940–941
13. Cavallo LM, Prevedello D, Esposito F, et al. The role of the endoscope in the transsphenoidal management of cystic lesions of the sellar region. Neurosurg Rev 2008;31:55–64, discussion 64
14. Schwartz TH, Anand VK. The endoscopic, endonasal transsphenoidal approach to the sella. In: Anand VK, Schwartz TH, eds. Practical Endoscopic Skull Base Surgery. San Diego: Plural Publishing; 2007:89–104
15. Catapano D, Sloffer CA, Frank G, Pasquini E, D' Angelo VA, Lanzino G. Comparison between the microscope and endoscope in the direct endonasal extended transsphenoidal approach: anatomical study. J Neurosurg 2006;104:419–425
16. Neal JG, Patel SJ, Kulbersh JS, Osguthorpe JD, Schlosser RJ. Comparison of techniques for transsphenoidal pituitary surgery. Am J Rhinol 2007;21:203–206
17. Koren I, Hadar T, Rappaport ZH, Yaniv E. Endoscopic transnasal transsphenoidal microsurgery versus the sublabial approach for the treatment of pituitary tumors: endonasal complications. Laryngoscope 1999;109:1838–1840
18. Cappabianca P, Cavallo LM, de Divitiis O, Solari D, Esposito F, Colao A. Endoscopic pituitary surgery. Pituitary, 2008;385–390
19. Nasseri SS, Kasperbauer JL, Strome SE, McCaffrey TV, Atkinson JL, Meyer FB. Endoscopic transnasal pituitary surgery: report on 180 cases. Am J Rhinol 2001;15:281–287
20. White DR, Sonnenburg RE, Ewend MG, Senior BA. Safety of minimally invasive pituitary surgery (MIPS) compared with a traditional approach. Laryngoscope 2004;114:1945–1948
21. Laufer I, Anand VK, Schwartz TH. Endoscopic, endonasal extended transsphenoidal, transplanum transtuberculum approach for resection of suprasellar lesions. J Neurosurg 2007;106:400–406
22. Schwartz TH, Anand VK. The endoscopic endonasal transsphenoidal approach to the suprasellar cistern. Clin Neurosurg 2007;54:226–235
23. Frank G, Pasquini E. Endoscopic endonasal approaches to the cavernous sinus: surgical approaches. Neurosurgery 2002;50:675
24. Frank G, Pasquini E. Endoscopic endonasal cavernous sinus surgery, with special reference to pituitary adenomas. Front Horm Res 2006;34:64–82
25. Cappabianca P, et al. Extended endoscopic endonasal transsphenoidal approaches to the suprasellar region, planum sphenoidale and clivus. In: de Divitiis E, Cappabianca P, eds. Endoscopic Endonasal Transsphenoidal Surgery. Vienna, New York: Springer-Verlag; 2003:176–188
26. Schwartz TH, Stieg PE, Anand VK. Endoscopic transsphenoidal pituitary surgery with intraoperative magnetic resonance imaging. Neurosurgery 2006;58(1, Suppl):ONS44–ONS51, discussion ONS44–ONS51
27. Cavallo LM, Dal Fabbro M, Jalalod'din H, et al. Endoscopic endonasal transsphenoidal surgery. Before scrubbing in: tips and tricks. Surg Neurol 2007;67:342–347
28. Dehdashti AR, Gentili F. Current state of the art in the diagnosis and surgical treatment of Cushing disease: early experience with a purely endoscopic endonasal technique. Neurosurg Focus 2007;23: E9
29. Fraser JF, Allen B, Anand VK, Schwartz TH. Three-dimensional neurostereoendoscopy: subjective and objective comparison to 2D. Minim Invasive Neurosurg 2009;52:25–31
30. Tabaee A, Anand VK, Fraser JF, Brown SM, Singh A, Schwartz TH. Three-dimensional endoscopic pituitary surgery. Neurosurgery 2009;64(5, Suppl 2):288–293, discussion 294–295
31. Brown SM, Tabaee A, Singh A, Schwartz TH, Anand VK. Three-dimensional endoscopic sinus surgery: feasibility and technical aspects. Otolaryngol Head Neck Surg 2008;138:400–402
32. Netea-Maier RT, van Lindert EJ, den Heijer M, et al. Transsphenoidal pituitary surgery via the endoscopic technique: results in 35 consecutive patients with Cushing's disease. Eur J Endocrinol 2006; 154:675–684
33. Couldwell WT, Weiss MH. Medical and surgical management of microprolactinoma. Pituitary 2004;7:31–32
34. Aho CJ, Liu C, Zelman V, Couldwell WT, Weiss MH. Surgical outcomes in 118 patients with Rathke cleft cysts. J Neurosurg 2005;102:189–193
35. Frank G, Sciarretta V, Mazzatenta D, Farneti G, Modugno GC, Pasquini E. Transsphenoidal endoscopic approach in the treatment of Rathke's cleft cyst. Neurosurgery 2005;56:124–128, discussion 129
36. Benveniste RJ, King WA, Walsh J, Lee JS, Naidich TP, Post KD. Surgery for Rathke cleft cysts: technical considerations and outcomes. J Neurosurg 2004;101:577–584
37. Kim JE, Kim JH, Kim OL, et al. Surgical treatment of symptomatic Rathke cleft cysts: clinical features and results with special attention to recurrence. J Neurosurg 2004;100:33–40
38. Jane JA Jr, Laws ER. Craniopharyngioma. Pituitary 2006;9:323–326

39. Teo C. Application of endoscopy to the surgical management of craniopharyngiomas. Childs Nerv Syst 2005;21:696–700
40. Maira G, Anile C, Albanese A, Cabezas D, Pardi F, Vignati A. The role of transsphenoidal surgery in the treatment of craniopharyngiomas. J Neurosurg 2004;100:445–451
41. Frank G, Pasquini E, Doglietto F, et al. The endoscopic extended transsphenoidal approach for craniopharyngiomas. Neurosurgery 2006;59(1, Suppl 1):ONS75–ONS83, discussion ONS75–ONS83
42. Schwartz TH, Fraser JF, Brown S, Tabaee A, Kacker A, Anand VK. Endoscopic cranial base surgery: classification of operative approaches. Neurosurgery 2008;62:991–1002, discussion 1002–1005
43. Liu AL, Wang C, Sun S, Wang M, Liu P. Gamma knife radiosurgery for tumors involving the cavernous sinus. Stereotact Funct Neurosurg 2005;83:45–51
44. Lucas-Morante T, García-Uría J, Estrada J, et al. Treatment of invasive growth hormone pituitary adenomas with long-acting somatostatin analog SMS 201-995 before transsphenoidal surgery. J Neurosurg 1994;81:10–14
45. Landolt AM, Haller D, Lomax N, et al. Octreotide may act as a radioprotective agent in acromegaly. J Clin Endocrinol Metab 2000; 85:1287–1289
46. Pollock BE, Nippoldt TB, Stafford SL, Foote RL, Abboud CF. Results of stereotactic radiosurgery in patients with hormone-producing pituitary adenomas: factors associated with endocrine normalization. J Neurosurg 2002;97:525–530
47. Caranci F, et al. The role of the neuroradiologist. In: de Divitiis E, Cappabianca P, eds. Endoscopic Endonasal Transsphenoidal Surgery. Vienna, New York: Springer-Verlag; 2003:61–81
48. Laine FJ, Smoker WR. The ostiomeatal unit and endoscopic surgery: anatomy, variations, and imaging findings in inflammatory diseases. AJR Am J Roentgenol 1992;159:849–857
49. Pimentel-Filho FR, Silva ME, Nogueira KC, Berger K, Cukiert A, Liberman B. Pituitary-adrenal dynamics after ACTH-secreting pituitary tumor resection in patients receiving no steroids post-operatively. J Endocrinol Invest 2005;28:502–508
50. Tabaee A, Placantonakis DG, Schwartz TH, Anand VK. Intrathecal fluorescein in endoscopic skull base surgery. Otolaryngol Head Neck Surg 2007;137:316–320
51. Placantonakis DG, Tabaee A, Anand VK, Hiltzik D, Schwartz TH. Safety of low-dose intrathecal fluorescein in endoscopic cranial base surgery. Neurosurgery 2007;61(3, Suppl):161–165, discussion 165–166
52. Cavallo LM, Messina A, Cappabianca P, et al. Endoscopic endonasal surgery of the midline skull base: anatomical study and clinical considerations. Neurosurg Focus 2005;19:E2
53. Oldfield EH, Vortmeyer AO. Development of a histological pseudocapsule and its use as a surgical capsule in the excision of pituitary tumors. J Neurosurg 2006;104:7–19
54. Tabaee A, Anand VK, Brown SM, Lin JW, Schwartz TH. Algorithm for reconstruction after endoscopic pituitary and skull base surgery. Laryngoscope 2007;117:1133–1137
55. Leng LZ, Brown S, Anand VK, Schwartz TH. "Gasket-seal" watertight closure in minimal-access endoscopic cranial base surgery. Neurosurgery 2008;62(5, Suppl 2):E342–E343, discussion E343
56. Hadad G, Bassagasteguy L, Carrau RL, et al. A novel reconstructive technique after endoscopic expanded endonasal approaches: vascular pedicle nasoseptal flap. Laryngoscope 2006;116:1882–1886
57. Hout WM, Arafah BM, Salazar R, Selman W. Evaluation of the hypothalamic-pituitary-adrenal axis immediately after pituitary adenomectomy: is perioperative steroid therapy necessary? J Clin Endocrinol Metab 1988;66:1208–1212
58. Chen JC, Amar AP, Choi S, Singer P, Couldwell WT, Weiss MH. Transsphenoidal microsurgical treatment of Cushing disease: postoperative assessment of surgical efficacy by application of an overnight low-dose dexamethasone suppression test. J Neurosurg 2003;98: 967–973
59. Locatelli M, Vance ML, Laws ER. Clinical review: the strategy of immediate reoperation for transsphenoidal surgery for Cushing's disease. J Clin Endocrinol Metab 2005;90:5478–5482
60. Krieger MD, Couldwell WT, Weiss MH. Assessment of long-term remission of acromegaly following surgery. J Neurosurg 2003;98: 719–724
61. Feelders RA, Bidlingmaier M, Strasburger CJ, et al. Postoperative evaluation of patients with acromegaly: clinical significance and timing of oral glucose tolerance testing and measurement of (free) insulin-like growth factor I, acid-labile subunit, and growth hormone-binding protein levels. J Clin Endocrinol Metab 2005;90:6480–6489
62. Amar AP, Couldwell WT, Chen JC, Weiss MH. Predictive value of serum prolactin levels measured immediately after transsphenoidal surgery. J Neurosurg 2002;97:307–314
63. Yoon PH, Kim DI, Jeon P, Lee SI, Lee SK, Kim SH. Pituitary adenomas: early postoperative MR imaging after transsphenoidal resection. AJNR Am J Neuroradiol 2001;22:1097–1104
64. Casler JD, Doolittle AM, Mair EA. Endoscopic surgery of the anterior skull base. Laryngoscope 2005;115:16–24
65. Cho DY, Liau WR. Comparison of endonasal endoscopic surgery and sublabial microsurgery for prolactinomas. Surg Neurol 2002;58: 371–375, discussion 375–376
66. Fatemi N, Dusick JR, de Paiva Neto MA, Kelly DF. The endonasal microscopic approach for pituitary adenomas and other parasellar tumors: a 10-year experience. Neurosurgery 2008;63(4, Suppl 2):244–256, discussion 256
67. Frank G, Pasquini E, Farneti G, et al. The endoscopic versus the traditional approach in pituitary surgery. Neuroendocrinology 2006;83:240–248
68. Tabaee A, Anand VK, Barrón Y, et al. Endoscopic pituitary surgery: a systematic review and meta-analysis. J Neurosurg 2009;111:545–554
69. Tabaee A, Anand VK, Barrón Y, et al. Predictors of short-term outcomes following endoscopic pituitary surgery. Clin Neurol Neurosurg 2009;111:119–122
70. Kabil MS, Eby JB, Shahinian HK. Fully endoscopic endonasal vs. transseptal transsphenoidal pituitary surgery. Minim Invasive Neurosurg 2005;48:348–354
71. Dehdashti AR, Ganna A, Karabatsou K, Gentili F. Pure endoscopic endonasal approach for pituitary adenomas: early surgical results in 200 patients and comparison with previous microsurgical series. Neurosurgery 2008;62:1006–1015, discussion 1015–1017

16 Clinical Pearls in Endoscopic Pituitary Surgery: A Neurosurgeon's Perspective

Paolo Cappabianca, Felice Esposito, Luigi M. Cavallo, and Isabella Esposito

The endoscopic endonasal approach to the sellar region is an evolution of the classical microsurgical transsphenoidal technique.[1] It is no longer considered a complement to microscopic surgery; rather, it has become "fully" endoscopic skull base surgery as the procedure is performed with the endoscope being the only optical device used to visualize the surgical target area.

The standard endoscopic endonasal approach to the sellar region has several benefits[2,3]:

- It avoids the need for the oral and the rhinoseptal submucosal nasal route; the special features of the telescopes used in this approach allow for a wider exposure of the operating field including the options of advancing toward the anatomical target area or inspecting the sphenoid sinus, sellar, supra-parasellar, and retroclival regions via a wide-angle panoramic view; the high-resolution close-up view of the anatomical structures enables a lesion arising from or involving such areas to be removed more safely, which, in turn, contributes to a reduced incidence of overall complications.
- It provides an improved postoperative course with less discomfort for the patient because there is no need to use the nasal speculum, and thus the risk of trauma to nasofacial structures is reduced. It avoids the need for postoperative nasal packing, thus minimizing breathing difficulties and discomfort for the patient.
- It reduces the duration of hospitalization and, therefore, the costs.

This approach includes the following steps, which involve a learning curve for the physician.[4] Acquiring the technique requires in-depth anatomical training to become familiar with the endoscopic view of the different nasal structures; this is dependent on the acquisition of specific endoscopic skills.[5] Use of specific instrumentation facilitates the readjustment process, but it takes times to achieve proficiency with the two-dimensional image provided by the endoscope. For instance, when first attempted, the restricted sensory feedback and loss of depth perception can cause slowing of surgical dexterity; a temporary difficulty in the hand-eye coordination abilities of the surgeon is usually noticeable. This temporary difficulty is overcome as the surgeon becomes increasingly confident viewing through a video monitor versus microscope oculars that are focused in the same direction as one's own hands.

Operating Room Setup and Patient Positioning

In the operating room, all of the equipment needed or recommended for the endoscopic surgery, that is, the cold light source, video camera, monitor, and video recording system, are placed ergonomically behind the head of the patient and in front of the operating surgeon, who is at the right side of the patient. The anesthesiologist and equipment are positioned at the left side of the patient at the level of the head. The second surgeon is at the left side of the patient, and the scrub nurse stays at the level of the patient's legs.

The use of image-guidance systems (IGSs), or neuronavigation, during the standard endoscopic approach is currently reserved for selected cases only, for example, patients with a conchal-type sphenoid sinus, or in certain recurrent cases previously operated transsphenoidally, or in patients with large lesions involving the para-suprasellar areas. When IGS is used, its monitor is usually put on the side of the main endoscopic monitor to allow the surgeon to see them both simultaneously.

The design of the operating room should reflect the philosophy of a team approach, and a dedicated integrated operating room helps to optimize teamwork and improve patient care.[6]

The patient's neurodiagnostic studies are reviewed. Besides the standard sellar contrast-enhanced magnetic resonance imaging (MRI), a computed tomography (CT) scan with coronal reconstructions has proven to be quite useful to show the relevant nasal structures involved in the procedure—the nasal septum and turbinates. Furthermore, the neurodiagnostic studies are of the utmost importance for studying the individual anatomical configuration of the sphenoid sinus septum, because they may help the surgeon's orientation while operating in the sphenoid sinus. Once the surgeon has gained sufficient confidence working with the endoscopic anatomy of the posterior wall of the sphenoid sinus or if the MRI scan already shows all septations inside the sinus, the preoperative CT scan of the nasal cavities may be no longer required.

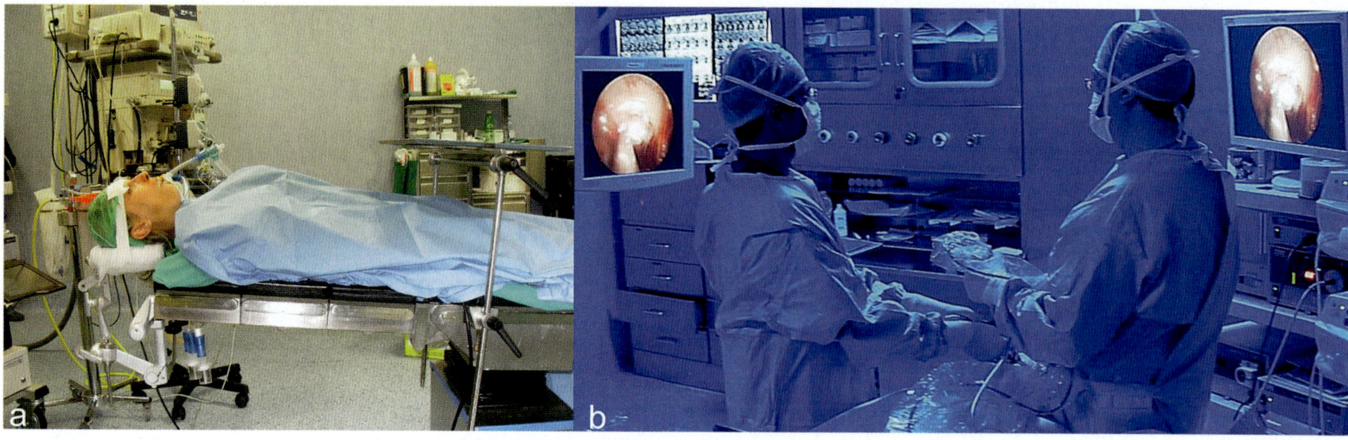

Fig. 16.1 Operating room setup. **(A)** Patient positioning. **(B)** Position of surgeons during the operation.

During the endoscopic approach to the sellar area the patient is positioned supine on the operating table with the trunk raised 10 degrees, and the head is placed in neutral position rotated 10 degrees toward the surgeon (**Fig. 16.1A**). The head is adequately secured in a horseshoe headrest without rigid three-pin fixation. The height of the table is adjusted so that the surgeon can work comfortably without having to hyperflex or extend the arms (**Fig. 16.1B**). The use of the Foley urinary catheter is not mandatory; however, it should be used if the operation is foreseen to last for more than 3 hours. The patient's body except for the neck and the face is covered with a thermal blanket. The eyes are protected with antibiotic eye ointment and covered with adhesive bandages to minimize the risk of injuries from use of the Betadine solution during the prepping of the nose and face.

Nasal Cavity

The operation can be performed through a single nostril. When a bi-nostril approach is performed, two or three operating instruments, depending on the specific needs and circumstances, plus the endoscope can be inserted through both nostrils, thus providing increased working space and improved maneuverability.[4]

Using a small Killian-type nasal speculum, cotton pledgets soaked in 50% polyvidone-iodine are placed along the floor of the nasal cavities and in the space between the nasal septum and the turbinates. They are allowed to take effect for approximately 5 minutes. We advise not using pure polyvidone-iodine antiseptic solution because it may irritate the nasal mucosa.

Before starting the surgical procedure, each component of the endoscopic apparatus (monitor, video camera, light source, light cable, endoscope, irrigation system, recording system, etc.) should be checked to be sure it is functioning correctly; the white balance of the video camera should also be checked.

During the first part of the procedure, a 0-degree telescope, 4 mm in diameter, 18 cm in length, is used freehand. Once the scope is introduced parallel to the floor of the nasal cavity, the first structure to come into view is the inferior turbinate. The scope is advanced along the floor of the nasal cavity, passing between the posterior end of the inferior turbinate and the nasal septum, to reach the choana, which is the true anatomical landmark of this step of the procedure and where the eustachian tube opens. The middle turbinate is above and posterior to the head of the inferior turbinate.

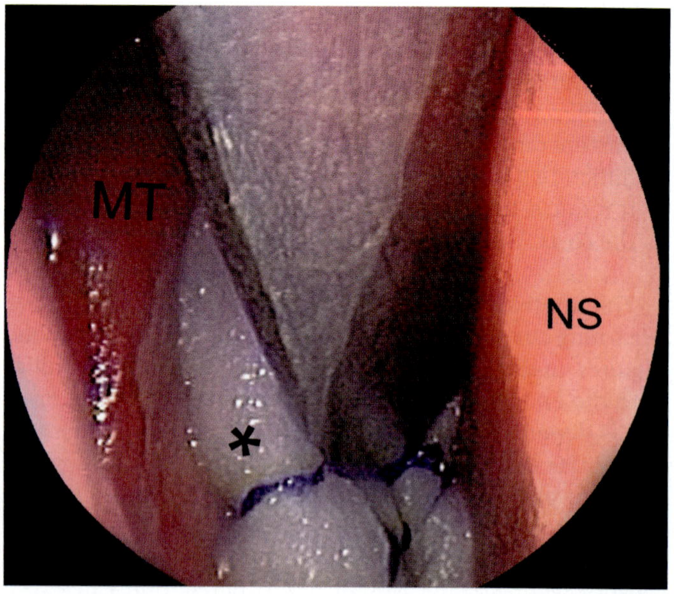

Fig. 16.2 Nasal step. Right nasal cavity. A cotton pledget soaked with diluted adrenaline protects the middle turbinate when pushing it laterally. MT, middle turbinate; NS, nasal septum; asterisk, cotton pledget.

In some cases, its head may be variously pneumatized (concha bullosa). Cotton pledgets, soaked in diluted adrenaline (1/10,000, 1:20 dilution) or xylometazoline hydrochlorate, are placed in the space between the middle turbinate and the nasal septum to achieve a vasoconstriction of the nasal mucosa (**Fig. 16.2**). The anesthesiologist should be notified of the use of the adrenaline as it might increase the patient's blood pressure and heart rate.

The middle turbinate is gently lateralized to widen the space between the nasal septum and the turbinate itself. Moving the endoscope forward between the middle turbinate and nasal septum, at a 30-degree upward angle relative to the floor of the nasal cavity, the sphenoethmoid recess is reached, extending between the roof of the choana and the natural sphenoid ostium (**Fig. 16.3A**). Such ostium varies in size and cannot always be viewed, as it may be hidden by the tail of the superior or the supreme turbinate. At this point, it is not necessary to visualize the sphenoid ostium because access to the sphenoid cavity can be gained by proceeding from the choana slightly upward for approximately 1.5 cm along the sphenoethmoid recess.

Sphenoid Sinus

The next step of the procedure begins with the decongestion or coagulation of the sphenoethmoid recess with the elevation of its mucosa, thus exposing the sphenoid prow (**Fig. 16.3B**). Subsequently, after having identified the sphenoid cavity, the nasal septum is detached from the anterior wall of the sphenoid sinus with a high-speed microdrill using a diamond bur of 5 mm in diameter and/or bone punches (**Fig. 16.3C**). The bone of the anterior sphenoid sinus wall is widely open either with the same microdrill and/or bone punches, proceeding circumferentially, taking care, while enlarging the opening in the inferolateral direction, of the

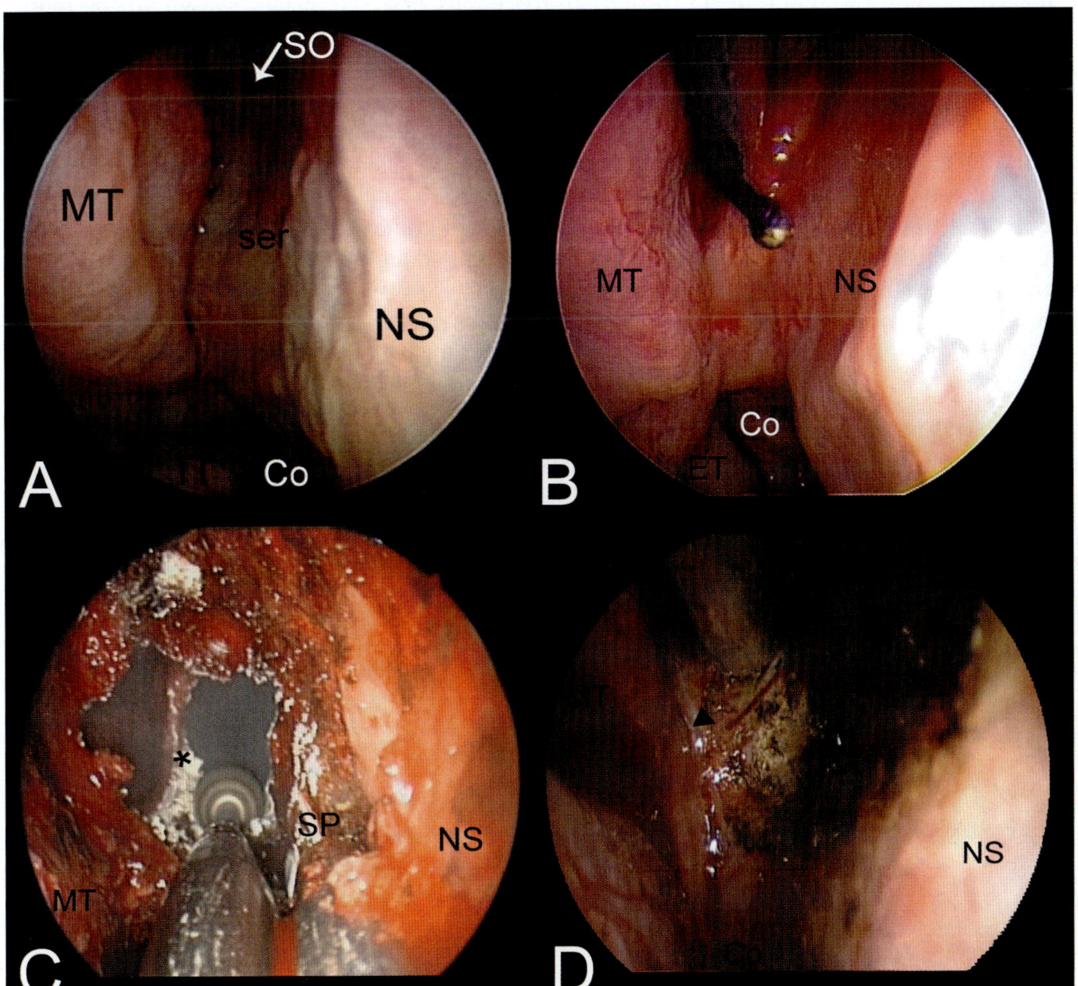

Fig. 16.3 Nasal step. Right nasal cavity. **(A)** Identification of the sphenoethmoid recess. **(B)** Monopolar coagulation. **(C)** Anterior sphenoidotomy. **(D)** Bleeding from a branch of the sphenopalatine artery. Co, choana; ET, eustachian tube; IT, inferior turbinate; MT, middle turbinate; NS, nasal septum; ser, sphenoethmoid recess; SO, sphenoid ostium; SP, sphenoid prow, asterisk, sphenoid septum; arrowhead, arterial bleeding.

sphenopalatine artery and its major branches. This artery is the terminal branch of the internal maxillary artery, which is, in turn, a branch of the external carotid artery. The sphenopalatine artery enters the nasal cavity through the sphenopalatine foramen, which is located topographically behind the tail of the middle turbinate. Within the nasal cavity the artery ramifies into two branches: one medial, the nasopalatine artery, which passes above the choana and vascularizes the nasal septum; and the other, the posterior nasal artery, which joins the lateral nasal wall to vascularize the turbinates.[7]

In case of arterial bleeding from a branch of the sphenopalatine artery, it is preferable to use bipolar coagulation because the monopolar coagulation has an increased risk of causing delayed hemorrhage (**Fig. 16.3D**).[7]

In some cases, a median or paramedian septum is present inside the sphenoid cavity, whereas in others multiple septa are found. If a CT scan of the nasal and paranasal structures has been obtained, the presence of such septa is already known. Particularly in cases of multiple septa, they may be located at the site of the optic or carotid prominence, a condition that requires the surgeon to pay particular attention during removal of these structures. The septa can be removed with through-cutting nasal forceps to avoid any elevation of the sphenoid mucosa.

At this point, the entire sellar region is in the field of vision. The endoscopic technique thus provides a panoramic view of the entire sphenoid cavity, with all the depressions and bony prominences that cover vulnerable neurovascular structures (i.e., the optic nerves and the carotid arteries) and allows identification of all anatomical landmarks, which is indispensable for gaining access to the sellar floor (optic and carotid protuberances, clivus, planum sphenoidale, and opticocarotid recess) (**Fig. 16.4A**).

Endoscopic Sella Opening

To free both of the surgeon's hands and allow for comfortable introduction of two instruments, the endoscope can be fixed to an adjustable holder, either mechanic or pneumatic. Another option is for the surgeon to operate two instruments through one or both nostrils bimanually, while the endoscope is held dynamically by a second surgeon (three- and four-hand technique).[4,8]

Prior to opening the sellar floor, it is fundamental to check that the endoscope has the proper orientation to ensure that all anatomical landmarks inside the sphenoid cavity are displayed in their appropriate position. In fact, operating with the 0-degree lens, if the camera is rotated with respect to the endoscope, the images shown on the monitor might be rotated as well. Creation of an opening in the sellar floor may be accomplished by several methods and with the use of various instruments, depending on the individual anatomical situation (intact, thinned out, eroded). The consistency of the sellar floor depends on the type of lesion present in the sellar cavity. It is nearly always intact in the case of microadenomas or Rathke's cleft cysts, whereas it is frequently thinned out or eroded in the case of pituitary macroadenomas.

Depending on its thickness, the sellar floor may be initially opened with a microdrill when intact or by means of a dissec-

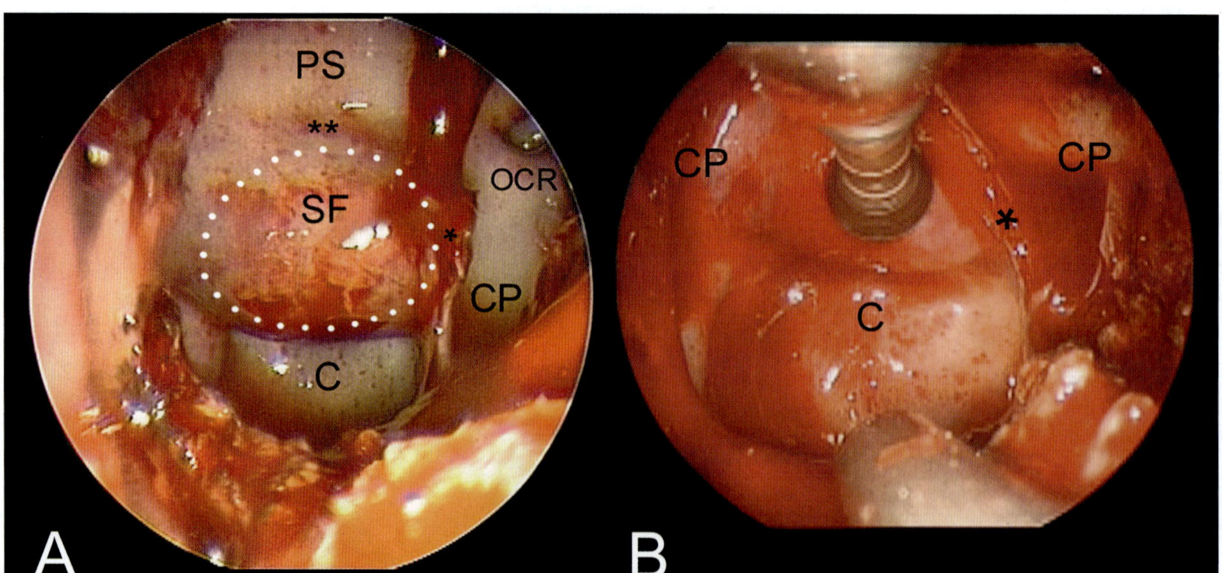

Fig. 16.4 Sphenoid step. **(A)** The anatomical landmarks that guide the sellar opening and the orientation of the surgeon are shown. **(B)** Drilling of the sellar floor. PS, planum sphenoidale; C, clivus; CP, carotid protuberance; OCR, opticocarotid recess; SF, sellar floor; asterisk, flattened sphenoid septum; double asterisk, tuberculum sellae; white dotted line: bone window.

tor when thinned out or eroded. A microdrill with diamond bur is used to create an opening in the sellar floor (**Fig. 16.4B**). With the help of a Kerrison bone punch, the fenestration is enlarged until the carotid prominences are visualized laterally, the planum sphenoidale above, and the clivus below.

Once the opening of the floor has been created, the dura mater may appear intact, thinned out, or infiltrated by the lesion. An ultrasound Doppler probe can be helpful for identifying the carotid arteries, thus allowing a safer sharp opening of the dura.

Particularly during the insertion of the knife in the nasal cavity, where it is not yet visible by the endoscope, there is the risk of iatrogenic trauma to the nasal mucosa. For such reason, we use a scalpel with telescopic blade, with the blade retracted before the tip enters the endoscope's field of vision, where the blade is extended. Once the dural incision has been made, the intrasellar lesion is removed by using variously angled and sized ring curettes and aspiration.

In the case of a macroadenoma, the inferior and lateral components of the lesion should be removed before the superior aspect. This step is necessary because if the superior part is removed first, the suprasellar cistern and the redundant diaphragma sellae will fall into the operative field, thus hiding the lateral portions of the lesion. In contrast, in the case of a microadenoma, one should attempt to identify a cleavage plane of the tumor pseudocapsule for an en-bloc excision, which, if possible, should be accomplished without compromising the residual pituitary gland tissue.

The entire procedure until this step is usually performed with a 0-degree telescope. The 30- or 45-degree telescopes can be helpful for inspecting the sellar cavity after tumor removal, evaluating the presence of some remnant, or identifying the point of cerebrospinal fluid (CSF) leakage over the cistern surface.

Upon completion of the endoscopic procedure, sellar reconstruction is required, mainly when an intraoperative CSF leak has occurred.[9–14] Autologous or heterologous materials, either resorbable or not, are used, if necessary, to achieve a safe and effective sellar reconstruction.[9–11] The aim of the repair is to guarantee a watertight closure, reduce the dead space, and prevent the descent of the chiasm into the sellar cavity.[11] This must be performed with care to avoid overpacking, which carries a risk of subsequent compression of the optic chiasm, possibly causing postoperative visual loss.

Different techniques are used (intra- or extradural closure of the sella, and packing of the sella with or without packing of the sphenoid sinus), depending on the size of osteodural defect and of the "dead space" inside the sella.

According to Kelly's paradigm, intraoperative CSF leaks are categorized based on size[11,15]:

- Grade 0: no leak observed
- Grade 1: small "weeping" CSF leak, confirmed by Valsalva maneuver, without a visible diaphragmatic defect
- Grade 2: moderate CSF leak, with definite diaphragmatic defect
- Grade 3: large diaphragmatic and/or dural defect

In our experience, the repair is based on the CSF leak grade as follows[9,16]:

- Grade 0: nothing inside the sella, or a collagen sponge only to reduce a large "dead" sellar space.
- Grade 1: collagen sponge placed over the exposed suprasellar cistern, followed by the filling of the sellar cavity with fibrin glue (Tisseel; Baxter, Deerfield, IL) and intra- or extradural closure of the sellar floor with a bone substitute (LactoSorb; Lorenz Surgical, Jacksonville, FL).
- Grade 2: the reconstruction starts from the management of the arachnoid defect. A small amount of fibrin glue is injected through the arachnoid defect and, if possible, the redundant arachnoid is then used to cover the defect (**Fig. 16.5A**). Different layers of collagen sponge are then placed over the cisternal surface, while fibrin glue (Tisseel) is used to fill the sellar cavity. Thereafter, the sellar floor is closed intra-, or better, extradurally with a bone substitute (**Fig. 16.5B**). Other layers of collagen sponge are positioned to cover the posterior wall of the sphenoid sinus which, lastly, is filled with fibrin glue (Tisseel) or synthetic glues (DuraSeal; Confluent Surgical, Waltham, MA) (**Fig. 16.5C**).
- Grade 3: this condition more often concerns the case of an extended approach for suprasellar lesions rather than standard pituitary surgery. Whichever approach is used, reconstruction proceeds in the same manner as for grade 2 up to the closure of the sellar floor, in this case performed with a single large layer of dural substitute in the extradural space. In addition, a sheet of resorbable solid material, tailored to conform to the size and grade of the defect, is then placed over the dural substitute and embedded in the extradural space dragging the dural substitute into overlay position.

This allows for the reconstruction becoming a sort of gasket seal,[14] or what we call "the grandma jam cap," as it resembles the extra layer of special paper or tissue that was put over the jar of marmalade and under the cap to secure the seal, avoiding outflow of the content or entrance of air into the container, thereby preserving the fruit for the whole winter season. Packing of the sphenoid sinus is then completed as for grade 2.

After sellar reconstruction, the surgical procedure is completed, checking the hemostasis and by putting back the middle turbinate, previously lateralized, to avoid obstruction of the ostium of the maxillary sinus and subsequent sinusitis.

At the end, the endoscope is removed from the nasal cavity and no nasal packing is used.

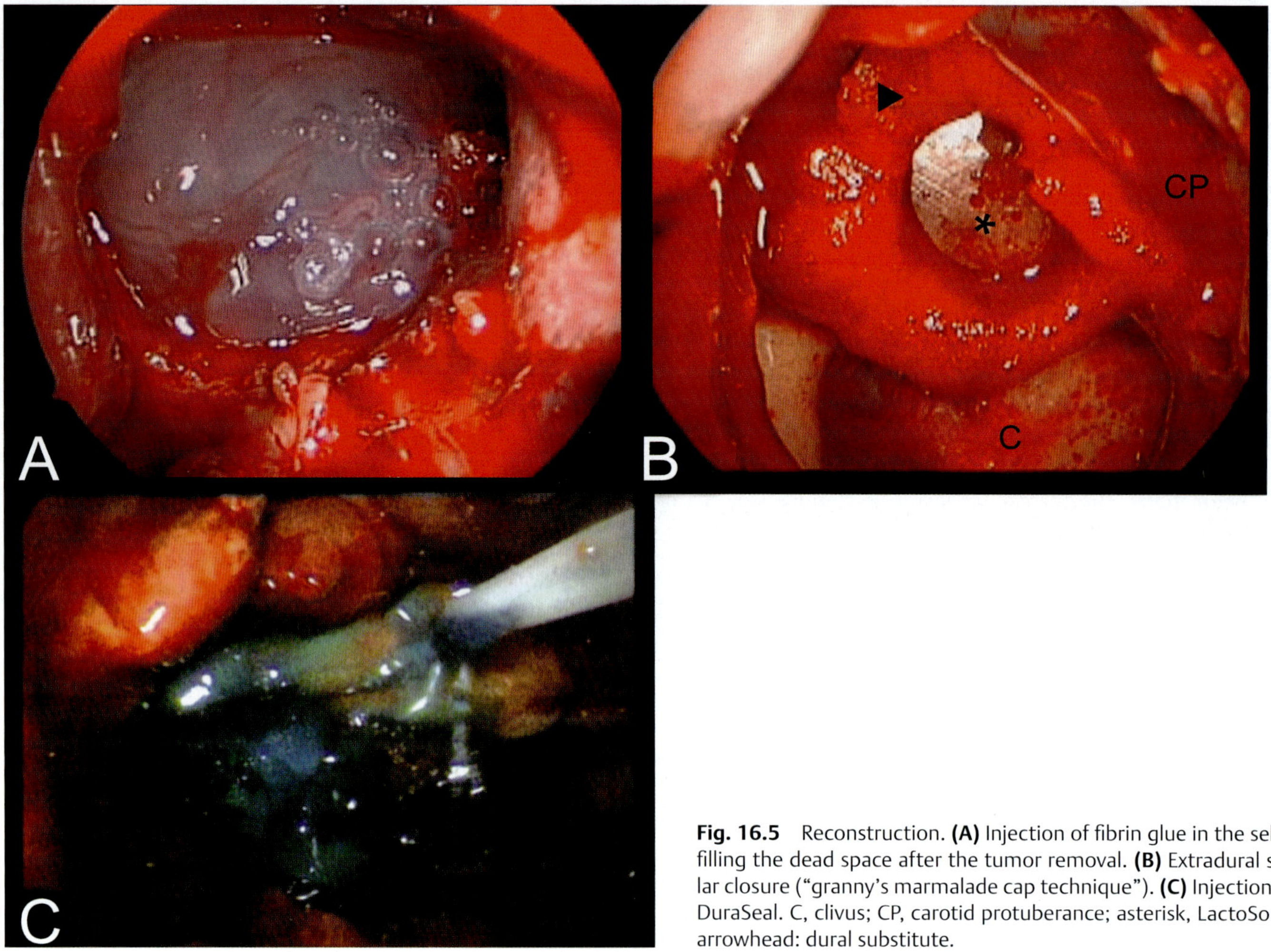

Fig. 16.5 Reconstruction. **(A)** Injection of fibrin glue in the sella, filling the dead space after the tumor removal. **(B)** Extradural sellar closure ("granny's marmalade cap technique"). **(C)** Injection of DuraSeal. C, clivus; CP, carotid protuberance; asterisk, LactoSorb; arrowhead: dural substitute.

The patient is awakened from anesthesia and transferred to the postanesthesia care unit for 1 to 3 hours. The patient then proceeds to the regular ward, and if the operation was uneventful (no intraoperative CSF leak or large bleedings), will ambulate a few hours later and have a light dinner.

Regarding the antibiotic therapy, it is our current policy to adopt a short-term prophylaxis with intravenous third-generation cephalosporins (ceftriaxone or ceftazidime), 30 minutes before starting the procedure and 6 hours after the first injection, with no increased risk for infectious complication. In the case of a grade 2 or 3 CSF leak, where a large communication exists with the subarachnoid compartment, we continue the prophylaxis for 3 days after the operation.

In cases of hormonally active adenomas, we advise checking the hormone levels on postoperative days 1 and 2. In fact, as demonstrated by previous studies, if the operation is successful, the pituitary hormones fall into the normal ranges or even in the subnormal ranges.[17–19]

The patient is observed for developing diabetes insipidus by checking the fluid balance.[20]

The patient is discharged from the hospital, usually on postoperative day 2 or 3, unless it is necessary to keep the patient in the hospital longer, and is instructed to contact the endocrinologist for the hormonal follow-up. The patient is instructed to return for a check of the serum sodium on postoperative days 4 to 6 to control for an incipient hyponatremia[21] that may be caused by the syndrome of inappropriate antidiuretic hormone secretion; this may be severe in some instances, requiring hospitalization. Typically, however, such hyponatremia is subclinical. The patient will then be seen in the outpatient clinic 3 months later for a postoperative sellar contrast-enhanced MRI. If a grade 2 or 3 CSF leak has occurred during the operation, or in the case of large lesions, the patient is scheduled as an outpatient for an endoscopic evaluation of the nasal and sphenoid sinus cavities to ensure that the mucosa is healing well and that there is no CSF leak.

References

1. Doglietto F, Prevedello DM, Jane JA Jr, Han J, Laws ER Jr. Brief history of endoscopic transsphenoidal surgery—from Philipp Bozzini to the

First World Congress of Endoscopic Skull Base Surgery. Neurosurg Focus 2005;19:E3

2. Cappabianca P, Cavallo LM, de Divitiis E. Endoscopic endonasal transsphenoidal surgery. Neurosurgery 2004;55:933–940, discussion 940–941
3. de Divitiis E, Cappabianca P, Cavallo LM. Endoscopic endonasal transsphenoidal approach to the sellar region. In: de Divitiis E, Cappabianca P, eds. Endoscopic Endonasal Transsphenoidal Surgery. Vienna, New York: Springer, 2003:91–130
4. Cavallo LM, Dal Fabbro M, Jalalod'din H, et al. Endoscopic endonasal transsphenoidal surgery. Before scrubbing in: tips and tricks. Surg Neurol 2007;67:342–347
5. Snyderman C, Kassam A, Carrau R, Mintz A, Gardner P, Prevedello DM. Acquisition of surgical skills for endonasal skull base surgery: a training program. Laryngoscope 2007;117:699–705
6. Cappabianca P, Cavallo LM, Esposito F, De Divitiis O, Messina A, De Divitiis E. Extended endoscopic endonasal approach to the midline skull base: the evolving role of transsphenoidal surgery. Adv Tech Stand Neurosurg 2008;33:151–199
7. Cavallo LM, Briganti F, Cappabianca P, et al. Hemorrhagic vascular complications of endoscopic transsphenoidal surgery. Minim Invasive Neurosurg 2004;47:145–150
8. Castelnuovo P, Pistochini A, Locatelli D. Different surgical approaches to the sellar region: focusing on the "two nostrils four hands technique." Rhinology 2006;44:2–7
9. Cappabianca P, Cavallo LM, Esposito F, Valente V, De Divitiis E. Sellar repair in endoscopic endonasal transsphenoidal surgery: results of 170 cases. Neurosurgery 2002;51:1365–1371, discussion 1371–1372
10. Esposito F, Cappabianca P, Fusco M, et al. Collagen-only biomatrix as a novel dural substitute. Examination of the efficacy, safety and outcome: clinical experience on a series of 208 patients. Clin Neurol Neurosurg 2008;110:343–351
11. Esposito F, Dusick JR, Fatemi N, Kelly DF. Graded repair of cranial base defects and cerebrospinal fluid leaks in transsphenoidal surgery. Neurosurgery 2007;60(4, Suppl 2):295–303, discussion 303–304
12. Kassam A, Carrau RL, Snyderman CH, Gardner P, Mintz A. Evolution of reconstructive techniques following endoscopic expanded endonasal approaches. Neurosurg Focus 2005;19:E8
13. Tabaee A, Anand VK, Brown SM, Lin JW, Schwartz TH. Algorithm for reconstruction after endoscopic pituitary and skull base surgery. Laryngoscope 2007;117:1133–1137
14. Leng LZ, Brown S, Anand VK, Schwartz TH. "Gasket-seal" watertight closure in minimal-access endoscopic cranial base surgery. Neurosurgery 2008;62(5, Suppl 2):E342–E343, discussion E343
15. Dusick JR, Esposito F, Kelly DF, et al. The extended direct endonasal transsphenoidal approach for nonadenomatous suprasellar tumors. J Neurosurg 2005;102:832–841
16. Cavallo LM, Messina A, Esposito F, et al. Skull base reconstruction in the extended endoscopic transsphenoidal approach for suprasellar lesions. J Neurosurg 2007;107:713–720
17. Chen JC, Amar AP, Choi S, Singer P, Couldwell WT, Weiss MH. Transsphenoidal microsurgical treatment of Cushing disease: postoperative assessment of surgical efficacy by application of an overnight low-dose dexamethasone suppression test. J Neurosurg 2003;98:967–973
18. Esposito F, Dusick JR, Cohan P, et al. Clinical review: early morning cortisol levels as a predictor of remission after transsphenoidal surgery for Cushing's disease. J Clin Endocrinol Metab 2006;91:7–13
19. Krieger MD, Couldwell WT, Weiss MH. Assessment of long-term remission of acromegaly following surgery. J Neurosurg 2003;98:719–724
20. Dumont AS, Nemergut EC II, Jane JA Jr, Laws ER Jr. Postoperative care following pituitary surgery. J Intensive Care Med 2005;20:127–140
21. Kelly DF, Laws ER Jr, Fossett D. Delayed hyponatremia after transsphenoidal surgery for pituitary adenoma. Report of nine cases. J Neurosurg 1995;83:363–367

17 Clinical Pearls in Endoscopic Pituitary Surgery: An Otolaryngologist's Perspective

Dharambir S. Sethi and Beng Ti Ang

Pituitary surgery has been traditionally performed using a sublabial transseptal transsphenoidal approach and the operating microscope.[1] Tumor dissection has been performed with the aid of the operating microscope, which provides excellent magnification, binocular vision, and a good depth of field essential for tumor removal, and transsphenoidal surgery has proven to be a safe and effective first-line therapy for most patients with sellar and suprasellar lesions. Since the description of endonasal resection of pituitary adenomas by Jankowski et al,[2] there has been a surge of interest in endonasal pituitary surgery. In the past decade, endonasal surgery for pituitary tumors has gained acceptance worldwide.[3–5] We started endonasal pituitary surgery at our institution in 1994. A cadaver study, in which 30 fresh frozen cadavers were endoscopically dissected to study the anatomy of the sphenoid sinus, sella turcica, cavernous sinus, and the parasellar region, formed the basis of this operation.[6] Working as a combined rhinology-neurosurgery team, we performed our first endoscopic pituitary surgery in October 1994. This has been a longstanding partnership in which almost 600 pituitary tumors have been operated on using direct endonasal techniques. Our initial approach was transseptal.[7] The transseptal approach had the major limitation of having to work through a narrow channel created by elevating bilateral mucoperichondrial flaps on the nasal septum. Instrumentation was often difficult, particularly when the situation required the combined efforts of two surgeons. To overcome these limitations, we modified our approach to a direct endonasal transsphenoidal approach, avoiding a septoplasty and its inherent complications. A common transnasal corridor is thus created, allowing the use of both hands and at times having four instruments in the operative field.[8,9] This chapter discusses the practical surgical aspects for those venturing into endonasal pituitary surgery.

■ Relevant Surgical Anatomy

The importance of cadaveric dissection for learning the endoscopic anatomy and becoming familiar with the endoscopic instrumentation cannot be overemphasized. The sphenoid sinus is subject to considerable variation in size and shape and in the degree of pneumatization.[10] Based on the extent of its pneumatization, the sphenoid sinus has been classified into three types: conchal, presellar, and sellar. In the conchal type the area below the sella is a solid block of bone without an air cavity. In the presellar type, the air cavity does not penetrate beyond a plane perpendicular to the sellar wall. The sellar type is the most common, occurring in 76% of individuals, and the air cavity extends into the body of the sphenoid below the sella and may extend as far posterior as the clivus. The conchal type is common in children under the age of 12 years, after which pneumatization begins within the sphenoid sinus. In the conchal type, which is infrequent in adults, the thickness of bone separating the sella from the sphenoid sinus is at least 10 mm.[11] A sellar-type pneumatized sphenoid sinus can be compared with a pyramid-shaped six-sided box, the larger side of which is facing forward and forms the anterior wall. The anterior wall is shaped like the keel of a ship and is termed the sphenoid rostrum. The sphenoid ostia are located in the anterior wall. The roof of the sphenoid sinus is flat and termed the planum sphenoidale. It is limited posteriorly by the sellar floor, laterally by the optic nerve prominences, and anteriorly by the anterior wall of the sphenoid sinus. The width of the planum sphenoidale anteriorly, between the lamina papyracea, has been measured in cadaver studies at 26 ± 4 mm and narrows to 16 ± 3 mm posteriorly at the posterior aspect of the tuberculum sella.[12] The posterior wall of the sphenoid sinus is made up of the sellar floor in the upper part and by the clivus in the lower part. It is limited laterally by the carotid prominences, superiorly by the roof or the planum sphenoidale, and inferiorly by the floor of the sphenoid sinus. The depth of the sphenoid sinus, defined as the distance from the ostium of the sphenoid sinus to the closest part of the sella, averages 17 mm (range 12–23 mm).[10,13] The lateral wall of the sphenoid sinus shows the prominence of the optic nerve anterosuperiorly and the cavernous carotid artery posteroinferiorly. The floor of the sphenoid sinus is formed by the clivus posteriorly and the sphenoid rostrum anteriorly. The extent to which the clivus participates in formation of the posterior wall or the floor of the sphenoid sinus depends on the pneumatization of the sphenoid sinus.

The ostium of the sphenoid sinus is located in the sphenoethmoid recess and varies in size from 1 to 4 mm. In most cases it can be identified medial to the nasal septum and lateral to the superior turbinate approximately 1.5 cm superior to the posterior choana. The septa within the sphenoid sinus vary greatly in size, shape, thickness, location, completeness, and relation to the sellar floor. The cavities within the sinus are seldom symmetrical and are often subdivided by irregular minor septa. A sphenoid sinus that has presellar pneumatization on one side and sellar type on the other side is not uncommon. A single major septum separating the sinus into two large cavities has been reported in only 68% of specimens and may be off the midline by as far as 8 mm.[11] The most common type of sphenoid sinus has multiple small cavities in the large paired sinuses. The smaller cavities are separated by septa oriented in all directions. These intersinus sinus septa or the accessory septa may terminate onto the carotid canal in 40% and onto the optic nerves in 4% of individuals.[10,13]

The lateral wall of the sphenoid sinus is related to the cavernous sinus that extends from the orbital apex to the posterior clinoid process. The cavernous sinus contains delicate venous channels; the cavernous part of the internal carotid artery; the third, fourth, and sixth cranial nerves; and fibrofatty tissue. The internal carotid artery is the most medial structure within the cavernous sinus and forms a discernible prominence on the posterolateral aspect of the lateral wall of the sphenoid sinus. This prominence is well identified when the sphenoid sinus is well pneumatized. The carotid prominence can be divided into three parts: the retrosellar, infrasellar, and presellar segments. The first part, the retrosellar segment, is located in the posterolateral part of the sinus. This segment of the prominence is present only in well-pneumatized sellar-type sinuses in which the air cavity extends laterally in the area below the dorsum. The second part, the infrasellar segment, is located below the sellar floor. The third part, the presellar segment, is located anterolateral to the anterior sellar wall. Of the 50 specimens examined, Rhoton[13] reported 98% had presellar, 80% had infrasellar, and 78% had retrosellar prominences. Any part of the prominence may be present and the others absent. If all three parts are present and connected, they form a serpiginous bulge marking the full course of the carotid artery.

The bone separating the artery and the sphenoid sinus is thinner over the anterior than the posterior parts of the carotid prominence and is thinnest over the part of the artery just below the tuberculum sellae. A layer of bone less than 0.5 mm thick separates the artery and sinus in nearly 90% of sinuses, and areas of absence of bone between the artery and the sinus may be present in nearly 10%. The proximity of the carotid prominences to the midline is an important consideration in pituitary surgery. The shortest distance between both carotid bulges into the sphenoid sinus is usually located at the level of the tuberculum sellae in 72%, at the level of the floor of the sella in 20%, and at the clivus in 8%.[10] On the anterosuperior aspect of the lateral wall of the sphenoid sinus is another bulge formed by the optic nerve as it traverses the optic canal from the optic chiasma to the orbital apex. There are areas where no bone separates the optic sheath and sinus mucosa. In nearly 80% of the optic nerves, less than 0.5 mm of bone separates the optic nerve and sheath from the sinus mucosa. In more than half the cases, both the optic nerve and the cavernous carotid artery are separated from the sphenoid sinus mucosa by bone 0.5 mm or less in thickness. The incidence of dehiscence of these structures has been noted to be 4% and 8%, respectively.[10]

The absence of such bony protection within the walls of the sinus may explain some of the cases of cranial nerve deficits and carotid artery injury after transsphenoidal operations.[14] The prominence of the internal carotid artery is separated from the bulge of the optic nerve by a pneumatized diverticulum on the lateral wall of the sphenoid sinus called the opticocarotid recess. The extent of pneumatization may vary and in some cases extend through the optic strut into the anterior clinoid process. In a well-pneumatized sphenoid sinus, the pterygoid canal and a segment of the maxillary division of the trigeminal nerve may be identified in the lateral recess of the sphenoid sinus. The trigeminal ganglion and the first and third trigeminal divisions are separated from the lateral wall of the sphenoid sinus by the carotid artery.

The roof of the sphenoid, the planum sphenoidale anteriorly, is in continuum with the roof of the ethmoid sinus. At the junction of the planum sphenoidale and the posterior wall of the sphenoid, the sphenoid bone is thickened to form the tuberculum sella. Inferior to the tuberculum sella, on the posterior wall, is the sella floor, which forms a midline bulge. The thickness of the anterior sellar wall ranges from 0.1 to 0.7 mm (mean, 0.4 mm) as compared with 0.3 to 1.5 mm (mean, 0.7 mm) for the presellar type.[11,15] Often the dura may be visible through this thin bone, imparting a bluish hue to the sellar floor that aids in its recognition. Removal of the sellar floor provides access to the sella turcica.

The main portion of the pituitary gland lies in the sella turcica and is connected to the brain by the infundibulum. The diaphragma sella forms the roof of the sella turcica. It covers the pituitary gland except for a small central opening in the center, which transmits the pituitary stalk. The diaphragma is more rectangular than circular, tends to be convex or concave rather than flat, and is thinner around the infundibulum and somewhat thicker at the periphery. It is frequently a thin, tenuous structure that would not be an adequate barrier for protecting suprasellar structures during transsphenoidal surgery.[11] The opening in the center of the diaphragm is large when compared with the size of the pituitary stalk. In front of the infundibulum, the upper aspect of the gland is related directly to the arachnoid and pia mater. An outpouching of arachnoid may protrude through the central opening in the diaphragma into the sella in about half the patients and may be inadvertently opened by probing instruments during tumor removal, causing cerebrospinal fluid leakage.[14] A deficiency of the diaphragma sella is assumed to be a precondition to formation of an empty sella.

Venous sinuses that interconnect the paired cavernous sinuses may be found in the margins of the diaphragma and around the pituitary gland. The intercavernous connections within the sella are named on the basis of their relationship to the pituitary gland; the anterior intercavernous sinuses pass anterior to the hypophysis, and the posterior intercavernous sinus pass behind the gland. These intercavernous connections may occur at any site along the anterior, inferior, or posterior surface of the gland, or all connections between the two sides may be absent. The anterior intercavernous sinus may cover the whole anterior wall of the sella. The anterior sinus is usually larger than the posterior sinus, but either or both may be absent. If the anterior and posterior connections coexist, the whole structure constitutes the "circular sinus."[11,13] Inadvertent entry into the anterior intercavernous connection that extends downward in front of the gland during transsphenoidal operation may produce brisk bleeding. However, this usually stops with temporary compression of the channel with hemostatic foam or with light coagulation, which serves to glue the walls of the channel together.

■ Working as a Multidisciplinary Team

Pituitary surgery lies within the realm of the neurosurgeon. For an otolaryngologist wishing to partake in pituitary surgery, it is extremely important to work closely with neurosurgeons. In the current era, the accumulated experience of endoscopic trained otolaryngologists may be used by neurosurgeons in providing endonasal access to the sphenoid sinus and the floor of the sella. The otolaryngologist's prime role during surgery is to provide a relatively bloodless unimpeded access to the sphenoid sinus through a wide midline sphenoidotomy and assist the neurosurgeon in tumor removal. Although it is possible for a single surgeon to perform this surgery, a team approach is preferred. Once the initial approach is complete, both the neurosurgeon and otolaryngologist can work together. In some situations it is important for the two surgeons to work together, the otolaryngologist providing manual manipulation of the endoscope to optimize visualization, particularly when angled scopes are used and the field of the view is constantly changing.

■ Working as Part of a Pituitary Service

Management of pituitary tumors requires a dedicated multidisciplinary treatment team. Inappropriate pituitary hormone secretion and visual field deficits are the most characteristic presenting features of pituitary adenomas. Therefore, our referral base comes mainly from departments of endocrinology and ophthalmology. Specialists from these departments are actively involved in perioperative care of patients with pituitary tumors. In addition, the neuroradiologist, neuroanesthesiologist, interventional radiologist, neuropathologist, and radiation oncologist form important members of the team. In our institution, we have formed a pituitary service that consists of dedicated specialists involved in the care of patients with pituitary tumors. In addition to the neurosurgeon, otolaryngologist, endocrinologists, ophthalmologist, radiologist, radiation oncologist, and interventional radiologist, the board also includes representatives from the service quality department. Pituitary board meetings are held on a 3-month or ad hoc basis. Complex cases, postoperative results, and complications are audited during these meetings.

■ Indications for Surgery

Surgery for pituitary tumors has proven to be effective therapy for both endocrine active and nonfunctioning pituitary adenomas. Indications for surgery include all nonsecreting and most secreting pituitary tumors except for prolactinomas, which are usually well controlled by medical therapy with a dopamine antagonist.[16] Indications for surgery also include failure of or resistance to medical treatment or intolerable side effects of medical therapy and recurrences, in combination or in association with the other therapeutic options, medical or radiotherapeutic.

Nonsecretory tumors may vary in size, expanding the sella and extending along the paths of least resistance, laterally into the cavernous sinuses, superiorly into the suprasellar cistern, and anteriorly into the sphenoid sinus. Some nonsecretory tumors may have very large suprasellar extension. These tumors are best managed surgically with a combined endonasal and transcranial approach either in the same setting or as staged operations. Residual tumor following maximal endonasal surgical debulking may be dealt with by a repeat endoscopic procedure or craniotomy or adjuvant stereotactic radiation therapy, depending on the evaluation of the patient. Most secretory tumors, presenting with features of acromegaly and Cushing's disease, are an indication for surgery. For prolactin-secreting tumors, surgery is considered for those tumors that do not respond to medical therapy or for patients who are unable to tolerate medical treatment or who have cystic tumors. Pituitary apoplexy may require emergent surgery, as these patients usually present with sudden and rapid deterioration of vision. For a surgeon embarking on pituitary surgery, it is recommended to start with small and soft tumors and after attaining adequate experience to advance to larger tumors with significant suprasellar extension or cavernous sinus invasion.

Operative Setup for Endoscopic Pituitary Surgery

The digital endoscopic video camera system (Karl Storz, Tuttlingen, Germany) is placed at the cephalic end of the table to enable both surgeons to view surgery on the video monitor. The neuroanesthesiologist is at the caudal end of the table. The scrub nurse and the instrument trolley are at the left cephalic end. Imaging studies are displayed for intraoperative reference. The otolaryngologist stands on the right side of the operating table and the neurosurgeon on the left side. The digital video camera is attached to the eyepiece of the telescope, and the entire procedure is monitored on a 19-inch LCD screen monitor. Video documentation of the surgical procedure is routinely done on a digital video recorder. A powered sinus dissection device is used for the sphenoidotomy. We use the microdebrider developed by Medtronic (Jacksonville, FL). A 4-mm bit with a serrated outer shaft is used for mucosal dissection.

Surgical Technique

Patient Positioning and Preparation

The nasal cavity is decongested by placing two neuropatties soaked in 4% cocaine in each side approximately 20 minutes prior to induction. The patient is placed under general anesthesia and administered antibiotics, glucocorticoids, and antihistamines. We routinely use cephazolin (2 g, intravenous), dexamethasone (10 mg, intravenous), and diphenylhydramine (50 mg, intravenous). Oral endotracheal intubation is used, and a pharyngeal pack is placed in the pharynx. A Foley urinary catheter is routinely inserted to monitor urinary output intraoperatively and postoperatively. The patient's head is placed on a horseshoe slightly extended, and turned slightly to the right. The head is elevated by approximately 30 degrees above the heart to facilitate venous drainage. Antiseptic solution (such as Povidine) is applied to the nose and mouth, and the area draped with sterile towels and a Steri-Drape. The lower abdomen is prepared and draped to obtain adipose tissue if necessary.

Nasal Preparation

The neuropatties that had been placed in the nasal cavity earlier are removed and discarded. The nasal cavity is once again decongested with topical application of cocaine. Sterile neuropatties soaked in 4% cocaine are endoscopically placed in the sphenoethmoid recess bilaterally. Allowing approximately 10 minutes for decongestion, the neuropatties are removed and the sphenoethmoid recess is infiltrated bilaterally, with 1% lidocaine with 1:80,000 epinephrine. A 21-gauge spinal needle is used for infiltration of the anterior wall of the sphenoid, sphenopalatine foramen, and the posterior part of the nasal septum.

Nasal Endoscopy and Identification of Sphenoid Ostia

After the nose has been adequately decongested, an endoscopic examination is performed using a 0- or 30-degree endoscope (Karl Storz). The sphenoid ostia are identified bilaterally. The ostium lies just above the sphenoethmoid recess, approximately 1.5 cm above the choana. The shape and size of the sphenoid ostia may vary but its location is almost constant. In some circumstances, the ostium is covered by a supreme turbinate, which can be gently retracted laterally or resected if necessary. Rarely, in the situation where the sphenoid ostium cannot be identified, entry into the sphenoid sinus can be gained using a blunt instrument or suction tip to exert controlled pressure to the anterior wall at the point of least resistance.

Midline Sphenoidotomy

Surgery is started on the side on which the sphenoid ostium is better visualized. Most of the time, we start on the right side. The microdebrider with a 4-mm bit with a serrated outer shaft is used to debride the mucosa in the sphenoethmoid recess around the sphenoid ostium, taking care not to traumatize the mucosa on the superior turbinates. The serrated blade of the microdebrider is directed medially and the outer sheath laterally, protecting the mucosa of the superior turbinate. The sphenoid ostium is widened inferiorly and medially down to the floor of the sphenoid sinus. Care is taken to avoid the septal branch of the sphenopalatine artery by not going too inferolaterally. Brisk bleeding may result if the septal branch of the sphenopalatine artery is encountered. This may be controlled by cauterizing the vessel with bipolar diathermy. In the rare situation where bleeding cannot be controlled, it may be necessary to expose and ligate the sphenopalatine artery at the sphenopalatine foramen, which is located in the superior meatus just posterior to the middle turbinate. Most endoscopic sinus surgeons are familiar with the technique.

If the bone of the sphenoid rostrum is thick, a 2-mm up- or down-biting Kerrison rongeurs may be used to extend the sphenoidotomy. Sometimes it may be necessary to use a firm but controlled tap of a hammer against the osteotome or a drill to remove the sphenoid rostrum. Mucosa is debrided from the posterior part of the vomer and the sphenoid rostrum. The sphenoidotomy is extended to the contralateral side by dislocating the attachment of the vomer from the sphenoid rostrum. The sphenoid ostium on the contralateral side is identified and the sphenoidotomy extended as far as the contralateral superior turbinate by removing the sphenoid rostrum. The sphenoid rostrum is removed with a strong septal forceps. A wide sphenoidotomy that extends superiorly to the roof of the sphenoid, inferiorly to the floor of the sphenoid sinus, and laterally to the superior turbinate on either side is fashioned.

Removal of the Posterior Nasal Septum

About 1 cm of the posterior part of the vomer is removed with a reverse-cutting forceps to facilitate the introduction of instruments from both nostrils. This step permits a panoramic view of the sphenoid sinus and provides the ability to use both hands by two surgeons, enabling introduction of up to four separate instruments, two through each nostril. The access to the sphenoid sinus is complete. For a very wide access, necessary in some patients with large tumors requiring an extended approach, the entire posterior bony nasal septum may be removed to facilitate instrumentation.

From this point onward, the neurosurgeon and otolaryngologist work as a team. The otolaryngologist manually manipulates the endoscope and assists the neurosurgeon in removal of tumor.

Identifying the Sphenoid Sinus Landmarks

The sphenoid sinus is next examined with 0-, 30-, and 70-degree 4-mm endoscopes, and the important anatomical landmarks within are noted. Of particular importance are the structures on the lateral wall. The carotid prominence, optic prominence, and opticocarotid recess can be well identified when the sphenoid sinus is well pneumatized. On the lateral recess of a well-pneumatized sphenoid sinus, the second branch of the trigeminal nerve (V2) and the vidian canal may be identified superolaterally and inferomedially, respectively.

On the posterior wall the tuberculum sella, the anterior wall of the sella, and the clivus are identified. The location of the intersinus septa, if any, is noted. If these septa have to be removed, extreme caution is exercised, as they often terminate on the carotid canal or the optic canal. It is safer to use Tru-cutting instruments to remove these septa. Injudicious avulsion of the septa with non–Tru-cutting instruments may cause fracture of the thin bone overlying the cavernous sinus or the optic nerve, with resultant hematoma, intractable bleeding, or even blindness. Caution is also exercised in not stripping the sphenoid mucosa, as this may result in considerable bleeding. Once a panoramic view of the entire sphenoid sinus and the surgical landmarks is obtained, the access to the sella turcica is complete.

The major landmarks for proper identification of the sellar floor are the planum sphenoidale above, the clivus below, and the carotid prominences bilaterally.

Fenestration of the Sellar Floor

Once the sellar floor has been identified, mucosa over the sellar floor is cauterized with bipolar diathermy to expose underlying bone. Extent of removal of the sellar floor will vary depending on the size and location of pathology. The thickness of the sellar floor may be assessed by gentle palpation with an instrument such as a ball probe. By direct visualization and tactile feedback, the thinnest part of the sellar floor is identified and gently fractured at the point of least resistance. A plane is developed between the dura and sellar floor with a right-angle hook. A 1-mm Kerrison punch or a curette may be used to delicately remove the sellar floor, exposing the dura. Boundaries of removal of the sellar floor are the planum sphenoidale superiorly, the clivus inferiorly, and the carotid prominence laterally.

If the anterior wall of the sella is thick, a high-speed diamond drill under constant irrigation may be used to thin the sellar floor to a point that the dura may be visualized, imparting a bluish hue through the thinned sellar floor. Care must be taken when removing the sellar floor over the intercavernous sinus to avoid tearing this vein, which can bleed profusely. In the event this takes place, the intercavernous sinus may be cauterized with bipolar diathermy.

Incision of the Dura

Bipolar diathermy is used for hemostasis over the dura before incising it. Incision may be made using a sickle knife, a scalpel with a retractable blade, or a 45-degree-angle alligator scissor. The type of incision made over the dura may vary depending on the surgeon's preference, the type and size of the tumor, and the exposure necessary to remove the tumor. The incision may be vertical, horizontal, cruciate, or diagonal, or made in the shape of a flap reflected inferiorly. Care is taken not to extend the vertical segment of the incision too superiorly, so as not to encounter the subarachnoid space or the anterior intercavernous venous sinus. The lateral extent of the horizontal incision is limited by the cavernous sinus on both sides, and great caution must be exercised to avoid the carotid artery in the far lateral corners of the exposure. Incising the dura on the diagonal from corner to corner provides a wider opening than a cruciate incision. The upper leaf of dura may be further incised in the midline if exposure over the top of the gland is needed.

Removal of Tumor

The delivery of the tumor depends on the consistency of tumor contents. A cystic tumor decompresses rapidly. Large gelatinous or semisolid tumors are usually under pressure and decompress on incising the tumor capsule. Tumor tissue is taken for histologic examination. Once we have sufficient tumor tissue for a histologic examination, the tumor is removed using a combination of blunt ring curettes and pituitary forceps. The otolaryngologist and neurosurgeon work in tandem at this point. While one surgeon removes the tumor with a ring curette, the other provides continuous suction enabling rapid removal. A systematic approach in removing the tumor is useful. Start to remove the tumor from the floor, work on the lateral extent next, and finally remove the suprasellar component if any. Often the tumor decompresses rapidly in areas where it is cystic or gelatinous. The diaphragma may descend rapidly in this region, giving the impression that the tumor has been completely removed, whereas in actual fact pockets of tumor where the tumor was more semisolid or adherent to the diaphragma may be left behind. Therefore, it is useful to attempt to control the descent of the diaphragma by systematic removal of the tumor.

It is extremely important to be gentle while working on the lateral aspect of the sella, as the medial layer of the cavernous sinus can be extremely thin. Arterial bleeding has been reported to result from carotid artery injury but may also arise from a tear in the arterial branch of the carotid, such as the inferior hypophyseal artery or by avulsion of a small capsular artery from the carotid artery.[13] Blunt curettes should be used, as the arachnoid can be extremely thin and cerebrospinal fluid (CSF) leakage may result even with gentle manipulation. If the diaphragma descends unequally, there may be a pocket of tumor left behind. In this situation it is useful for one surgeon to gently retract the diaphragma away to enable visualization of and removal of the retained tumor by the other surgeon.

Endoscopic Inspection of the Sellar Cavity

Once the tumor has been removed, a 4-mm angled endoscope, 30-, 45-, or 70-degree, is used to view the sellar cavity and suprasellar cistern to ensure absence of residual tumor. Lateral visualization with angled endoscopes enables exploration of the medial wall of the cavernous sinus. The extent to which the neurovascular structures in the cavernous sinus are encased by the pathology must be carefully assessed. Although encasement is not a contraindication to this approach, surgeons must judge their ability to safely dissect the tumor off the carotid artery and should keep in mind the possibility of radiosurgery and fractionated radiation to control the growth of residual unresectable tumor. In some cases, what appears to be tumor encasement of a vessel on preoperative magnetic resonance imaging (MRI) scan turns out to represent a vessel coursing along the capsule of the tumor that can be separated by an excellent arachnoid plane.

Sellar Hemostasis

Once the tumor has been completely removed, minor oozing from the sella is controlled by packing the sella with neuropatties providing tamponade for approximately 5 minutes. Upon removal of the neuropatties, the sella is once again endoscopically examined and any localized oozing is controlled with placement of Surgicel (Johnson & Johnson, New Brunswick, NJ) over the area. In the situation, where oozing from sella persists despite above measures, it may be controlled by application of thrombin-infused gelatin matrix[17] (FloSeal; Baxter, Deerfield, IL).

Management of Cerebrospinal Fluid Leak

In the event a CSF leak is recognized intraoperatively, the defect is plugged with a pad of abdominal fat sandwiched between Surgicel squares and sealed with fibrin matrix (Tisseel; Baxter, Deerfield, IL). In our practice, for the standard transsphenoidal approach to pituitary lesions, a lumbar drain is not routinely placed for intraoperative leaks.

Nasal Hemostasis

Once the surgery is concluded, nasal hemostasis is ensured. Any minor mucosal oozing or bleeding from the septal branch of the sphenopalatine artery (SPA) is controlled with bipolar diathermy. If the bleeding from the septal branch of the SPA is persistent, it may be necessary to expose the SPA at the sphenopalatine foramen and ligate the vessel by applying arterial clips.

Nasal Packs

To facilitate postoperative mucosal healing, ensure the bone of the sphenoid rostrum is not exposed and is adequately covered in mucosa; 8-cm nasal Merocels (Medtronic Xomed Surgical Products, Jacksonville, FL) are placed in the nasal cavity on either side and hydrated with saline to expand. These are removed after 24 hours.

Modifications to the Technique

The technique described above is used for most lesions confined to the sella turcica. However, modifications to the approach may be necessary in certain situations where there is considerable extension of the sellar lesion through the diaphragma sella into the suprasellar cistern. Removal of the tuberculum sella and part of the planum sphenoidale is required in such cases to visualize and remove the tumor from the suprasellar cistern.

For wider access to the sphenoid sinus and wider exposure of the planum sphenoidale, the approach may be combined with bilateral ethmoidectomies and removal of the entire posterior bony nasal septum. The wide exposure of the sphenoid and the skull base provides excellent access to the planum sphenoidale and tuberculum sella. With this exposure the removal of the sellar floor can be extended

A–C

D–F

G–I

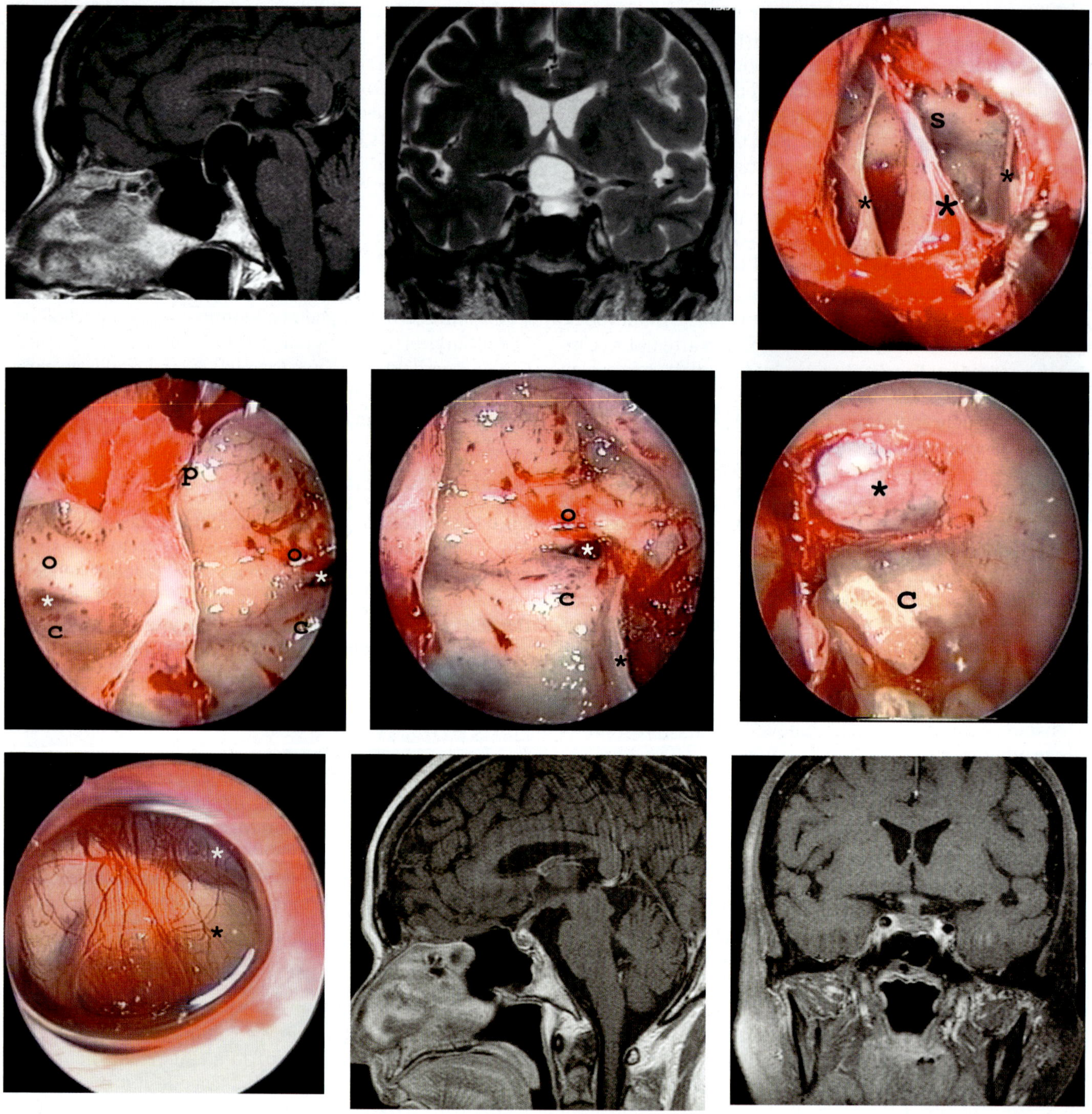

Fig. 17.1 Case 1. **(A)** T1-weighted gadolinium-enhanced magnetic resonance imaging (MRI) sequence showing a bilobed cystic mass occupying and enlarging the sella and extending to the suprasellar region through the diaphragm. **(B)** T2-weighted MRI sequence (coronal section). **(C)** Endoscopic view with 0-degree endoscope showing the midline sphenoidotomy providing access to the sphenoid sinus. *Large asterisk* indicates the intersinus septum terminating onto the anterior wall of the sella (s). *Small asterisks* indicate the accessory septa terminating laterally onto the carotid artery. **(D)** Sphenoid anatomy viewed with a 70-degree endoscope. The planum sphenoidale (p) forms the roof. Superiorly on the lateral wall are the optic nerves (o) and inferiorly the bulge of the carotid arteries (c). The recess between the two structures (*white asterisks*) is the opticocarotid recess. **(E)** Endoscopic view of the left lateral wall showing the optic nerve (o), carotid artery (c), and the opticocarotid recess (*white asterisk*). Note the left accessory septum (*black asterisk*) terminating onto the carotid artery. **(F)** The sellar floor has been removed, exposing the dura (*black asterisk*). The position of the clivus (c) is inferior to the sella. **(G)** Intraoperative endoscopic view (30-degree endoscope) of the diaphragm and the infundibulum following removal of the tumor. The *white asterisk* indicates the thin arachnoid membrane and the *black asterisk* the gyrus. **(H,I)** Two-month postoperative MRI scans showing good suprasellar decompression.

superiorly to remove the tuberculum sella and part of the planum sphenoidale. Incision of the dura provides excellent visualization of the suprasellar cistern, enabling more complete removal of sellar lesions that extend through the diaphragma sella into the suprasellar cistern. The approach may also be used for some purely suprasellar prechiasmal and postchiasmal lesions that rest above a normal-sized sella. This endoscopic extended transsphenoidal approach to the suprasellar cistern has been reported by several authors.[18–20]

Postoperative Care

Once the surgery is complete, the patient is extubated and brought to the recovery room, where the patient's vital signs are monitored. For the next 24 hours the patient is monitored in the neurosurgical intensive care unit, particularly for diabetes insipidus and for visual deterioration. A fasting morning cortisol level is obtained on the morning of the second postoperative day, and cortisol replacement is initiated only if the level is abnormally low. Nasal packing is removed on the first postoperative day. If no lumbar drain has been placed, patients ambulate on the second postoperative day and may be and discharged on the third postoperative day or as soon as they are ambulating and eating well. During the postoperative period, the patient is monitored for any CSF leak or symptoms and signs of meningitis or any hemorrhage. Antibiotic and analgesics are routinely prescribed. The patient is examined following the removal of the packs. Any blood clots in the nasal cavity are aspirated under endoscopic guidance.

The first office visit is scheduled after a week following the surgery. After application of topical 4% cocaine, blood clots are endoscopically removed from the nasal cavity and sphenoid sinus. The sella is carefully examined for any bleeding or CSF leakage. The patient is seen on a weekly basis by the otolaryngologist for the first 3 weeks and then every 3 weeks for the next two appointments. Healing usually takes approximately 3 to 6 weeks. Further appointments are scheduled as necessary. Postoperative follow-up is also provided by the endocrinologist, ophthalmologist, and neurosurgeon.

Demonstration Cases

Four cases of different sellar pathology are presented to demonstrate the surgical technique and results.

Case 1

A 60-year-old hypertensive woman presented with bitemporal hemianopia. The patient's MRI scans show a bilobed cystic mass occupying and enlarging the sella and extending to the suprasellar region through the diaphragma (**Fig. 17.1A,B**). Intraoperative pictures of the endonasal transsphenoidal approach are shown. A midline sphenoidotomy has been achieved by extending bilateral sphenoidotomies to the midline and removing part of the posterior nasal septum (**Fig. 17.1C**). Note the midline intersinus septum inserting onto the sellar floor and bilateral accessory intersinus septi.

Figure 17.1D provides a panoramic view of the sphenoid sinus with a 70-degree endoscope. Note the intersinus septum inserting on the tuberculum sella and planum sphenoidale. The optic nerves and the carotid artery prominences are visualized on the lateral wall. In **Fig. 17.1E** note the accessory intersinus septum inserting on the optic nerve and the carotid artery. The sellar floor has been removed (**Fig. 17.1F**). **Figure 17.1G** shows the intraoperative view of the diaphragma and the infundibulum. The contents of the mass were mucoid secretion, consistent with a Rathke's cyst. An intraoperative CSF leakage resulted from the thin arachnoid membrane. This was repaired with adipose tissue and fibrin glue. The MRI scans status 2 months postsurgery show that the chiasm has been decompressed (**Fig. 17.1H,I**).

Case 2

A 47-year-old woman presented with severe headaches. An MRI scan (**Fig. 17.2A**) shows a 1.5- × 1.2-cm sellar lesion with a suprasellar convex component elevating and mildly compressing the anterior aspect of optic chiasm. Her preoperative endocrine evaluation was normal. Intraoperatively soft whitish adenoma was removed. The diaphragma has descended following removal of the tumor (**Fig. 17.2B**). Histology confirmed a pituitary adenoma. Immunohistochemistry was negative for secretory tumors. Postoperative coronal and sagittal MRI scans showed complete removal of the tumor with some postsurgical changes in the sella (**Fig. 17.2C,D**).

Case 3

A 49-year-old woman presented with headaches and diplopia of 2 weeks' duration. A preliminary computed tomography (CT) of the brain showed a sellar lesion. Subsequent MRI studies show a uniformly enhancing mass within the sella extending into the suprasellar cistern, compressing and elevating the optic chiasms (**Fig. 17.3A–C**).

Intraoperative pictures show the left optic nerve, carotid artery, and the opticocarotid recess (**Fig. 17.3D**). A cruciate incision was made on the dura (**Fig. 17.3E**), and **Fig. 17.3F** depicts the intrasellar view of the descended diaphragma. Intraoperatively heavily blood-stained fluid with infracted pituitary tissue was removed from the sella. Findings were consistent with that of pituitary apoplexy. Histopathology confirmed a hemorrhagic infracted pituitary adenoma. MRI

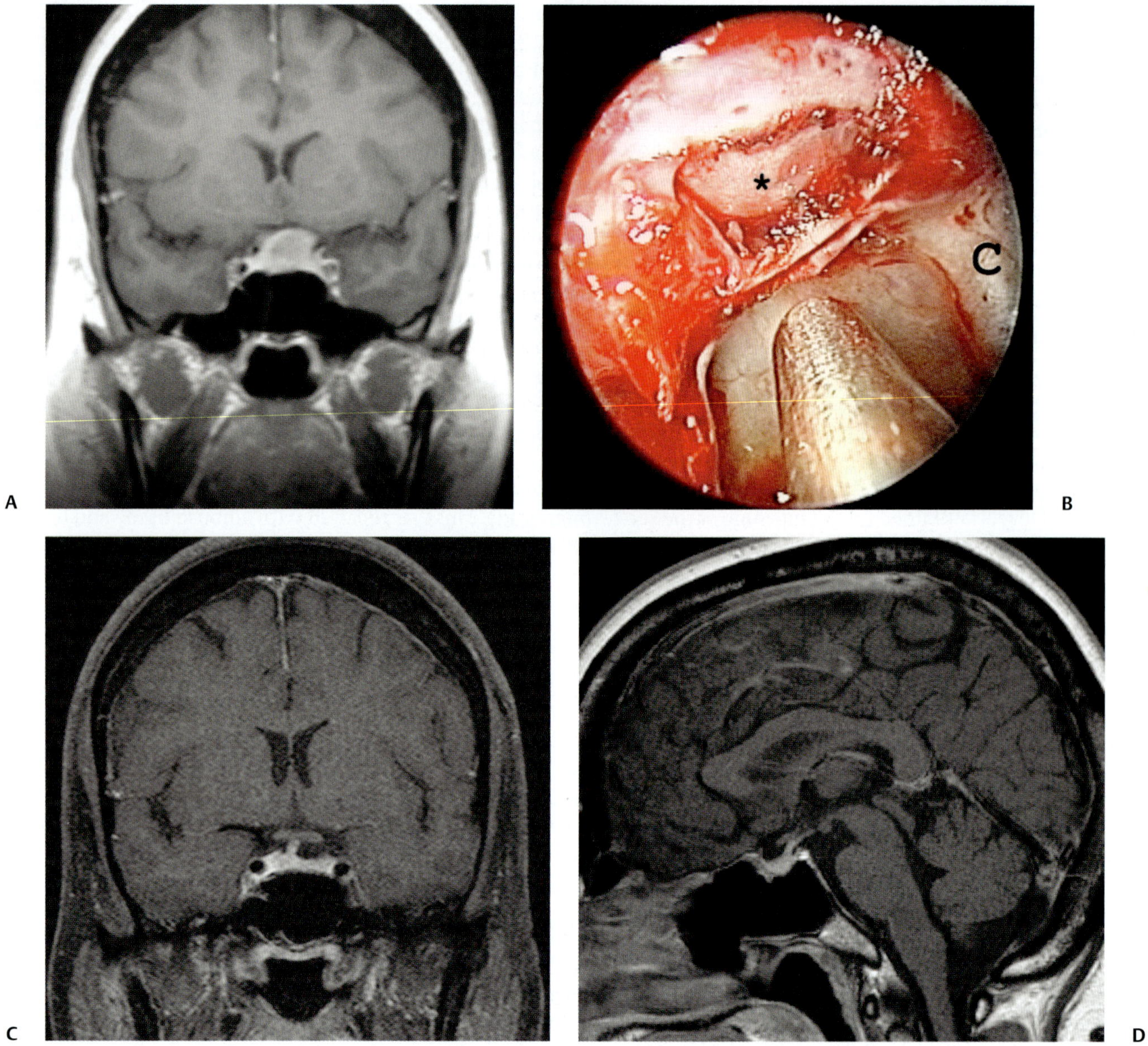

Fig. 17.2 Case 2. **(A)** T1-weighted gadolinium-enhanced MRI scan. **(B)** Intraoperative endoscopic view of the exposed dura (*black asterisk*) following removal of the sellar floor. Note the position of the paraclival part of the left internal carotid artery (C). **(C,D)** Three-month postoperative MRI scans.

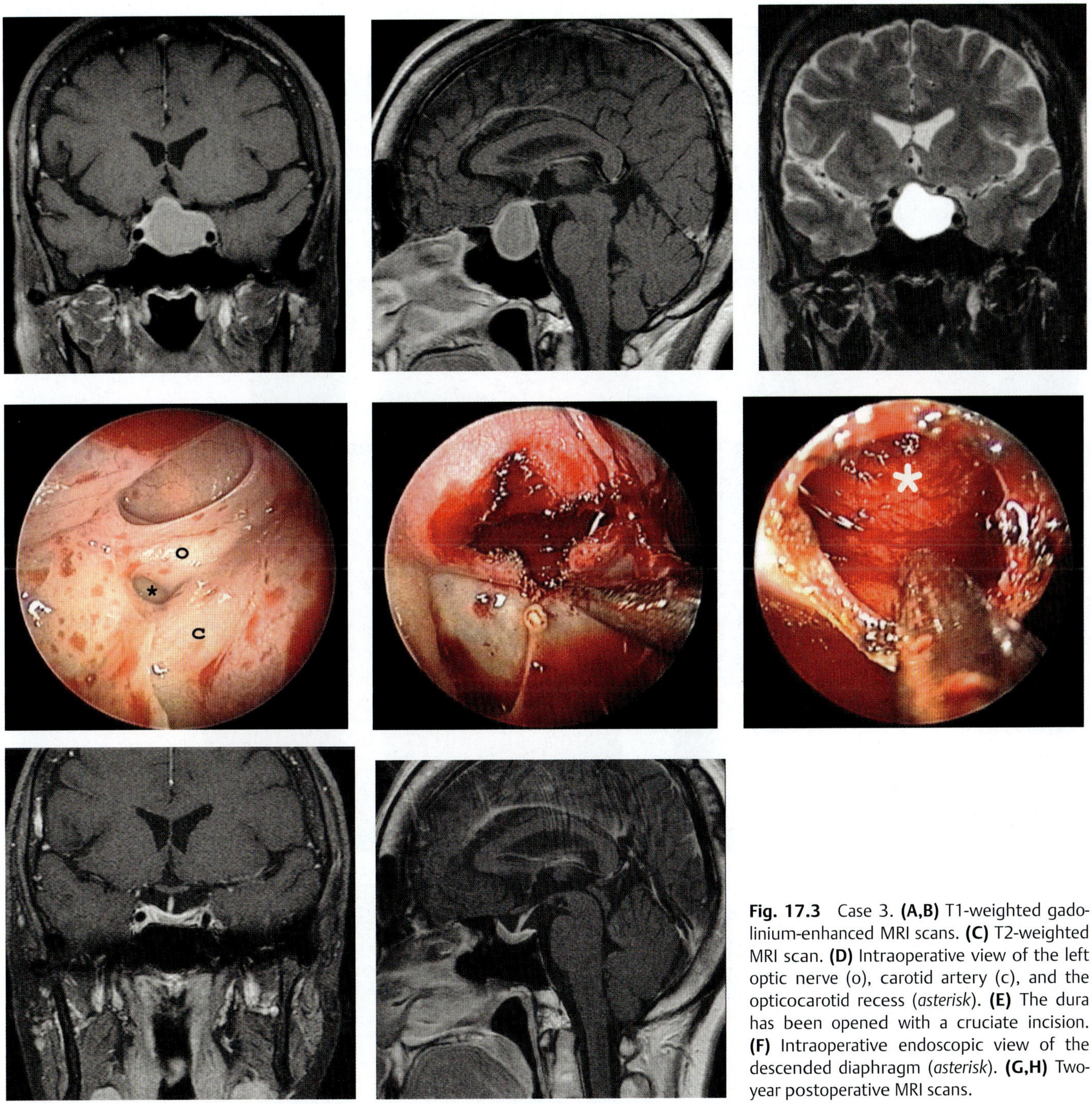

Fig. 17.3 Case 3. **(A,B)** T1-weighted gadolinium-enhanced MRI scans. **(C)** T2-weighted MRI scan. **(D)** Intraoperative view of the left optic nerve (o), carotid artery (c), and the opticocarotid recess (*asterisk*). **(E)** The dura has been opened with a cruciate incision. **(F)** Intraoperative endoscopic view of the descended diaphragm (*asterisk*). **(G,H)** Two-year postoperative MRI scans.

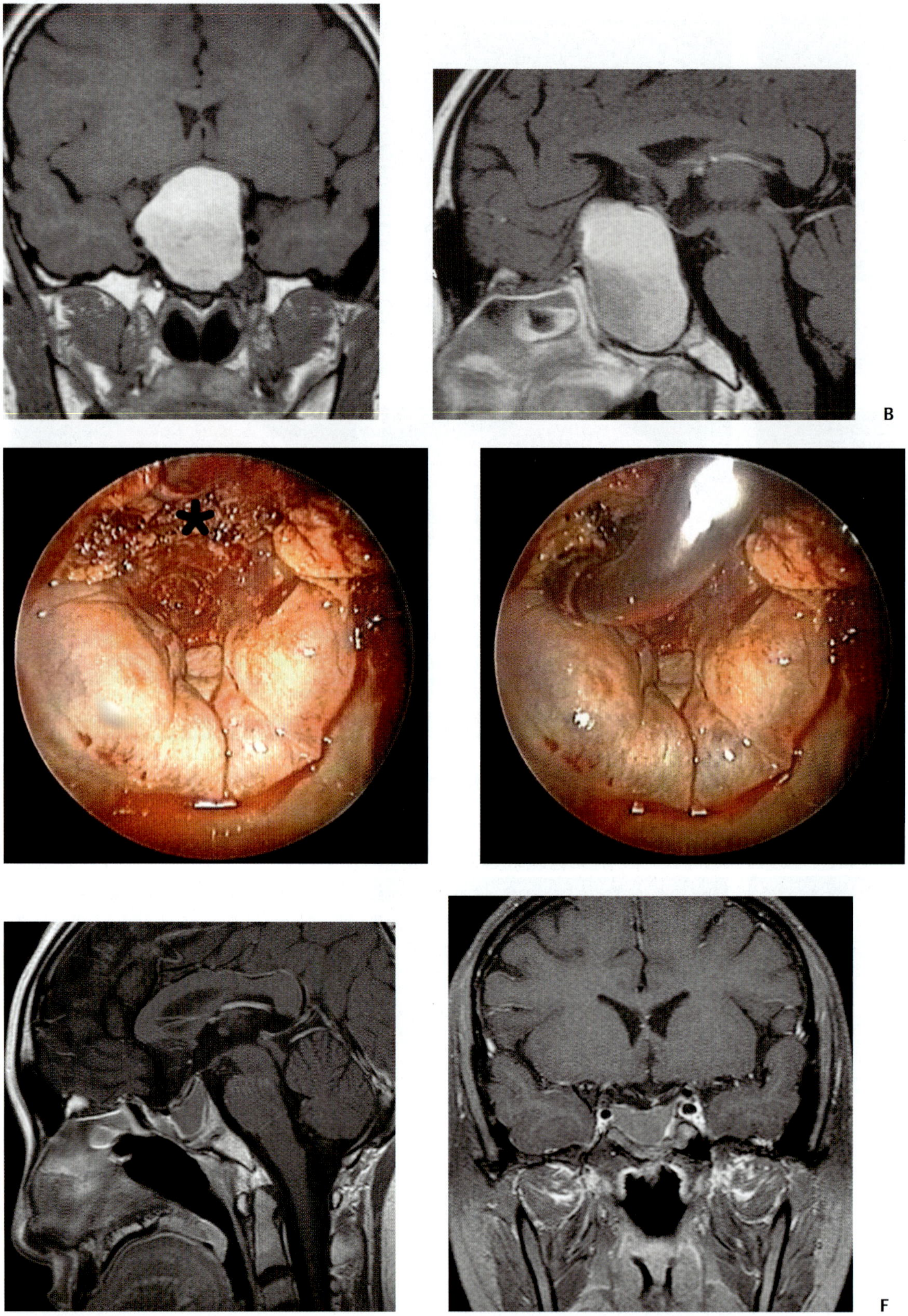

A B C D E F

Fig. 17.4 Case 4. **(A,B)** T1-weighted gadolinium-enhanced MRI scans. **(C)** A 70-degree endoscopic view of the undescended diaphragm with some residual tumor (*asterisk*). **(D)** The residual tumor is being removed aided by a 70-degree endoscope and long 3-mm curved olive cannula suction. **(E,F)** Two-year postoperative MRI scans showing some postoperative changes.

scans 2 years postsurgery show postsurgical changes. Normal enhancing pituitary tissue is still seen on the right side of the fossa. The pituitary stalk also shows normal enhancement (**Fig. 17.3G,H**).

Case 4

A 24-year-old woman presented with panhypopituitarism. An MRI study showed a mildly enhancing large 4.8- × 3.6- × 2.6-cm mass with mixed cystic and solid components occupying the pituitary fossa (**Fig. 17.4A,B**). The lesion extended inferiorly into the sphenoid sinus and superiorly into the suprasellar cistern displacing the optic chiasm.

Intraoperatively, the tumor was noted to be mainly soft, yellowish, and solid in some areas. **Figure 17.4C** shows the view of the diaphragma with a 70-degree endoscope after the tumors had been removed. Some remnant tumor adherent to the anterior aspect of the diaphragma was visualized. The remnant tumor was removed with a long curved olive-shaped canula aided with a 70-degree endoscope (**Fig. 17.4D**). Histopathology of the tumor was reported as a craniopharyngioma. Postoperative changes in the sella were seen 2 years later (**Fig. 17.4E,F**). The large tumor has been removed and is replaced with a small cystic lesion with postoperative changes. This is being monitored with serial MRI scan.

Managing Complications

It is imperative that the operating surgeon be familiar with the complications that can take place and be prepared to handle these complications.

The most common intraoperative complication is CSF leakage. The usual cause of CSF rhinorrhea is trauma to the diaphragma resulting from instruments such as the curette, forceps, or suction. The diaphragma may often be very thin and susceptible to trauma. Extreme caution must be exercised when removing tumor from this delicate structure. It is also important to remember that in front of the infundibulum, the upper aspect of the gland is related directly to arachnoid and pia, and the subarachnoid space here extends below the diaphragm and may be inadvertently breached while removing tumor. When a CSF leak is identified intraoperatively, the intrasellar defect should be identified. Precaution should be taken not to make it worse or larger, and surgery should be completed by working around it. At the conclusion of the surgery the defect should be repaired with intrasellar placement of abdominal fat and fibrin matrix (Tisseel). In some cases the CSF leak may be due to a minor "weeping" defect from the arachnoid when the vertical component of the cruciate incision is extended superiorly. In these patients, the weeping defect is repaired with a small amount of adipose tissue placed on the defect and fixing it with fibrin matrix (Tisseel).

Intraoperative bleeding may result from inadequate nasal decongestion prior to surgery, trauma to the SPA, inadvertent stripping of sphenoid mucosa, cavernous sinus trauma, intercavernous sinus injury, or trauma to the cavernous part of the internal carotid artery.

Decongesting the nasal mucosa preoperatively and intraoperatively, the use of bipolar diathermy on the tumor capsule and the dura prior to incising it, and taking the precaution of not stripping the sphenoid mucosa are the key points in reducing intraoperative bleed. Tumor tissue tends to bleed. Quick removal of tumor ensures early hemostasis. If bleeding continues from the sellar cavity, endoscopic examination with a 30-degree telescope is particularly useful in identifying the bleeding point or residual tumor. The bleeding point can then be controlled with application of tamponade, bipolar diathermy, or a thin layer of Surgicel.

Cavernous sinus bleeding should be suspected when venous bleeding fills the surgical field; it can be repaired with Surgicel, fibrin matrix, or application of FloSeal.

Perhaps the most feared complication is trauma to the cavernous carotid artery. Bleeding from the carotid artery should be suspected if the surgeon is working laterally. Tamponade by promptly packing the nose and the sinus cavity is the initial measure to be taken. Meanwhile, the patient's condition is assessed. Replacement of blood loss should be expedient. At the same time arrangements are made for angiography and an occlusion test. If the packing holds and the patient passes the occlusion test, the internal carotid artery may be occluded with a balloon. However, if the patient fails the occlusion test, a bypass procedure is necessary prior to occluding the internal carotid artery. If the packing is unable to hold the bleeding, emergent measures such as occlusion of the internal carotid artery in the neck or a craniotomy may have to be undertaken.

Significant postoperative hemorrhage may be due to oozing from the nasal mucosa at the site of the sphenoidotomy or active bleeding from one of the branches of the sphenopalatine artery. Profuse bleeding that is difficult to control should alert one to the possibility of intracranial vascular trauma and warrant an angiogram.

Transient or permanent worsening of vision may occur as a result of intrasellar hematoma or direct damage to optic nerve. Intrasellar hematoma should be suspected when patients complain of deteriorating vision after surgery. Emergency CT scan of the brain and immediate surgical evacuation of the hematoma should be performed if intrasellar hematoma is suspected.

Conclusion

The endoscopic transsphenoidal approach is the most direct and least invasive method for reaching the sellar floor and is now widely accepted in most institutions around the world. However, it is emphasized that detailed knowledge of the surgical anatomy and endoscopic techniques is essential prior to undertaking this surgery. This surgery should always be performed with a neurosurgeon and only by surgeons with significant experience in both transsphenoidal and endoscopic surgery, preferably after considerable practice on cadaver specimens. With experience the technique may be extended to encompass lesions extending to the suprasellar cistern or located purely in the suprasellar cistern with an intact sella.

This surgery not only is a partnership between the neurosurgeons and the otolaryngologist but also should be partnership among all specialists involved in management of pituitary tumors.

References

1. Hardy J. Transsphenoidal hypophysectomy. J Neurosurg 1971;34: 582–594
2. Jankowski R, Auque J, Simon C, Marchal JC, Hepner H, Wayoff M. Endoscopic pituitary tumor surgery. Laryngoscope 1992;102:198–202
3. Jho HD, Carrau RL. Endoscopic endonasal transsphenoidal surgery: experience with 50 patients. J Neurosurg 1997;87:44–51
4. Nasseri SS, Kasperbauer JL, Strome SE, McCaffrey TV, Atkinson JL, Meyer FB. Endoscopic transnasal pituitary surgery: report on 180 cases. Am J Rhinol 2001;15:281–287
5. Cappabianca P, Alfieri A, de Divitiis E. Endoscopic endonasal transsphenoidal approach to the sella: towards functional endoscopic pituitary surgery (FEPS). Minim Invasive Neurosurg 1998;41:66–73
6. Sethi DS, Stanley RE, Pillay PK. Endoscopic anatomy of the sphenoid sinus and sella turcica. J Laryngol Otol 1995;109:951–955
7. Sethi DS, Pillay PK. Endoscopic surgery for pituitary tumors. Op Tech Oto-Head Neck Surg 1996;7:264–268
8. Sethi DS, Leong JL. Endoscopic pituitary surgery. Otolaryngol Clin North Am 2006;39:563–583, x
9. Sethi DS, Kumar K. Endoscopic pituitary surgery. Op Tech Otolaryngol Head Neck Surg 2007;18(1):57–64
10. Fujii K, Chambers SM, Rhoton AL Jr. Neurovascular relationships of the sphenoid sinus. A microsurgical study. J Neurosurg 1979;50: 31–39
11. Renn WH, Rhoton AL Jr. Microsurgical anatomy of the sellar region. J Neurosurg 1975;43:288–298
12. Jho HD, Ha HG. Endoscopic endonasal skull base surgery: part 1—the midline anterior fossa skull base. Minim Invasive Neurosurg 2004;47:1–8
13. Rhoton AL Jr. Anatomy of the pituitary gland and sellar region. In: Thapar K, Kovacs K, Scheithauer BW, Lloyd RV, eds. Diagnosis and Management of Pituitary Tumors. Totowa, NJ: Humana Press; 2000:13–40
14. Laws ER Jr, Kern EB. Complications of trans-sphenoidal surgery. Clin Neurosurg 1976;23:401–416
15. Rhoton AL Jr, Hardy DG, Chambers SM. Microsurgical anatomy and dissection of the sphenoid bone, cavernous sinus and sellar region. Surg Neurol 1979;12:63–104
16. Molitch ME. Medical treatment of prolactinomas. Endocrinol Metab Clin North Am 1999;28:143–169, vii
17. Ellegala DB, Maartens NF, Laws ER Jr. Use of FloSeal hemostatic sealant in transsphenoidal pituitary surgery: technical note. Neurosurgery 2002;51:513–515, discussion 515–516
18. Schwartz TH, Anand VK. The endoscopic endonasal transsphenoidal approach to the suprasellar cistern. Clin Neurosurg 2007;54: 226–235
19. de Divitiis E, Cavallo LM, Cappabianca P, Esposito F. Extended endoscopic endonasal transsphenoidal approach for the removal of suprasellar tumors: part 2. Neurosurgery 2007;60:46–58, discussion 58–59
20. Laufer I, Anand VK, Schwartz TH. Endoscopic, endonasal extended transsphenoidal, transplanum transtuberculum approach for resection of suprasellar lesions. J Neurosurg 2007;106:400–406

18 Virtual Endoscopy in Endoscopic Pituitary Surgery

Stefan Wolfsberger and André Neubauer

Because of its outstanding imaging quality, endoscopy is gaining increasing acceptance for the transsphenoidal approach to sellar lesions. Due to a steep learning curve, however, special training and preoperative planning are mandatory for the safe application of this technique.

Virtual endoscopy is a concept allowing the user to navigate through computationally reconstructed patient anatomy using a virtual camera, mimicking a real endoscopic approach. It fuses radiologic imaging with advanced three-dimensional (3D) computer graphic techniques to produce views that closely reflect those obtained during physical endoscopy.

Virtual endoscopy can visualize the nasal anatomy and its variations, the location of the sphenoid ostium, the sphenoid sinus septations, and the chambers for improved intraoperative orientation. The pituitary gland, tumor, and adjacent vascular structures can be concurrently demonstrated in relation to the sphenoid sinus landmarks for planning a tailored opening of the sellar floor and tumor removal.

This chapter describes the simulator for transsphenoidal endoscopic pituitary surgery (STEPS), which is based on virtual endoscopy. The system is designed as a tool for training and planning of the endonasal transsphenoidal approach. It has been our experience that virtual endoscopy may increase the safety of the procedure by preoperative visualization of anatomical variations in the individual patient.

At present, the microscopic transsphenoidal approach is considered worldwide the standard neurosurgical technique for the removal of most sellar tumors. Although it has been well established for decades, incomplete tumor resection is not uncommon even for experienced pituitary surgeons.[1] Invasive growth with extension into perisellar regions beyond the microscopic field of view may be possible causes of tumor tissue being left behind during surgery.

The use of endoscopes[1] ensures excellent illumination due to light emission close to the region of interest[2]; offers a high-resolution, close-up, and wide-angle view of the anatomy due to the proximity of the lens to the region of interest[3]; offers the possibility to look "around the corner" by the application of endoscopes at different angles, enabling direct visualization of the removal of tumor remnants in the parasellar compartments[4]; and offers extended maneuverability of the surgical instruments, as movements are not hindered by a rigid nasal speculum.[2] Therefore, the endoscopic technique may increase the extent of tumor removal and the safety of the procedure compared with the standard microscopic transsphenoidal approach.

Although Guiot et al[3] made the first attempts to use an endoscope for surgery of sellar pathologies as early as 1963, it was not until recently that a group of neurosurgeons reconsidered and popularized the technique of the purely endoscopic transsphenoidal pituitary approach.[4,5] This technique, however, has certain disadvantages, which contribute to its steep learning curve.[6] Neurosurgeons are usually well accustomed to the operating microscope but often are unfamiliar with the handling of an endoscope. Furthermore, the endoscope provides a different view of the surgical anatomy due to its two-dimensional image, peripheral barrel distortion, high magnification, and unusual viewing angles.

To overcome these possible risk factors associated with the new technique, teaching and training of the endoscopic transsphenoidal approach are essential for the novice. Endoscopic training, including handling and anatomical viewing skills, is currently provided in workshops at different centers throughout the world. However, cadaver training is costly and often not easily accessible.

Therefore, beginning in 2004, we developed the STEPS prototype based on virtual endoscopy.[7] For training purposes, it has since been successfully applied at our workshop facility. In the clinical setting the simulator has proved to be beneficial to the experienced endoscopic surgeon in preoperative planning of surgical cases.[8] STEPS has continually been improved by ongoing discussion among trainees, surgeons, and engineers.[9,10] This chapter describes our experience with the application of STEPS, its benefits and drawbacks, as well as techniques of visualization and current developments.

■ Virtual Endoscopy

Virtual endoscopy enables the user to navigate through computationally reconstructed patient anatomy using a virtual camera, mimicking a real endoscopic approach. It fuses radiologic imaging with advanced 3D computer graphic techniques to produce views that closely reflect those obtained during physical endoscopy. Depending on the application, virtual endoscopy can be used either instead of physical endoscopy or as an addition.

David Vining, who was the first to assess computer-generated images of the interior of the colon,[11] is often referred to as the inventor of virtual endoscopy. Soon after, various areas of application were presented, including examination of the carotid arteries[12] and virtual endoscopy in stereotactic neurosurgery.[13] On the basis of this early work, virtual endoscopy became an active area of research, and every year a substantial number of researchers, from both the medical and the technical community, present and assess new techniques and applications. Supported by this wide field of collected knowledge, virtual endoscopy is now making its way from preclinical research into clinical practice.

Virtual colonoscopy was first introduced by Vining[11] as a reliable, cost-effective, and less invasive diagnostic alternative to physical colonoscopy. At present, virtual endoscopy is most commonly used in the clinical setting for the detection of colonic polyps. It has proven be an effective technique for finding colonic polyps and has the potential to limit the application of physical colonoscopy specifically to cases in which either a suspicious polyp was found or that were inconclusive in virtual colonoscopy. Another popular area of application is virtual bronchoscopy. It can locate lesions, detect carcinoma, and reliably evaluate airway stenoses.[14] Virtual endoscopy has been applied in blood vessels as virtual angioscopy,[15,16] for example, in the assessment of abdominal or cerebral aneurysms, carotid stenoses, and atherosclerotic plaques, as well as in the coronary blood vessels, to assess abnormalities of myocardial dynamics.[17] Furthermore, virtual endoscopy is currently applied in the small intestines, the stomach, the urinary tract, and the cerebral ventricles.

Some work has been presented on virtual endoscopy in the nose and paranasal sinuses.

Morra et al[18] claim that virtual endoscopy provides clear visualization of the anatomical structures of the nasal cavity and sinuses, producing images that are similar to those of conventional endoscopy. Moreover, virtual endoscopy visualizes those paranasal sinuses that are not accessible in conventional endoscopy. The authors state that the main limitations of virtual endoscopy are the arbitrary choice of reconstruction parameters and the scalarization resulting in homogenization of different tissue densities.

Bisdas et al[19] claim that in comparison to looking at plain radiographs, virtual endoscopy enables physicians to better understand the complex and varied intracranial structures. They tested virtual endoscopy in 50 patients with the diagnosis of an acute or chronic nasal obstructive disease. The 3D images provided a clear demonstration of the various pathologies within their anatomical contexts. However, this group also experienced difficulties arising from inflexible reconstruction parameters. For example, they point out that their virtual endoscopy software proved inadequate when the nasal cavities were totally filled with soft tissue, such as in extensive acute inflammation or a heavily obstructive disease.

Rogalla[20] reported a prospective study in which two radiologists assessed coronal reconstructions and virtual endoscopy with respect to the ease of finding pathologies. In 30 patients, the surgeons were asked to rank the degree of assistance of the preoperative virtual endoscopy. A high degree of similarity between virtual endoscopy and intraoperative aspect was reported.

Due to inflexible surface reconstruction, however, certain anatomical structures (e.g., upper nasal conchae) were not displayed, and the maxillary sinuses could not be approached. Still, virtual endoscopy was found applicable as a preoperative assistance for the surgeon.

Virtual endoscopy for preoperative planning of transsphenoidal pituitary surgery was first presented by Talala et al.[21] In addition to standard virtual endoscopy software, nonperspective visualization of the sphenoid anatomy, in which the pre-segmented carotid arteries were displayed, was generated. The authors state that even this nonperspective viewing, which significantly deviates from what is seen during real endoscopic interventions, increases the safety of the procedure.

In recent years, technical advances have led to considerable improvements of processing capabilities of personal computers. This has resulted in enhanced potential for virtual endoscopy software. Motivated by these advancements, we have developed a software package that is not impaired by the aforementioned shortcomings of prior efforts. The STEPS system is described in the following section.

The STEPS System

The STEPS virtual endoscopy system is used for preoperative planning and training of endoscopic pituitary surgery. It is integrated in the commercially available Impax EE PACS system (Agfa-Gevaert Group, Vienna, Austria).

Image Data

Prior to the surgical intervention, standard radiologic images that are used for routine preoperative workup and intraoperative neuronavigation are generated and can be used for virtual endoscopy. Thus, the application of STEPS does not cause additional patient discomfort, radiation hazard, or financial expense.

Due to its high resolution and superior air/mucosa/bone delineation, as compared with magnetic resonance imaging (MRI), a computed tomography (CT) scan is used for reconstruction of the virtual cavities and bony anatomy of the nose and skull base. The CT images used comply with the following protocol: axial plane, 0-zero gantry tilt, 512 × 512 matrix, starting just inferior to the nares and advancing at 1-mm slice thickness.

An MRI is performed for the visualization of anatomical objects of interest. The T1-weighted contrast-enhanced images are used for delineation of the sellar pathology, the pituitary gland, the optochiasmatic structures, and adjacent arachnoid spaces. The proposed sequence at 1.5 tesla is a T1-weighted turbo field echo scan with 20-millisecond repetition time and 4.6-millisecond echo time, one excitation, 25-degree flip angle, 256 × 256 matrix, 2-mm slice thickness. A magnetic resonance angiography (MRA) scan is performed for optimal delineation of the parasellar internal carotid arteries: contrast-enhanced 3D time-of-flight MRA, 512 × 512 matrix, 1.4-mm slice thickness on a 1.5-tesla magnetic resonance (MR) scanner.

For preprocessing of image data, CT and MR scans are stored on the hard disk of the virtual endoscopy workstation.

Software and Workflow (Figs. 18.1 and 18.2)

In addition to the standard virtual endoscopy functionality, the STEPS software package offers the following features:

1. *Object processing:* Anatomical objects of interest can be segmented by the user and then displayed behind the semitransparent walls of the virtual endoscopy nasal cavity to enhance the information given. Objects of interest are extracted (segmented) from the MR images. Because the visualization of the boundaries of the investigated cavities is based on CT-derived data, the two data sets must be geometrically aligned (registered) to ensure exact correlation of object locations.

   Registration is performed automatically by the Impax EE PACS workstation. After registration, objects of interest can be segmented in the MR image and displayed at correct positions during the CT-based virtual fly-through.

   Segmentation is mainly performed manually, supported by thresholding techniques. Although time-consuming, manual segmentation is necessary for exact definition of the sellar pathology, pituitary gland, optochiasmatic system, and arachnoid spaces on T1-weighted MRI. Semiautomatic segmentation via threshold settings can be used for the arteries of the circulus arteriosus on MRA. Segmented anatomical structures are stored as objects on the disk.

   To display the segmented background objects during the virtual fly-through, each object must be reconstructed from its binary segmentation mask. This is not a trivial problem because the resulting object should have a natural-looking surface while remaining faithful to the segmentation result. In **Fig. 18.1A** (left), a resulting object that was directly reconstructed from the segmentation mask without any filtering is shown. This is an accurate representation of the segmentation result, but it is of little utility because the sharp edges look quite unnatural. In **Fig. 18.1A** (middle), the opposite extreme is shown; in this case, the object was filtered without taking care to preserve its features. It is clearly visible that important features are lost, which is inappropriate for a surgical planning application. In **Fig. 18.1A** (right), the result of applying a reconstruction algorithm we developed for this project is shown; this algorithm preserves all volume elements when filtering the inside-outside classification. Thus, although the resulting object appears acceptably smooth, it still accurately corresponds to the segmentation result.
2. *Fast and flexible reconstruction:* The virtual endoscopic images are generated using two different reconstruction techniques, one for rendering the standard virtual endoscopy views (the foreground) and one for rendering the background objects. Both techniques are highly optimized in terms of speed and flexibility.

   For every frame of the animation sequence, two images, one for the foreground and one for the background, are generated. In a second step, the two images are fused to a single result image. In image fusion, a simple trick is used to improve depth perception. In **Fig. 18.1B** (left), only the foreground sphenoid sinus anatomy is depicted. The image displayed in **Fig. 18.1B** (middle) shows the foreground and background objects and was generated using constant foreground transparency. In **Fig. 18.1B** (right), the transparency was dependent on the distance between the foreground and background, which significantly increases depth perception. Of course, the user can switch to constant transparency at any time to view the whole set of background objects.

   The user may also wish to obtain more information about what is behind the surface. STEPS offers a feature that displays surface rigidity, giving information, for example, about whether there is bone directly behind the mucosa. This aids navigation and helps the user to mentally connect the reconstructed image with the real anatomy. Three modes are offered: The fastest is simple color-coding. The second mode is double iso-surfacing, where a second surface is displayed beyond the primary foreground surface, representing firm structures (bone) that are nearby. The slowest, but visually most attractive, method is local direct volume rendering (**Fig. 18.3E**, middle).
3. *Simulation of the surgical procedure:* The user can simulate a complete endoscopic intervention, from the nasal to the sellar phase. The process of advancing the endoscope through the narrow nasal cavities and finding the correct way to the sphenoid sinus can be simulated as well as the process of widening the sphenoid ostium, the removal of sphenoid septa, and, one of the most crucial parts of the actual surgical operation, the process of opening the sellar floor. Simulation is used mainly for training purposes but can also provide information about accessibility and

the risks and obstacles to expect, which makes it useful also for preoperative planning. For the simulation, it is important to model the degrees of freedom and constraints experienced when working with a rigid endoscope as accurately as possible. Thus the user is confronted with similar challenges as in the real procedure.

During the simulation, the user's range of view is very limited. It can, as in real endoscopy, be enhanced by switching to an angled endoscope. However, this is often not sufficient to acquire a complete picture of the current state of the simulation, which would be useful especially for training purposes. STEPS provides the possibility of suspending the simulation, in which case the simulation is frozen and the application switches to a temporary free-flight mode. During suspension of the simulation, the endoscope is added to the rendered scene as an additional background object. The user can view the current situation and assess the state of the simulation from arbitrary view points (**Fig. 18.3F**, right).

The STEPS system provides a virtual surgical instrument that simulates the effect of a bone punch or drill. It can be used to enlarge the sphenoid ostium (**Fig. 18.3E**, right), to remove septa inside the sphenoid sinus, and to open the sellar floor (**Figs. 18.4C**, left, and **18.5C**, right). The instrument is operated using the mouse, and a preview of the effect is always given. As in reality, the diameter and depth of the punch can be selected by the user.

If a background object is very close to the surgical site, it will be shown in the preview. In the example in **Fig. 18.1C** (right), the distance between the tumor, color-coded in gray, and the surface is somewhat smaller than the depth of the punch. This is important, especially when the internal carotid artery (ICA) is close to the opening site.

To further increase the realism of the simulation, it is possible to add barrel distortion (**Fig. 18.1C**, left and middle), to use angled optics, and to introduce depth shading,

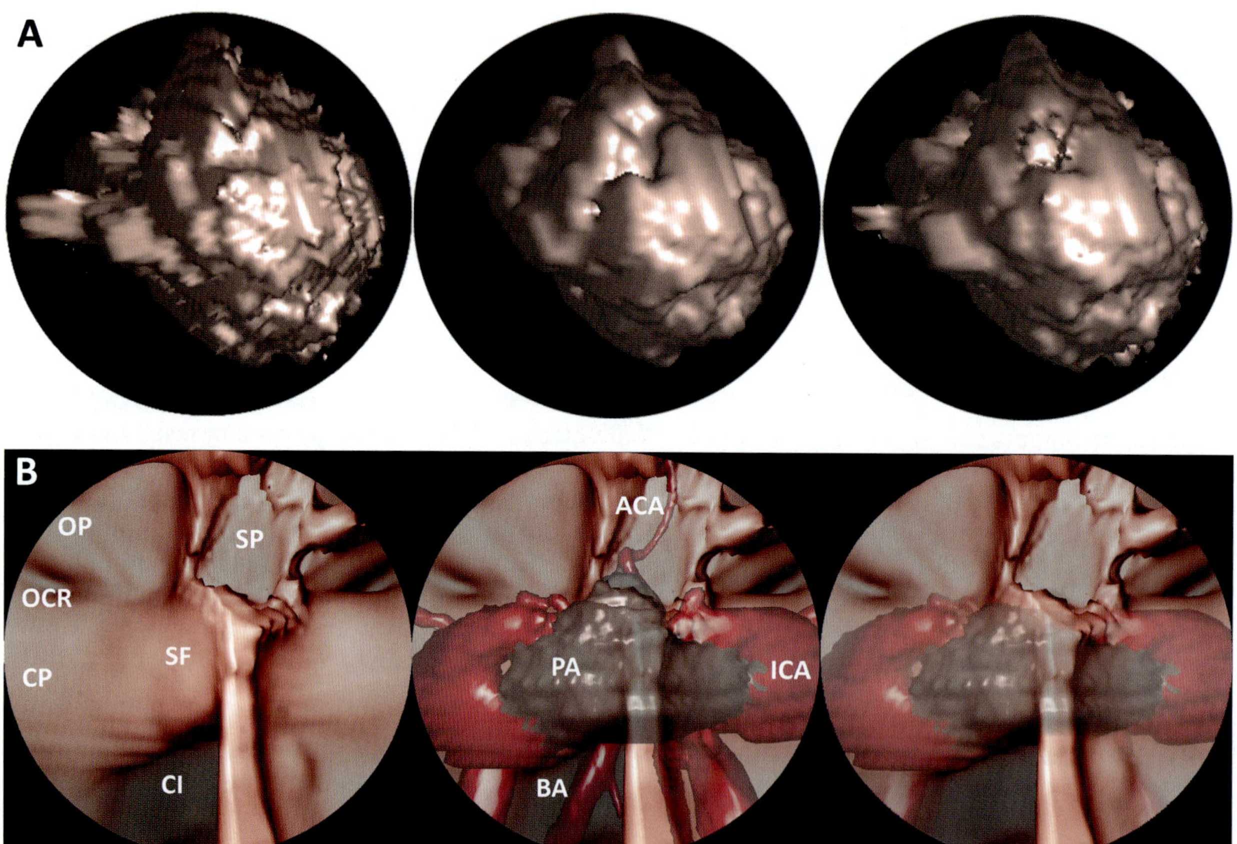

Fig. 18.1 Software features. **(A)** Object reconstruction algorithm. Left: Direct reconstruction of the segmentation mask without filtering. Middle: Filtering without preservation of object features. Right: The developed filtering algorithm preserves all volume elements during filtering the inside-outside classification. **(B)** Enhanced depth information. Left: Only the foreground sphenoid sinus anatomy is shown. Middle: Using constant foreground transparency, all background objects are visible. Right: To improve depth perception, the transparency is set dependent on the distance between the foreground and background objects.

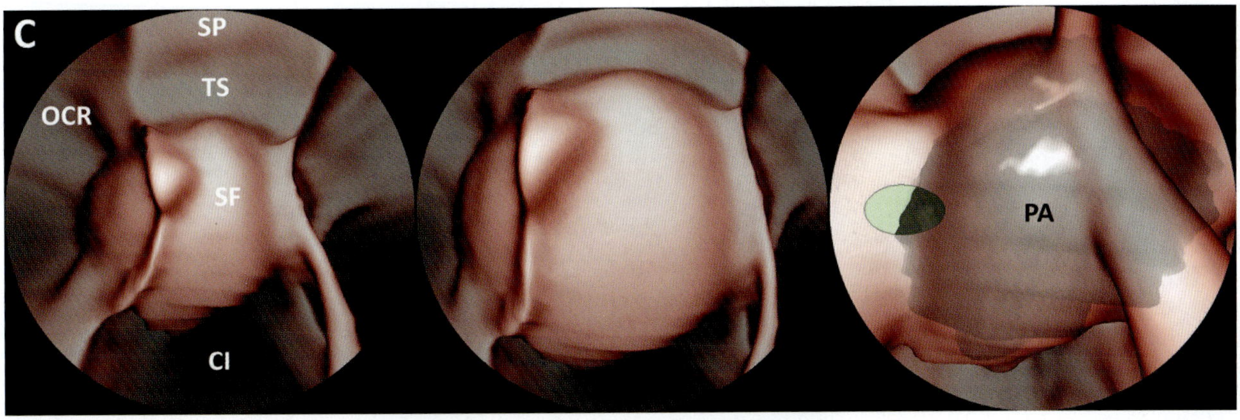

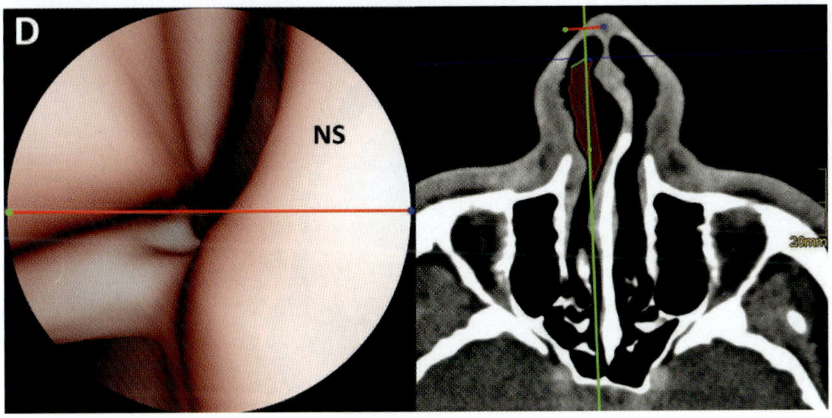

Fig. 18.1 (*Continued*) **(C)** Left and middle: The peripheral barrel distortion can be adjusted by the user to best match the image of the individual type of endoscope used. Right: Preview of the virtual surgical instrument simulating a bone punch or drill. **(D)** The virtual endoscopic image (left) is linked to the images of the multiplanar reconstruction (axial view, right) by color-coded lines and dots to enhance orientation. ACA, anterior cerebral artery; BA, basilar artery; CI, clival indentation; CP, carotid prominence; NS, nasal septum; OCR, opticocarotid recess; OP, optic protuberance; PA, pituitary adenoma; SF, sellar floor; SP, sphenoid plane; TS, tuberculum sellae.

simulating the limited light range of endoscopes observed in reality.

4. *Navigation aids:* Especially for an inexperienced surgeon, it is often hard to find the correct route through the nasal cavities to the sellar floor. Therefore, navigation aids are required. In physical endoscopy, navigation aids can be provided by a navigation system that tracks the position of the endoscope camera or a pointing device and displays it in a multiplanar reconstruction (MPR). In virtual endoscopy, this can be achieved more easily and more accurately because the exact endoscope position is always known. The MPR displayed by STEPS provides a feasible means of increasing the understanding of the relationship between original data and reconstructed 3D images. The user can link any of the section views to the 3D view, as illustrated in **Fig. 18.1D**, a snapshot from a simulated intervention. If a section view

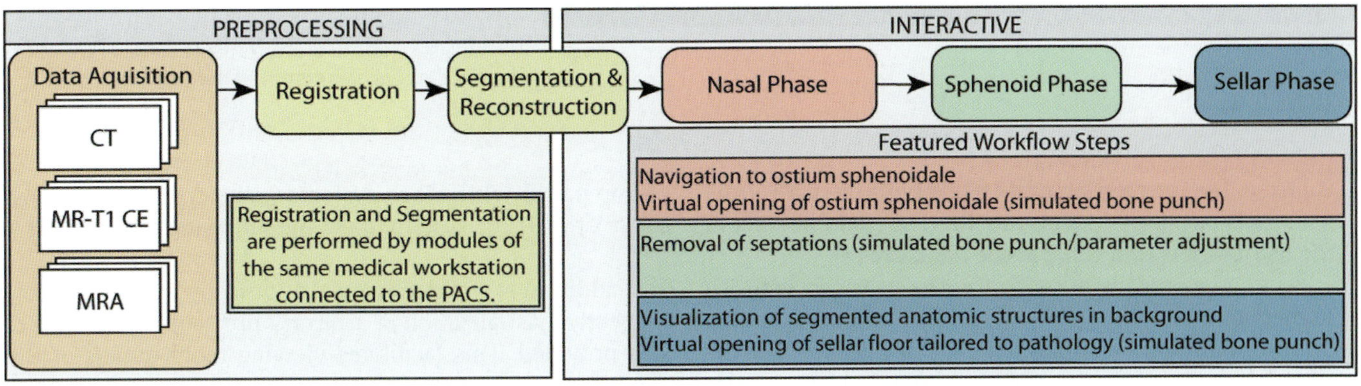

Fig. 18.2 Workflow of a virtual endoscopic transsphenoidal approach. CT, computed tomography; MRA, magnetic resonance angiography; MR-T1 CE; T1-weighted contrast-enhanced magnetic resonance imaging.

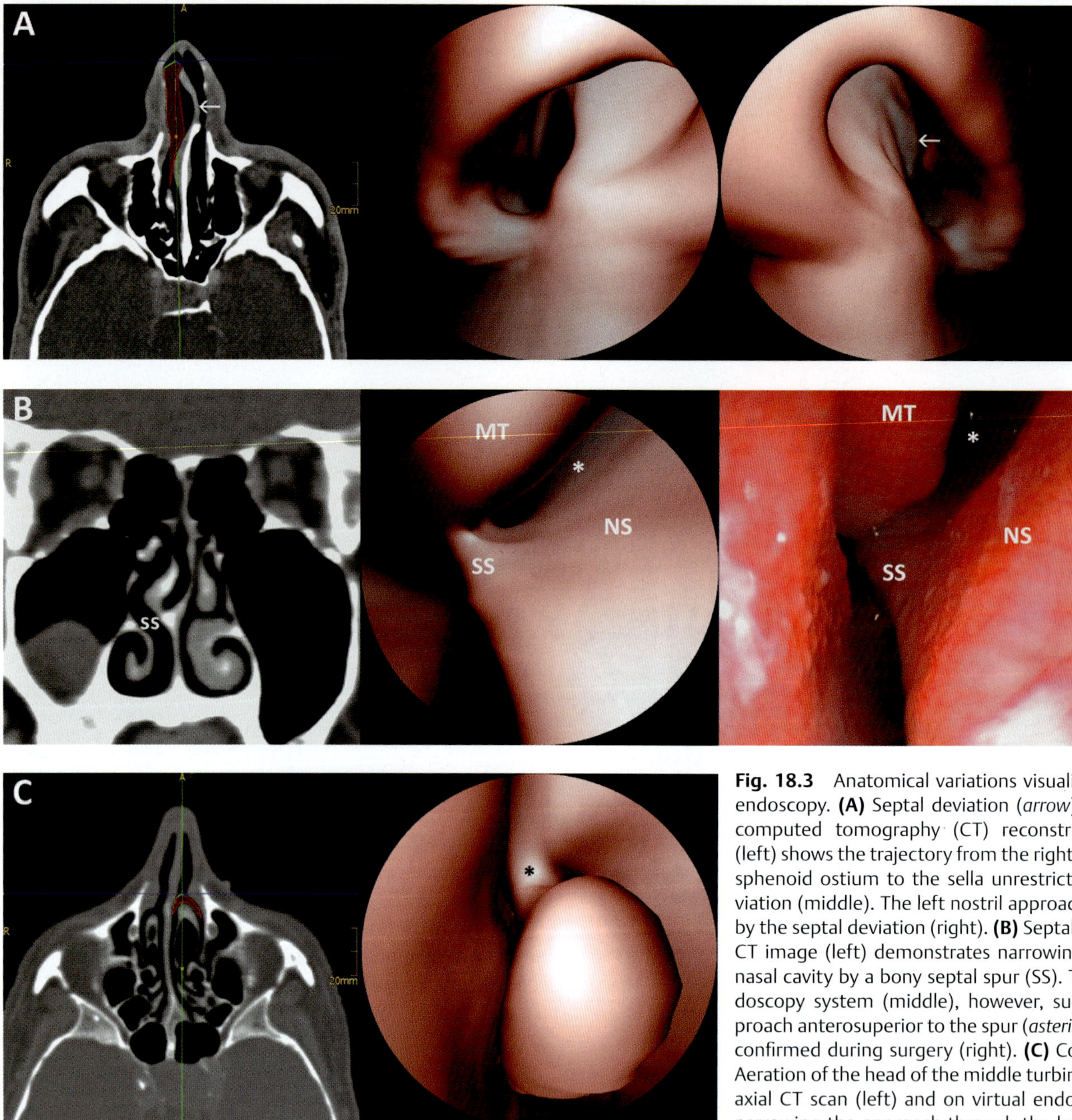

Fig. 18.3 Anatomical variations visualized by virtual endoscopy. **(A)** Septal deviation (*arrow*). The oblique computed tomography (CT) reconstruction image (left) shows the trajectory from the right nostril via the sphenoid ostium to the sella unrestricted by the deviation (middle). The left nostril approach is narrowed by the septal deviation (right). **(B)** Septal spur. Coronal CT image (left) demonstrates narrowing of the right nasal cavity by a bony septal spur (SS). The virtual endoscopy system (middle), however, suggests an approach anterosuperior to the spur (*asterisk*), which was confirmed during surgery (right). **(C)** Concha bullosa. Aeration of the head of the middle turbinate is seen on axial CT scan (left) and on virtual endoscopy (right), narrowing the approach through the left nasal cavity to the sella. Note the attachment (*asterisk*) by which the middle concha is removed during turbinectomy.

is linked, the intersection of its plane with the part of the mucosa is displayed in both the 3D view (red line) and in the section view (red curve inside nasal cavity).

As another means of guidance, the user can define a target point (e.g., the sphenoid ostium), and the direction to this point will be displayed in the 3D view during the simulation. Furthermore, the background objects can be displayed at any time by switching to constant transparency, which points out the principal direction to follow.

Compared with other systems (see Virtual Endoscopy, above), the STEPS system offers the following advantages:

1. In addition to standard virtual endoscopy, interactive perspective visualization of arbitrary pre-segmented objects is provided. This facilitates viewing more details of the patient anatomy, potentially increasing the safety of the procedure.
2. It provides simulation of the complete procedure.

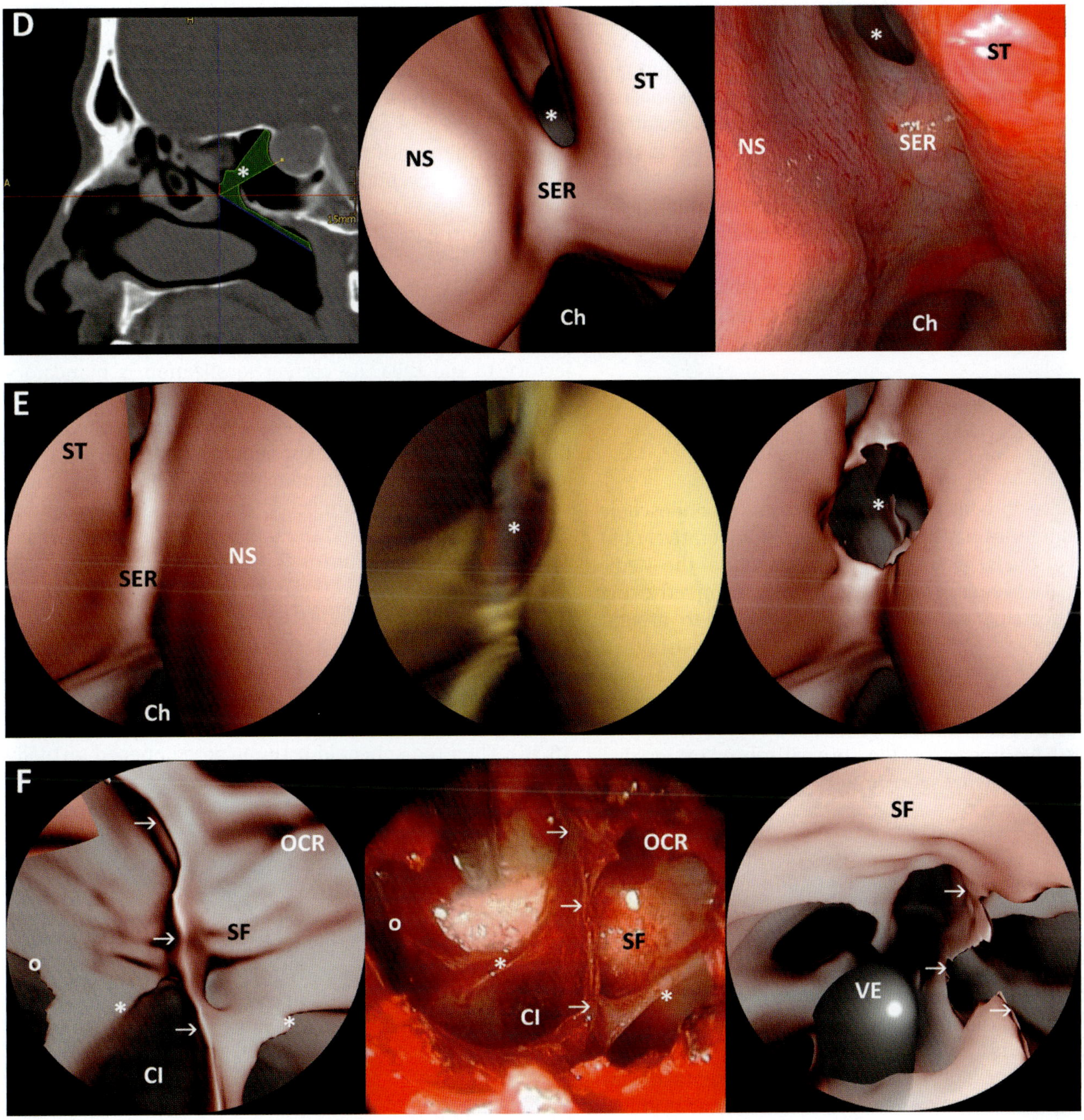

Fig. 18.3 (*Continued*) **(D)** Sphenoid ostium. Sagittal CT reconstruction reveals a visibly open left sphenoid ostium (*asterisk*). This was confirmed by virtual endoscopy preoperatively and during surgery. **(E)** Occult sphenoid ostium. In this case, the right sphenoid ostium is not directly visualized (left) but covered by a thin layer of mucosa (*asterisk*). Volume-rendering mode can demonstrate the density of the underlying structures, such as mucosa only (*red*) and the surrounding bone (*yellow*, middle). Virtual enlargement of the sphenoid ostium is possible using a simulated bone punch (right). **(F)** Multiseptated sphenoid sinus. Virtual endoscopy may enhance intraoperative orientation by visualizing complete (*arrows*) and incomplete (ring, *asterisks*) septations before surgery. The suspended-simulation mode (right) shows the current position of the virtual endoscope through the sphenoid ostium and inside the multiseptated sphenoid sinus, in this view from above. Ch, choana; Cl, clival indentation; MT, middle turbinate; NS, nasal septum; OCR, opticocarotid recess; SER, sphenoethmoid recess; SF, sellar floor; SS, septal spur; ST, superior turbinate; VE, virtual endoscope. (Parts B and F from Wolfsberger S, Neubauer A, Bühler K, et al. Advanced virtual endoscopy for endoscopic transsphenoidal pituitary surgery. Neurosurgery 2006;59:1005. Reprinted with permission.)

3. It provides flexible reconstruction. The graphical reconstruction is not performed only once at the beginning of the examination but is renewed after every user interaction. This enables adjustment of the reconstruction parameters according to the situation. During simulation, for example, continuous adjustments are required to keep the visual output close to reality.
4. Optional navigation aids have been implemented, facilitating the handling of the software especially for less experienced users.
5. It provides display of surface rigidity, which facilitates navigation and the mapping of virtual to real anatomy.

Clinical Experience with the STEPS System

Since its development in 2004, more than 100 endoscopic pituitary surgeries have been simulated preoperatively using STEPS at the Department of Neurosurgery of the Medical University Vienna. The time expenditure for retrieving and preprocessing image data has decreased to around 20 minutes per case. Prior to the surgery, the neurosurgeon routinely uses STEPS to display the patient anatomy and its specific variations to enhance the surgical planning. In our experience, STEPS visualizes the various anatomical structures that have impact on the surgical procedure, as discussed in the following subsections.

Nasal Phase

With the standard microscopic technique, the side of the approach is typically chosen contralaterally to the maximum parasellar extension of the pituitary adenoma because of the angle at which the nasal speculum is inserted. With the endoscopic technique, however, the side of the approach depends more on considerations of the nasal anatomy. Therefore, STEPS can assist in preoperatively depicting the wideness of the nasal corridor, the septal deviations and spurs, the bullous conchae, and other anatomical variations.

Intraoperatively, the nasal cavities are initially narrow slit-like spaces, and the actual size of the working corridor is observed only after decongestion of the nasal mucosa by, for example, diluted epinephrine or cocaine introduced on cottonoids. STEPS simulates the task of nasal decongestion by manual adjustment of the reconstruction parameters.

Strong anterior to middle septal deviation may decrease the width of the working corridor; thus the opposite nasal cavity may be considered (**Fig. 18.3A**). Similarly, a septal spur may be encountered, and either it has to be removed before the endoscope can be advanced or the contralateral approach needs to be chosen (**Fig. 18.3B**). The trajectory of the endoscopic approach to the sphenoid ostium is via the inferior angle of the head of the middle turbinate. Enlargement of this bullous portion of the middle turbinate due to aeration, termed concha bullosa, is not uncommon (8 to 53%[22–24]) and is of particular interest as it can substantially diminish the width of the working corridor (**Fig. 18.3C**). Furthermore, a septal deviation to the contralateral side is commonly associated with concha bullosa,[8,23] making the narrow contralateral nasal cavity less inviting for an endoscopic approach. Thus, the neurosurgeon can plan to perform a middle turbinectomy if a concha bullosa is found on virtual endoscopy.

The sphenoid ostium is the next checkpoint for the trajectory to the sella. Its correct localization is mandatory because enlarging the ostium by bone punch or high-speed diamond drill permits a safe entrance into the sphenoid sinus. Especially for the inexperienced endoscopic surgeon, locating the sphenoid ostium may be challenging. The opening may be partly or completely covered by mucosa and is commonly hidden behind the tail of the superior turbinate. Anatomically, the ostium is located approximately 5 mm lateral to the midline,[22] 10 mm above the end of the tail of the superior turbinate, and 10 mm below the frontal skull base.[25] With STEPS, the exact position of the sphenoid ostium can be visualized (**Fig. 18.3D**), and, using the local volume rendering mode (see Software and Workflow, above), the state of occlusion by mucosa can be displayed (**Fig. 18.3E**). Then the sphenoid ostium can be opened virtually using a circular bone punch at various depths and diameters (**Fig. 18.3E**, right). Therefore, the neurosurgeon can plan the size of opening the ostium and the amount of removal of the posterior septum necessary to gain sufficient insight into the sphenoid sinus.

If the user defines the nares and the sphenoid ostium as the starting and ending point of the trajectory, the flight mode of STEPS displays the nasal anatomy of this corridor. This is particularly valuable, as not every nasal anatomical variation is relevant to the endoscopic approach (**Fig. 18.3B**).

Sphenoid Phase

Inside the sphenoid sinus, STEPS can preoperatively visualize the bony anatomical landmarks (**Figs. 18.1B,C** and **18.4B**): the carotid and optic prominences cover the ICA and optic nerve, respectively. The opticocarotid recess, between the two prominences, corresponds to the indentation of the anterior clinoid process with varying degrees of pneumatization. Superior to the sella, the indentation of the tuberculum sellae may be encountered, and inferior to the sella, the clival indentation.

Depending on the degree of pneumatization, the configuration of the sphenoid sinus may vary in size from the smallest conchal type presellar and sellar, to the largest postsellar

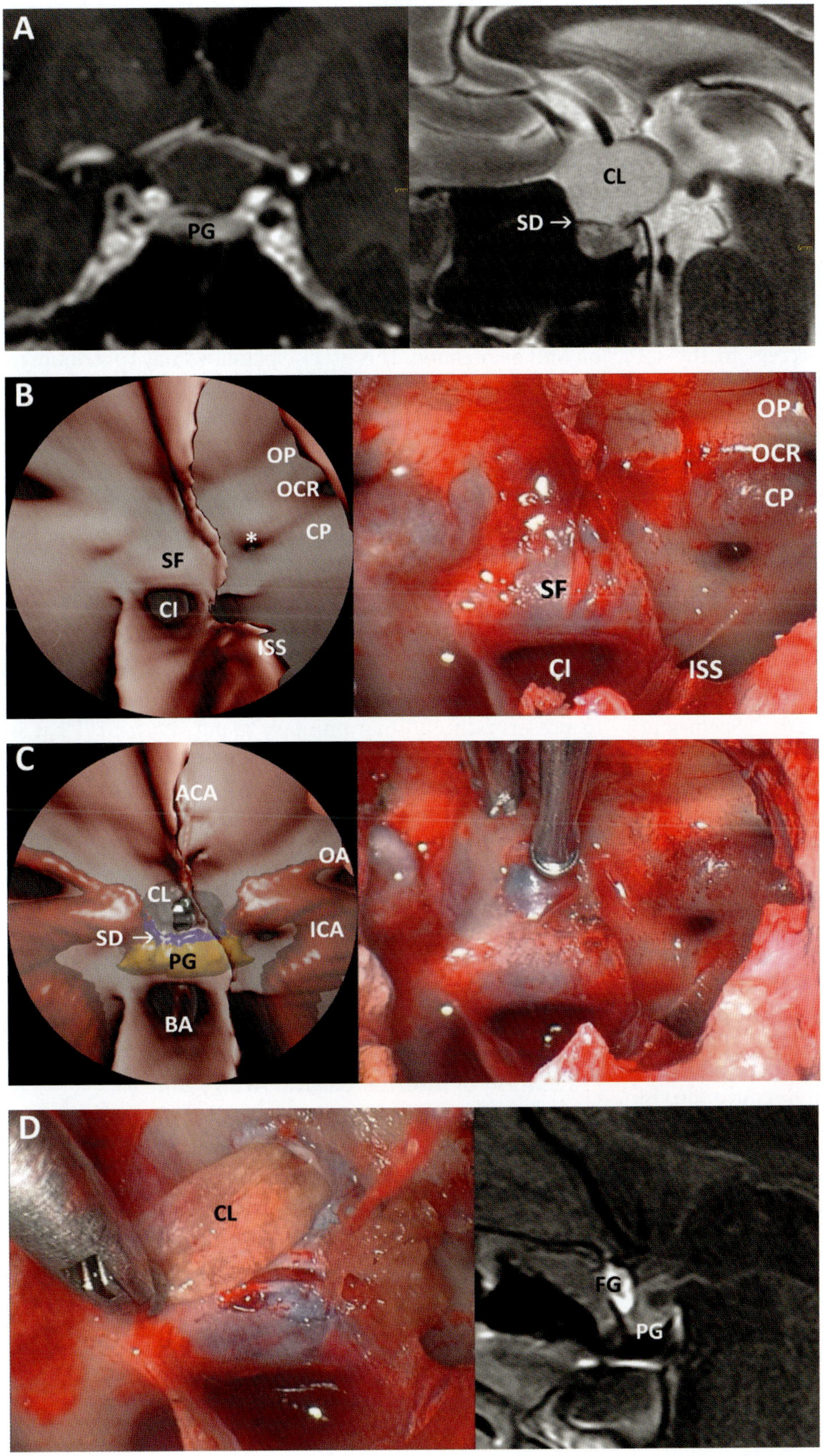

Fig. 18.4 Case 1: cystic supradiaphragmatic lesion. **(A)** T1-weighted contrast-enhanced coronal MR image (left), obtained from a 61-year-old man with visual deterioration, depicts a lesion with peripheral enhancement superior to the pituitary gland. The cystic configuration is shown on T2-weighted sagittal MR image (right). Note the sellar diaphragm as a low-intensity line between the pituitary gland and the cyst. **(B)** Endoscopic anatomy of the sphenoid sinus as simulated by virtual endoscopy and its correlation with the intraoperative view. The optic and carotid protuberances and the well-pneumatized opticocarotid recess as the invagination of the anterior clinoid process are visualized on both sides. As a variant, a further invagination is observed in the left carotid siphon (*asterisk*). **(C)** Opening of the sellar floor. Using virtual endoscopy, anatomical objects of interest, such as the pituitary gland, cystic lesion, sellar diaphragm, and internal carotid artery (ICA), can be visualized in the background to plan the optimal opening of the sellar floor superficial to the supradiaphragmatic cyst. Note the emerging of the ophthalmic artery from the ICA and the position of the anterior cerebral artery superior to the cyst on the virtual endoscopy image. **(D)** Intraoperative endoscopic view of the removal of the lesion (left). The cyst wall was easily detachable and removed safely through a small dural opening. Histology revealed a craniopharyngioma. Postoperative T1-weighted contrast-enhanced sagittal magnetic resonance image (right). The infundibulum is now observed behind the fat graft covering the dural defect. The patient did not suffer any pituitary hormone insufficiencies. ACA, anterior cerebral artery; CI, clival indentation; CL, cystic lesion; CP, carotid protuberance; FG, fat graft; ISS, intersinus septum; OA, ophthalmic artery; OCR, opticocarotid recess; OP, optic protuberance; PG, pituitary gland; SD, sellar diaphragm; SF, sellar floor; SP, sphenoid plane; TS, tuberculum sellae.

type. In the rare cases of a conchal type (3%[22]) and a presellar-type sinus (11 to 24%[22]), the familiar anatomical landmarks inside the sphenoid sinus are commonly missing. STEPS can visualize the configuration and anatomy of the sphenoid sinus preoperatively. This information can enhance intraoperative orientation and be used for planning, whether or not and wherever exact drilling will be required.

Sphenoid septations show considerable variation in number and completeness. In addition to the most frequently encountered median intersinus septum that divides the sphenoid sinus in two separate chambers, multiple other septations may exist in the region of the synchondroses of the sphenoid bone.[22] To gain sufficient access to the sellar floor, the complete septations need to be removed. Incomplete septations can serve as anatomical landmarks for orientation inside the sphenoid sinus and correct opening of the sellar floor. STEPS can visualize the sphenoid septations, their variations, and their number preoperatively (**Fig. 18.3F**). Therefore, the virtual endoscopic images can be employed for planning the opening of the sellar floor, specifically tailored to the pathology. Further, STEPS allows a virtual removal of the septations, using adjustment of reconstruction parameters (**Fig. 18.5B**) and a virtual bone punch before surgery.

The intersinus septum often deviates from the midline and attaches to the protuberances of the ICAs.[26] Such an insertion has to be respected when removing the septum to prevent damage to the underlying ICA. STEPS can prospectively depict such an anatomical situation before surgery.

Horizontal septations can be particularly challenging to the endoscopist because they may be mistaken for the sphenoid plane and left in place. Such an incomplete opening of the sphenoid sinus may consequently prevent full access to the sellar floor. Horizontal septations are encountered in posterior ethmoid air cells (Onodi cell, **Fig. 18.5B**), which have been reported to occur in approximately 12% of patients[22] and increase the risk of surgical complications.[27] Preoperative knowledge of a horizontal septum by virtual endoscopy may maximize access to the sellar floor and reduce the risk of an inadvertent opening of the sphenoid plane, with its consequent complications, such as cerebrospinal fluid (CSF) leak, bleeding, and infection.

Sellar Phase

Using volume-rendering techniques (see previous section "Software and Workflow"), STEPS can visualize the consistency of the sellar floor. Thus, decisions about whether a thick bony sellar floor needs to be removed with a high-speed drill, or an eroded sellar floor can be opened solely with a punch, can be made preoperatively.

The exact location and size of the opening of the sellar floor are usually tailored to the configuration of the specific underlying pathology. For drainage of Rathke's cleft cysts and removal of microadenomas, a partial and selective opening may be sufficient. Large macroadenomas usually require maximum opening of the sellar floor. STEPS can aid in planning the sellar floor opening preoperatively by visualizing the sphenoid sinus anatomical landmarks. The lateral extension of the opening may be defined by the carotid arteries that are displayed and the by the insertions of (incomplete) septations at the carotid protuberances. The superior extension of the sellar floor removal will be limited by the opticocarotid recess, optic protuberance, and indentation of the tuberculum sellae, and by arachnoid cisterns herniating below the diaphragm sellae level that have been segmented on MRI beforehand. This precise planning may contribute to the lower incidence of CSF leaks intraoperatively.

Preoperative visualization of the pre-segmented anatomical objects of interest behind the semitransparent walls of the sphenoid sinus can aid in planning the adenoma resection, avoiding injury to the normal pituitary gland and ICA, and at the same time maximizing the exposure of the adenoma tissue.

Preservation of Normal Pituitary Gland

In cases of microadenomas, the bony sellar floor may be removed selectively superficial to the underlying adenoma to preserve the normal pituitary gland. With STEPS it is possible to plan such an individually tailored opening beforehand, as it visualizes the adenoma with its relation to the pituitary gland and the overlying sphenoid landmarks (**Fig. 18.5**).

If the endosellar lesion is anteriorly covered by the pituitary gland, such as in Rathke's cleft cysts, a transpituitary approach is needed. The optimal position for incising the gland can be preoperatively planned using STEPS. Thus, the incidence of postoperative pituitary failures may be reduced further.

Prevention of Internal Carotid Artery Injury

Intraoperative ICA injury has been reported to occur in less than 0.2% of patients in large series of microscopic transsphenoidal surgeries.[28,29] As this number, however, is taken from centers with very experienced pituitary surgeons, it probably underestimates the frequency of this life-threatening complication. In a national survey on complications of transsphenoidal surgery, Ciric et al[30] included 958 pituitary surgeons of varying degree of expertise. They reported a rate of 1.1% of ICA injury.

Although infrequently encountered,[31] ICA injury may occur more commonly with a newly employed surgical technique and in cases of distorted anatomy, such as reoperations.[29] Visualization of the ICA (segmented from MRA) in relation to the pituitary adenoma (segmented from T1-weighted MRI), behind the semitransparent walls of the

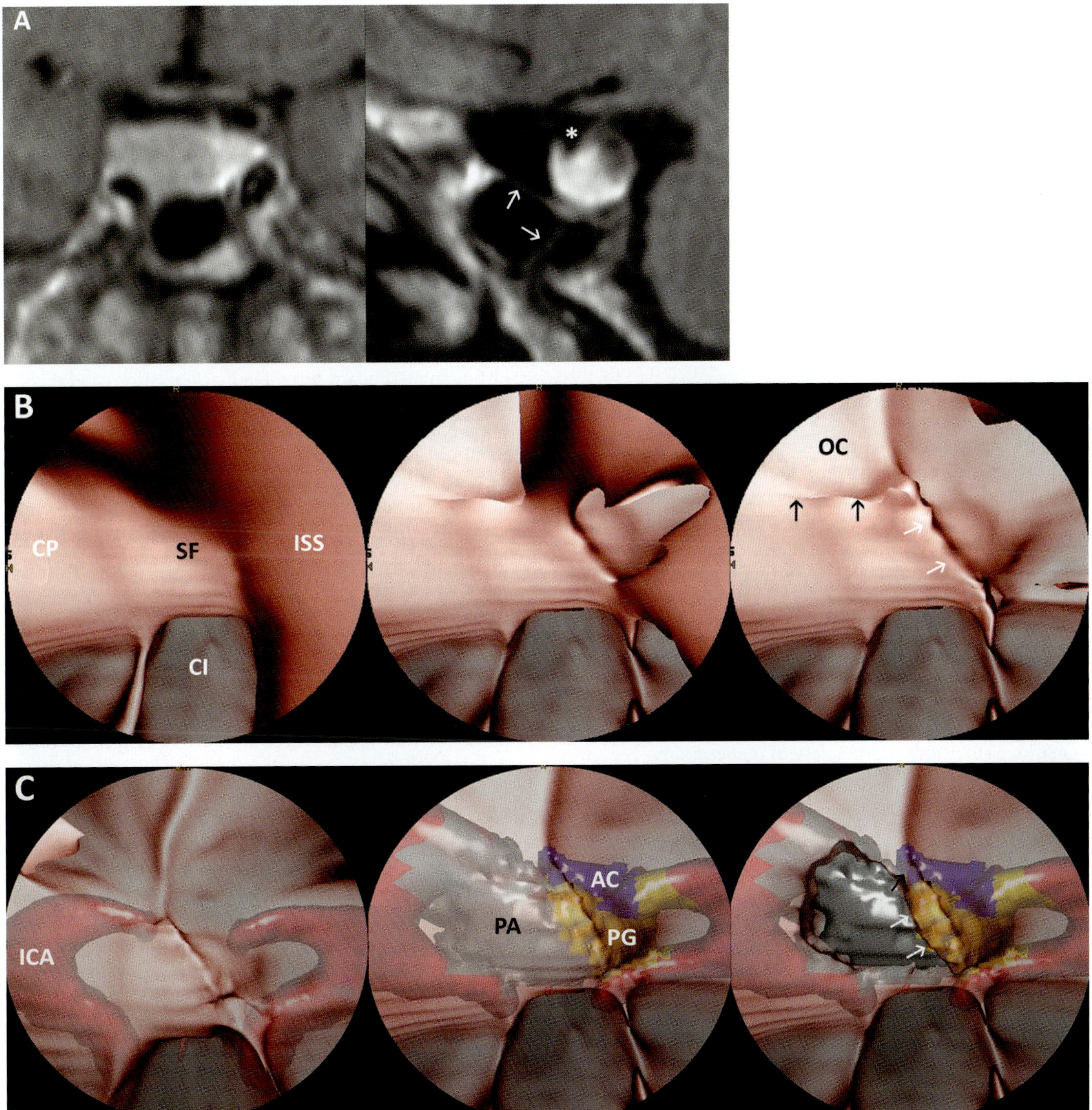

Fig. 18.5 Case 2: right endosellar microadenoma. **(A)** T1-weighted contrast-enhanced magnetic resonance images (MRI) obtained from a 42-year-old man with acromegaly (basal growth hormone level 50 ng/mL). The coronal MRI scan depicts a right-sided macroadenoma with extension into superior cavernous sinus compartment (left). The sagittal MRI scan (right) reveals a multiseptated sphenoid sinus (*arrows*) and a large hypophyseal cistern (*asterisk*). **(B)** The virtual endoscopic images visualize the individual anatomy during preoperative planning. The sphenoid septations are removed by adjusting the threshold of the ray-casting algorithm to computed tomography Hounsfield units. Note an oblique intersinus septum (*white arrows*) and a horizontal septum (*black arrows*) detaching an Onodi cell from the right sphenoid sinus chamber. **(C)** The anatomical objects of interest are visible through the transparent walls of the sphenoid sinus (left and middle). Using the virtual rongeur, the removal of the sellar floor can be simulated (right). This allows planning of the exact extension of opening to protect the ICA and pituitary gland (*white arrows*) and to prevent a cerebrospinal fluid leak (*black arrow*). AC, arachnoid cistern; CI, clival indentation; CP, carotid prominence; ICA, internal carotid artery; OC, Onodi cell; PA, adenoma; PG, pituitary gland; SF, sellar floor. (From Wolfsberger S, Neubauer A, Bühler K, et al. Advanced virtual endoscopy for endoscopic transsphenoidal pituitary surgery. Neurosurgery 2006;59;1006. Reprinted with permission.)

sphenoid sinus, provides preoperative knowledge about the anatomical variations in the patient that may be fraught with risk for vascular injury:

1. Septal deviations that insert at the carotid prominences may mislead the midline approach. If not respected, inadvertent ICA laceration may occur when removing such an oblique septum.
2. Absence of the bone covering the ICA prominences may cause inadvertent ICA injury when opening the sellar floor laterally.[32] Such bony dehiscence was reported to occur in 5 to 15% of cadaver and radiologic studies.[26] In our experience, this not only is a feature of elderly patients, due to bone erosion, but also can occur in the young as well. STEPS can preoperatively visualize such a bone defect by a stronger coloration of the parts of the ICA that are not covered.
3. A narrow intercarotid distance may be potentially hazardous when opening the sellar floor or the basal sellar dura and during tumor removal. It has been reported as low as 4 mm in the literature,[33,34] even when contacting the opposite side artery as in "kissing carotids."[35] The virtual endoscopic tool can depict such a situation preoperatively.
4. In recurrent adenomas, the normal sphenoid anatomy is usually distorted from previous removal of bone and consequent scarring. Therefore, these patients are at higher risk for inadvertent injury to the ICA when opening the sellar floor.[29] By depicting the position of the ICA behind the scar tissue and its relation to the remaining landmarks, STEPS adds to the safety of reoperations.

Experience with STEPS as a Training Device

At present, endoscopic handling and anatomical viewing skills are trained at cadaver workshops, which are given by different centers throughout the world. However, this type of training is costly and often not easily accessible. Although the haptic experience of handling an endoscope cannot be simulated at present, STEPS provides the possibility for the novice of endoscopic pituitary surgery to study the endoscopic anatomy. Surpassing cadaver training, the virtual endoscopy tool can be used to prepare for a teaching operation by studying the patient anatomy in an endoscopic view before live surgery. This may increase the safety of the procedure and reduce operation time.

A STEPS workstation has been available at the yearly endoscopic pituitary workshops at the Department of Anatomy of the Medical University Vienna since 2004. According to the feedback from the trainees, the virtual endoscopy system is a beneficial teaching and training tool for beginners in endoscopic pituitary surgery.

Benefits and Drawbacks

One of the major benefits of this virtual endoscopy system is its possibility of being hosted by a standard PC without the need for expensive hardware for its fast real-time 3D reconstruction. Furthermore, the image quality has been enhanced dramatically throughout the ongoing development so that it now features a near-realistic visualization of the nasal and paranasal sinus anatomy. As automated image registration and manual and threshold segmentation tools have been integrated into the Impax system, the time necessary for preprocessing of image data has been reduced to around 20 minutes, mainly depending on image data retrieval and storage.

Although a standard force-feedback joystick can be connected, no sophisticated input device simulating the haptics of a real endoscope is available yet. Further, the simulation of bleeding and hemostasis, which can pose a major challenge to the novice endoscopist, is missing. Concerning virtual instruments, only a rongeur with variable diameter and depth is presently available. Finally, the system is not commercially available at present.

Future Developments

Intraoperative Tracking

Currently, the use of STEPS is restricted to the preoperative planning of endoscopic procedures. Connected to an intraoperative tracking device, such as a navigation system that is routinely used during transsphenoidal endoscopic surgery, the actual coordinates of the endoscope could be transferred to the STEPS workstation and the virtual endoscopic image that is displayed would ideally match the intraoperative view. On the semitransparent virtual image, however, the anatomical background objects of interest could be displayed to the neurosurgeon. If the tip of the instrument was concurrently tracked and displayed as a point on the virtual endoscopy screen, the surgeon could always perceive potentially hazardous situations. By delineating the oncoming anatomy, STEPS might maximize the safety of the procedure. As well, the tumor extensions in relation to the ICA could always be displayed on the virtual screen to maximize tumor removal.

The intraoperative use of STEPS, however, is restricted by tissue deformation and tissue removal, which at present cannot sufficiently be simulated by the software.

Virtual Ventriculoscopy

The STEPS software can be used for other fields of virtual endoscopy. For paranasal sinus surgery, no major adaptions are needed. For neurosurgery, virtual ventriculoscopy may aid in preoperative planning of third ventriculostomy or intraventricular tumor biopsy.[36-39] In contrast to endonasal virtual endoscopy, where the nasal cavity is derived from CT data, the ventricular walls have to be reconstructed from MR image data, and thus slight adaptations of the STEPS software are necessary. The basilar artery, pre-segmented from an MRA scan, and the dorsum sellae, pre-segmented from a CT scan, can then be displayed as background objects through the semitransparent third ventricular floor. Using the existing virtual punch, the opening of the third ventricular floor can be planned and simulated. A ventricular tumor, pre-segmented from T1-weighted MRI, can be also be displayed. An extension of the software for planning the optimal trajectory would be necessary.

Conclusion

One of the strongest criticisms of endoscopic transsphenoidal pituitary surgery addresses the steep learning curve encountered when using an endoscope as opposed to the microscope. The virtual endoscopy software STEPS tackles this problem. For the novice, STEPS may be a valuable tool for learning the endoscopic anatomy and for simulating simple surgical tasks in a virtual setting. Although the use of STEPS does not obviate the need for a thorough anatomical training using the endoscope in laboratory dissections to become comfortable and familiar with this type of surgery, it allows the novice to understand the actual surgical anatomy of a given case.

For the experienced pituitary surgeon, STEPS can visualize the individual anatomy of the patient and may thus improve intraoperative orientation. Furthermore, by providing a preview of unpredictable anatomical variations, STEPS may increase the safety of the procedure.

References

1. Thapar K, Laws ER Jr. Pituitary surgery. In: Thapar K, Kovacs K, Scheithauer BW, Lloyd RV, eds. Diagnosis and Management of Pituitary Tumors. Totowa, NJ: Humana Press; 2001:225–246
2. de Divitiis E, Cappabianca P. Endoscopic Endonasal Transsphenoidal Surgery. Vienna: Springer, 2003
3. Guiot G, Bouche J, Hertzog E, Vourc'H G, Hardy J. [Hypophysectomy by trans-sphenoidal route.]. Ann Radiol (Paris) 1963;6:187–192
4. Cappabianca P, Alfieri A, de Divitiis E. Endoscopic endonasal transsphenoidal approach to the sella: towards functional endoscopic pituitary surgery (FEPS). Minim Invasive Neurosurg 1998;41:66–73
5. Jho HD, Carrau RL. Endoscopy assisted transsphenoidal surgery for pituitary adenoma. Technical note. Acta Neurochir (Wien) 1996;138:1416–1425
6. Koc K, Kenan K, Anik I, et al. The learning curve in endoscopic pituitary surgery and our experience. Neurosurg Rev 2006;29:298–305, discussion 305
7. Wolfsberger S, Forster MT, Donat M, et al. Virtual endoscopy is a useful device for training and preoperative planning of transsphenoidal endoscopic pituitary surgery. Minim Invasive Neurosurg 2004;47:214–220
8. Wolfsberger S, Neubauer A, Bühler K, et al. Advanced virtual endoscopy for endoscopic transsphenoidal pituitary surgery. Neurosurgery 2006;59:1001–1009, discussion 1009–1010
9. Neubauer A, Wolfsberger S, Forster MT, Mroz L, Wegenkittl R, Bühler K. Advanced virtual endoscopic pituitary surgery. IEEE Trans Vis Comput Graph 2005;11:497–507
10. Neubauer A, Wolfsberger S, Forster MT, Mroz L, Wegenkittl R, Buhler K. STEPS—an application for simulation of transsphenoidal endonasal pituitary surgery. In: Proceedings of the IEEE Symposium on Visualization. 2004:513–520
11. Vining DJ, Gelfand DW. Noninvasive colonoscopy using helical CT scanning 3D reconstruction. SGR Scientific Program 1994; 70:1994
12. Lorensen WE, Jolesz FA, Kikinis R. The exploration of cross-sectional data with a virtual endoscope. In: Satava RM, Sieburg HB, Mattheus R, Christensen JP, eds. Interactive Technology and the New Paradigm for Healthcare. Amsterdam; Washington, DC: IOS Press; 1995:221–230
13. Kikinis R, Langham Gleason P, Jolesz FA. Surgical planning using computer-assisted three-dimensional reconstructions. In: Taylor R, Lavalle S, Burdea G, Mosges R, eds. Computer Integrated Surgery. Cambridge, MA: MIT Press; 1995:147–154
14. Summers RM, Aggarwal NR, Sneller MC, et al. CT virtual bronchoscopy of the central airways in patients with Wegener's granulomatosis. Chest 2002;121:242–250
15. Bartz D. Virtual endoscopy in research and clinical practice. Eurographics State-of-the-Art-Reports 2003;S4
16. Davis CP, Ladd ME, Romanowski BJ, Wildermuth S, Knoplioch JF, Debatin JF. Human aorta: preliminary results with virtual endoscopy based on three-dimensional MR imaging data sets. Radiology 1996;199:37–40
17. Bartz D, Gürvit Ö, Lanzendorfer M, Kopp A, Küttner A, Straßer W. Virtual endoscopy for cardiovascular exploration. Proc Comput Assist Radiol Surg 2001;(CARS 01):960–964
18. Morra A, Calgaro A, Cioffi V, Pravato M, Cova M, Pozzi Mucelli R. [Virtual endoscopy of the nasal cavity and the paranasal sinuses with computerized tomography. Anatomical study]. Radiol Med (Torino) 1998;96:29–34
19. Bisdas S, Verink M, Stieve M, Lazakidou A, Ebangelou I, Becker H. Three dimensional imaging of the nasal cavity and paranasal sinuses. In: Proceedings of the Special Mini-Symposium BIOHEMED '04 within the Context of the 4th WSEAS International Conference ISA '04. 2004:138
20. Rogalla P. Virtual endoscopy: An application snapshot. Medicamundi 1999;43:17–23
21. Talala T, Pirilä T, Karhula V, Ilkko E, Suramo I. Preoperative virtual endoscopy and three-dimensional imaging of the surface landmarks of the internal carotid arteries in trans-sphenoidal pituitary surgery. Acta Otolaryngol 2000;120:783–787
22. Lang J. Clinical Anatomy of the Nose, Nasal Cavity and Paranasal Sinuses. A Basis for Diagnosis and Surgery. New York: Thieme; 1998
23. Stallman JS, Lobo JN, Som PM. The incidence of concha bullosa and its relationship to nasal septal deviation and paranasal sinus disease. AJNR Am J Neuroradiol 2004;25:1613–1618

24. Zinreich SJ, Mattox DE, Kennedy DW, Chisholm HL, Diffley DM, Rosenbaum AE. Concha bullosa: CT evaluation. J Comput Assist Tomogr 1988;12:778–784
25. Kim HU, Kim SS, Kang SS, Chung IH, Lee JG, Yoon JH. Surgical anatomy of the natural ostium of the sphenoid sinus. Laryngoscope 2001;111:1599–1602
26. Unal B, Bademci G, Bilgili YK, Batay F, Avci E. Risky anatomic variations of sphenoid sinus for surgery. Surg Radiol Anat 2006;28:195–201
27. Kantarci M, Karasen RM, Alper F, Onbas O, Okur A, Karaman A. Remarkable anatomic variations in paranasal sinus region and their clinical importance. Eur J Radiol 2004;50:296–302
28. Fahlbusch R, Buchfelder M. Surgical complications. In: Landolt AM, Vance ML, Reilly P, eds. Pituitary Adenomas. New York: Churchill Livingstone; 1996:395–408
29. Laws ER Jr. Vascular complications of transsphenoidal surgery. Pituitary 1999;2:163–170
30. Ciric I, Ragin A, Baumgartner C, Pierce D. Complications of transsphenoidal surgery: results of a national survey, review of the literature, and personal experience. Neurosurgery 1997;40:225–236, discussion 236–237
31. Cappabianca P, Briganti F, Cavallo LM, de Divitiis E. Pseudoaneurysm of the intracavernous carotid artery following endoscopic endonasal transsphenoidal surgery, treated by endovascular approach. Acta Neurochir (Wien) 2001;143:95–96
32. Oskouian RJ, Kelly DF, Laws ER. Vascular injury and transsphenoidal surgery. In: Laws ER, Sheehan JP, eds. Pituitary Surgery—A Modern Approach. Basel: Karger; 2006:256–278
33. Lang J. Skull Base and Related Structures. Stuttgart: Schattauer; 1995
34. Renn WH, Rhoton AL Jr. Microsurgical anatomy of the sellar region. J Neurosurg 1975;43:288–298
35. Pereira Filho AdeA, Gobbato PL, Pereira Filho GdeA, Silva SB, Kraemer JL. Intracranial intrasellar kissing carotid arteries: case report. Arq Neuropsiquiatr 2007;65:355–357
36. Burtscher J, Dessl A, Bale R, et al. Virtual endoscopy for planning endoscopic third ventriculostomy procedures. Pediatr Neurosurg 2000;32:77–82
37. Freudenstein D, Bartz D, Skalej M, Duffner F. New virtual system for planning of neuroendoscopic interventions. Comput Aided Surg 2001;6:77–84
38. Jödicke A, Accomazzi V, Reiss I, Böker DK. Virtual endoscopy of the cerebral ventricles based on 3-D ultrasonography. Ultrasound Med Biol 2003;29:339–345
39. Krombach A, Rohde V, Haage P, Struffert T, Kilbinger M, Thron A. Virtual endoscopy combined with intraoperative neuronavigation for planning of endoscopic surgery in patients with occlusive hydrocephalus and intracranial cysts. Neuroradiology 2002;44: 279–285

19 3D Stereoendoscopic Pituitary Surgery*

Seth Brown, Vijay K. Anand, Jonathan Roth, and Theodore H. Schwartz

Recent years have seen a rapidly growing interest in both endoscopic and robotic surgery, not only in neurosurgery and otolaryngology, but also in nearly every surgical field. Advances have facilitated increasing surgical precision and decreasing operative times in select procedures. The early results of endoscopic pituitary surgery, in terms of length of stay, tumor control, and complications, compare favorably with microscopic surgery.[1–6] Additionally, endoscopic pituitary surgery allows for preservation of important nasal structures including the turbinates, the olfactory fibers, and the anterior septum to maximize sinonasal function postoperatively. Neurosurgeons performing endoscopic pituitary surgery are quite familiar with the excellent visualization an endoscope provides because of the ability to bring light to the source of the lesion, as well as the ability to look "around the corner" via angled scopes. Essentially, the endoscope addresses some of the limiting factors of traditional transsphenoidal surgery: the long, narrow operative corridor, which limits the field of view, and the inability to adequately assess extension of the pathology behind and around critical neurovascular structures. Despite these advances, conversion of many neurosurgeons to this technology has been limited, due partly to the nature of monocular vision of endoscopes. Monocular endoscopes create a two-dimensional (2D) image that impairs the surgeon's perception of depth, spatial relations, and the size of the anatomical structures.[7,8]

The majority of practicing neurosurgeons were trained to perform transsphenoidal surgery with the aid of a microscope, allowing for binocular vision. Using an endoscope requires surgeons to train their hand–eye coordination to respond to visual cues received by the interaction of the operative instruments within the environment to accurately understand the relative depth of structures in the 2D projection. This leads to steeper learning curves for trainees, such as residents and neurosurgeons, attempting neuroendoscopic procedures.

There is little debate that depth perception is of the utmost importance in many surgeries. Depth perception is thought to be critical to precise motor movement. This has been demonstrated in one study that showed the primary cause of error in laparoscopic surgery is secondary to a visual perceptual illusion.[9] Perhaps the best device would be one that has the capacity of the endoscope to provide a minimally invasive approach to the tumor with a panoramic viewing capacity, yet provides the surgeon with depth perception to judge tumor size and location in reference to surrounding structures. This would more closely mimic direct vision, which remains the gold standard in task completion.[8]

The distinct aspects of the control of fine surgical movements involve initiation of a gross movement in the general desired direction, followed by multiple correctional movements that are modified based on a combination of visual cues.[10] The number of required movements and accuracy of each movement are affected by the clarity of the visual feedback and experience of the surgeon. In endoscopic surgery, tactile cues must be obtained via long instruments. This, combined with 2D visualization, represents a significant barrier to efficient and accurate movements. The acquisition of endoscopic skills inherently involves the ability to translate a 2D image into a mental three-dimensional (3D) representation of a given area. This occurs partially through monocular signals, including variations in color, size, and overlap between the various displayed objects. Trained surgeons also learn to infer spatial relations from haptic cues and surgical movements. Despite these compensatory factors, 2D visualization does not match the depth perception afforded by binocular cues, including vergence, stereopsis, and vertical disparities.[11] Studies of human kinematics have demonstrated the negative consequences of monocular vision, including longer movement times and a tendency to underestimate distances between objects.[12]

Initial studies comparing 2D to 3D in surgical task completion have been performed based on laparoscopic procedures. In using direct vision as a baseline, researchers have found a significant decrease in the "endoscopic handicap" both in novice and experienced surgeons using 3D as compared with 2D endoscopes.[8] Furthermore, even physicians used to 2D surgery are able to complete motor skill tasks faster with binocular vision.[13] Studies have also shown that 3D vision reduces performance time and error rates in surgical tasks for both resident and attending surgeons[7,14] This appears to be more sensitive as tasks increase in complexity.[15] In looking at vascular anastomosis, 3D vision was found to facilitate quicker and more precise movements, reducing surgical times.[16] Other studies have demonstrated a benefit in speed, efficiency, and learn-

* In order to properly view the 3D images in this chapter, please use the glasses included inside the back cover of this book.

ing when using the 3D as compared with the 2D scopes.[7,8,17] These findings of reduced surgical times and improved efficiency have been replicated in a study comparing 2D and 3D endoscopic visualization in a model of endoscopic skull base surgery using a group of practicing skull base surgeons and residents performing surgical tasks designed to simulate the transsphenoidal surgery environment.[18]

Nevertheless, surgeons with significant experience in 2D endoscopic surgery overcome these limitations by using visual and tactile cues. Hence, as demonstrated in other studies, the 3D stereoendoscope makes a more significant difference for novice users.[8,14,17–21] Likewise, several independent laboratories and clinical studies using experienced laparoscopic surgeons reported improved subjective depth perception but failed to identify any difference in task performance using 2D versus 3D visualization.[22–24] Therefore, it is likely that the greatest impact of a 3D stereoendoscope would be in decreasing the learning curve for new users. In fact, experienced 2D endoscope users may actually find the 3D scopes disorienting if they are used to working with 2D scopes. For these reasons, it can be difficult to find any objective significant endpoints when comparing experienced user outcomes between 2D and 3D scopes.

Although stereoendoscopes exist, their use in neurosurgery has been limited based on the larger diameter and poor resolution of earlier generations.[7,8,17] Consequently, only one report exists of using stereoendoscopes in neurosurgery and only as an adjunct to the microscope.[25] It appears that this technology, though slow to enter the mainstream due to some of the limitations described previously, could become the wave of the future for all endoscopic procedures if designed with some minor changes in specifications.

Three-Dimensional Technology

There are several current technologies available that create stereoscopic 3D images. The most widely available is based on dual-channel technology, which incorporates information from two distinct perspectives to render a single 3D view, similar to human vision. Dual-channel video is used by the DaVinci robotic system (Intuitive Surgical, Sunnyvale, CA), in which a dual-channel optical scope is connected to two video cameras to deliver two pictures to the viewer on a stereoscopic display. Another version of this is dual chip-on-the-tip, similarly using a dual-channel video generated by two video chips on a single camera. The main disadvantage that exists with dual-camera technology is related to user side effects, such as fatigue, headache, dizziness, and eye strain, resulting from viewing two images that differ slightly in picture angle, brightness, color, optical distortion, and sharpness.[26] Another method of creating 3D images is by using shutter mechanism. This relies on the principle that the camera is never absolutely still and thus renders a 3D view from slight angle changes created by continuous movement of the camera.

Perhaps the newest technology to enter the 3D medical market is based on "insect-eye" technology. This works by placing a microscopic array of lenses in front of a single video chip on the end of the scope.[26] This technology may have the most promise in neuroendoscopy and has been reported on in nasal and sinus surgery and tested in neurosurgical procedures.[27] The 3D visualization in "insect eye" technology is based on a dual pupil imaging objective and an image sensor coated by an array of microlenses (a plenoptic camera), which functions like a compound "insect eye" (**Fig. 19.1**). The image is created by using a dual pupil objective that splits light into two paths and a single lens that then multiplexes these two paths and focuses them onto an array of microlenses that then focuses the light onto an array of pixels. These data are processed through a single video source to reconstruct a 3D image. The spatial relations are conveyed by the single video chip and charge-coupled device (CCD) incorporated into the endoscope. By generating an image from a single CCD and thus avoiding two separate image sources such as that which dual-camera technologies require, side effects are negated related to ocular strain.

In simple terms, by using a microarray of lenses, the technology creates multiple small images that are then divided into simultaneous left and right images. The viewers' eyes then simultaneously pick up two slightly different images of the same object. This provides a natural stereoscopy, which is the two-eyed ability to judge depth, volume, or distance accurately.

Although the optical resolution of well-designed lenses is generally greater than the resolution of digital image

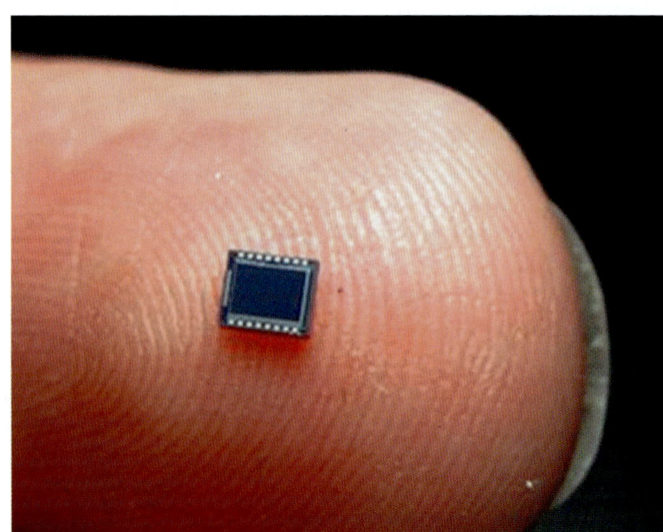

Fig. 19.1 Photograph demonstrating the relative size and construction of the "insect eye" endoscopic lens.

sensors, the plenotopic camera takes advantage of certain limitations inherent in endoscope design that traditionally limit the optical resolution. Endoscopes must have a small lens with a high depth of field and a wide field of view. These constraints limit their resolution by creating a blur spot that cannot be improved regardless of the pixel resolution of the sensor.[28] For this reason, the resolution of the digital 3D plenoptic endoscope can be superior to a 2D endoscope because it is not constrained by the blur spot.

The system currently being used at our institution was created by Visionsense (Petach Tikva, Israel). On this system, the endoscope and camera unit and separate light carrier connect directly to the tower and monitor. The resolution of this camera is 800 × 400 pixels with a refresh rate of 50 frames per second. The depth of field is 15 to 70 mm with a field of view of 70 degrees. The virtual interpupillary distance is 0.8 mm. The images are displayed using a Planar (Beaverton, OR) stereoscopic dual-flatscreen system, which uses a coated mirror to overlay right and left images. Simple polarizing glasses are worn for 3D visualization; the system does not require complex or heavyweight goggles (**Fig. 19.2A**). Furthermore, the endoscope is of similar profile to typical 2D endoscopes and is not more massive or cumbersome to handle (**Fig. 19.2B**). The variance in the image by the lens array allows for a 3D rendering of the displayed object. The system also calculates volumetric information that can be used to create hybrid images with other data sets including radiographic studies.

Previous 3D endoscopes have found little use in nasal surgery due to a variety of technical limitations, namely their large diameter, the lack of angled endoscopes, the decreased resolution compared with 2D endoscopes, and the need to wear 3D glasses that permit 3D sensation at only certain viewing angles and result in eye strain. Recent technologic advances have addressed many of these obstacles. The initial endoscopes created with this technology were designed for use in laparoscopic surgery and have been approved by the Food and Drug Administration for such use. As a result, the endoscopes were available only as 0-degree endoscopes with a diameter of 6.5 mm. With excellent initial results in nasal and sinus surgery, the endoscopes have decreased in size to 4.7 mm and soon to 4.0 mm to rival traditional endoscopes used in the nose.[27] Furthermore, angled endoscopes, specifically 30-degree endoscopes, are now available. Finally, the glasses will soon be replaced by 3D monitors that display the images in 3D space.

Additional studies are ongoing to test the 3D endoscope in neuroendoscopy. To date, this has been performed

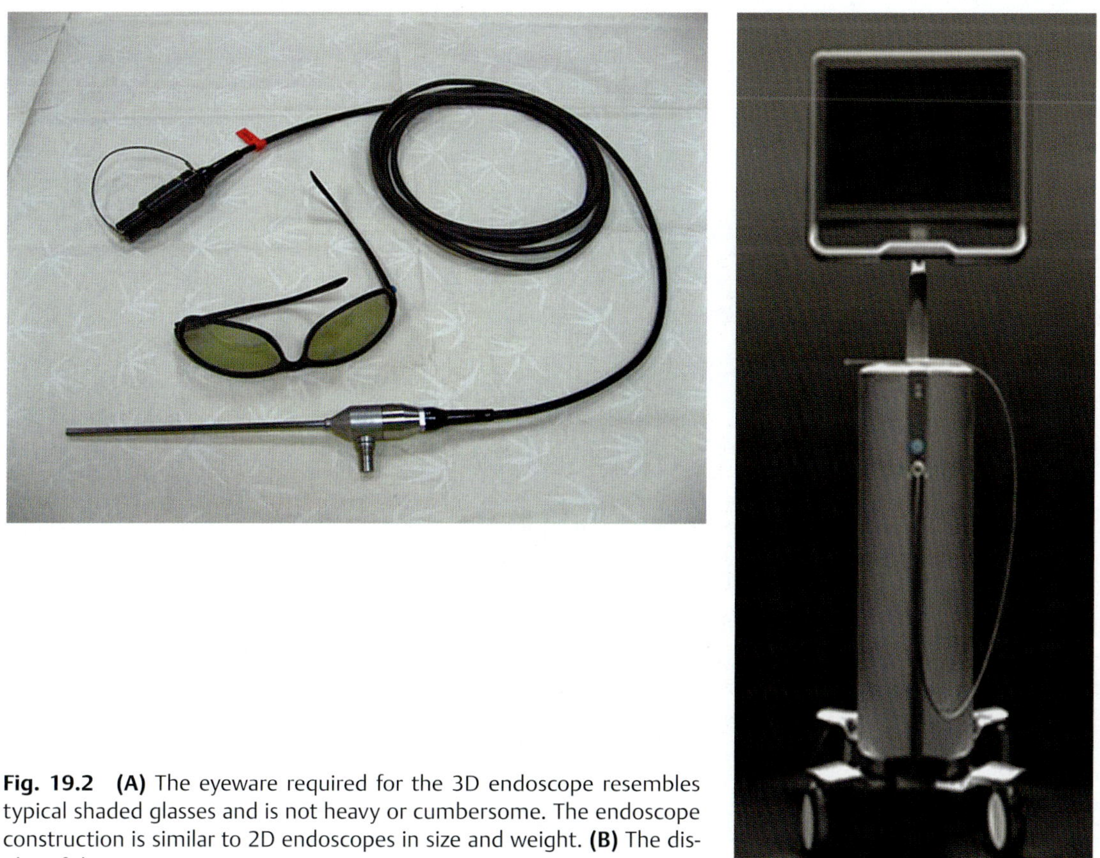

A

B

Fig. 19.2 **(A)** The eyeware required for the 3D endoscope resembles typical shaded glasses and is not heavy or cumbersome. The endoscope construction is similar to 2D endoscopes in size and weight. **(B)** The display of the Visionsense system.

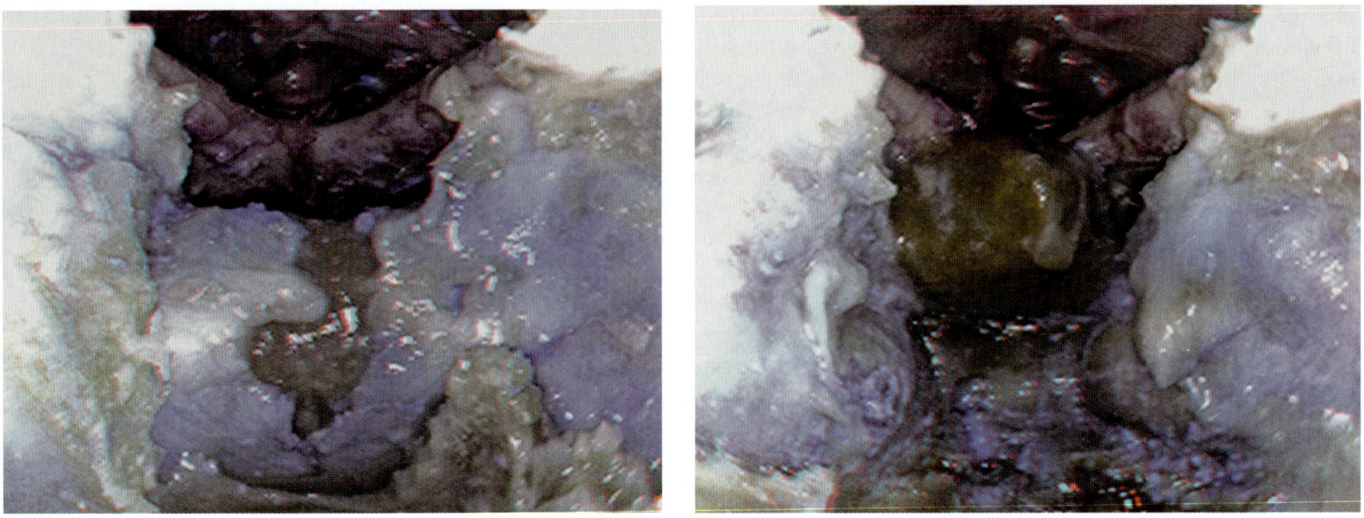

A B

Fig. 19.3 An example of a 3D cadaveric dissection is shown, representing a 3D endoscopic transsphenoidal approach to the pituitary. **(A)** Dissection of the sphenoid sinus to expose the sella with the optic chiasm seen above. **(B)** Removal of the bone of the sella and dura reveals the pituitary and its infundibulum with the optic chiasm above.

successfully in cadavers (**Figs. 19.3** and **19.4**) and in nearly 20 actual cases of pituitary surgery including suprasellar dissection (**Figs. 19.5** and **19.6**).[29,30] The initial results have been promising, with the surgeons who have used the system reporting increased tissue understanding and depth of the lesion. Furthermore, although little advantage appears when transitioning from a 2D endoscope to 3D, when converting back to 2D the surgeons have noticed a significant decrease in visualization. Future studies will help to better define the advantages of systems such as the one created by Visionsense as well as the potential shortcomings.

Future Developments

Perhaps the most exciting potential of 3D vision is the ability to see anatomy that is present but not yet visible (i.e., structures deep to the plane of dissection or lying behind

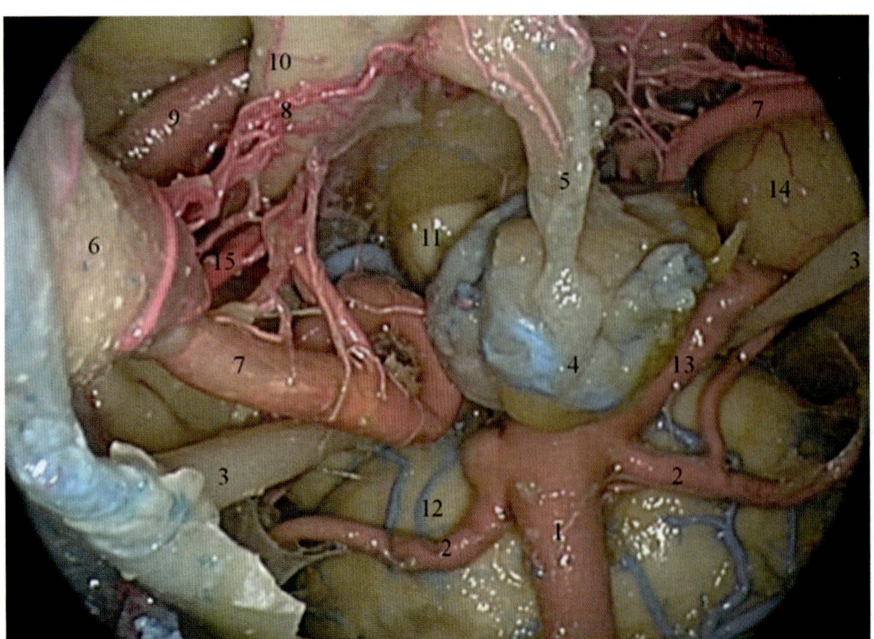

Fig. 19.4 Cadaver dissection with a 2D panoramic picture of the retrosellar/retroclival area. The pituitary gland was dissected from the surrounding dura, and the inferior hypophyseal arteries were cut. Posterior clinoids and upper clivus were drilled. 1, basilar artery (BA); 2, superior cerebellar artery (SCA) (with incidental right SCA aneurysm); 3, cranial nerve III; 4, pituitary gland; 5, pituitary stalk; 6, supraclinoid internal carotid artery (ICA); 7, posterior communicating artery; 8, superior hypophyseal arteries; 9, A1 segment of the anterior cerebellar artery (ACA); 10, optic chiasm and proximal tract; 11, mamillary body; 12, pons; 13, P1 segment of PCA; 14, temporal uncus; 15, anterior choroidal artery.

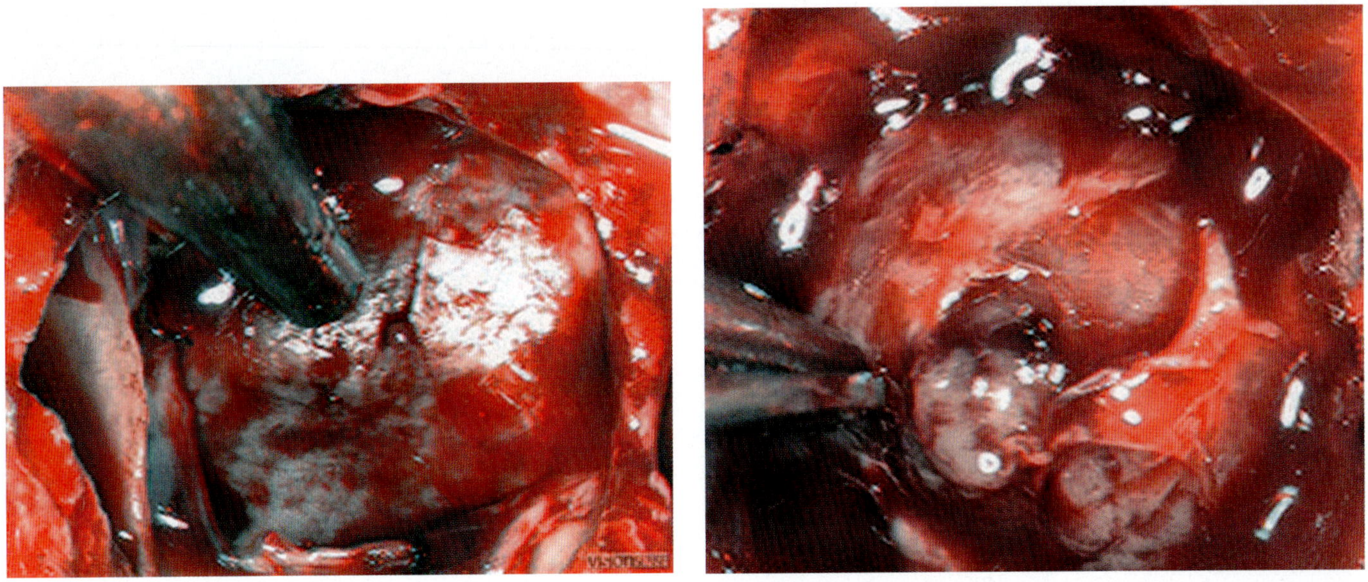

A B

Fig. 19.5 Illustrative case of pituitary adenoma resection. **(A)** The bone of the sella floor is being removed. **(B)** The dura has been incised, and the tumor is herniating through the dural opening.

bone). This would be invaluable in pituitary surgery where critical structures are at potential risk without being in the field of vision. Specifically, knowing where the internal carotid artery, cavernous sinus, and optic nerve are at all times could add an extra level of safety to these procedures. Currently available technology such as image-guided navigation systems and micro-Dopplers can assist in these endeavors. However, the potential exists to be able to see beyond the bone. This would be accomplished by mapping out these structures preoperatively on an image-guided system and then merging this on the monitor, so that the exact location of a structure, such as the internal carotid artery, can be seen in 3D behind the bone. This type of image overlay provided through fusion of endoscopic and neuronavigation technology is currently becoming available and is in its early application to the clinical setting (**Fig. 19.7**). This may allow

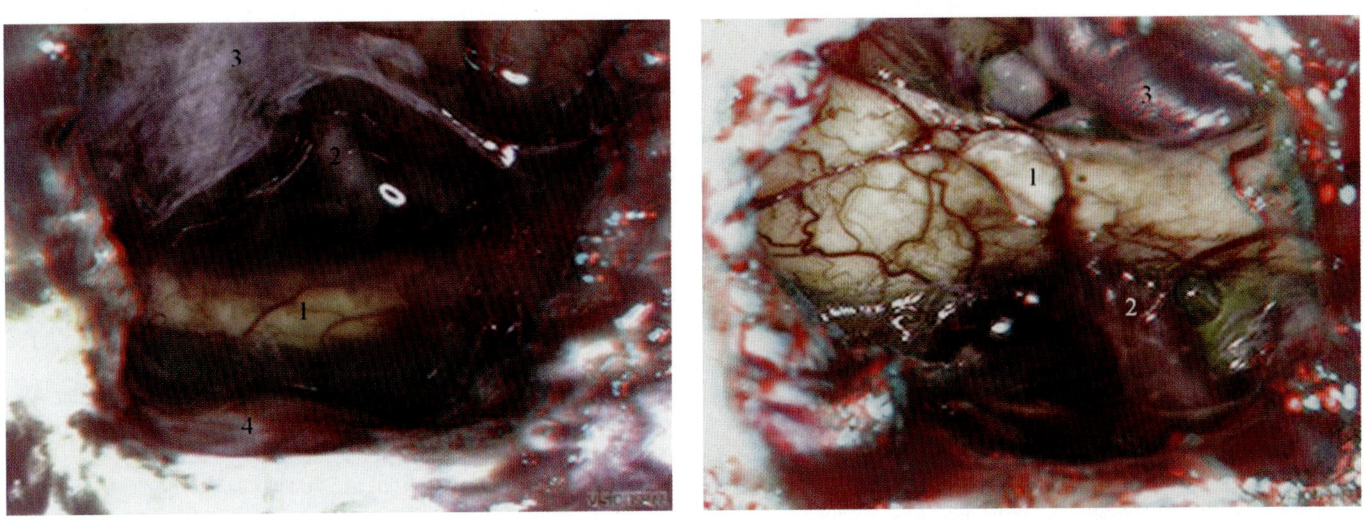

A B

Fig. 19.6 Intraoperative 3D photographs of a patient undergoing an extended transplanum, transtuberculum approach to the suprasellar cistern. **(A)** 1, optic chiasm; 2, anterior communicating artery (ACA) complex; 3, arachnoid over the interhemispheric fissure; 4, diaphragma sella. **(B)** 1, optic chiasm; 2, pituitary stalk and superior hypophyseal arteries; 3, A1 segment of left ACA.

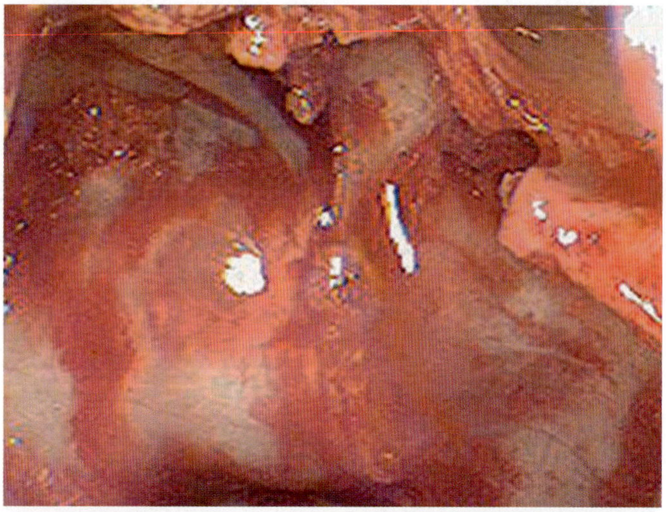

A

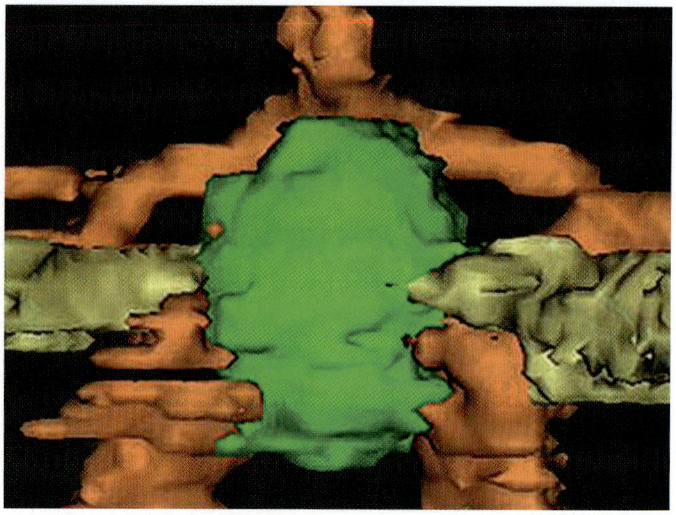

B

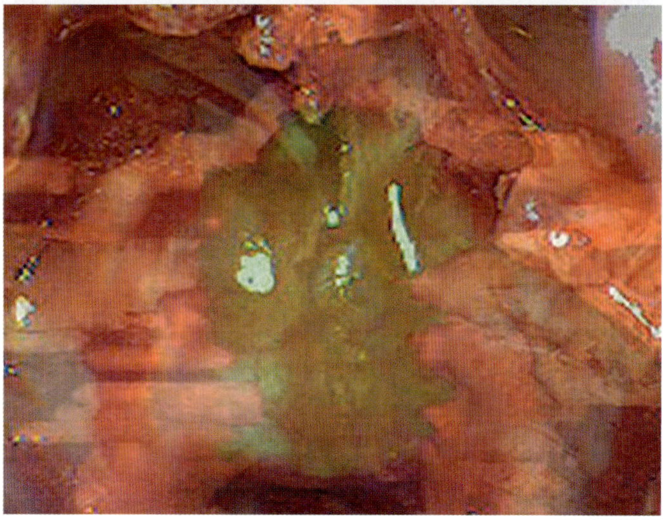

C

Fig. 19.7 Example of 3D and neuronavigation overlay. The 3D endoscopic image **(A)** and the designated object renderings in the neuronavigation software **(B)** (carotid arteries, circle of Willis, and tumor in this case) are combined to form the real-time endoscopic image overlay **(C)**.

surgeons to continue to expand minimally invasive surgery intracranially.

Three-dimensional endoscopy may represent the next technologic frontier in endoscopic anterior skull base and pituitary surgery. The ability to judge depth can only assist in understanding the location of critical structures. Furthermore, it will ultimately allow the surgeon to gain better recognition of the depth of the tumor to obtain a more complete resection. Finally, in addition to improvement in task completion, it will likely decrease the barrier of entry into endoscopy by surgeons used to microscopic binocular vision.

References

1. Tabaee A, Anand VK, Barrón Y, et al. Endoscopic pituitary surgery: a systematic review and meta-analysis. J Neurosurg 2009;111:545–554
2. Cappabianca P, Cavallo LM, Colao A, de Divitiis E. Surgical complications associated with the endoscopic endonasal transsphenoidal approach for pituitary adenomas. J Neurosurg 2002;97:293–298
3. Cappabianca P, Cavallo LM, de Divitiis E. Endoscopic endonasal transsphenoidal surgery. Neurosurgery 2004;55:933–940, discussion 940–941
4. Frank G, Pasquini E, Farneti G, et al. The endoscopic versus the traditional approach in pituitary surgery. Neuroendocrinology 2006;83:240–248
5. Jho HD. Endoscopic transsphenoidal surgery. J Neurooncol 2001;54:187–195
6. Laufer I, Anand VK, Schwartz TH. Endoscopic, endonasal extended transsphenoidal, transplanum transtuberculum approach for resection of suprasellar lesions. J Neurosurg 2007;106:400–406
7. Badani KK, Bhandari A, Tewari A, Menon M. Comparison of two-dimensional and three-dimensional suturing: is there a difference in a robotic surgery setting? J Endourol 2005;19:1212–1215
8. Taffinder N, Smith SG, Huber J, Russell RC, Darzi A. The effect of a second-generation 3D endoscope on the laparoscopic precision of novices and experienced surgeons. Surg Endosc 1999;13:1087–1092
9. Way LW, Stewart L, Gantert W, et al. Causes and prevention of laparoscopic bile duct injuries: analysis of 252 cases from a human factors and cognitive psychology perspective. Ann Surg 2003;237:460–469

10. Chua R, Carson RG, Goodman D, Elliott D. Asymmetries in the spatial localization of transformed targets. Brain Cogn 1992;20:227–235
11. Goodale MA, Meenan JP, Bülthoff HH, Nicolle DA, Murphy KJ, Racicot CI. Separate neural pathways for the visual analysis of object shape in perception and prehension. Curr Biol 1994;4:604–610
12. Servos P, Goodale MA, Jakobson LS. The role of binocular vision in prehension: a kinematic analysis. Vision Res 1992;32:1513–1521
13. Falk V, Mintz D, Grünenfelder J, Fann JI, Burdon TA. Influence of three-dimensional vision on surgical telemanipulator performance. Surg Endosc 2001;15:1282–1288
14. Byrn JC, Schluender S, Divino CM, et al. Three-dimensional imaging improves surgical performance for both novice and experienced operators using the da Vinci Robot System. Am J Surg 2007;193:519–522
15. Birkett DH, Josephs LG, Este-McDonald J. A new 3-D laparoscope in gastrointestinal surgery. Surg Endosc 1994;8:1448–1451
16. Gulbins H, Boehm DH, Reichenspurner H, Arnold M, Ellgass R, Reichart B. 3D-visualization improves the dry-lab coronary anastomoses using the Zeus robotic system. Heart Surg Forum 1999;2:318–324, discussion 324–325
17. Blavier A, Gaudissart Q, Cadière GB, Nyssen AS. Comparison of learning curves and skill transfer between classical and robotic laparoscopy according to the viewing conditions: implications for training. Am J Surg 2007;194:115–121
18. Fraser JF, Allen B, Anand VK, Schwartz TH. Three-dimensional neurostereoendoscopy: subjective and objective comparison to 2D. Minim Invasive Neurosurg 2009;52:25–31
19. Perez-Cruet MJ, Foley KT, Isaacs RE, et al. Microendoscopic lumbar discectomy: technical note. Neurosurgery 2002;51(5, Suppl):S129–S136
20. Sidhu RS, Tompa D, Jang R, et al. Interpretation of three-dimensional structure from two-dimensional endovascular images: implications for educators in vascular surgery. J Vasc Surg 2004;39:1305–1311
21. Votanopoulos K, Brunicardi FC, Thornby J, Bellows CF. Impact of three-dimensional vision in laparoscopic training. World J Surg 2008;32:110–118
22. Chan AC, Chung SC, Yim AP, Lau JY, Ng EK, Li AK. Comparison of two-dimensional vs three-dimensional camera systems in laparoscopic surgery. Surg Endosc 1997;11:438–440
23. Hanna GB, Shimi SM, Cuschieri A. Randomised study of influence of two-dimensional versus three-dimensional imaging on performance of laparoscopic cholecystectomy. Lancet 1998;351:248–251
24. McDougall EM, Soble JJ, Wolf JS Jr, Nakada SY, Elashry OM, Clayman RV. Comparison of three-dimensional and two-dimensional laparoscopic video systems. J Endourol 1996;10:371–374
25. Chen JC, Levy ML, Corber Z, Assifi MM. Concurrent three dimensional neuroendoscopy: initial descriptions of application to clinical practice. Neurosurg Focus 1999;6:e12
26. Szold A. Seeing is believing: visualization systems in endoscopic surgery (video, HDTV, stereoscopy, and beyond). Surg Endosc 2005;19:730–733
27. Brown SM, Tabaee A, Singh A, Schwartz TH, Anand VK. Three-dimensional endoscopic sinus surgery: feasibility and technical aspects. Otolaryngol Head Neck Surg 2008;138:400–402
28. Yaron A, Shechterman M, Horesh N. Blur spot limitations in distal endoscope sensors. In: Stereoscopic Displays and Virtual Reality Systems XIII. SPIE–International Society for Optical Engine San Jose, CA: 2006
29. Roth J, Singh A, Nyquist G, et al. Three-dimensional and 2-dimensional endoscopic exposure of midline cranial base targets using expanded endonasal and transcranial approaches. Neurosurgery 2009;65:1116–1128, discussion 1128–1130
30. Tabaee A, Anand VK, Fraser JF, Brown SM, Singh A, Schwartz TH. Three-dimensional endoscopic pituitary surgery. Neurosurgery 2009;64(5, Suppl 2):288–293, discussion 294–295

20 Endoscope-Assisted Transsphenoidal Surgery

Joshua R. Dusick, Manoel de Paiva Neto, Nasrin Fatemi, and Daniel F. Kelly

The direct endonasal transsphenoidal approach for removal of pituitary adenomas was described over two decades ago.[1,2] Although initially a technique performed solely with the operating microscope, in recent years this approach has been increasingly performed with endoscopy either as the sole source of visualization or as providing assistance. The panoramic vision provided by the endoscope allows one to visualize and access parasellar areas not possible with the operating microscope. Effective endoscopic assistance in endonasal pituitary adenoma removal can translate into a more complete tumor removal in a widened sella, the cavernous sinus, and the suprasellar space. This chapter describes the technique of endoscopic-assisted endonasal pituitary surgery and methods of complication avoidance.

Transsphenoidal surgery emerged into the microsurgical era in the early 1970s with the advent of the operating microscope[3,4] and the technique of selective adenomectomy as described by Hardy.[5] Additional experience by many in the 1970s and early 1980s further improved the safety and efficacy of transsphenoidal surgery.[6–14] Griffith and Veerapen[2] in 1987 and Cooke and Jones[1] in 1994 subsequently described the direct endonasal approach, which minimizes patient discomfort associated with the sublabial approach.[1–3,15–19] This approach, which requires minimal posterior nasal mucosal dissection and no turbinate removal, is now commonly used with the operating microscope and endoscopic assistance.[1,2,20–27] Advances in the technique have resulted largely from better instrumentation, surgical navigation, and, most importantly, endoscopy.[28–32] The expanded visualization provided by the endoscope enables the surgeon to see into areas of the parasellar space that are not possible to see with the tunnel vision of the operating microscope. Regardless of the technique used, the surgical goal for patients with pituitary adenomas should be a selective adenomectomy with preservation or improvement of pituitary gland function. This goal is best achieved by performing a wide and tall sphenoidotomy and complete sellar bony opening to maximize sellar exposure and instrument maneuverability.[33] Herein we provide a technical description of the direct endonasal approach with the operating microscope and endoscope assistance for removal of pituitary adenomas.

Surgical Technique

Patient Preparation

Endonasal pituitary surgery is performed as originally described by Griffith and Veerapen[2] with additional modifications as described below and in our recent publications.[2,26,27,34,35] Preoperative antibiotics (typically cefazolin) are given and continued for 24 hours. In patients with normal preoperative adrenal function or those with Cushing's disease, no preoperative glucocorticoids are administered.[36] Those with adrenal insufficiency or borderline adrenal function are given 100 mg of intravenous hydrocortisone.

Patient Positioning and Room Setup

The endotracheal tube emerges from the left corner of the mouth, and anesthesia equipment is positioned on the left side of the patient. An arterial line and Foley catheter are placed. The patient is placed supine with the head resting freely in the horseshoe head-holder and angled approximately 30 degrees toward the left shoulder as originally described by Laws,[37] which allows the surgeon to stand comfortably on the patient's right side. The patient's head is typically inclined in a neutral plane (0 degrees) relative to the floor for most pituitary adenomas. For lesions with marked suprasellar extension, 10 to 15 degrees of neck extension is used. The nostrils and the perinasal and right lower abdominal areas are prepped and draped in standard fashion. Topical or injected mucosal decongestants are not used.

Surgical Navigation

Surgical navigation for trajectory guidance is recommended for all endonasal transsphenoidal surgeries, unless one is highly experienced with the approach. For most patients with a pituitary adenoma, C-arm fluoroscopy is simple and effective for giving excellent trajectory guidance in the sagittal plane. Frameless stereotactic surgical navigation based on either a preoperative magnetic resonance imaging (MRI) or computed tomography (CT) scan provides significantly more data than fluoroscopy. It is particularly helpful in patients with prior surgery or large invasive tumors with markedly distorted anatomical landmarks. If fluoroscopy is used, the base of the operating microscope is placed just outside the arc of the C-arm above the patient's head, with the microscope to the patient's right side.

Endoscopic Equipment and Setup

The endoscope video monitor and tower are placed above the patient's head on the patient's left side to allow for comfortable viewing by the surgeon and the assistant who will be standing on the patient's right side. Standard 4-mm rigid endoscopes (18 cm long) with 0-, 30-, and 45-degree angled lenses should be available. An endoscope holder, which is often helpful, can also be positioned with the insertion device fixed to the leftmost cephalad aspect of the operating table.

Surgical Instrumentation

Given the narrow working space of the endonasal approach, all instruments should be as low profile as possible with angled or bayoneted handles to minimize visual obstruction and to maximize instrument maneuverability. For example, Cottle dissectors, microdissectors, ring curettes, and microblades are on bayoneted handles, whereas microscissors and tumor forceps are of a single-shaft pistol-grip construction to minimize visual obstruction. High-speed drills and ultrasonic aspirators are also of the lowest possible diameter with angled hand-pieces. A micro-Doppler probe is also used for all cases to localize the cavernous carotid arteries prior to dural opening.[29] Short (60- to 70-mm) endonasal speculums also enhance maneuverability and increase exposure compared with longer speculums as shown in **Fig. 20.1**.[30]

Nasal Approach and Sphenoidotomy

The initial portion of the procedure is performed with the operating microscope and a handheld speculum. The nostril chosen for the approach is based largely on tumor location as defined by the patient's preoperative MRI. For tumors projecting more to one side of the sella, the contralateral nostril is used, given that exposure across the midline to the contralateral sella and cavernous sinus (CS) area is consistently wider than to the ipsilateral side. This rule also applies in the great majority of patients with septal deviations. In patients with relatively midline tumors, the right nostril is used, given that the surgeon stands on the patient's right side, and this affords a more comfortable operating position. A relaxing alar incision, although used occasionally early in our experience to accommodate the endonasal speculum, has not been used in more than 550 cases given the availability of smaller and thinner speculums.

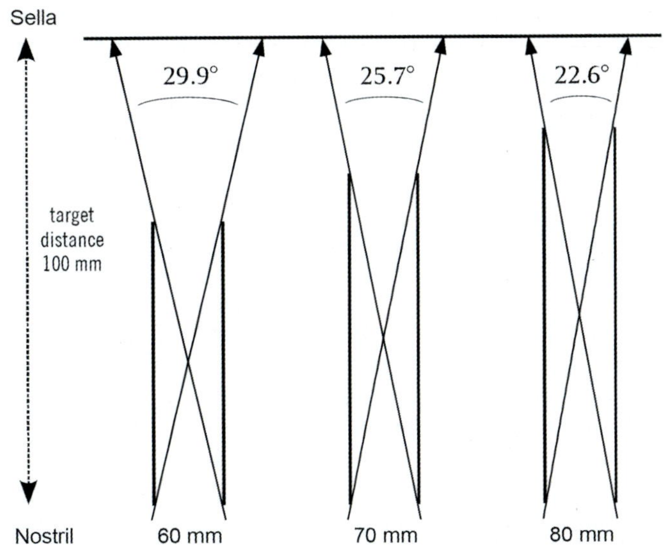

Fig. 20.1 Line drawings comparing the 60-mm, 70-mm, and 80-mm speculums depicted as parallel lines with 16 mm proximal and distal openings and a target distance of 100 mm from the nostril to the sellar target. Note the increase in the angle of exposure for the 60-mm speculum. The width of exposure at the 100-mm target is 37 mm for the 60-mm speculum compared with 30 mm for the 70-mm speculum and 24 mm for the 80-mm speculum. (From Fatemi N, Dusick JR, Malkasian D, et al. Instrumentation assessment: short trapezoidal speculums for suprasellar and infrasellar exposure in endonasal transsphenoidal surgery. Neurosurgery 2008;62(5 Suppl 2):ONS325–329; discussion ONS329–330. Reprinted with permission.)

The handheld speculum is passed into the anterior nostril to identify the inferior and middle turbinates. The speculum is then gently passed along the trajectory of the middle turbinate with care being taken to minimize trauma to the anterior and midnasal septum and turbinates. The speculum blades gently displace the middle turbinate laterally and pass further into the nasal cavity to expose the junction of the keel of the sphenoid and the posterior nasal septum. After confirming the correct trajectory to the sella with fluoroscopy or surgical navigation, the posterior septal mucosa is cauterized with a bipolar cautery in a vertical swath, and a vertical mucosal incision of approximately 2 cm is made with a Cottle elevator. The mucosa is reflected laterally to expose the midline sphenoid keel and ipsilateral sphenoid ostium, which is typically superolateral to the equator of the keel at the 10 o'clock or 2 o'clock positions. The posterior nasal septum is then displaced off the midline by the distal tips of the handheld speculum to allow exposure of the contralateral side of the keel and the contralateral ostium. The Cottle elevator can also be used to further reflect this contralateral mucosa.

After the sphenoid keel and ostia are exposed, the handheld speculum is replaced by a self-retaining endonasal speculum, typically 60 to 70 mm long (Mizuho America, Beverly,

MA).[30] The distal speculum blades should straddle the sphenoid keel, with the ostia visualized bilaterally, and the nasal end of the speculum should be flush with the nostril. If the ostia are seen higher than the 10 o'clock and 2 o'clock positions, the speculum trajectory is likely to be too far inferior and should be re-angled more superiorly and confirmed with fluoroscopy or surgical navigation. The added exposure from the use of a shorter speculum is shown in **Fig. 20.1.**

A wide and tall sphenoidotomy is next performed with pituitary and Kerrison rongeurs. Sphenoid bone and mucosal removal should extend beyond the lateral edges of the ostia bilaterally and allow visualization of the tuberculum sella and sellar floor. To maximize maneuverability of instruments during the endoscopic phase of the procedure (described below), removing bone up close to the ethmoid roof and down to a level flush with the floor of the sphenoid sinus is recommended. As we have recently shown, a smaller and less complete sphenoidotomy will otherwise restrict maneuverability and visualization and has been associated with incomplete tumor removal (**Fig. 20.2**).[33]

Because the sphenopalatine arteries run in the posterior inferior nasal mucosa at approximately the 8 o'clock and 4 o'clock positions, it is best to displace this mucosa laterally with the speculum or to cauterize it prior to removing it to avoid injuring the vessels with the rongeurs. This bleeding, however, can be stopped relatively easily with bipolar or monopolar cautery.

Sellar Bony Opening and Carotid Localization

After the sphenoidotomy, the sellar face is identified and the operative view of intrasphenoidal bony septations should be correlated with those septations seen on the patient's preoperative MRI. Septations ending on the sellar face are removed with a rongeur down to the sella; those that end over a carotid artery should be removed with care, and excessive torquing of the bone fragments should be avoided. Mucosa over the sella is removed, but sphenoid sinus mucosa in the lateral aspects and roof of the sphenoid sinus can be left undisturbed. The sellar bone is then removed from CS to CS and from the sellar floor inferiorly to the tuberculum sella superiorly with a Kerrison rongeur or in some instances with a high-speed diamond bit drill. In patients with large invasive tumors, the sellar bone may be markedly thinned or absent and tumor may be directly under the mucosa or under an attenuated or absent sellar dura.

After the sellar bone removal and before dural opening, a micro-Doppler probe is used to localize the cavernous carotid arteries (10-MHz ES-100X MiniDop with NRP-10H bayonet probe [Koven, St. Louis, MO] or 20-MHz Surgical Doppler [Mizuho America]). As previously described and

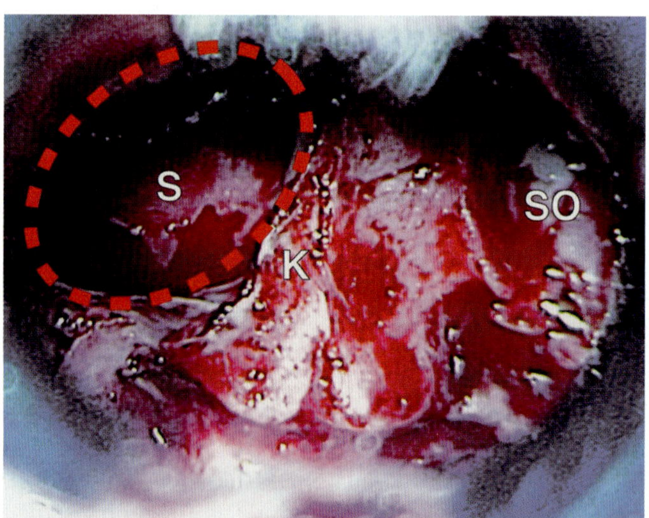

A

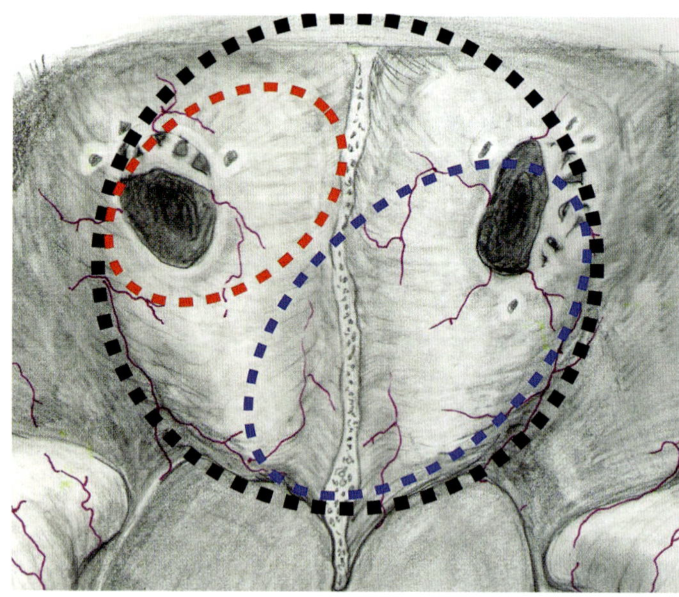
B

Fig. 20.2 **(A)** Intraoperative photograph of the sphenoid keel in a patient with prior endonasal surgery showing that at the original surgery, only bone to the right of the keel had been removed, whereas the midline keel and left half of sphenoid bone and sphenoid ostium were left intact. K, sphenoid keel; S, prior opening into sphenoid sinus; SO, sphenoid ostium. **(B)** Drawing of variations on the restricted sphenoid keel openings seen at reoperation shown as shaded circles and ovals. The *red oval* represents the extent of bone removal in the patient in **A**, whereas the *blue oval* demonstrates an example of other openings seen previously. The *black circle* indicates the optimal bony removal of the sphenoid keel to provide maximal exposure into the sphenoid sinusfi. (From Mattozo CA, Dusick JR, Esposito F, et al. Suboptimal sphenoid and sellar exposure: a consistent finding in patients treated with repeat transsphenoidal surgery for residual endocrine-inactive macroadenomas. Neurosurgery 2006;58:857–865. Reprinted with permission.)

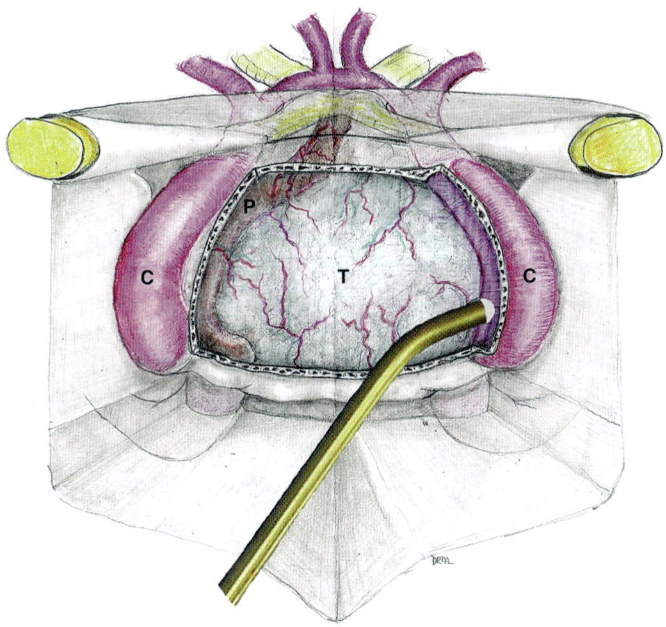

Fig. 20.3 Illustration depicting a view of the sella containing a macroadenoma as seen from a right endonasal approach. The sellar bone has been removed and, as is often the case, the contralateral bone removal on the left is somewhat more extensive than on the right, leaving the medial edge of the left cavernous internal carotid artery (ICA) exposed. The micro-Doppler probe is being used to localize the left cavernous ICA and to guide the appropriate location for dural opening. C, cavernous ICA; P, pituitary gland; T, tumor. (From Dusick JR, Esposito F, Malkasian D, Kelly DF. Avoidance of carotid artery injuries in transsphenoidal surgery with the Doppler probe and micro-hook blades. Neurosurgery 2007;60(4, Suppl 2)322–328, discussion 328–329. Reprinted with permission.)

shown in **Fig. 20.3**, the probe is placed initially at the edge of the bony opening at 90 degrees to the dura.[29] If only faint or no audible flow is present, the probe is angled more laterally under the bone edge. In most patients, this angulation results in the carotid flow becoming louder. The probe is then moved superiorly and inferiorly to further determine the carotid course. Typically, the carotids have their most medial course superiorly near the tuberculum sella just before they pass through the dural ring to enter the subarachnoid space. If no flow is evident, then additional bone can be removed laterally to enlarge sellar exposure. If audible flow is still absent, consideration should be given to whether the probe is malfunctioning, which can occur on occasion.

Dural Opening and Tumor Removal

The sellar dural opening is performed with a straight microblade (Mizuho America) in a U-shaped fashion, avoiding the area of greatest audible Doppler flow.[29] An attempt should be made not to transgress the pituitary gland or adenoma with the initial dural opening. After the initial opening, angled microdissectors are used to separate the dura from the underlying tumor and pituitary gland. As shown in **Fig. 20.4**, the dural opening is then enlarged superiorly, inferiorly, and laterally as needed with the use of angled microhook blades or curved microscissors that allow the blade's cutting force to be directed away from the sellar and CS structures.[29] Care should be taken in extending the dural opening too far superiorly in patients with microadenomas who often have a shallow sella and low-lying diaphragma sella; such an opening can result in an early cerebrospinal fluid (CSF) leak. Laterally, the opening should generally extend to within 1 to 2 mm of the medial wall of the CS. Low-pressure CS venous bleeding can generally be easily controlled using hemostatic agents such as Surgifoam (Ethicon; Johnson & Johnson, Piscataway, NJ) or Gelfoam (Pfizer, Brooklyn, NY) and applying gentle pressure with a cottonoid.

Selective adenomectomy with preservation of normal gland function should be the surgical goal. In some patients with grossly invasive adenomas, for example, into the CS, an effective debulking with decompression of the optic apparatus and complete intrasellar adenoma removal is a reasonable and prudent goal. As discussed further below, with endoscopic assistance it is often possible to remove

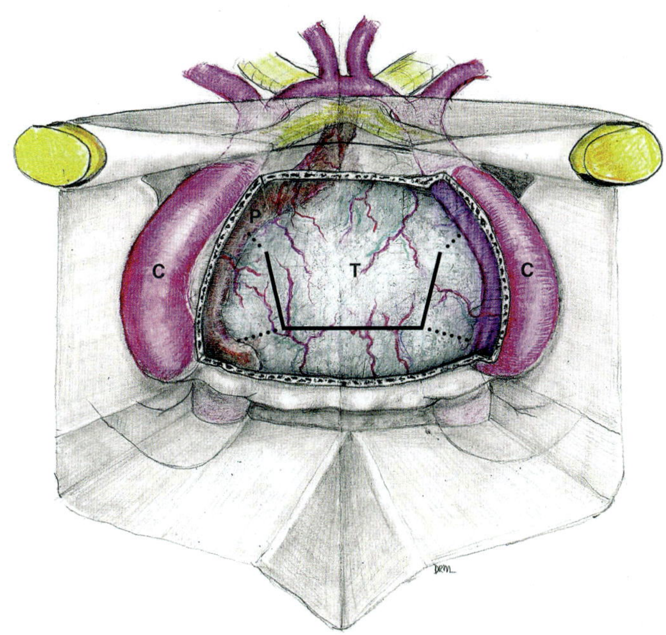

Fig. 20.4 Illustration demonstrating the initial sellar dural opening in a U-shaped fashion (*solid line*) which is performed with a straight microblade as shown in **Fig. 20.5**, and the subsequent lateral dural openings (*dashed lines*) that may be used for additional exposure, which should be performed with a right-angled microhook blade or angled microscissors. C, cavernous internal carotid artery; P, pituitary gland; T, tumor. (From Dusick JR, Esposito F, Malkasian D, Kelly DF. Avoidance of carotid artery injuries in transsphenoidal surgery with the Doppler probe and micro-hook blades. Neurosurgery 2007;60(4, Suppl 2)322–328, discussion 328–329. Reprinted with permission.)

additional tumor beyond that obtainable with the operating microscope alone, particularly tumor with CS invasion as well as fibrous or rubbery tumors with suprasellar extension.

In many instances, the tumor pseudocapsule can be identified and a plane established between the adenoma and normal gland. Using microdissectors, irrigation, and gentle traction on the pseudocapsule, such adenomas can often be removed completely with preservation of the pseudocapsule, as described by Oldfield et al.[38] However, many large macroadenomas are soft and require initial internal debulking with ring curettes and suction. Next, the tumor "rind" with an intact pseudocapsule can often be gently separated away from the normal gland and diaphragma sellae. For firm or rubbery adenomas, initial debulking with curved and straight pistol-grip microscissors may be needed. Adenomas with suprasellar extension should be debulked inferiorly first, followed by removal of the suprasellar component, which allows the suprasellar tumor to deliver itself from above and may minimize the chances of causing an early CSF leak. For large macroadenomas, it is essential to confirm the descent of the diaphragma sellae as an indication that a complete tumor removal has been accomplished. Probing the folds of the diaphragma with up-angled ring curettes will help dislodge residual tumor remnants. To further encourage downward descent of the suprasellar tumor, the anesthesiologist can induce a Valsalva maneuver to transiently increase intracranial pressure.

For tumors with CS invasion, one should attempt to visualize the medial CS wall. A microscopic view of the CS contralateral to the nostril of approach can often be achieved. However, such visualization typically requires use of a short (60- to 70-mm) endonasal speculum.[30] To gain full advantage of this speculum, 1 to 2 cm of the posterior nasal septum should be removed, the sphenoidotomy should be widened on the contralateral side, and adequate contralateral sellar bone must be removed.

In some instances, what appeared to be CS invasion on MRI may only be tumor compression of the medial CS wall.[39,40] However, often, after the sellar adenoma has been removed, a defect in the medial CS wall is visualized. Tumor in the medial CS can often be removed or effectively debulked using gentle suction and angled ring curettes. Given the potential for injury to the cavernous carotid and the abducens nerve lateral to the carotid, aggressive removal or grasping of tumor along or lateral to the carotid artery should be minimized.

Endoscopic Assistance to Maximize Tumor Removal

Once tumor removal is as complete as possible with the microscope, the 0-, 30-, and 45-degree angled endoscopes can be used to search for residual tumor. This endoscopic look is particularly important in patients with macroadenomas extending into the CS and in those with suprasellar extension when the diaphragma sellae or a thin rim or normal pituitary gland has not descended fully into the sella. In the majority of such cases, the endoscope will reveal additional suprasellar tumor hindering a full descent of the diaphragma. If residual tumor is visualized, one can attempt to remove it under microscopic visualization with angled ring curettes. However, it is typically more effective to perform such tumor removal under endoscopic visualization using angled suctions and tumor-grasping forceps or ring curettes. Tumor removal from the medial CS can also be accomplished under direct visualization in similar fashion using a 30- or 45-degree angled lens. As discussed in Case 3, later, endoscopy in this setting typically allows tumor removal in these areas that was not visualized or was inaccessible with the tunnel vision of the operating microscope. This removal is often best facilitated by using a three-hand technique in which the assistant holds and drives the endoscope and the surgeon holds the suction and a ring curette or tumor-grasping forceps. Alternatively, one can use the endoscope holder as the third hand, but this provides less maneuverability and slows the change of position otherwise possible with an assistant. Finally, to maximize maneuverability of the endoscope and to minimize instrument congestion within the nasal cavity, the endonasal speculum can be removed. This removal also allows a bi-nostril approach. In most instances, this bi-nostril approach requires making an opening in the contralateral posterior nasal mucosa over the previously performed sphenoidotomy to allow easy passage of the instruments into the sphenoid sinus.

Intrasellar Hemostasis

After tumor removal, hemostasis is obtained with Surgifoam and full-strength hydrogen peroxide. The peroxide can be irrigated directly into the sphenoid sinus and sella for up to 5 minutes. Its use appears to be safe in terms of pituitary hormonal function, as we have recently demonstrated, and it may have additional tumoricidal effects on residual microscopic foci of adenoma.[41] However, it should not be used if there is a large diaphragmatic defect that would allow it to track into the subarachnoid space. In cases in which there is persistent oozing, one should further inspect the sella with the endoscope to look for residual tumor.

Sellar Reconstruction and Cerebrospinal Fluid Leak Repair

As previously described,[42] sellar reconstruction is performed with microscopic visualization and tailored to the size of the CSF leak and dural defect. Prior to reconstruction, the size of the diaphragmatic defect is assessed. If no obvious CSF leak is seen, a Valsalva maneuver is induced to help visualize an occult or small (grade 1) CSF leak emanating through a small diaphragmatic defect. All repairs involve use of collagen sponge (Duragen, Helistat, or Instat) as part of the repair as a scaffolding for fibroblast in-growth.[43–46] In patients with no CSF leak (grade 0), a single layer of minimally moistened collagen sponge placed over the exposed diaphragma sellae, pituitary gland, and sellar dura is typically used as the only repair material. For most small (grade 1) CSF leaks, the repair includes intrasellar collagen sponge with an intrasellar, extradural buttress of titanium mesh or Medpor TSI (Transsphenoidal Sellar Implant; Porex Corp., Fairburn, GA) and a second layer of collagen placed over the buttress and adjacent sellar and sphenoid bone. The repair can be further reinforced and held in position with a small amount of tissue glue. For grade 2 CSF leaks or grade 1 leaks with a large intrasellar dead space, an intrasellar abdominal fat graft is placed followed by a layer of collagen sponge and a buttress of titanium mesh or Medpor placed in the intrasellar extradural space. Additional fat is placed over the sella followed by another layer of collagen; the construct is held in position with tissue glue such as DuraSeal (Confluent Surgical, Waltham, MA). In some recent cases of grade 1 and 2 leaks, no buttress has been used and instead the repair with collagen sponge, with or without a fat graft, has been reinforced only with tissue glue. Such patients can also be placed on Diamox (acetazolamide) 250 mg every 8 hours for 48 hours after surgery to diminish CSF production. To further assess the adequacy of the repair, prior to placing tissue glue, the anesthesiologist is asked to perform a Valsalva maneuver to raise the patient's intracranial pressure; if either movement of the buttress or significant leakage of CSF is observed, the repair should be revised.

For the large (grade 3) defects, typically seen with extended suprasellar approaches, the repair is similar to a grade 2 repair with the addition of a lumbar drain for CSF diversion for 48 hours. Grade 3 leaks, however, are uncommon after adenoma removal unless the tumor is extensively invasive above the diaphragma sellae. It is important to note that tissue glue in this repair paradigm is not for stopping egress of CSF per se, but to prevent migration of the repair materials (fat and collagen) away from the sella.[42]

Nasal Closure

Once sellar reconstruction is complete, the speculum is removed and the handheld speculum is used to explore both nasal cavities bilaterally. In most cases, there may be mild venous oozing from along the nasal septum, inferior turbinate, or middle turbinate, which can be controlled with Surgifoam or bipolar cautery. Nasal hemostasis should be relatively complete to minimize blood being swallowed during the first few hours after surgery, which can lead to nausea and vomiting. The middle turbinate on the side of the approach, which is out-fractured by the speculum at the start of the procedure, is medialized to minimize chances of a postoperative maxillary sinus mucocele. Finally, using the handheld speculum, the nasal septum is returned to the midline. Nasal packing is not used; a small gauze dressing is placed over the nostrils. To minimize nasal epistaxis or intrasellar bleeding, excessive coughing or "bucking" on the endotracheal tube should be avoided during extubation, and blood pressure should be carefully controlled in the early postoperative period.

Postoperative Care

Postoperatively, most patients undergoing adenoma removal do not require intensive care unit admission and are admitted instead to a regular ward. For the first postoperative night, patients are given a humidified face tent and decongestants are available. Saline nasal spray is provided for a week after surgery and used based on patient preference. The Foley catheter is removed the morning of postoperative day 1, and patients are ambulated. All patients are followed in-hospital by an endocrinologist and are monitored for diabetes insipidus based on urine output and urine specific gravity. Adrenal function is monitored by measuring morning serum cortisol and adrenocorticotropic hormone (ACTH) levels on the mornings of postoperative days 1 and 2. For patients with acromegaly, a prolactinoma, or Cushing's disease, growth hormone, prolactin, and cortisol/ACTH levels are followed on postoperative days 1 and 2 to document early remission based on subnormal hormone levels.[27,35] Most patients are discharged on postoperative day 2 and have a serum sodium level checked on postoperative day 4 or 5 to assess for hyponatremia.[47,48] The first postoperative visit is within 2 to 3 weeks of surgery, and a follow-up visit occurs 3 months after surgery, including a complete pituitary hormonal evaluation. An early postoperative MRI or CT scan is typically performed within 2 days of surgery for patients with macroadenomas or other larger tumors, and a follow-up MRI is usually performed at 3 months after surgery.

Illustrative Cases

Case 1: Adrenocorticotropic Hormone–Secreting Microadenoma

A 52-year-old man with a 5-year history of hypertension and weight gain was diagnosed with Cushing's disease based on elevated 24-hour urinary free cortisols, elevated serum ACTH and cortisols, and petrosal sinus sampling with corticotropin-releasing hormone stimulation. His pituitary MRI showed a 3- × 6-mm hypoenhancing lesion in the central and left inferior aspect of the pituitary gland. He underwent endonasal selective adenomectomy. His postoperative day 1 serum cortisol level was unmeasurable, and he remains in remission on glucocorticoid replacement therapy 8 months after surgery (**Fig. 20.5**).

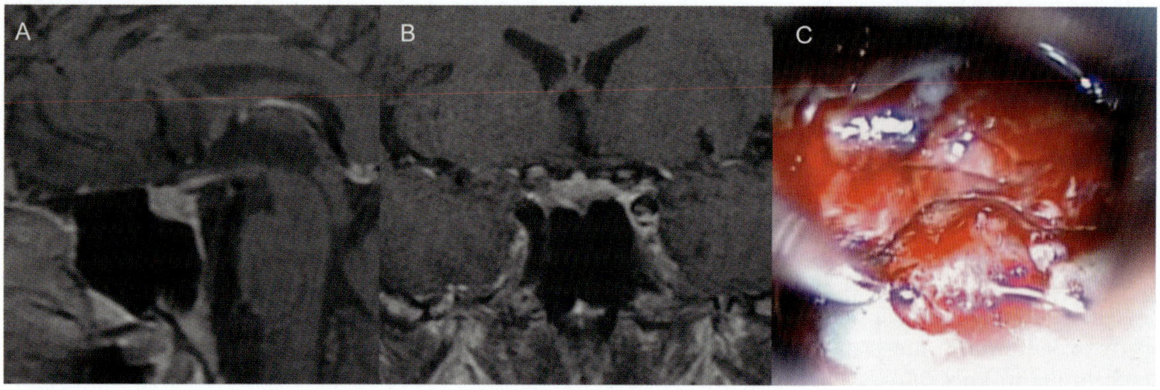

Fig. 20.5 Case 1. Preoperative sagittal **(A)** and coronal **(B)** postgadolinium sellar magnetic resonance imaging showing a 3- × 6-mm hypoenhancing inferior central and left-sided microadenoma. **(C)** Microscopic view of the resection cavity after a total tumor removal.

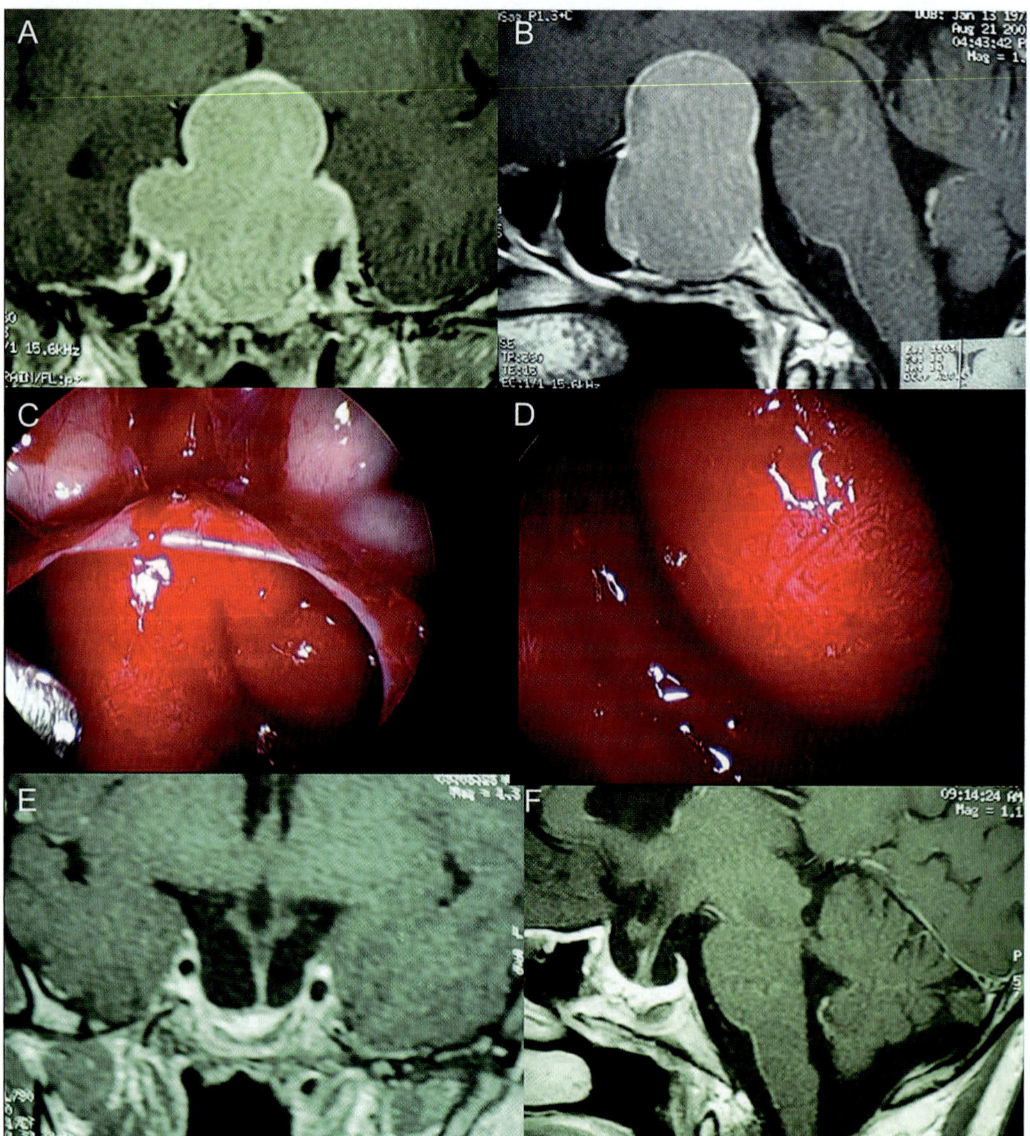

Fig. 20.6 Case 2. Preoperative coronal **(A)** and sagittal **(B)** postgadolinium sellar MRI showing a 4- × 5-cm cystic and solid sellar mass with marked suprasellar extension, chiasmal compression, and gland compression and elevation. **(C)** Endoscopic inspection after microscopic tumor removal with a 0-degree lens showing the inversion of the diaphragma sellae. **(D)** Endoscopic inspection of the right sellar space with a 30-degree endoscope. Coronal **(E)** and sagittal **(F)** postgadolinium MRI showing total tumor removal 4 months after surgery.

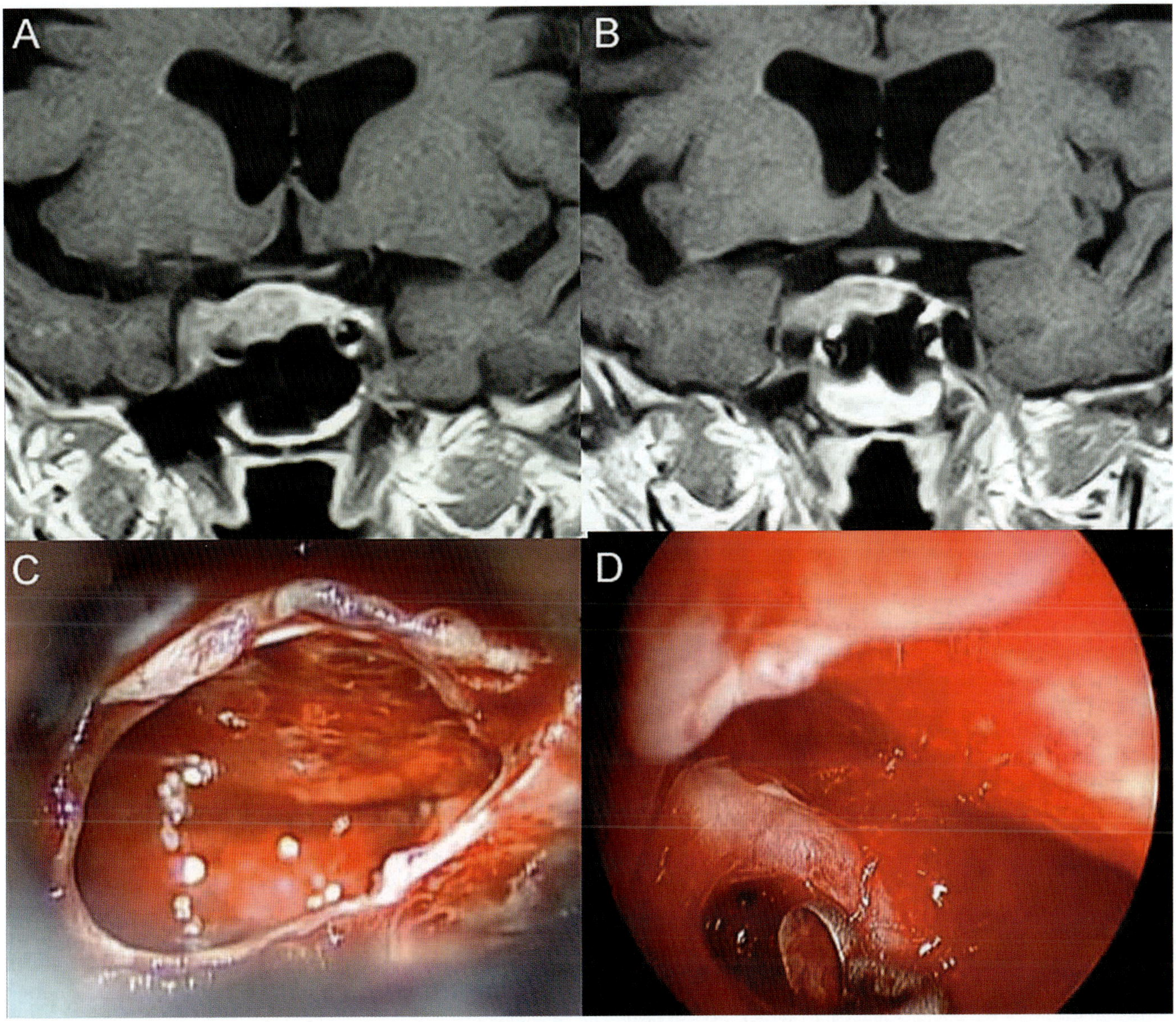

Fig. 20.7 Case 3. **(A,B)** Preoperative coronal postgadolinium views showing invasive macroadenoma with right CS invasion and normal gland compression to left and superiorly. **(C)** Microscopic intraoperative view of the sella after sellar tumor resection. **(D)** Endoscopic view (30-degree lenses) of a right cavernous sinus wall defect and additional tumor resection using ring curettes.

Case 2: Giant Endocrine-Inactive Macroadenoma with Apoplexy

A 34-year-old woman developed abrupt left vision decline during pregnancy that worsened until she delivered her baby. An MRI performed after the delivery showed a 5- × 4-cm cystic and solid sellar/suprasellar causing severe chiasmal compression and pituitary gland compression. She had central hypothyroidism, hypoadrenalism, and hypogonadism with a minimal elevation in prolactin. She underwent right endonasal adenoma removal with endoscope assistance. She had transient diabetes insipidus that resolved 1 week after surgery; however, she still requires anterior hormone replacement therapy. Her vision has returned to normal. Her MRI at 4 months after surgery shows no residual or recurrent tumor (**Fig. 20.6**).

Case 3: Endocrine-Inactive Adenoma with Right Cavernous Sinus Invasion

An 81-year-old woman with a known endocrine inactive macroadenoma had serial MRIs showing progressive tumor enlargement with right CS invasion. She underwent left extended endonasal tumor removal with endoscope assistance and near-complete total tumor removal (**Fig. 20.7**).

Conclusion

Direct endonasal microscopic tumor removal is a well-established, safe, and effective treatment for the great majority of patients with pituitary adenomas. The addition of endoscopic visualization assistance is recommended for all endonasal adenomectomy procedures, particularly for patients with larger tumors, suprasellar extension, or CS invasion.

References

1. Cooke RS, Jones RA. Experience with the direct transnasal transsphenoidal approach to the pituitary fossa. Br J Neurosurg 1994;8:193–196
2. Griffith HB, Veerapen R. A direct transnasal approach to the sphenoid sinus. Technical note. J Neurosurg 1987;66:140–142
3. Liu JK, Das K, Weiss MH, Laws ER Jr, Couldwell WT. The history and evolution of transsphenoidal surgery. J Neurosurg 2001;95:1083–1096
4. McDonald TJ, Laws ER Jr. Historical aspects of the management of pituitary disorders with emphasis on transsphenoidal surgery. In: Laws ER Jr, Randall R, Kern E, eds. Management of Pituitary Adenomas and Related Lesions: With Emphasis on Transsphenoidal Microsurgery. New York: Appleton-Century-Crofts; 1982:1–13
5. Hardy J. Transsphenoidal microsurgery of the normal and pathological pituitary. Clin Neurosurg 1969;16:185–217
6. Black PM, Zervas NT, Candia GL. Incidence and management of complications of transsphenoidal operation for pituitary adenomas. Neurosurgery 1987;20:920–924
7. Ciric I, Mikhael M, Stafford T, Lawson L, Garces R. Transsphenoidal microsurgery of pituitary macroadenomas with long-term follow-up results. J Neurosurg 1983;59:395–401
8. Ebersold MJ, Quast LM, Laws ER Jr, Scheithauer B, Randall RV. Long-term results in transsphenoidal removal of nonfunctioning pituitary adenomas. J Neurosurg 1986;64:713–719
9. Fahlbusch R, Buchfelder M, Müller OA. Transsphenoidal surgery for Cushing's disease. J R Soc Med 1986;79:262–269
10. Kern EB, Pearson BW, McDonald TJ, Laws ER Jr. The transseptal approach to lesions of the pituitary and parasellar regions. Laryngoscope 1979;89(5 Pt 2, Suppl 15):1–34
11. Randall RV, Laws ER Jr, Abboud CF, Ebersold MJ, Kao PC, Scheithauer BW. Transsphenoidal microsurgical treatment of prolactin-producing pituitary adenomas. Results in 100 patients. Mayo Clin Proc 1983;58:108–121
12. Weiss MH. Surgery of the pituitary gland. Bull Los Angeles Neurol Soc 1977;42:190–200
13. Wilson CB. A decade of pituitary microsurgery. The Herbert Olivecrona lecture. J Neurosurg 1984;61:814–833
14. Wilson CB, Dempsey LC. Transsphenoidal microsurgical removal of 250 pituitary adenomas. J Neurosurg 1978;48:13–22
15. Ciric I, Ragin A, Baumgartner C, Pierce D. Complications of transsphenoidal surgery: results of a national survey, review of the literature, and personal experience. Neurosurgery 1997;40:225–236, discussion 236–237
16. Eisele DW, Flint PW, Janas JD, Kelly WA, Weymuller EA Jr, Cummings CW. The sublabial transseptal transsphenoidal approach to sellar and parasellar lesions. Laryngoscope 1988;98:1301–1308
17. Schoem SR, Khan A, Wilson WR, Laws ER. Minimizing upper lip and incisor teeth paresthesias in approaches to transsphenoidal surgery. Otolaryngol Head Neck Surg 1997;116(6 Pt 1):656–661
18. Sharma K, Tyagi I, Banerjee D, Chhabra DK, Kaur A, Taneja HK. Rhinological complications of sublabial transseptal transsphenoidal surgery for sellar and suprasellar lesions: prevention and management. Neurosurg Rev 1996;19:163–167
19. Sherwen PJ, Patterson WJ, Griesdale DE. Transseptal, transsphenoidal surgery: a subjective and objective analysis of results. J Otolaryngol 1986;15:155–160
20. Badie B, Nguyen P, Preston JK. Endoscopic-guided direct endonasal approach for pituitary surgery. Surg Neurol 2000;53:168–172, discussion 172–173
21. Das K, Spencer W, Nwagwu CI, et al. Approaches to the sellar and parasellar region: anatomic comparison of endonasal-transsphenoidal, sublabial-transsphenoidal, and transethmoidal approaches. Neurol Res 2001;23:51–54
22. Kawamata T, Iseki H, Ishizaki R, Hori T. Minimally invasive endoscope-assisted endonasal trans-sphenoidal microsurgery for pituitary tumors: experience with 215 cases comparing with sublabial trans-sphenoidal approach. Neurol Res 2002;24:259–265
23. Koren I, Hadar T, Rappaport ZH, Yaniv E. Endoscopic transnasal transsphenoidal microsurgery versus the sublabial approach for the treatment of pituitary tumors: endonasal complications. Laryngoscope 1999;109:1838–1840
24. Nasseri SS, Kasperbauer JL, Strome SE, McCaffrey TV, Atkinson JL, Meyer FB. Endoscopic transnasal pituitary surgery: report on 180 cases. Am J Rhinol 2001;15:281–287
25. Sheehan MT, Atkinson JL, Kasperbauer JL, Erickson BJ, Nippoldt TB. Preliminary comparison of the endoscopic transnasal vs the sublabial transseptal approach for clinically nonfunctioning pituitary macroadenomas. Mayo Clin Proc 1999;74:661–670
26. Dusick JR, Esposito F, Mattozo CA, Chaloner C, McArthur DL, Kelly DF. Endonasal transsphenoidal surgery: the patient's perspective-survey results from 259 patients. Surg Neurol 2006;65:332–341, discussion 341–342
27. Zada G, Kelly DF, Cohan P, Wang C, Swerdloff R. Endonasal transsphenoidal approach for pituitary adenomas and other sellar lesions: an assessment of efficacy, safety, and patient impressions. J Neurosurg 2003;98:350–358
28. Cavallo LM, Prevedello D, Esposito F, et al. The role of the endoscope in the transsphenoidal management of cystic lesions of the sellar region. Neurosurg Rev 2008;31:55–64, discussion 64
29. Dusick JR, Esposito F, Malkasian D, Kelly DF. Avoidance of carotid artery injuries in transsphenoidal surgery with the Doppler probe and micro-hook blades. Neurosurgery 2007;60(4, Suppl 2):322–328, discussion 328–329
30. Fatemi N, Dusick JR, Malkasian D, et al. Instrumentation assessment: short trapezoidal speculums for suprasellar and infrasellar exposure in endonasal transsphenoidal surgery. Neurosurgery 2008;62(5 Suppl 2):ONS325–329; discussion ONS329–330
31. Jagannathan J, Prevedello DM, Ayer VS, Dumont AS, Jane JA Jr, Laws ER. Computer-assisted frameless stereotaxy in transsphenoidal surgery at a single institution: review of 176 cases. Neurosurg Focus 2006;20:E9
32. Prevedello DM, Doglietto F, Jane JA Jr, Jagannathan J, Han J, Laws ER Jr. History of endoscopic skull base surgery: its evolution and current reality. J Neurosurg 2007;107:206–213

33. Mattozo CA, Dusick JR, Esposito F, et al. Suboptimal sphenoid and sellar exposure: a consistent finding in patients treated with repeat transsphenoidal surgery for residual endocrine-inactive macroadenomas. Neurosurgery 2006;58:857–865, discussion 857–865
34. Dusick JR, Esposito F, Kelly DF, et al. The extended direct endonasal transsphenoidal approach for nonadenomatous suprasellar tumors. J Neurosurg 2005;102:832–841
35. Fatemi N, Dusick JR, de Paiva Neto M, Kelly DF. The endonasal microscopic approach for pituitary adenomas and other parasellar tumors: a 10-year experience. Neurosurgery 2008;63(ONS Suppl 2):244–256
36. Esposito F, Dusick JR, Cohan P, et al. Clinical review: Early morning cortisol levels as a predictor of remission after transsphenoidal surgery for Cushing's disease. J Clin Endocrinol Metab 2006;91:7–13
37. Laws ER. Transsphenoidal approach to pituitary tumors. In: Schmidek H, Sweet W, eds. Operative Neurosurgical Techniques: Indications, Methods, and Results, Vol 1, 3rd ed. Philadelphia: WB Saunders; 1995:283–292
38. Oldfield EH, Vortmeyer AO. Development of a histological pseudocapsule and its use as a surgical capsule in the excision of pituitary tumors. J Neurosurg 2006;104:7–19
39. Yokoyama S, Hirano H, Moroki K, Goto M, Imamura S, Kuratsu JI. Are nonfunctioning pituitary adenomas extending into the cavernous sinus aggressive and/or invasive? Neurosurgery 2001;49:857–862, discussion 862–863
40. Yoneoka Y, Watanabe N, Matsuzawa H, et al. Preoperative depiction of cavernous sinus invasion by pituitary macroadenoma using three-dimensional anisotropy contrast periodically rotated overlapping parallel lines with enhanced reconstruction imaging on a 3-tesla system. J Neurosurg 2008;108:37–41
41. Mesiwala AH, Farrell L, Santiago P, Ghatan S, Silbergeld DL. The effects of hydrogen peroxide on brain and brain tumors. Surg Neurol 2003;59:398–407, discussion 407
42. Esposito F, Dusick JR, Fatemi N, Kelly DF. Graded repair of cranial base defects and cerebrospinal fluid leaks in transsphenoidal surgery. Neurosurgery 2007;60(4, Suppl 2):295–303, discussion 303–304
43. Kelly DF, Oskouian RJ, Fineman I. Collagen sponge repair of small cerebrospinal fluid leaks obviates tissue grafts and cerebrospinal fluid diversion after pituitary surgery. Neurosurgery 2001;49:885–889, discussion 889–890
44. Kleinman HK, Klebe RJ, Martin GR. Role of collagenous matrices in the adhesion and growth of cells. J Cell Biol 1981;88:473–485
45. Narotam PK, Van Dellen JR, Bhoola K, Raidoo D. Experimental evaluation of collagen sponge as a dural graft. Br J Neurosurg 1993;7: 635–641
46. Narotam PK, van Dellen JR, Bhoola KD. A clinicopathological study of collagen sponge as a dural graft in neurosurgery. J Neurosurg 1995;82:406–412
47. Kelly DF, Laws ER Jr, Fossett D. Delayed hyponatremia after transsphenoidal surgery for pituitary adenoma. Report of nine cases. J Neurosurg 1995;83:363–367
48. Zada G, Liu CY, Fishback D, Singer PA, Weiss MH. Recognition and management of delayed hyponatremia following transsphenoidal pituitary surgery. J Neurosurg 2007;106:66–71

21 Endoscopic Pituitary Surgery in the Cavernous Sinus

Giorgio Frank and Ernesto Pasquini

The history of surgical treatment of cavernous sinus (CS) tumors has had an alternating evolution; in beginning the CS was considered to be a "no-man's land," and all surgical approaches were avoided. In the 1960s, with the advent of the transcranial approach,[1] a 20-year-long phase of enthusiasm began. Disappointment, arising from the elevated morbidity of this type of surgery, resulted in another refusal to operate on the CS.[2] With the recent introduction of minimally invasive surgical techniques, combined with the changing mentality regarding the management of benign tumors of this area, our thinking is again changing. The goal is to resolve symptoms and control tumor progression without causing additional neurologic deficit. Radical removal, if associated with significant postoperative deficits, is no longer acceptable. It is better to implement a multimodal treatment strategy in which surgery, together with radiation and pharmacologic therapy, contributes to the final result.

The endoscope represents the most recent adjunct in the century-long evolution of the transsphenoidal approach, which began by using the naked eye, evolved to incorporate magnifying glasses, and, finally in the 1970s, together with the microscope, became the approach of choice. The endoscope, thanks to its angled view and the flexibility of its surgical trajectories, has improved surgical results and has renewed interest in approaches to the CS. The endoscope improves the possibility of accessing, through an extracranial route, the lateral extension of the tumor thanks to the panoramic and angled view and peripheral magnification.[3] In an anatomical study in 2001, Alfieri and Jho[4] demonstrated the feasibility and the advantages of the endoscope in the endonasal approach to the CS. Three types of approaches—paraseptal, middle turbinectomy, and middle meatal—have been described, which are tailored according to the mediolateral extension of the tumor.

The Bologna group reported the first surgical series,[5,6] proposing a "far-lateral" approach, the ethmoido-pterygosphenoidal endoscopic approach (EPSEA), which is appropriate for tumors also invading the lateral compartment of the CS. Another extreme lateral approach may be considered, namely the trans-maxillo-pterygoid approach, which is indicated for tumors extending from the CS through the foramen rotundum to the pterygomaxillary fossa, or vice versa. Therefore, multiple endoscopic endonasal approaches are currently available, and they should be selected and tailored according to the CS compartments involved by the tumor.

In this chapter we report our experience in endoscopic endonasal CS surgery in pituitary adenomas. We focus our attention on pituitary adenomas because they are the most representative and homogeneous group of pathologies invading the CS, and there are well-established criteria to evaluate the results, making the present series comparable with previously reported series.

Indications for Endoscopic Endonasal Cavernous Sinus Surgery

In agreement with many authors,[1,7] we believe that the CS is an extradural vascular venous structure, in continuity with other similar structures along the craniospinal axis. Following the general surgical rule of removing extradural tumors using an extradural approach, we believe that endoscopic endonasal CS surgery should be used in CS tumors having an extradural location. The advantages of an extradural approach are multiple; it is extracerebral, avoiding any brain manipulation; the CS is penetrated through the medial wall in its sellar or sphenoidal part, which is devoid of any cranial nerves; the operation proceeds through surgical corridors with no risk (medial and posterosuperior compartments) or little risk (anteroinferior or lateral compartments) of cranial nerve damage. If there is an intradural growth, a transcranial approach, or a combined or multistaged craniotomy and endoscopic approach, is preferred.

It is of paramount importance to have adequate instrumentation and to plan the approach according to the CS compartments involved by the tumor.

Instrumentation

The instrumentation used in the endoscopic technique is a Xenon 300-W cold-light fountain source, an endoscopic video camera, and a video recorder. The endoscopes are 0-, 30-, and 45-degree Hopkins telescopes (Karl Storz, Tuttlingen, Germany), 4 mm in diameter, and 18 mm long. A cleaning system with pedal control is used to reduce the necessity of extracting the telescope from the nose every time vision becomes unclear. At the end of the approach phase and during the tumor removal phase, we use a mechanical holder for the endoscope to allow the surgeon to work with both hands. The camera zoom allows a better definition of the anatomical features, and positioning the endoscope further away from the surgical field reduces the possibility of contamination of the tip of the telescope by blood.

Technical Adjuncts

Computer-assisted navigation and the micro-Doppler help to precisely localize the internal carotid artery (ICA) before the incision in the CS wall and during the tumor debulking. Modern navigation systems using a magnetic field to localize the pointer are especially suitable for endoscopy. They allow more continuous navigation, avoiding line-of-site obstruction from the body of the surgeon, or the endoscope itself coming between the pointer and the camera.

Intraoperative magnetic resonance imaging (MRI) or computed tomography scans may be extremely useful. We believe that they should be adjuncts to, and not substitutes for, the navigation system and the Doppler.

Surgical Technique

Surgery is performed with the patient under general anesthesia using orotracheal intubation; the patient is placed in a half-sitting position with the head turned toward the surgeon resting freely in the horseshoe head-holder. The oropharynx is packed with moist gauze to prevent blood and secretions from the operative site from reaching the stomach. The nose and face are cleaned with soap and aqueous solutions. The nasal mucous membranes are decongested with 5% Xylocaine. The periumbilical abdomen is routinely prepared for the eventual harvest of a free fat graft.

Different surgical approaches can be used for pituitary adenomas involving the CS: either the midline transsphenoidal endoscopic approach (MTEA) or the EPSEA.

The approach is selected according to the compartments involved by the tumor. An MTEA is adequate when the invasion is confined to the medial and posterosuperior compartments (**Figs. 21.1, 21.2,** and **21.3**). When the tumor invades the anteroinferior and lateral compartments of the CS or invades the entire CS, the EPSEA is required (**Figs. 21.4, 21.5,** and **21.6**).

Midline Transsphenoidal Endoscopic Approach

The surgical procedure can be divided into three stages: approach, tumor removal, and closure.

Stage I: Approach

The lateral dislocation of the middle and upper turbinate allows the localization of the sphenoethmoidal recess and the natural ostium of the sphenoid sinus.

The opening of the sphenoid sinus starts with the enlargement of the natural ostium. The anterior sphenoidotomy should be wide, extending from the roof to the floor of the sphenoid sinus vertically and exceeding the sphenoidal ostia laterally. To gain access to the surgical field from both nostrils, 1 cm of the posterior end of the nasal septum has to be removed, using a back-biting forceps.

All the sphenoidal septa should be removed. The sphenoidal mucosa may be preserved because the wide opening of the natural ostia avoids the risk of postoperative mucocele; preserving the mucosa permits faster postoperative stabilization of the sphenoid cavity with decreased incidence of sphenoidal inflammatory sequel.

The opening of the sellar floor is performed using a drill and is enlarged using a Kerrison rongeur; it should be wide, from the superior to the inferior inter-CS and from one CS to the other (**Fig. 21.7A**). The bone overlying the invaded CS must be carefully removed from the opticocarotid recess to the paraclival carotid protuberance vertically and 1 cm laterally to the sella, exposing the main bulge of the parasellar carotid artery (**Fig. 21.7B**). This bone removal later increases the capacity of inspection of the CS content by gently displacing the anterior membranous CS wall laterally.

Stage II: Tumor Removal

The dural opening starts in the sellar area. The sellar component of the tumor is removed first. Subsequently, the medial compartment of the CS is entered, either enlarging the opening of the medial wall created by the tumor itself or (more rarely) making an incision into the medial wall in a safe area (normally located in the posterior two thirds of the medial wall of the CS) (**Fig. 21.7B**). Recognition of this "safe" area requires the identification of the bulging of the tumor and an accurate mapping of the course of the ICA (using direct vision, micro-Doppler, and neuronavigation) (**Figs. 21.1** and **21.6**) The removal of the tumor inside the medial and posterosuperior compartments of the CS is performed under direct view and has no risk of neural damage due to the absence of cranial nerves in this location (**Fig. 21.8**). Usually, a 0-degree endoscope is adequate for the procedure.

Stage III: Final Exploration and Closure of the Surgical Field

Hemostasis is obtained by packing with a cottonoid. At the end of the removal stage, free-hand exploration into the surgical field using angled 30- and 45-degree optic scopes is recommended.

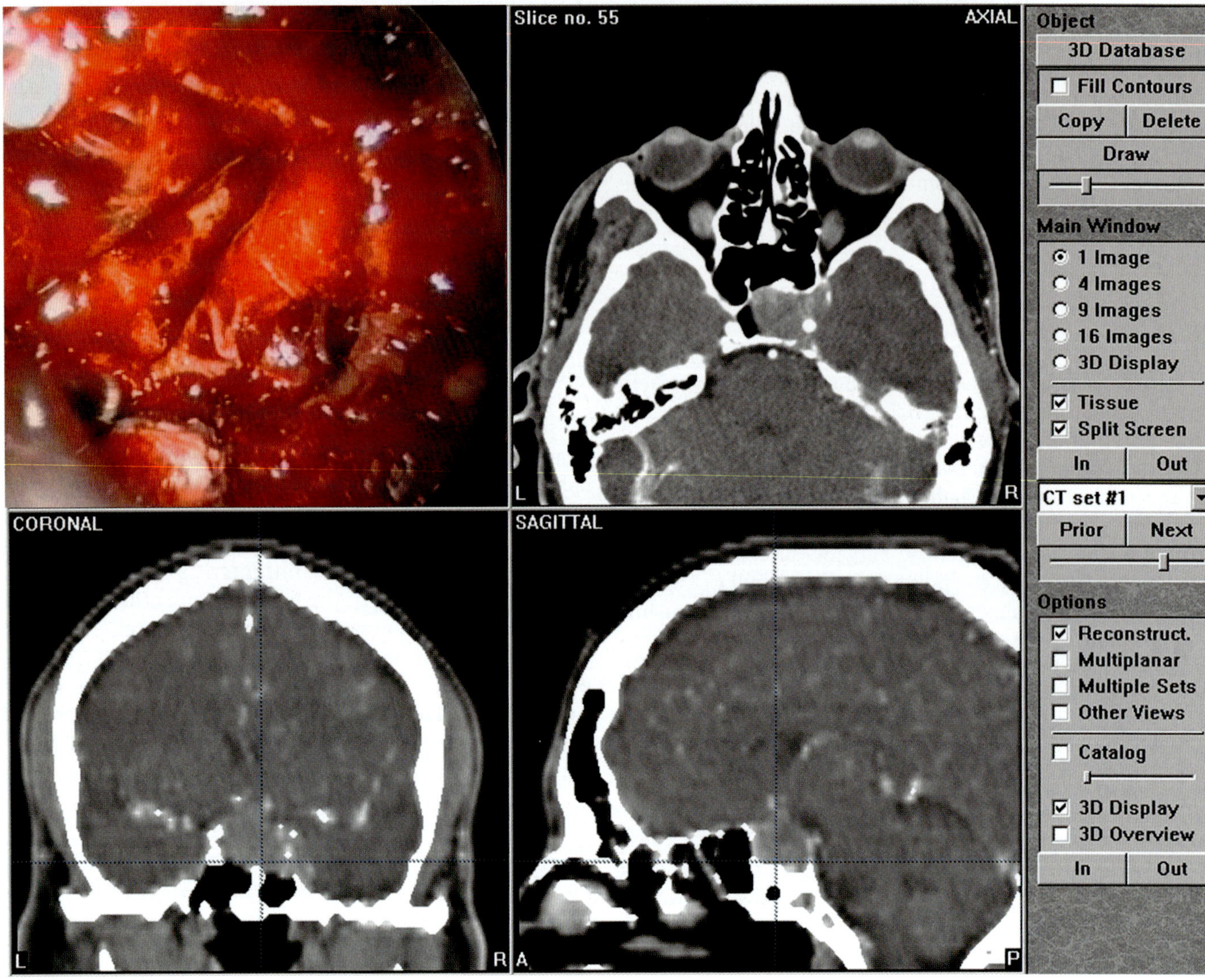

Fig. 21.1 Patient C.E. with adrenocorticotropic hormone adenoma invading the left cavernous sinus (CS) (anteroinferior compartment) and compressing the right CS. (From Fatemi N, et al. Instrumentation assessment: short trapezoidal speculums for suprasellar and infrasellar exposure in endonasal transsphenoidal surgery. Neurosurgery 2008; 62(5 Suppl2):ONS325–329. Reprinted with permission. Copyright 2008 Lippincott Williams & Wilkins.)

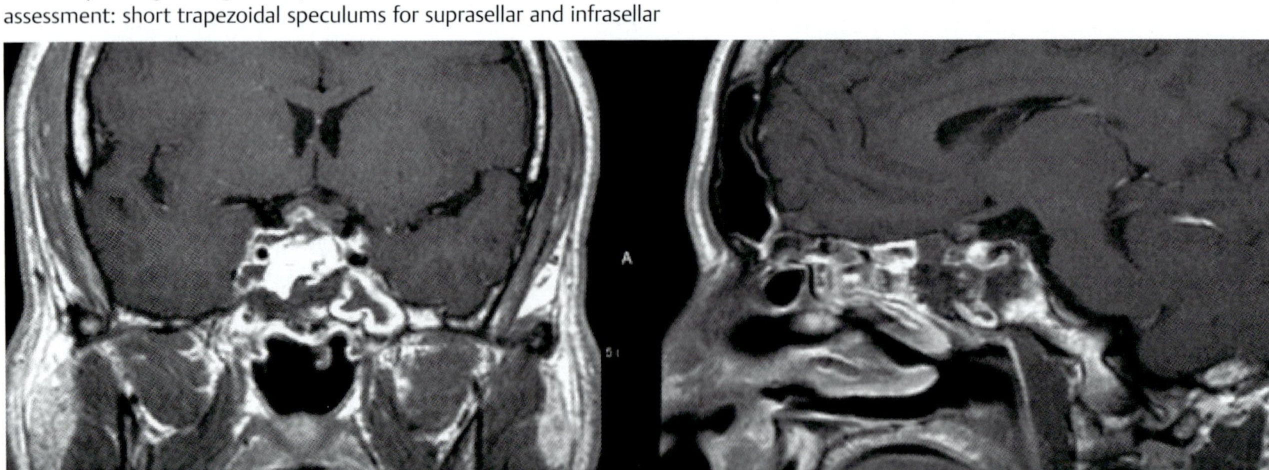

Fig. 21.2 Magnetic resonance imaging at 2-day follow-up in patient C.E. Tumor removal from the sella cavity and the anteroinferior compartment of left cavernous sinus is clearly visible. (From Mattozo CA, et al. Suboptimal sphenoid and sellar exposure: a consistent finding in patients treated with repeat transsphenoidal surgery for residual endocrine-inactive macroadenomas. Neurosurgery 2006;58:5. Reprinted with permission. Copyright 2006 Lippincott Williams & Wilkins.)

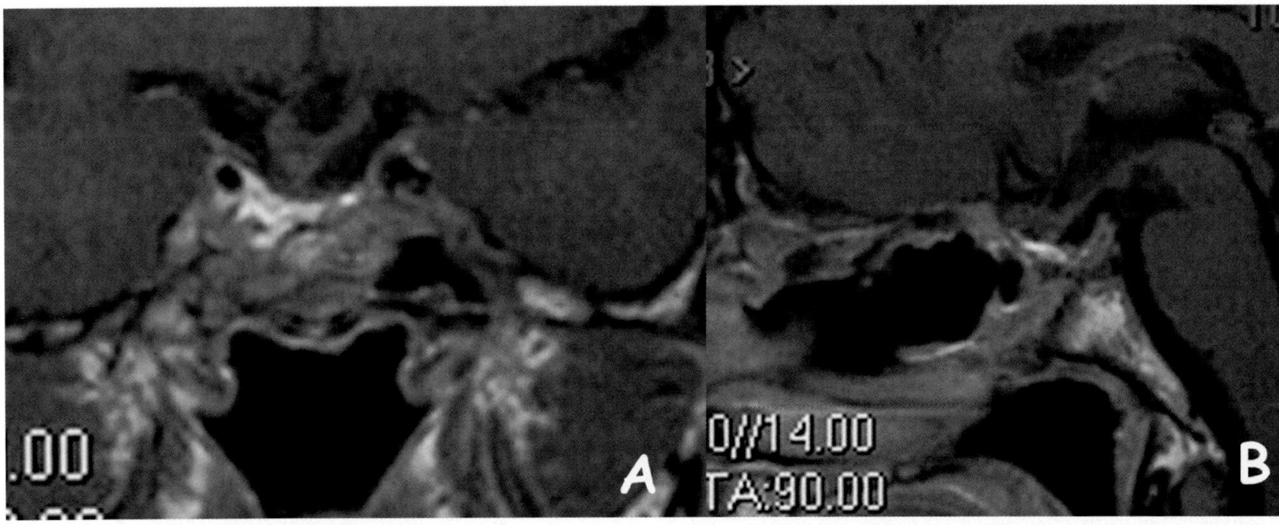

Fig. 21.3 **(A,B)** Magnetic resonance imaging at 6-month follow-up in patient C.E.; no residual tumor. The fat is subtotally reabsorbed and the pituitary gland is sloped downward. (From Dusick Jr, et al. Avoidance of carotid artery injuries in transsphenoidal surgery with the Doppler probe and micro-hook blades. Neurosurgery 2007;60:ONS Suppl 5. Reprinted with permission. Copyright 2006 Lippincott Williams & Wilkins.)

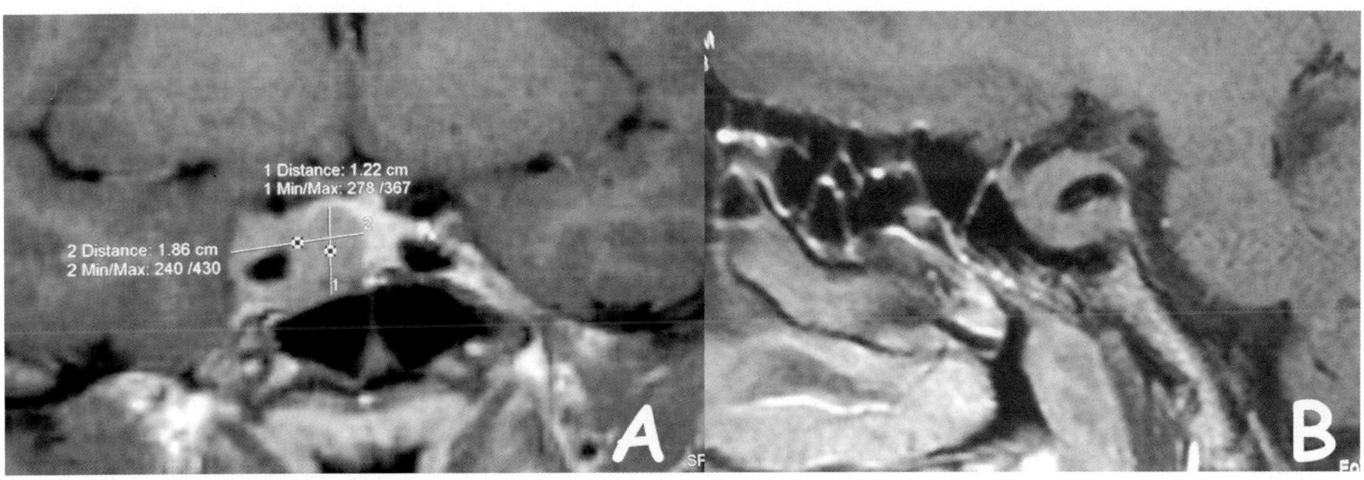

Fig. 21.4 Patient A.F. with growth hormone adenoma involving the anteroinferior and posterosuperior compartment of the right cavernous sinus (CS). The tumor displaces the lateral wall of CS laterally with subtotal encasement of the internal carotid artery. **(A)** An MRI coronal view clearly shows the sellar and CS components of the adenoma. **(B)** A sagittal view shows the involvement of the posterosuperior and anteroinferior compartments. (From Dusick Jr, et al. Avoidance of carotid artery injuries in transsphenoidal surgery with the Doppler probe and micro-hook blades. Neurosurgery 2007;60:ONS Suppl 5. Reprinted with permission. Copyright 2006 Lippincott Williams & Wilkins.)

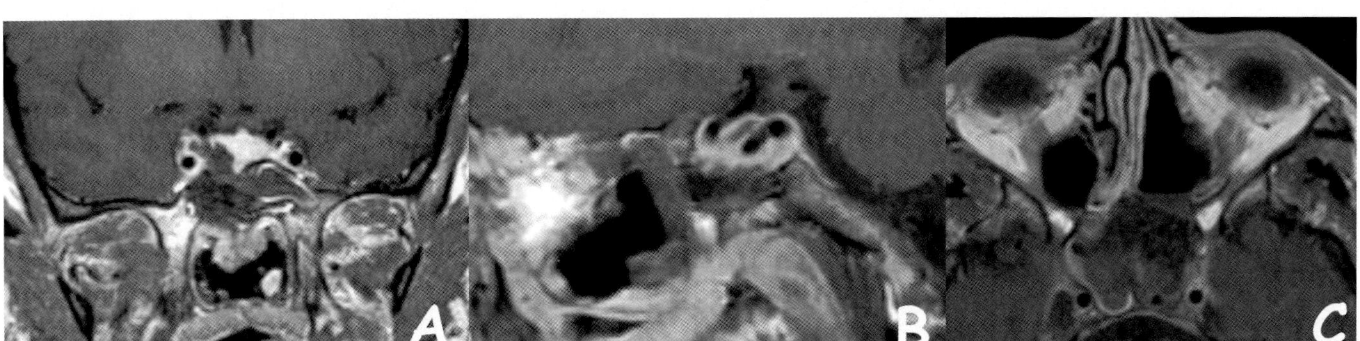

Fig. 21.5 Three-day postsurgical MRI in patient A.F. Tumor removal from the cavernous sinus (CS) **(A–C)** and preservation of the pituitary gland **(A)** are clearly visible. An axial view **(C)** shows the ethmoido-pterygo-sphenoidal endoscopic approach with the right ethmoidectomy and middle turbinectomy and with the frontal exposition of the right CS.

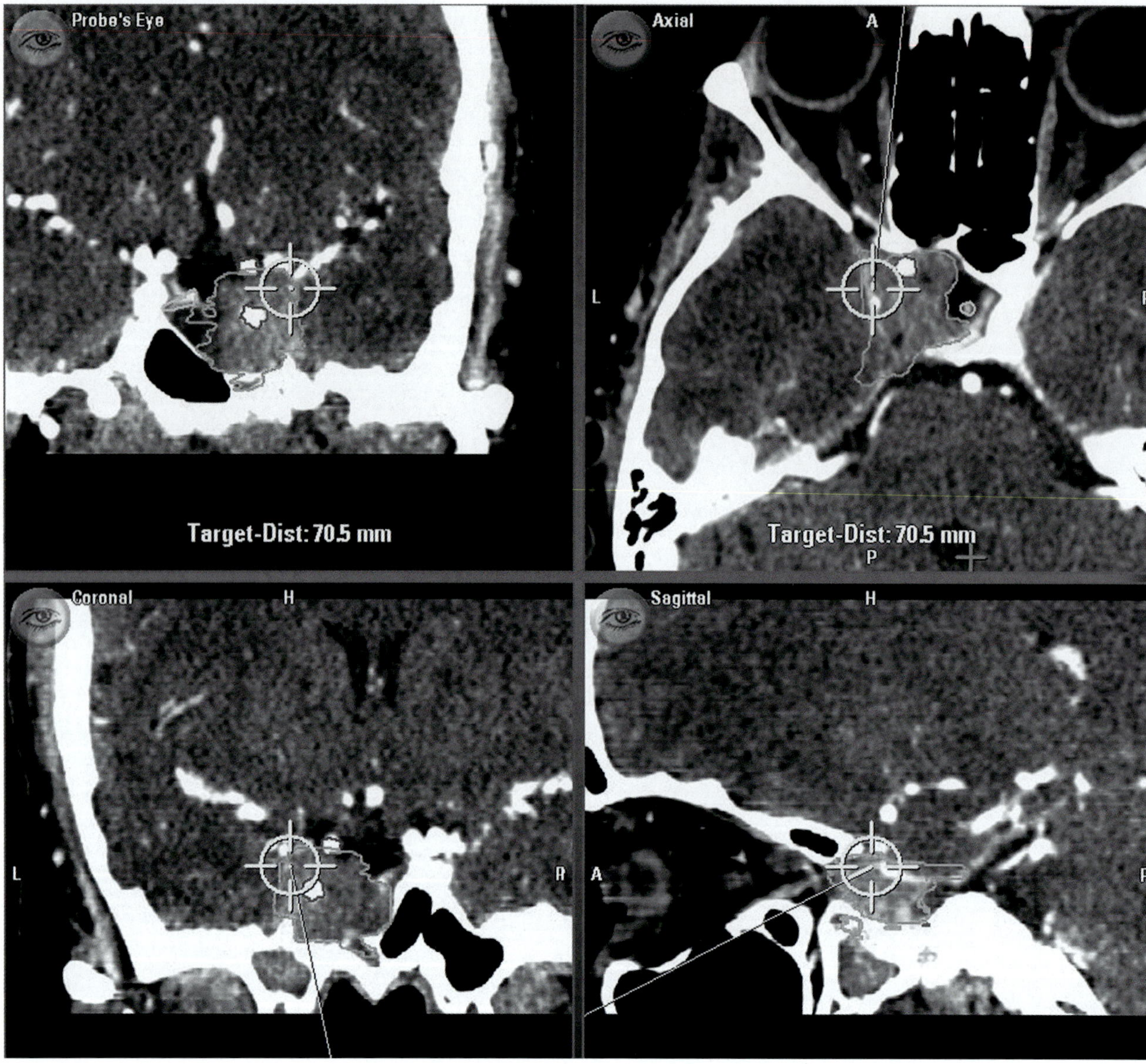

Fig. 21.6 Intraoperative computed tomography images as seen by the neuronavigator. The tumor encases the internal carotid artery (ICA) of the left cavernous sinus (CS). The pointer shows the surgical trajectory lateral to the ICA and as a tangent to the lateral wall of the CS.

In the absence of cerebrospinal fluid (CSF) leaks, the surgical cavity is simply packed with Gelfoam. If a CSF leak is detected or suspected, a multilayer plastic repair is performed by applying autologous fat in the cavity, a piece of bone or cartilage (if available) extradurally, and a mucoperiosteal flap overlay (from the middle turbinate or from the septum). It is important to remember that, to have a viable graft, it is necessary to remove the mucosa and to apply the graft directly over the bleeding surface.

The sphenoid sinus is packed with Gelfoam and, finally, the middle turbinate is medially displaced to its original position. Nasal packing is not routinely required. Lumbar drainage is not used.

Ethmoido-Pterygo-Sphenoidal Endoscopic Approach

The EPSEA is used for tumors invading the anteroinferior or lateral compartments of the CS or for tumors invading the entire CS. This procedure is the most versatile, allowing the total exposition of the CS with the possibility of simultaneous direct control of all compartments of the CS

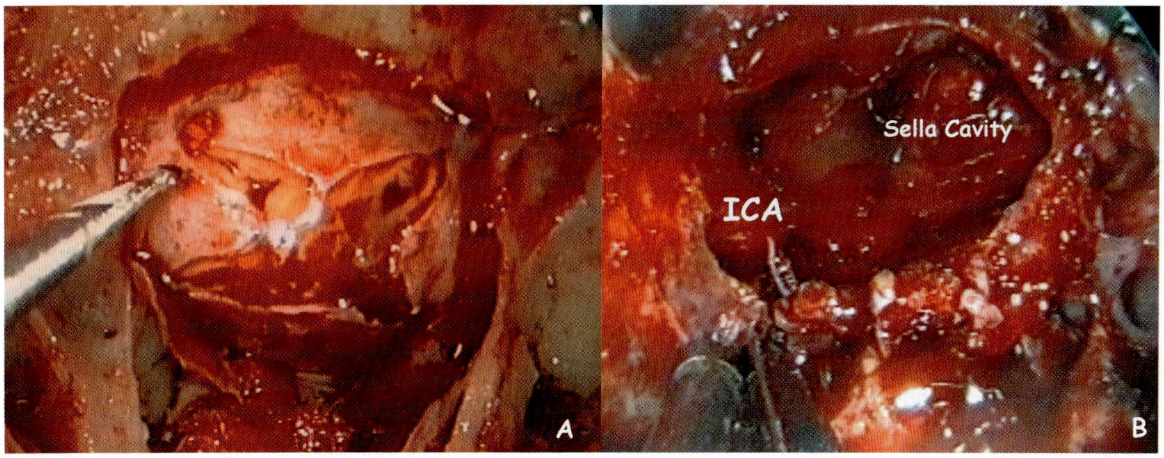

Fig. 21.7 Intraoperative view. **(A)** The opening of the sellar floor should be wide extending from the superior to the inferior intercavernous sinus and from one cavernous sinus (CS) to the other. **(B)** The bone overlying the invaded CS is removed between the opticocarotid recess to the paraclival carotid protuberance. The medial wall of the right CS in its anteroinferior portion is opened and the tumor is removed.

(**Figs. 21.4, 21.5,** and **21.6**). The procedure can be schematically divided into three stages.

Stage I: Approach

An ethmoidal route is used and a complete sphenoethmoidectomy with a wide meatotomy and subtotal resection of middle turbinate is performed. The medial portion of the posterior wall of the maxillary sinus is resected to expose the posterior wall of the maxillary antrum and the vertical process of the palatine bone. After ligation of the sphenopalatine artery, the superior portion of the medial pterygoid process is drilled out. Resection of the medial pterygoid process permits the exposition of the inferolateral portion of the CS (**Fig. 21.5C**). A partial resection of the pterygoid process is performed, taking into account the degree of pneumatization of the lateral recess of the sphenoid and the need for visualization of the lateral and inferior walls of the sphenoid sinus.

Stage II: Opening of the Cavernous Sinus and Removal of the Tumor

To expose the anterior CS, it is necessary to remove part of the bone of the posterolateral wall of the sphenoid sinus. The bone to be removed is a quadrilateral-shaped structure located between the opticocarotid recess and the paraclival carotid protuberance medially and the orbital apex and the trigeminal nerve protuberance laterally. The vidian canal on the floor of the sphenoidal sinus is a useful landmark

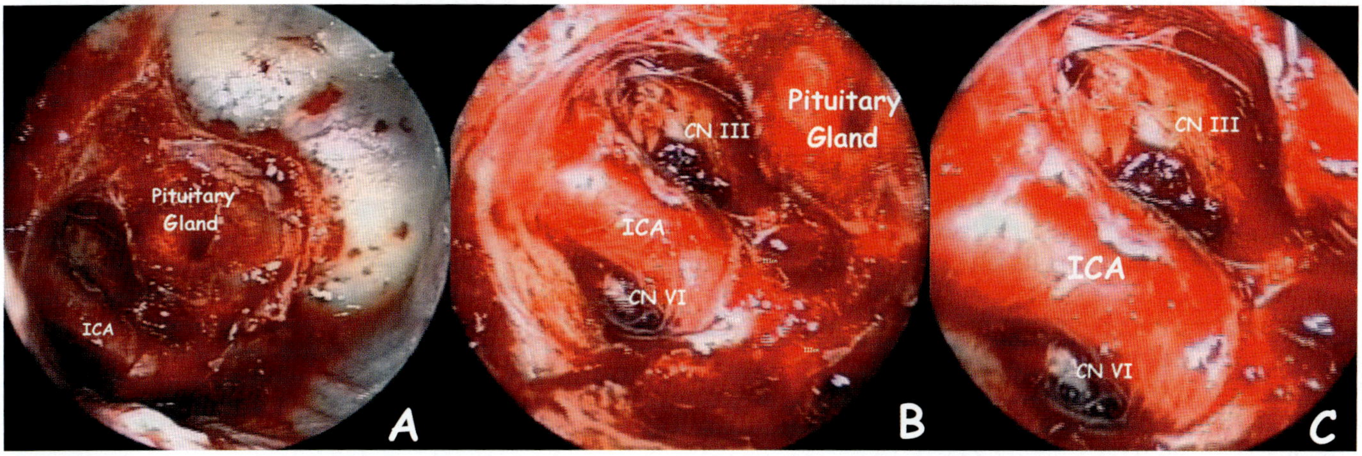

Fig. 21.8 **(A–C)** Intraoperative endoscopic view of the right cavernous sinus (CS) after the removal of a tumor having multifocal invasion. The medial wall of the CS is totally absent, and the internal carotid artery (ICA), the pituitary gland, and partially cranial nerves (CNs) III and VI in the lateral and anteroinferior compartments area of CS, respectively, are well visible.

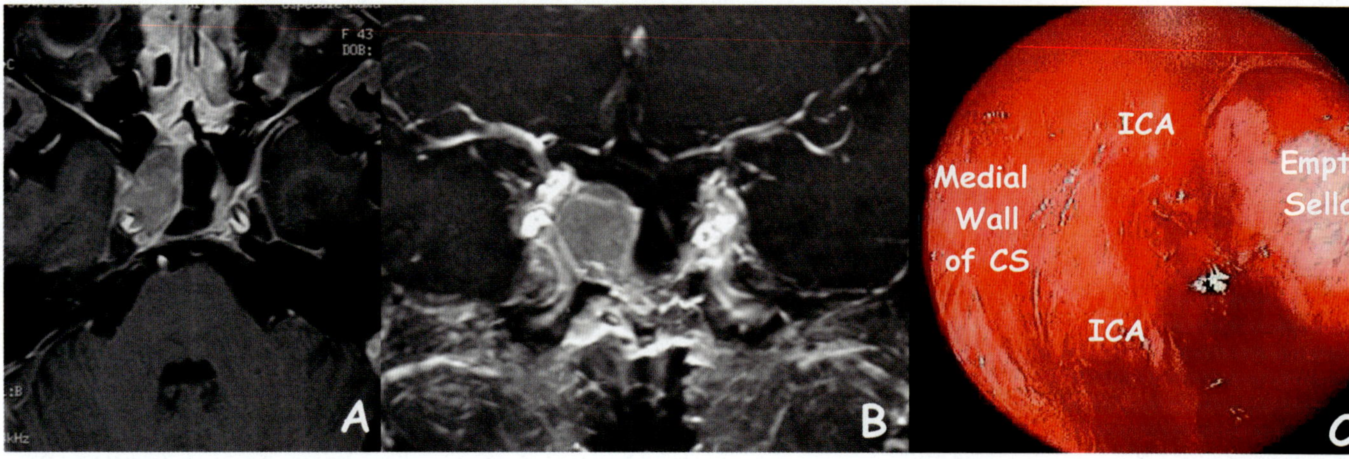

Fig. 21.9 **(A–C)** Recurrent nonfunctioning (NF) adenoma compressing the right cavernous sinus (CS). **(A,B)** Preoperative MRI: the tumor displaces posterosuperiorly the internal carotid artery, laterally to the empty sella. **(C)** An intraoperative view shows the integrity of the medial wall of the CS. The CS is compressed but not invaded.

because it indicates the junction of the horizontal petrosal part of the carotid artery with the ascending paraclival segment of the vessel, and therefore it is a guide to the inferior portion of the CS.[8]

The precise site of the opening of the inferior CS wall (or sphenoidal part of the medial wall) depends on the displacement that the tumor produces along the course of the carotid artery and should be performed in a safe area away from the carotid artery. When the tumor displaces the ICA medially or laterally, the incision of the wall is to be performed laterally or medially to the vessel, respectively. In cases of lesions involving the anteroinferior compartment of the CS, the ICA is generally displaced backward; in this case, the lesion covers the vessel, making the opening of the dura less dangerous. Conversely, in cases of lesions involving the posterosuperior compartment, the ICA is displaced forward and is in close contact with the anterior wall of the CS. In the latter circumstance, before any dura incision, it is mandatory to locate the position of the ICA exactly, with the combined use of neuronavigation and the micro-Doppler (**Figs. 21.1, 21.2, 21.3, 21.4, 21.5,** and **21.6**).

With the exception of a tumor exclusively located in the lateral compartment of the CS, the dural opening is made in the sellar region and progressively enlarged following the tumor from its medial to its lateral and inferior portion. As pointed out earlier, maximal care is required during the sectioning of the dura in front of the carotid artery to avoid injury to the vessel, but also to avoid injury to the abducens nerve, which, in the inferior portion of the CS, runs close to the dura in a inferolateral direction toward the superior orbital fissure (**Fig. 21.9**).

The tumor is removed piece by piece, gradually gaining an increasingly larger working area and obtaining good visual control of the contents of the CS.

Stage III: Final Exploration and Closure of the Surgical Defect

Venous bleeding is usually insignificant. It may be more evident after tumor removal and is well controlled with Gelfoam or FloSeal (Baxter, Deerfield, IL) and cotton packing.

At the end of the tumor resection, inspection of the surgical field with 30- and 45-degree angled endoscopes permits the detection and removal of remnants.

Nasal packing with a single Merocel (Medtronic Xomed Surgical Products, Jacksonville, FL) is usually kept in place for 2 days.

Material and Methods

Our study included all consecutive patients referred to our center having pituitary adenomas with intraoperative invasion of the CS. Between May 1998 and January 2008, a

Table 21.1 Number and Percentage of Intraoperative Cavernous Sinus Invasion in the Series of Patients Operated on for Functioning or Nonfunctioning Pituitary Adenomas

Type of Tumor	No. of Cases	Percent
GH	27/154	17.5
PRL	15/91	16.5
ACTH	7/97	7.2
TSH	2/10	20
NF	56/329	17
Total	**107/681**	**15.7**

ACTH, adrenocorticotropic hormone; GH, growth hormone; NF, nonfunctioning; PRL, prolactin; TSH, thyroid-stimulating hormone.

Table 21.2 Knosp's Classification and Intraoperative Cavernous Sinus Invasion (ICSI) Index in Patients with a Pituitary Adenoma Invading the CS

MRI Knosp	ICSI		
	Focal Extension	Multifocal Extension	Total ICA Encasement
0	4		
1	2		
2	20	11	
3	12	21	4
4		19	14
Total	38 (35.5%)	51 (47.7%)	18 (16.8%)

ICA, internal carotid artery; MRI, magnetic resonance imaging.

total of 681 patients affected by pituitary adenomas were treated at Bellaria Hospital of Bologna, of whom 107 (15.7%) had an intraoperative invasion of one or both CSs; 59 (55%) were men and 48 (45%) were women. Pituitary adenomas compressing and not invading the CS were excluded (**Table 21.1**). Age ranged from 18 to 77 years (mean, 50; median, 51). There was at least a 6-month follow-up (range, 6 to 102; mean, 30; median, 23).

The Knosp classification[9] was used to describe CS involvement as evidenced by MRI (**Table 21.2**).

We performed an intraoperative evaluation of CS invasion in every case, which was then classified in one of five grades: 0, no involvement; 1, compression/invagination of the medial wall with no invasion (**Fig. 21.9**); 2, focal extension through one or more little pit holes of the medial wall; 3, multifocal invasion without encasement of the ICA (**Fig. 21.8**); and 4, total encasement of the ICA (**Fig. 21.6**).

The patients included in this study had an Intraoperative Cavernous Sinus Invasion (ICSI) Index of 2 or more.

The tumors were classified into three groups according to consistency: tumors with soft consistency (easily removable using suction), tumors with intermediate consistency (partially removable, with difficulty, using suction), and tumors with hard consistency (not removable using suction but excised en bloc or piece by piece using scissor).

Pituitary adenomas were histologically and immunohistochemically investigated. They are classified as functioning (growth hormone [GH], prolactin [PRL], adrenocorticotropic hormone [ACTH]-secreting adenomas), or nonfunctioning (NF) adenomas in relation to the clinical activity. The proliferative index (K_i-67) was measured in all cases; p53 was measured in only some patients and was therefore not included in the overall results.

Endocrinologic cure was defined as follows. In GH adenomas, remission was defined by a normal sex- and age-adjusted insulin-like growth factor-1 level, and GH nadir <1 ng/mL after an oral glucose tolerance test.[10] In PRL-secreting adenomas, remission is defined as having normal serum PRL levels (<30 ng/mL in women, <15 ng/mL in men) at their latest checkup, without having previously had dopaminergic therapy for at least 2 months.[11] In ACTH adenomas, remission is defined by an early morning cortisol level <50 nmol/L requiring substitutive therapy and then by the normalization of 24-hour urinary free cortisol levels.[12]

The results were evaluated for each surgical procedure at a 3-month follow-up with respect to the entity of tumor removal at MRI and to the evaluation of clinical symptoms or endocrinological status.

The overall results of the multimodal management of the individual patients were classified in the comprehensive evaluation comparing the MRI and clinical data at a 6-month or longer follow-up.

The entity of tumor removal was judged on the basis of MRI imaging: 1, radical—no evidence of residual tumor; 2, subtotal—residual tumor less than 20%; 3, partial—residual tumor less than 50%; and 4, insufficient—residual tumor of 50% or more.

We defined the clinical parameters as follows: 1, cure—symptom resolution in NF adenomas and endocrinologic remission in functioning adenomas; and 2, no cure—no symptom resolution.

Finally, the comprehensive evaluation was defined as follows: 1, cured—radical removal and clinical cure; 2, controlled without subsequent postoperative therapy—subtotal removal with symptom resolution (normally for NF adenomas), radical removal with amelioration of symptoms (normally for functioning adenomas); 3, controlled with subsequent postoperative therapy; and 4, not cured—residual tumor with persistent symptoms.

Statistical analysis was performed using the Fisher's exact test.

Table 21.3 Referral Symptoms in Functioning and Nonfunctioning (NF) Pituitary Adenomas

	Incidental Findings	Endocrinologic Disturbances	Hypopituitarism Partial/Total	Visual Disturbances	Neurologic Deficit
Functioning	1	41	7	11	7
NF	9	6	25	37	8
Total	10 (9%)	47 (44%)	32 (30%)	48 (45%)	15 (14%)

Table 21.4 Pituitary Adenomas and Surgical Approaches

Type of Tumor	Surgical Approaches	
	MTEA	EPSEA
GH	21	6
PRL	5	10
ACTH	3	4
TSH	2	
NF	30	26
Total	**61** **57%**	**46** **43%**

ACTH, adrenocorticotropic hormone; EPSEA, ethmoido-pterygo-sphenoidal endoscopic approach; GH, growth hormone; MTEA, midline transsphenoidal endoscopic approach; NF, nonfunctioning; PRL, prolactin; TSH, thyroid-stimulating hormone.

Table 21.5 Surgical Results: Gross Tumor Removal at 3-Month MRI Follow-Up

Type of Tumor	Follow-Up MRI at 3 Months			
	Radical	<20%	<50%	≥50%
GH	17 (63.0%)	8	2	
PRL	7 (46.7%)	7	1	
ACTH	3 (42.9%)	3	1	
TSH	1 (50%)	1		
NF	37 (66%)	13	5	1
Total	**65 (60.7%)**	**32 (29.9%)**	**9 (8.4%)**	**1 (0.9%)**

ACTH, adrenocorticotropic hormone; GH, growth hormone; MRI, magnetic resonance imaging; NF, nonfunctioning; PRL, prolactin; TSH, thyroid-stimulating hormone.

Results

All patients harbored macroadenomas invading the CS. The referral symptoms are shown in **Table 21.3**.

The MTEA was used in 61 patients, whereas in the remaining 46 the EPSEA approach was performed (**Table 21.4**).

Median surgical time was 50 minutes (range, 35 to 90 minutes) for the MTEA and 90 minutes (range, 60 to 180 minutes) for the EPSEA.

There was no perioperative mortality. Patient hospital stay was between 2 and 91 days (median: 4 days).

Surgical Results

The surgical results for individual procedures were evaluated with the entity of the gross tumor removal as shown by MRI and the resolution of the clinical or biohumoral signs at 3 months.

Gross Tumor Removal

The 3-month follow-up MRI showed that macroscopic radical removal of the tumor was obtained in 65 (60.7%) procedures, 32 (29.9%) were subtotal, nine (8.4%) were partial, and only in one patient was the tumoral debulking deemed insufficient (**Table 21.5**).

Endocrinologic Results

Table 21.6 shows the short-term (≤3 months) results for individual procedures. Ten of 27 (37.0%) acromegalics were in remission after surgery. Three of 15 (20%) patients with PRL-secreting adenomas who were operated on due to resistance to medical therapy achieved endocrinologic remission. Three of seven (42.9%) patients with ACTH-secreting adenomas was cured. One of two thyroid-stimulating hormone (TSH) adenomas was in remission. Finally, five of six (83.3%) NF adenomas with preoperative hyperprolactinemia (<120 ng/mL) showed a normal PRL level in the postoperative analysis.

None of 32 patients with preoperative hypopituitarism recovered pituitary functionality.

Visual and Neurologic Outcome

Visual disturbances and neurologic deficits (**Table 21.7**) were observed in 55 (51%) patients. Visual function recovered in the majority of patients (42 of 51 [82.4%]), improved in four (7.8%) cases, and was unchanged in four (7.8%) cases. In one case, visual worsening, due to overpacking of the surgical cavity, occurred, and it was only partially corrected by early surgical revision.

All preoperative neurologic symptoms (**Table 21.7**) resolved themselves after surgery in all but two patients: one case of trigeminal neuralgia, which was controlled by medical

Table 21.6 Surgical Results: Endocrinologic Results at 3-Month Follow-Up

Type of Tumor	Endocrinologic Results at 3 Months		
	No.	1	2
GH	27	10 (37.0%)	17
PRL	15	3 (20%)	12
ACTH	7	3 (42.9%)	4
TSH	2	1 (50%)	1
NF	6	5 (83.3%)	1
Total	**57**	**22 (38.6%)**	**35 (61.4%)**

ACTH, adrenocorticotropic hormone; GH, growth hormone; NF, nonfunctioning; PRL, prolactin; TSH, thyroid-stimulating hormone.

Table 21.7 Surgical Results: Visual and Neurologic Deficits at 3-Month Follow-Up

Visual and Neurologic Deficits		Remission	Improved	Unchanged/Worsened*	Total
Functioning	**None**				36
	Neurol.	2	1	1+1*	4
	Visual	8			8
	Both	3			3
	Total	**13/15** **87%**			
Nonfunctioining	**None**				16
	Neurol.	2		1	3
	Visual	27	3	2	32
	Both	4		1	5
	Total	**33/40** **83%**			

therapy, and one with complete ophthalmoplegia, which was resolved only partially. There was one additional cranial nerve III palsy after surgery; this patient is listed in **Table 21.7** with an asterisk in the unchanged/worsened group.

Comprehensive Evaluations

The parameters in **Table 21.8** describe the overall results for patients treated surgically with and without other postoperative therapy at a 6-month or longer follow-up (mean, 31; median, 24; range, 6 to 102 months).

Findings at Statistical Analysis

Each category of outcome data (e.g., gross tumor removal, clinical outcome, and comprehensive evaluation) was analyzed using the following parameters: age, sex, previous surgery, tumor consistency, intraoperative CS invasion, and proliferative index (K_i-67). The results are summarized in **Table 21.9**. To perform the contingency table analyses, we divided each outcome data group into two subgroups; gross tumor removal was subdivided into total and nontotal tumor removal; clinical outcome into remission and nonremission; and comprehensive evaluation into surgically controlled and nonsurgically controlled.

Sex

We did not find any association between the sex variable and each category of outcome data.

Age

The age variable was analyzed and the patients were subdivided into two groups: 40 years and older and under 40 years of age. We found only a slightly ($p = .0279$) significant correlation

Table 21.8 Comprehensive Evaluation

Tumor	Remission	Controlled Without Other Therapy	Controlled with Other Therapy	Not Controlled
	Surgically Controlled		**Not Surgically Controlled**	
GH	9		16	1
PRL	3	1	8	1
ACTH	2		1	3
TSH	1		1	
NF	33	9	10	
Total	**48** **58 (59%)**	**10**	**36** **41 (41%)**	**5**

Note: Results refer to patients treated with only surgical therapy (remission and controlled without other therapy) or treated with other therapies (medical therapy and/or radiotherapy). The last column indicates the number of patients still presenting an uncontrolled disease despite a multimodal treatment.
ACTH, adrenocorticotropic hormone; GH, growth hormone; NF, nonfunctioning; PRL, prolactin; TSH, thyroid-stimulating hormone.

Table 21.9 Findings at Statistical Analysis: Contingency Tables Using the Fisher's Exact Test

Variables	Parameters			Gross Tumor Removal	Endocrine Results	Comprehensive Evaluation
				Statistical Significance		
Age (yr)	<40	vs	≥40	$p = 0.002$	NS	$p = 0.03$
Sex	Male	vs	Female	NS	NS	NS
Previous treatment	No therapy	vs	Therapy	NS	NS	NS
Type of tumor	Funct.	vs	NF	NS	$p < 0.0001$	$p < 0.00001$
Consistency	Soft	vs	Hard	$p = 0.007$	NS	NS
ICSI	Focal	vs	Diffuse	$p = 0.0010$	$p = 0.008$	$p = 0.0015$
K_i-67	<3%	vs	≥3%	$p = 0.0012$	NS	$p = 0.019$

ICSI, Intraoperative Cavernous Sinus Invasion; NS, not significant.

with the variables of gross tumor removal and comprehensive evaluation; no correlation was found with clinical outcome. Based on a long-term follow-up, it seems that, in patients under 40 years of age, there was less control of the disease.

Previous Surgical Treatment

We did not find any significant correlation between previous surgical treatment (no patient underwent radiosurgery as a first treatment) and the outcome variables.

Consistency

We analyzed the consistency subdivided into two groups: soft tumors and hard tumors (intermediate and hard consistency, respectively). The two-sided *p*-value shows a significant correlation ($p = .0758$) only with gross tumor removal. Patients having hard tumors have a lower probability of total tumor removal, but this did not affect control of the symptoms.

Type of Tumors

The correlation between functioning and nonfunctioning adenomas was extremely significant in the clinical outcome and in the comprehensive evaluation ($p < .0001$) but not significantly correlated with the gross tumor removal variable. Patients having functioning pituitary adenomas had the same chance of gross tumor removal but a poorer chance of clinical and surgical control of the disease. These data stress the endpoint of biohumoral control of the disease in functioning adenomas rather than only an MRI evaluation as in NF adenomas. On the other hand, it is easy to resolve the mass effect symptomatology compared with the endocrinologic syndrome.

Intraoperative Cavernous Sinus Invasion

We divided the ICSI parameters into focal and diffuse infiltration (multifocal and ICA encasement) (**Table 21.10**).

The correlation between the ICSI and the outcome variables was very significant in all the analyses ($p = .0010$). Patients with focal invasion had a better chance of disease control also at long-term follow-up. In our opinion, these data probably mean that focal invasion does not necessarily correspond to invasive behavior of the adenoma but is more likely caused by an extension through the medial wall of the CS.

Histopathologic Findings: Proliferative Index

The K_i-67 proliferative index was measured in every surgical specimen; in the majority of cases (72%), it was less than 3%, and in 25 (28%) cases it was between 3 and 10% (**Table 21.10**).

We found a proliferative index higher than 10% in nine cases. Two out of these nine cases were both positive for p53 and developed metastases (one after 3 months and one after 7 years) and died from the disease. In one, the disease has not been controllable even after craniotomy and radiotherapy. One patient with a PRL adenoma nonresponsive to medical therapy died 2 years after surgery as a result of vascular problems not correlated with the disease.

The proliferative index of the tumors was not statistically associated with the ICSI (Fisher's exact test: $p = .461$).

Table 21.10 Proliferative Index and Intraoperative Cavernous Sinus Invasion (ICSI)

	Proliferative Index (K_i-67)				
	Low		High		
ICSI	**Neg.**	**<3%**	**≥3%**	**>10%**	**Total**
Focal	9	21	7	1	38
Diffuse	15	23	7	6	51
Total encasement	1	11	4	2	18
Total	**25**	**55**	**18**	**9**	**107**

Table 21.11 Surgical and Endocrinologic Complications

Surgical Complications		
Postoperative CSF leak	4	3.7%
Epistaxis	1	0.9%
Hematoma	2	1.9%
CN III palsy (no EPS)	1	0.9%
Overpacking	1	0.9%
Endocrinologic Complications		
Adrenocortical insufficiency	2	1.9%
Transient diabetes insipidus	2	1.9%
Permanent diabetes insipidus	2	1.9%

CN, cranial nerve; CSF, cerebrospinal fluid; EPS, exophthalmos producing substance.

When the K_i-67 proliferative index was matched with gross tumor removal (p = .0012) and comprehensive evaluation (p = .0191), the two-sided p-value was very significant (**Table 21.9**); patients having pituitary adenomas with a proliferative index of less than 3% had a better chance of gross tumor removal and surgical control of the disease at a 6-month or longer follow-up.

Complications

Surgical and endocrinologic complications are summarized in **Table 21.11**.

In 26 (24%) cases, there was intraoperative evidence of a CSF leak that necessitated reconstruction with the use of abdominal fat or fascia lata together with the mucoperiosteum of the middle turbinate. Four patients experienced delayed postoperative CSF leaks that required reintervention.

In one case, a worsening of a visual deficit was observed; it was related to overpacking of the sella and was only partially corrected by early surgical revision. One patient who underwent partial removal of his tumor was reoperated with a transcranial approach for residual tumor and hemorrhagic infarction in the temporal lobe. One delayed (18 days after surgery) epistaxis was observed, and it required intraoperative coagulation of the sphenopalatine artery after emergency nasal packing.

Among the medical complications, there were two ACTH insufficiencies that required replacement therapy and two transient and two permanent diabetes insipidus.

One patient died 3 months after surgery from tumor progression; multiple brain metastases were discovered at autopsy. One patient died after 2 years from unrelated myocardial ischemia. One patient, 6 years after surgery, developed multiple brain metastases; he underwent a retrosigmoid approach for removal of symptomatic clival lesions and died 1 year later due to progression of the disease.

Discussion

Cavernous sinus surgery is one of the most debated topics in neurosurgery. The contemporary philosophy is the culmination of a long history of contradictory points of view; in the beginning, the CS was considered to be a "no-man's land," that is, territory not suitable for surgical management. After the 1960s, with the introduction of the transcranial approach to the parasellar area,[1] there was a period of enthusiasm for this surgery, which lasted 20 years. Disappointment with the elevated morbidity from the extreme surgical aggressiveness resulted in continued refusal to perform this type of surgery. The current phase reflects an extremely cautious attitude but weighs the surgical risk in proportion to the possible advantages for the patient. The indications are more selective, and approaches are preferred that minimize the trauma, maximize the resection, and optimize tumor control through pharmacologic or complementary radiotherapy. Multiple different intra- and extracranial approaches are available; they are selected and tailored according to the characteristics (location, extension, biologic character) of the tumor.

The transsphenoidal approach is definitely the preferable anterior extracranial approach, and it has long been used for sellar tumors with parasellar extension. The main drawback of this approach in CS surgery is the strictly median access, which is risky during the blind use of curettes when the lateral sellar compartment is not adequately exposed. This is the reason why variations in the classic microscopic transsphenoidal approach were sought with the aim of improving the surgical exposure of the CS. In 1979, Laws et al[13] proposed a cross-court approach using a contralateral transethmoidal-transsphenoidal approach, which provided improved exposure of the contralateral medial compartment of the CS. Lalwani et al[14] accessed this route using a Lynch incision and combined this with a medial maxillectomy when necessary. Arita et al,[15] using a slightly modified speculum, proposed another "cross-court" approach. Fraioli et al,[16] based on the anatomical study by Inoue et al,[17] suggested an inferomedial exposure of the CS by adding a maxillary osteotomy or by fracturing the medial wall of the maxillary sinus in the standard transsphenoidal approach with the use of a modified speculum. A distant lateral inferomedial route combined with a transmaxillary transsphenoidal approach was proposed by Sabit et al[18] to allow a safe extradural lateral to medial passage in the parasellar region. Kitano and Taneda[19] suggested an extended microscopic transsphenoidal approach with a submucosal posterior ethmoidectomy. In spite of the wider exposure allowed by these different approaches, the surgical route to the CS remains narrow and rigid, with limited lateral visualization due to the use of the speculum and the optical features of the microscope.

More recently, the endoscope has been introduced into the neurosurgical armamentarium and has renewed interest in the extended approaches to the CS, encouraged by the peripheral view given by the endoscope and by the avoidance of any rigid retractor. Detailed anatomic studies[4,20] have shown the feasibility and efficacy of the endoscope in exploring the lateral sellar compartment. Alfieri and Jho[4] have described three different endoscopic routes to the CS in their cadaveric dissections: the paraseptal as a median approach, the middle turbinectomy as a lateral approach, and the middle meatal as a far lateral approach.

The Bologna group has had experience with a large surgical series of pituitary adenomas invading the CS that were treated by endoscopic endonasal surgery.[6] Only pituitary adenomas invading the CS without major intradural extension were considered for this procedure. They represent 15.7% of the pituitary adenomas operated on in our center. The surgical procedures were performed using two different endoscopic endonasal approaches: MTEA or EPSEA. The choice of approach was based on the grade and type of CS invasion. When invasion is confined to the medial and posterosuperior compartment, an MTEA may be sufficient. When the tumor also invades the anteroinferior and lateral compartments of the CS, an EPSEA is required. If the tumor also invades the upper structure, it is necessary to open a supradiaphragmatic corridor (two cases) or enlarge the opening toward the clivus in case of downward extension. An additional approach to the CS, never used for pituitary adenomas, is worth mentioning, namely, the trans-maxillo-pterygoid approach, which is indicated in tumors extending from the CS through the foramen rotundum to the pterygo-maxillary fossa, or vice versa, used more frequently for neurinomas and meningiomas.

The complication rate in our series of pituitary adenomas invading the CS appears to be low (**Table 21.11**). Our data are better than those reported in the literature for microscopic procedures.[21,22] Moreover, with respect to the report of Kitano et al,[22] we rarely had the necessity to use a hemotrasfusion (3%), and we had only one case of cranial nerve III palsy due to a blind curettage in an MTEA approach in a hard tumor invading the posterosuperior compartment of the CS.

Related to our own experience, as well as the experience of others in the recent literature,[22] we suggest revaluating the role of surgery in the management of pituitary adenomas invading the CS because it allows the surgeon to directly view and diagnose CS invasion, make a precise histopathologic diagnosis, perform tumoral debulking, and, in many cases, also the cure of the patient.

Definition of True Cavernous Sinus Involvement

Numerous studies have dealt with the predictive value of preoperative neuroimaging of CS invasion. Knosp et al[9] suggested a specific classification of CS invasion[6] based on the position of the lateral portion of the tumor in relation to the ICA (**Table 21.10**). Knosp's classification shows an incremental rate of risk of real involvement of the CS, but in analyzing all our pituitary adenoma cases, we did not find any correlation comparing the ICSI with Knosp's classification. (Correlation coefficient $[r] = -0.341$, $p = .1204$.) This finding confirms the reports of other authors[23–25] regarding a low predictive value of the preoperative MRI of the real tumoral extension to the CS. We have indeed experienced CS invasion when none was expected from neuroradiologic study (0.8%) and found no invasion when the MRI was highly suggestive of CS invasion (2.5%), and, in the more frequent MRI situation (Knosp classification 2), the predictive value is not indicative (~50%).

The limits of neuroradiologic studies are due to their present inability to clearly demonstrate the medial wall of the CS; it may appear as a fine line interposed between the medial venous compartment and the sellar content. However, when the tumor compresses the venous compartment, it may be absolutely indistinct from the wall of the carotid artery. On the other hand, there are situations where tumors that are completely enclosed in the sella area with a potentially high probability of surgical cure could be considered invasive and denied for surgical treatment. In our opinion, surgical inspection still remains the only way to ascertain the presence or absence of CS invasion.

Curing the Patient

The ideal goal in the management of pituitary adenomas is tumor removal with a long-term regression of the compressive symptoms or hormonal oversecretion without adjunctive alteration of pituitary functionality. Even if this target is thought to be very difficult to attain in tumors invading the CS, we obtained surgical cure in 48 (48%) of the patients (63% in NF adenomas and 31% in functioning adenomas). The success rate is lower than that reported by Kitano et al,[22] and this difference may be explained by the lower number of patients considered in their series. These data probably confirm that CS invasion is often a tumoral extension through the mesh of the medial wall of the CS more than real aggressiveness.[24,25] According to this observation, we found an extremely significant correlation ($p = .0009$) between the ICSI (focal invasion versus diffuse invasion of the CS) and the possibility of curing the patient.

Tumor Debulking

If tumor behavior did not permit radical removal of the tumor, the surgical goal was to debulk the tumor to achieve resolution of the compressive symptoms or to improve the efficacy of the postoperative medical therapy or radiotherapy.

As reported by other authors,[26] the mass effect symptoms, visual or neurologic deficits (**Table 21.7**), may improve or regress completely with surgical decompression, even with long-lasting duration. We obtained complete regression of the compressive symptoms in 83.6% of the cases (87% in functioning and 82% in NF adenomas).

Furthermore, tumor volume reduction plays an important role in the response of the tumor to adjuvant therapy. Tumor debulking is important for increasing the safety and efficacy of radiation therapy because it reduces the tumor residual volume and increases the distance from radiosensitive structures, such as the optic nerves and the chiasm.[27,28]

Petrossians et al[29] and Colao et al[30] have reported that tumor debulking increases the likelihood of achieving biochemical disease control with somatostatin analogues in acromegalic patients with adenomas who were not amenable to complete surgical resection and in whom primary somatostatin analogue therapy was unable to achieve good biochemical control.

When surgery alone is not able to obtain control of the disease, a multimodal approach is mandatory; medical therapy, radiotherapy, craniotomy, or additional revision endoscopic surgery could be used. With this type of management, an extra 36% (**Table 21.8**) of disease control can be obtained. This type of disease control could not be considered a surgical success but rather correct multimodal treatment of this complex pathology, and it justifies the necessity of centers where all types of competency are available.

In spite of multimodal management, six patients (6%) still remain noncontrolled and three of them subsequently died from brain invasion or distant metastasis (**Table 21.8**).

Histopathologic Evaluation

Precise histopathologic and immunohistochemical diagnoses are the cornerstone for the management of pituitary adenomas. Wolfsberger et al[31] did not find any differences in the specimens obtained from the sella and those from the CS in a study of patients treated for pituitary adenomas. In pituitary adenomas, the value of some immunohistochemical markers, such as K_i-67, is still debatable. In our experience, we found a significant correlation (p = .0182) between K_i-67 and the possibility of obtaining remission of the symptoms or controlling the tumor progression (**Table 21.9**).

In our series, a high value of K_i-67 (>10%) was associated with a poorer outcome; only one patient of nine is in remission, two developed metastasis and died from the pathology, and one is in rapid disease progression despite surgery and radiotherapy. Therefore, in our opinion, this index should be included among the factors that influence the postoperative treatment of the patient (i.e., radiosurgery will also be justified in small asymptomatic residual tumors having a high proliferative index).

■ Conclusion

In our experience, the endoscopic endonasal approach allows safe and effective management of pituitary adenomas with CS extension. MTEA may be adequate for a minor extension limited to the medial or posterosuperior compartments.

For a major extension having lateral or anteroinferior involvement of the CS, the extended approach (EPSEA) is preferable.

The aim of surgery is to confirm CS invasion, to reach a histologic diagnosis, which should include the measurement of the proliferative index, and to remove the tumor as radically and safely as possible. Radical removal may allow the patient to be cured even in secreting adenomas, but this result is possible only in a reduced percentage of cases and mainly when focal invasion occurs. When radical removal is not possible, debulking of the tumor may give satisfactory results because it allows clinical improvement and facilitates the effectiveness of the multimodal management controlling the tumor.

References

1. Parkinson D. A surgical approach to the cavernous portion of the carotid artery. Anatomical studies and case report. J Neurosurg 1965;23:474–483
2. Sekhar LN, Goel A, Sen CN. Cavernous sinus tumours. In: Apuzzo MLJ, ed. Brain Surgery: Complication Avoidance and Management. New York: Churchill Livingstone; 1993:2197–2218
3. Jho HD, Carrau RL. Endoscopic endonasal transsphenoidal surgery: experience with 50 patients. J Neurosurg 1997;87:44–51
4. Alfieri A, Jho HD. Endoscopic endonasal approaches to the cavernous sinus: surgical approaches. Neurosurgery 2001;49:354–360, discussion 360–362
5. Frank G, Pasquini E, Calbucci F. Endoscopic approach to the cavernous sinus via an ethmoido-pterygo-sphenoidal route. Presented at the 5th European Skull Base Society Congress, Copenhagen Denmark, June 15–17, 2001 (additional abstract, p009b)
6. Frank G, Pasquini E. Endoscopic endonasal cavernous sinus surgery, with special reference to pituitary adenomas. Front Horm Res 2006;34:64–82
7. Taptas JN. [The parasellar osteo-dural chamber and the vascular and neural elements that traverse it. An anatomical concept that would replace the cavernous sinus of classical anatomy]. Neurochirurgie 1990;36:201–208
8. Kassam AB, Vescan AD, Carrau RL, et al. Expanded endonasal approach: vidian canal as a landmark to the petrous internal carotid artery. J Neurosurg 2008;108:177–183
9. Knosp E, Steiner E, Kitz K, Matula C. Pituitary adenomas with invasion of the cavernous sinus space: a magnetic resonance imaging classification compared with surgical findings. Neurosurgery 1993;33:610–617, discussion 617–618
10. Giustina A, Barkan A, Casanueva FF, et al. Criteria for cure of acromegaly: a consensus statement. J Clin Endocrinol Metab 2000;85:526–529
11. Losa M, Mortini P, Barzaghi R, Gioia L, Giovanelli M. Surgical treatment of prolactin-secreting pituitary adenomas: early results and long-term outcome. J Clin Endocrinol Metab 2002;87:3180–3186

12. Nishizawa S, Oki Y, Ohta S, Yokota N, Yokoyama T, Uemura K. What can predict postoperative "endocrinological cure" in Cushing's disease? Neurosurgery 1999;45:239–244
13. Laws ER Jr, Onofrio BM, Pearson BW, McDonald TJ, Dirrenberger RA. Successful management of bilateral carotid-cavernous fistulae with a trans-sphenoidal approach. Neurosurgery 1979;4:162–167
14. Lalwani AK, Kaplan MJ, Gutin PH. The transsphenoethmoid approach to the sphenoid sinus and clivus. Neurosurgery 1992;31:1008–1014, discussion 1014
15. Arita K, Kurisu K, Tominaga A, et al. Transsphenoidal "cross court" approach using a slightly modified speculum to reach pituitary adenomas with lateral growth. Acta Neurochir (Wien) 2000;142:1055–1058
16. Fraioli B, Esposito V, Santoro A, Iannetti G, Giuffrè R, Cantore G. Transmaxillosphenoidal approach to tumors invading the medial compartment of the cavernous sinus. J Neurosurg 1995;82:63–69
17. Inoue T, Rhoton AL Jr, Theele D, Barry ME. Surgical approaches to the cavernous sinus: a microsurgical study. Neurosurgery 1990;26: 903–932
18. Sabit I, Schaefer SD, Couldwell WT. Extradural extranasal combined transmaxillary transsphenoidal approach to the cavernous sinus: a minimally invasive microsurgical model. Laryngoscope 2000; 110(2 Pt 1):286–291
19. Kitano M, Taneda M. Extended transsphenoidal approach with submucosal posterior ethmoidectomy for parasellar tumors. Technical note. J Neurosurg 2001;94:999–1004
20. Cavallo LM, Cappabianca P, Galzio R, Iaconetta G, de Divitiis E, Tschabitscher M. Endoscopic transnasal approach to the cavernous sinus versus transcranial route: anatomic study. Neurosurgery 2005; 56(2, Suppl):379–389, discussion 379–389
21. Couldwell WT, Weiss MH, Rabb C, Liu JK, Apfelbaum RI, Fukushima T. Variations on the standard transsphenoidal approach to the sellar region, with emphasis on the extended approaches and parasellar approaches: surgical experience in 105 cases. Neurosurgery 2004;55:539–547, discussion 547–550
22. Kitano M, Taneda M, Shimono T, Nakao Y. Extended transsphenoidal approach for surgical management of pituitary adenomas invading the cavernous sinus. J Neurosurg 2008;108:26–36
23. Enseñat J, Ortega A, Topcewski T, et al. [Predictive value of the Knosp classification in grading the surgical resection of invasive pituitary macroadenomas. A prospective study of 23 cases]. Neurocirugia (Astur) 2006;17:519–526
24. Roux FX, Obreja C, Moussa R, et al. [Intracavernous extension of hypophyseal macroadenomas: infiltration or invagination?]. Neurochirurgie 1998;44:344–351
25. Yokoyama S, Hirano H, Moroki K, Goto M, Imamura S, Kuratsu JI. Are nonfunctioning pituitary adenomas extending into the cavernous sinus aggressive and/or invasive? Neurosurgery 2001;49:857–862, discussion 862–863
26. Fahlbusch R, Buchfelder M. Transsphenoidal surgery of parasellar pituitary adenomas. Acta Neurochir (Wien) 1988;92:93–99
27. Shin M, Kurita H, Sasaki T, et al. Stereotactic radiosurgery for pituitary adenoma invading the cavernous sinus. J Neurosurg 2000;93(Suppl 3):2–5
28. Liu JK, Schmidt MH, MacDonald JD, Jensen RL, Couldwell WT. Hypophysial transposition (hypophysopexy) for radiosurgical treatment of pituitary tumors involving the cavernous sinus. Technical note. Neurosurg Focus 2003;14:e11
29. Petrossians P, Borges-Martins L, Espinoza C, et al. Gross total resection or debulking of pituitary adenomas improves hormonal control of acromegaly by somatostatin analogs. Eur J Endocrinol 2005;152:61–66
30. Colao A, Pivonello R, Galderisi M, et al. Impact of treating acromegaly first with surgery or somatostatin analogs on cardiomyopathy. J Clin Endocrinol Metab 2008;93:2639–2646
31. Wolfsberger S, Kitz K, Wunderer J, et al. Multiregional sampling reveals a homogenous distribution of Ki-67 proliferation rate in pituitary adenomas. Acta Neurochir (Wien) 2004;146:1323–1327, discussion 1327–1328

22 Microscopic versus Endoscopic Transsphenoidal Pituitary Surgery

Jonathan H. Sherman, Stephen J. Monteith, Edward R. Laws Jr., and John A. Jane Jr.

Historical Perspective

Surgical approaches to the sella turcica have interested both the neurosurgeon and otolaryngologist since the early 1900s. Davide Giordano initially proposed a transglabellar-nasal approach to the sella turcica using anatomical studies.[1,2] Based on the work of Giordano, Hermann Schloffer performed the first successful transsphenoidal resection of a pituitary tumor in 1907 via a three-stage lateral rhinotomy approach.[3,4] In this approach, Schloffer performed a nasal skin incision that extended to the glabella and allowed for the nose to be reflected laterally. This approach was modified in 1909 by Theodor Kocher, who performed a submucosal resection of the nasal septum. Kocher's technique included a complicated external nasal incision that resulted in improved cosmetic results as compared with those of his predecessors. Since the endonasal approach was initially described by Oskar Hirsch, the utility of the transsphenoidal approach to both sellar and parasellar lesions has grown in analogous fashion to our understanding of the tumor pathology as well as to advances in technology.[4,5]

Hirsch fashioned his endonasal surgical technique, avoiding the external nasal incision, after his mentor M. Hajek, who described a surgical approach to treat sphenoid sinusitis. In 1910, Hirsch performed his first endonasal approach on a patient with visual loss secondary to a pituitary lesion. The surgical resection of the lesion was performed over 5 weeks and in five different stages, each under local anesthesia, that included a middle turbinectomy, resection of the ethmoid air cells, an anterior sphenoidotomy, resection of the sellar floor, and finally resection of the pituitary lesion with subsequent improvement in vision.[6,7] Hirsch subsequently modified his approach based on the submucosal technique of Kocher to decrease the operative time. In addition, he added the nasal speculum to both retract the mucosal flaps laterally and maintain exposure.[4,5]

Harvey Cushing's first transsphenoidal operation used a modified version of Schloffer's approach in a patient with acromegaly. The approach resembled a technique that was later described by Ottokar Chiari in 1912, in which an external incision was performed in the superomedial aspect of the orbit followed by a wide ethmoidectomy.[8,9] Cushing later modified his technique based on the surgical approach described by Albert E. Halstead (**Fig. 22.1**). In 1912, Halstead described a sublabial gingival incision to allow for increased exposure of the sphenoid sinus.[8,10] In 1921 Cushing stated, "It is certain that no method is applicable for all conditions of pituitary tumor and that for some no satisfactory procedure has been devised."[3,11] Despite success with the transsphenoidal approach, Cushing exclusively used the transfrontal approach by 1929 for pituitary lesions, noting that chiasmal compression was more effectively relieved under the direct vision provided by the latter procedure.[3]

Following Cushing's example, the majority of neurosurgeons followed suit in abandoning the transsphenoidal approach. Hirsch, however, continued to defend the role of transsphenoidal surgery in treating pituitary lesions.[5] Norman Dott learned the transsphenoidal approach from Cushing and continued to operate on pituitary lesions via the transsphenoidal route long after his mentor had abandoned the approach. In 1956, Gerard Guiot observed Dott performing the transsphenoidal resection of a pituitary lesion in two patients. Based on this experience as well as a review of Dott's results with the approach, Guiot adopted the transsphenoidal approach in his own surgical practice and introduced an invaluable adjunct, intraoperative radiologic control.[7]

The resurgence of the transsphenoidal approach in North America was closely related to the work of Jules Hardy, who worked for 1 year under the tutelage of Guiot and during that time developed an appreciation for the transsphenoidal approach. To improve intraoperative visualization, Hardy introduced the surgical microscope to provide both illumination and magnification.[7] Based on this improved visualization, he was able to identify a cleavage plane between the tumor and the normal gland. Using this plane, he introduced the concept of the selective microadenomectomy in which removal of such a lesion could be accomplished without affecting the function of the normal gland. With the combination of the microscope and intraoperative fluoroscopic guidance, Hardy was able to remove a variety of sellar and parasellar lesions with less morbidity and mortality than that seen with the transcranial approach.[8]

The first neurosurgeon to use the endoscope in a transsphenoidal approach was Guiot, who abandoned the instrument secondary to inadequate visualization.[8] The use of the endoscope to assist in microscopic transsphenoidal surgical

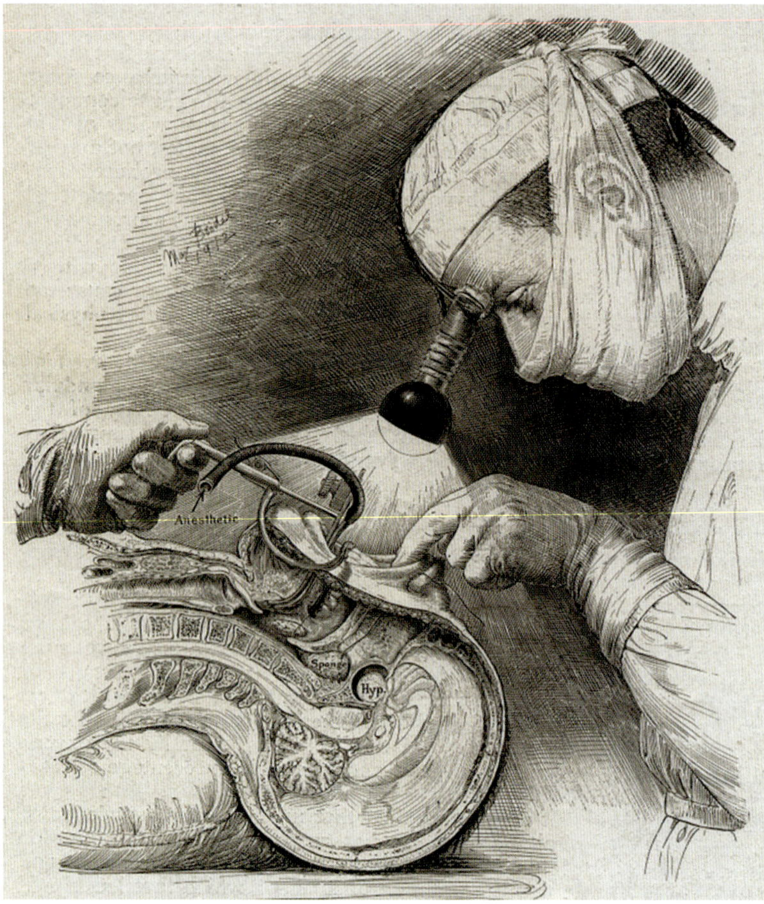

Fig. 22.1 The sublabial approach of Harvey Cushing. Original drawing by Max Brodel displaying a mouth gag, a sponge in the posterior nasopharynx to prevent aspiration, and a tongue depressor apparatus to administer ether anesthesia. (From Cushing H. Surgical experiences with pituitary disorders. JAMA 1921;76:1721–1726. Reprinted with permission.)

procedures was not again reported until 1977 by Apuzzo et al[12] and soon thereafter by Bushe and Halves[13] in 1978. Jankowski et al[14] subsequently reported in 1992 the role of a pure endoscopic transsphenoidal approach to the sella turcica. The pioneers of the latter technique for resecting pituitary adenomas include Hae Dong Jho, a neurosurgeon, and Ricardo Carrau, an otolaryngologist, at the University of Pittsburgh Medical Center (UPMC). In addition, Amin Kassam, a neurosurgeon at UPMC, has looked to expand the role of the endoscope for the resection of skull base lesions outside of the sella turcica. Significant contributions to both the surgical technique as well as the surgical instruments for the pure endoscopic approach are attributed to neurosurgeons and otolaryngologists in North America and Europe.[15]

Sinonasal Anatomy

The goal of any surgical procedure is to minimize morbidity while maximizing surgical success. An understanding of the sinonasal anatomy is critical in reaching this goal. Effective mucociliary movement is critical for maintaining mucous flow toward the sinus ostia and onto the nasopharynx. Blockage of this flow can result in stagnation of mucus within the sinus and subsequent sinusitis.[16]

The corridor to access the sphenoid sinus is between the middle turbinate and the nasal septum. Anterior to the middle turbinate, the drainage sites for the frontal, anterior ethmoid, and maxillary sinuses converge. The sphenoethmoidal recess is located between the rostrum of the sphenoid sinus and the inner aspect of the middle turbinate and serves as the confluence of drainage for the posterior ethmoid and sphenoid sinuses. Consequently, preservation of the anatomy anterior and lateral to the middle turbinate is critical to maintaining the normal drainage pathways of the paranasal sinuses. Therefore, both the approach used to access the sphenoid sinus and the manner of closure are important in minimizing morbidity.[16]

Endonasal Pituitary Surgery

The transsphenoidal approach has continued to be developed to allow for maximal tumor resection with minimal morbidity and mortality. The primary goals in resecting functioning pituitary microadenomas include eliminating tumor mass and minimizing risk of recurrence, normalization of hormone hypersecretion, and preservation of pituitary function. The resection of pituitary macroadenomas has similar goals, with the addition of removing mass effect on vital structures, such as the optic chiasm.[17] The aforementioned goals can best be accomplished by using an operative approach that minimizes the morbidity secondary to the surgical approach while at the same time maximizing the visualization of the sellar and parasellar regions. The operative microscope has been a key component to the successful resection of a variety of these sellar and parasellar lesions by providing three-dimensional visualization of the surgical field.[18] In an effort to improve visualization, the endoscope has become a valuable tool in transsphenoidal resection of pituitary lesions.

Patient Positioning

Patients are positioned such that the surgeon can comfortably access the sphenoid sinus and sella turcica and minimize intraoperative bleeding. Although a variety of positions are used, we advocate a lawn-chair–type position for both the endoscopic and microscopic approaches. Venous congestion is consequently minimized, allowing for increased venous drainage and decreased bleeding. The traditional position used by the otolaryngologist places the surgeon at the head of the table with the patient positioned supine. Although this improves surgeon comfort, this supine position does not allow for the reduced venous congestion offered by the lawn-chair–type position.[19]

The patient's head is positioned in a Mayfield horseshoe headrest and flexed laterally. For ease in producing an accurate lateral radiograph with intraoperative fluoroscopy, the bed is positioned such that the patient's head is parallel to the walls of the room and the nasal dorsum is parallel to the floor. In addition, the bed is placed in reverse Trendelenburg position such that the thorax is situated at approximately a 30-degree angle above the horizontal. The bed is also tilted slightly to the surgeon, both to prevent the surgeon from leaning over the patient and to improve the patient's lateral neck rotation (**Fig. 22.2**). As the patient's head is not fixed to the operative table, this position can be subtly manipulated intraoperatively. This is more pertinent in microscopic surgery in which the surgeon can rotate the head to look laterally instead of moving the microscope.[19]

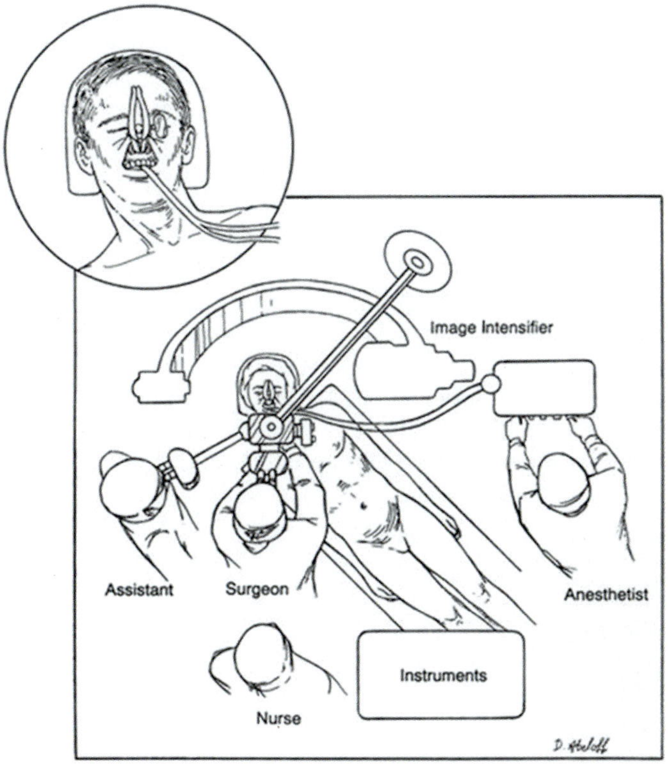

Fig. 22.2 Operating room setup and patient positioning for the microscopic transsphenoidal approach. The magnified drawing of the patient's head displays the sublabial approach with the nasal speculum in place. (From Elias WJ, Laws ER Jr. Transsphenoidal approaches to lesions of the sella. In: Schmidek HH, Sweet WH, eds. Operative Surgical Techniques: Indications, Methods, and Results, Vol 1, 4th ed. Philadelphia: WB Saunders, 2000:373–384. Reprinted with permission.)

Nasal Preparation

The nasal preparation begins preanesthesia with intranasal oxymetazoline sprays. Once the patient is in the operating room, immediately after intubation and prior to positioning, additional oxymetazoline should be applied intranasally. After the patient is positioned, the nares and maxilla are first washed with chlorhexidine antiseptic solution. The middle turbinate and septum may be injected with 1:200,000 epinephrine. In the sublabial approach, the mucosa overlying the maxilla is also injected. Cotton patties, soaked in either oxymetazoline or epinephrine, are placed between the middle turbinate and the septum for the purpose of hemostasis. Following draping, the patties are removed. For the endoscopic approach, the nasal preparation is perhaps more important as even small amounts of bleeding can make the exposure difficult.

Surgical Approaches

The manner in which the surgeon accesses the sphenoid sinus can be broadly divided into endonasal and sublabial approaches. Traditionally, both endonasal and sublabial approaches were performed using submucosal tunnels. Some surgeons have advocated an endonasal direct sphenoidotomy.[20] This approach and its variants have the benefit of fewer anterior septal complications and a more rapid access to the sphenoid sinus. However, the width of the exposure (and therefore the field of view and maneuverability of instruments) progressively decreases from the sublabial to the endonasal transseptal to the endonasal direct sphenoidotomy.[19,21]

Following exposure of the sphenoid sinus and completion of the anterior sphenoidotomy, the surgeon must decide the required sellar and parasellar exposure to adequately resect the tumor. The traditional microscopic exposure involves only removal of the anterior wall of the sella turcica. A chisel and mallet or drill may be used to gain initial access to the sellar dura followed by use of the Kerrison punch. Often the sellar bone has been thinned by the tumor and can be easily out-fractured. The goal of bony removal is to expose the dura just medial to the medial surface of the cavernous segment of the carotid artery bilaterally. As the carotid protuberances most often cannot be completely visualized with the microscopic approach, this bony removal requires the combination of direct visualization and surgical feel with the Kerrison punch (**Fig. 22.3**). Inferiorly the bone forming the sellar floor should be removed and superiorly the bony opening should reach the inferior border of the superior intercavernous sinus. For larger tumors extending toward the anterior cranial fossa, an extended transsphenoidal approach can be of value. In this approach, the bony opening is extended beyond the anterior wall of the sella turcica to include the planum sphenoidale.[21–23]

Our pure endoscopic technique has evolved over time from attempting to recapitulate a mononostril microscopic approach to a more practical binostril approach. There has also been a shift from using an endoscope holder to using a three-hand technique. One of the primary advantages of using the latter approach is the pseudo–three-dimensional surgical view that can be generated by movement of the endoscope during the operation.[24]

For initial exposure, the surgeon uses a two-hand technique (**Fig. 22.4**) with the 0-degree short endoscope for dissection to the sphenoid ostia. The right nostril is typically used for this purpose, unless a septal deviation significantly decreases the working room, requiring use of the left nostril. The middle turbinate is then identified and carefully lateralized with the use of a suction spatula. The surgeon must be careful to minimize damage to the normal mucous drainage pathway as described above.[24]

There are several techniques that may be employed to perform the initial sphenoidotomy. The sphenoid ostium is identified typically at the inferior third of the superior turbinate. The mucosa at the keel of the sphenoid bone adjacent to the ostium is then either incised with a Cottle elevator or coagulated with the suction Bovie. The Cottle elevator can then be used to reflect the posterior wall of the nasal septum and expose the contralateral sphenoid ostium. The bone beyond the two ostia can then be removed, which provides the initial sphenoidotomy. A soft tissue shaver is then used to efficiently remove the mucosa over the anterior wall of the sphenoid sinus. The shaver in combination with backbiting instruments can then be used to produce a posterior septectomy, an essential component to the binasal approach. The surgeon can then use the endoscope to look into the contralateral nostril, lateralize the middle turbinate, and gain access to the exposed sphenoid sinus.[24]

The mucosa overlying the inferolateral portion of the anterior sphenoid wall should be elevated to expose the bony surface. The posterior branch of the sphenopalatine artery runs in this mucosa such that resection of the bone and the mucosa together can lead to damage to the artery. If the source of bleeding is not adequately appreciated and hemostasis is not effectively achieved intraoperatively, bleeding from this artery can continue postoperatively and lead to epistaxis and possible reoperation. The anterior sphenoidotomy is then performed such that the opticocarotid recess is visualized superolaterally and the clivus is identified inferiorly, displaying a significant improvement in visualization as compared with the microscopic approach (**Fig. 22.5**). To take advantage of this improved visualization, we have found that the endoscopic sphenoidotomy must be larger that what is typically performed during a microscopic approach. The sphenoidotomy required for an endoscopic approach must

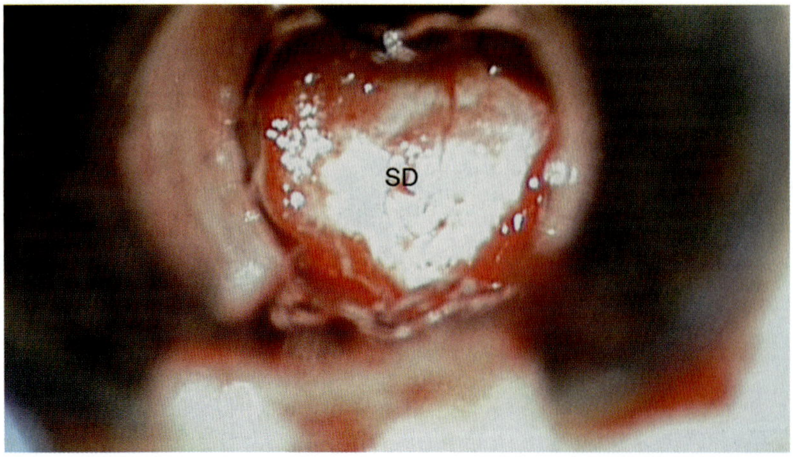

Fig. 22.3 Microscopic operative view following an anterior sphenoidotomy. The sellar dura (SD) is exposed to the cavernous sinus bilaterally; however, the microscope's line of sight limits direct lateral visualization.

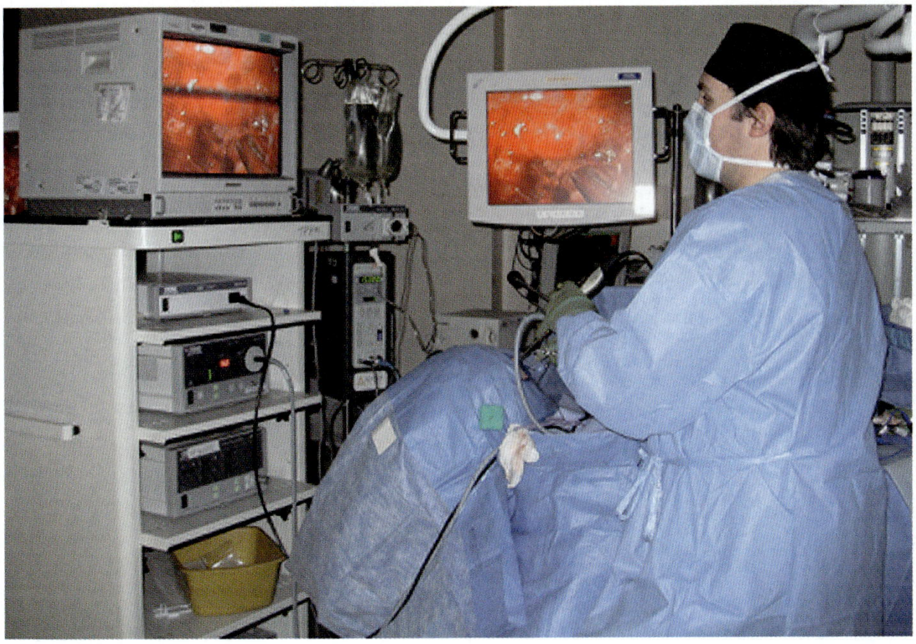

Fig. 22.4 Initial endoscopic exposure of the sphenoid sinus and sella turcica using a two-hand surgical technique. The surgeon is using the 0-degree short endoscope for this portion of the approach.

be large enough to accommodate not only the usual instruments (suction, curette) but also the endoscope.[24]

We advocate switching to a three-hand technique prior to opening the bony sella. This confirms an adequate degree of exposure prior to removing tumor. If the surgeons note a conflict of instruments with the endoscope, then a larger sphenoidotomy is needed. It is better if this is recognized prior to tumor resection than during the actual resection. The surgeon is then able to use both hands for tumor resection through a binasal approach (**Fig. 22.6**). The sphenoid mucosa is first removed only over the anterior wall of the sella turcica. A fine chisel and mallet or drill is then used to remove the anterior wall of the sella turcica to the same extent as seen in the microscopic approach. The planum sphenoidale can also be removed for an extended approach for resecting lesions that extend outside the confines of the sella turcica.[24,25] Through the work of Kassam and colleagues from UPMC, an expanded endonasal approach can also be used to resect lesions extending toward the clivus, petrous bone, and middle cranial fossa.[26,27]

The opening of the sella using the endoscope does not differ in dimension compared with the microscopic approach. However, because the intrasphenoidal anatomy is often better visualized endoscopically, a more precise opening of the sella can be performed. Most often the anatomy is seen well enough to forgo an intraoperative x-ray. An exception is in

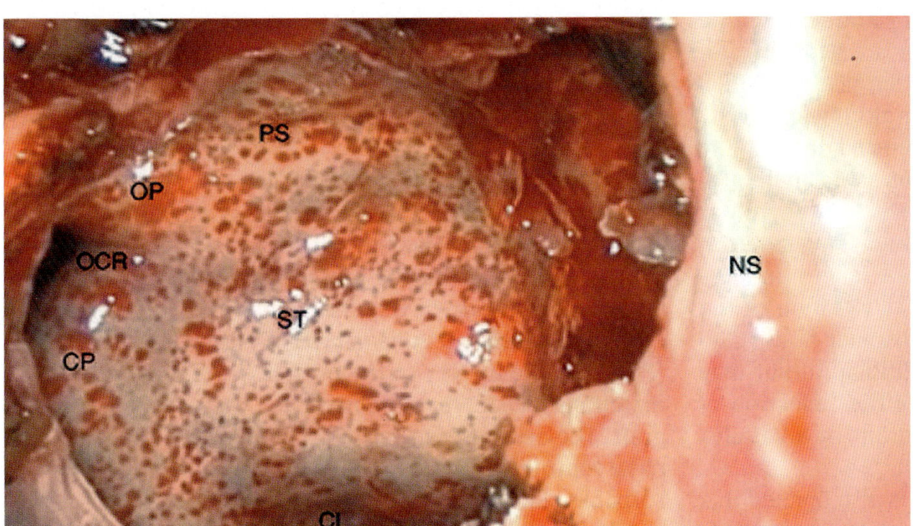

Fig. 22.5 Endoscopic operative view of the sphenoid sinus anatomy following the anterior sphenoidotomy and posterior septectomy. The optic protuberance (OP) overlying the optic nerve and the carotid protuberance (CP) overlying the cavernous carotid are readily visible, as is the opticocarotid recess (OCR). The view provided by the endoscope can also aid in delineating between the sella turcica (ST), the clivus (Cl), and the planum sphenoidale (PS). The nasal septum (NS) is also seen is this figure.

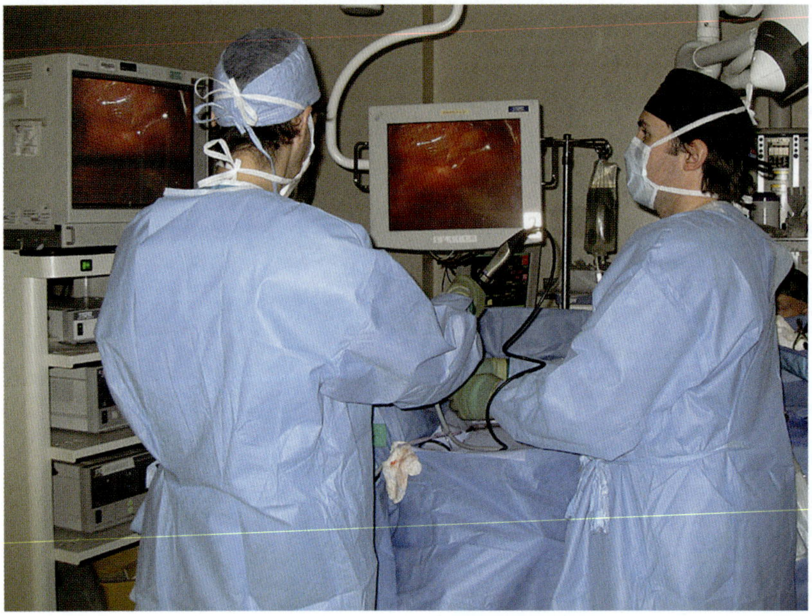

Fig. 22.6 Three-handed endoscopic technique for opening of the anterior wall of the sella turcica and tumor resection. The assistant surgeon can use the 0-, 30-, or 45-degree long endoscopes for this portion of surgical procedure.

patients with conchal and presellar sphenoid anatomy in whom the confines of the sella may be difficult to assess. In these patients, frameless image guidance can be helpful.

Tumor Resection

In the microscopic approach, the operative microscope should be adjusted prior to incising the dura such that the objective distance is approximately 375 mm to allow for adequate space for both the operative instruments and the surgeon's hands. In addition, the magnification should be set such that the sellar dura fills the entire field of view. The dura is then typically opened with a surgical blade. In macroadenomas, an uncauterized window of dura can be removed as a pathologic specimen to evaluate for dural tumor invasion. A nerve hook is then used to generate a plane between the inner dural layer and the tumor/pituitary gland surface. The lateral and inferior aspects of the tumor are generally removed prior to the superior portion. This surgical technique can allow for the tumor to fall into the surgical field.

The operative microscope can be adjusted to partially visualize the medial wall of the cavernous sinus bilaterally. However, the lateral and superior portions of the tumor most often are removed by blind pass of blunt ring curettes, relying on the surgeon's experience to feel for residual tumor and minimize complications, such as violation of the diaphragm sella and subsequent cerebrospinal fluid (CSF) leak. To assist with tumor resection, additional tumor may be delivered into the surgical field via either injection of 10 mL of air or saline through a lumbar drain, by a Valsalva maneuver, or by jugular vein compression.[19]

In the endoscopic approach, the dura is also opened in a similar fashion to that of the microscopic approach. However, because there is no speculum in place, the surgeon must take care not to injure mucosa when placing the blade intranasally. To obviate the risk of mucosal injury, the surgeon may also use a knife with a retractable blade as designed by Paolo Cappabianca. The tumor is also resected in the same sequential manner as in the microscopic technique, first generating a plane between the dura and the tumor. Subsequently, the tumor is removed inferiorly, laterally, and then superiorly. After tumor resection the 30- and 45-degree endoscopes can be used to better visualize the cavernous sinus wall and diaphragm sella. The primary difference in an endoscopic removal of a tumor is that the tumor is removed under direct visualization instead of by feel. Tumor can be seen being removed from the cavernous sinus walls and the diaphragm more directly. This improves the surgical efficiency and provides a more certain removal of tumor. Of course, some tumors (i.e., those with cavernous sinus invasion) will not be completely removed regardless of whether a microscope or endoscope is used.[24]

Closure

In our view, regardless of whether an endoscopic or microscopic approach has been employed, the method of closure primarily depends on the presence or absence of an intraoperative CSF leak. In the absence of a leak in the microscopic approach, the sella is typically packed with Gelfoam (Pfizer, Brooklyn, NY). In the presence of a small hole in the diaphragm sellae, the sella is packed with an abdominal fat graft. The sella is then reconstructed with either the bony nasal septum with the transseptal approach or with a bioabsorbable plate with the direct sphenoidotomy approach. As autologous bone or cartilage is unavailable, a bioabsorbable plate must be used to reconstruct the anterior sellar wall. However, with a large diaphragmatic defect the sphenoid sinus mucosa is removed and both the sella and sphenoid sinus are typically packed with abdominal fat. Nasal packing is used at closure to prevent a septal hematoma after transseptal approaches but is not necessary after the direct microscopic or endoscopic approaches.[21,28,29]

Although our basic algorithms are the same, the repair of intraoperative CSF leaks following the endoscopic or microscopic approach is not precisely the same. The primary difference is that after an endoscopic technique the defect is larger. Not only is the bony anterior sphenoidotomy larger in all directions, unlike the microscopic transseptal approach, but also the nasal mucosa overlying the sphenoid is completely removed during the approach. Therefore, one of the barriers typically present after the microscopic approach is absent. Also because a speculum is not used, the fat graft can be more difficult to place during an endoscopic approach.

Microscopic Versus Endoscopic Surgical Outcomes

The microscopic transsphenoidal approach has been the most common technique for resecting pituitary lesions over the past 40 years. Consequently, the majority of large surgical series include patients with tumors primarily resected via this approach. In addition, many of the older series do not differentiate among those patients treated via the microscopic, endoscopic-assisted, or pure endoscopic approach. Over the past 10 years, larger case series have been published reporting the surgical results using the pure endoscopic approach alone. The most comprehensive studies as described below show the efficacy of the transsphenoidal approach with a significantly higher remission rate for noninvasive microadenomas as compared with invasive macroadenomas.

Microscopic Approach

Laws and Jane[21] reported their series of 4020 transsphenoidal operations in which the majority of cases used the microscope approach alone. Of patients presenting with nonfunctioning adenomas and preoperative visual loss, 87% displayed postoperative visual improvement. Patients with growth hormone (GH)-secreting adenomas displayed an 88% remission rate with microadenomas and a 65% remission rate with macroadenomas. Requirements for remission included normalization of insulin-like growth factor-1 (IGF-1) levels, a random GH level less than 2.5 ng/mL, and a nadir GH level less than 1 ng/mL during an oral glucose tolerance test (OGTT). Acromegalic symptoms were improved in 95% of patents with a 10-year recurrence risk of only 2%. Of patients with medically unresponsive prolactin (PRL)-secreting tumors, 87% with microadenomas and 56% with macroadenomas displayed normalization of prolactin levels postoperatively. Of patients with adrenocorticotropic hormone (ACTH)-secreting tumors, a 91% remission rate was achieved for those with microadenomas, with a 65% remission rate for those with macroadenomas.

Several smaller series have also been reported looking at outcomes with individual tumor subtypes. Tyrrell et al[30] reported the results of 219 female patients who underwent microsurgical resection of prolactinomas. The study evaluated patients treated between 1976 and 1979 and those treated between 1998 and 1992 to assess the role of surgery before (group 1) and during (group 2) the era of dopamine agonist therapy for medical management. Of patients with preoperative PRL levels ≤100 ng/mL, 91% of patients with microadenomas and between 80 and 88% of patients with either intrasellar or suprasellar macroadenomas displayed initial remission. Patients with PRL values >200 ng/mL with larger and more invasive tumors displayed a much lower initial remission rate of between 37 and 41%. The authors reported a 82% continued remission rate with a median follow-up of 15.6 years in group 1 and an 88% continued remission rate with a median follow-up of 3.2 years in group 2.

With regard to Cushing's disease, Pouratian et al[31] reported the outcomes in 111 patients with the diagnosis of Cushing's disease without postoperative pathologic confirmation. Surgical remission was defined in this study as a drop in serum cortisol levels to 2 µg/mL or lower within 72 hours of surgery. The authors reported that 50% of patients achieved postoperative remission as compared with 79% for the 490 total transsphenoidal operations for Cushing's disease performed by this chapter's senior author.

Understanding the effect of microscopic dural invasion of pituitary adenomas is an important aspect for decreasing recurrence of nonsecretory adenomas and achieving remission in secretory adenomas. Meij et al[32] analyzed 354 dural specimens with the diagnosis of a pituitary adenoma for tumor cell invasion. Of the specimens, 161 contained tumor cell invasion and 192 displayed no evidence of invasion. In addition, 291 specimens were from primary transsphenoidal resection and 55 specimens were from repeat transsphenoidal resection. The neuropathologist identified dural invasion in 41% of the former group and in 69% in the latter group. Of patients who underwent primary resection, tumor size correlated with tumor invasion such that 70% of tumors greater than 4 cm displayed dural tumor cell invasion. In addition, dural invasion was noted in 50% of nonsecretory tumors and in 30 to 35% of the secretory tumors. The incidence of residual tumor was significantly higher and the remission rate was significantly lower in patients with invasive tumors undergoing primary tumor resection as compared with patients without invasive tumors.

Laws et al studied the outcomes in 56 patients using the extended transsphenoidal skull base technique, as first described by Weiss.[33] Although the majority of tumors were craniopharyngiomas (54%), the report provides insight in the role of the transsphenoidal approach for lesions extending outside of the sella turcica. Of the 44 patients with preoperative visual decline, 64% displayed postoperative visual improvement. Postoperative CSF leakage and meningitis occurred in 12.5% of patients. All patients responded to repeat transsphenoidal closure of the leakage and appropriate antibiotic therapy for meningitis. The authors felt that as compared with traditional craniotomy approaches, the results were satisfactory for these large, difficult-to-treat lesions.[22]

Endoscopic Approach

The nuances of the endoscopic approach have been well described in the literature, including such details as the anatomical considerations as well as the essential endoscopic instruments.[25,29,34–37] Over the past 10 years, reports detailing the surgical outcomes following the endoscopic resection of pituitary adenomas have emerged. These reports have subsequently allowed for a comparison between the microscopic and endoscopic techniques.

Kabil et al[38] evaluated the surgical outcomes of 300 patients treated via a pure endoscopic approach. The tumor subtypes included 54% nonsecretory adenomas, 21% PRL-secreting adenomas, 16% GH-secreting adenomas, and 9% ACTH-secreting adenomas. The authors compared their results to numerous microscopic transsphenoidal surgical series using the mean remission rate between series. They also compared complication rates to the rates reported by Ciric et al,[39] generated via a national survey evaluating surgeons using a transseptal-transsphenoidal approach. For nonsecretory adenomas, complete surgical resection was confirmed via postoperative magnetic resonance imaging in 93% of cases using the pure endoscopic approach and in 82% of cases using the microscopic approach. An improved initial remission rate for secretory tumors was also seen in comparing the pure endoscopic versus microscopic approach such that ACTH-secreting adenomas displayed a 86% versus 81% remission rate, PRL-secreting tumors displayed a 89% versus 66% remission rate, and GH-secreting tumors displayed a 85% versus 77% remission rate. A decreased rate of postoperative complications was also seen for surgeons performing the pure endoscopic approach. In comparing the microscopic transseptal versus the pure endoscopic approach, nasal septal perforations decreased from 6.7% to 0.7%, postoperative epistaxis decreased from 10% to 1.3%, diabetes insipidus decreased from 17.8% to 5.3%, and CSF leak decreased from 3.9% to 1.7%.[39]

Frank et al[40] also reported similar surgical outcomes in comparing the pure endoscopic approach versus the microscopic approach. They also compared their surgical results with microscopic surgical results as reported in the literature. They analyzed 381 patients including 208 secretory adenomas and 173 nonsecretory adenomas. For GH-secreting tumors, they defined remission as normalization of serum IGF-1 and found comparable results to microscopic resection with 69.2% versus 70%. Normalization of serum PRL in patients with PRL-secreting adenomas was reported at 85.7% in microadenomas and 68.5% in macroadenomas. In ACTH-secreting adenomas, the authors found a similar remission rate between microadenomas and macroadenomas reported at 67.7% and 68%, respectively. Finally, the authors reported a 76.9% rate of complete resection for nonsecretory macroadenomas. In comparing the microscopic versus the endoscopic approach, epistaxis decreased from 1.7% to 0.7%, sinusitis decreased from 6.0% to 0%, septum perforation decreased from 4.6% to 0%, and CSF leak decreased from 2.8% to 1.2%.

Comparison Between the Microscopic and Endoscopic Approach

In assessing any surgical lesion, the surgeon must always consider what surgical approach can best be utilized to maximally resect the tumor while minimizing morbidity and morbidity. As reported by Ciric et al,[39] the surgeon's experience with the transsphenoidal approach directly correlated with a decreased complication rate. Although the report analyzed only the microscopic approach, the results can likely be extrapolated to the endoscopic approach as well.

There are distinct advantages to the microscopic adenomectomy. The operative microscope is a standard part of many neurosurgical operations from spinal to intracranial procedures. Consequently, most neurosurgeons are familiar with how to manipulate the microscope to obtain an ideal three-dimensional view. In addition, the microscope can easily be positioned such that the manipulation of surgical instruments is not impeded. The microscopic approach uses a nasal speculum, potentially allowing for decreased injury to the nasal mucosa. In addition to mucosal protection, once its position is confirmed by image guidance, the speculum provides a constant safe trajectory to the sella. Finally, in many centers the microscopic approach can be safely performed in less time as compared with the endoscopic approach.[24]

Although numerous advantages exist for the microscopic approach, the technique is not without disadvantages. The field of view is narrow, restricting the view of anatomical landmarks within the sphenoid sinus. The carotid protuberances and opticocarotid recesses, which are not usually visualized in the microscopic approach, are helpful landmarks to identify the surgical midline. Thus, this approach relies on such adjuncts as intraoperative fluoroscopy to assist with the approach to the sella turcica. In addition, the microscope limits the surgical view by line of sight. With regard to tumor resection, the sellar floor and cavernous sinus walls are rarely fully visible. The optic chiasm is also rarely visible, limiting direct confirmation that it is adequately decompressed. Finally, the transseptal microscopic approach typically requires postoperative nasal packing.[24]

Compared with the microscopic technique, the endoscopic approach offers unique advantages to the surgeon. Unlike the limitations imposed by the microscope's line of sight, the endoscope provides a panoramic view to identify the key landmarks of interest. The endoscope allows for a superior view of the nasal anatomy for identification of the sphenoid sinus. Consequently, fluoroscopic guidance is not necessary for safely reaching the sphenoid ostia. Once inside the sphenoid sinus, the limits of the sella turcica can be accurately determined via identification of such anatomical landmarks as the carotid protuberance and the opticocarotid recess. An exception is noted with a presellar or conchal sphenoid sinus in which image guidance is still helpful. With regard to tumor resection, the endoscope provides a magnified view of the tumor–gland interface. Identification of this interface can potentially lead to improvement in both the degree of tumor resection as well as preservation of normal pituitary gland function. In addition, the 0- and 30-degree endoscopes can visualize the sellar floor, the cavernous sinus wall, and the optic chiasm and decrease the risk of leaving residual tumor. Finally, this approach rarely requires nasal packing, which has been shown to correlate with improved patient comfort and satisfaction. Perhaps the most significant advantage is that during resection the surgeon removes a greater portion of the tumor under direct visualization, providing a more certain and efficient resection.[24,41]

Although the endoscopic approach offers many advantages, it also has disadvantages. Most neurosurgeons are not familiar with the endoscope, and a steep learning curve exists for a safe and effective endoscopic surgical tumor resection. As such, many neurosurgeons may choose to ask an otolaryngologist to perform the approach. For the otolaryngologist, the endoscopic approach demands more time in the operating room than does the microscopic approach. With the microscopic transsphenoidal approach, the otolaryngologist performs the exposure and the closure. With the endoscopic approach, the otolaryngologist must be present throughout the operation. The operative time is typically longer than that seen in the microscopic approach, especially when the approach is performed by a neurosurgeon. The focus and zoom features are also limited with the endoscope camera and require a facile assistant to maintain visualization on the region of interest.[24]

In addition, the use of endoscopic instruments poses three main issues. First, the nasal mucosa is not protected by the nasal speculum, as in the microscopic approach. This mucosa can subsequently be injured via instrument insertion and removal throughout the surgical procedure. Second, the assistant driving the endoscope must be constantly aware of the endoscope's position so that it does not interfere with the surgical instruments and does not rotate, providing incorrect information regarding the anatomical orientation. Finally, and as a corollary to this second issue, the surgeon must maximize the exposure of the sella turcica to provide enough room for both the endoscope and endoscopic instruments. Consequently, the binasal endoscopic exposure is larger than the microscopic exposure.[24]

Conclusion

The transsphenoidal resection of pituitary lesions has a rich history that dates to the beginning of the 20th century. The surgical approach has continually evolved over this time period. The contributors to this evolution have all based their unique contributions on the same goals. These goals include maximizing surgical resection of the lesion while minimizing morbidity and mortality. As the neurosurgeon gains experience with any modification to the surgical approach, complications will continue to decrease as surgical outcomes equal and perhaps surpass those achieved by previous techniques. The microscopic and endoscopic approaches to the sella are both safe and effective techniques in which a pituitary lesion may be resected. As neurosurgeons gain experience with the latter technique, surgical outcomes can be more accurately compared with those obtained with the microscope.

References

1. Artico M, Pastore FS, Fraioli B, Giuffrè R. The contribution of Davide Giordano (1864–1954) to pituitary surgery: the transglabellar-nasal approach. Neurosurgery 1998;42:909–911, discussion 911–912
2. Liu JK, Cohen-Gadol AA, Laws ER Jr, Cole CD, Kan P, Couldwell WT. Harvey Cushing and Oskar Hirsch: early forefathers of modern transsphenoidal surgery. J Neurosurg 2005;103:1096–1104
3. Cohen-Gadol AA, Laws ER, Spencer DD, De Salles AA. The evolution of Harvey Cushing's surgical approach to pituitary tumors from transsphenoidal to transfrontal. J Neurosurg 2005;103:372–377
4. Kanter AS, Dumont AS, Asthagiri AR, Oskouian RJ, Jane JA Jr, Laws ER Jr. The transsphenoidal approach. A historical perspective. Neurosurg Focus 2005;18:e6
5. Lanzino G, Laws ER Jr. Pioneers in the development of transsphenoidal surgery: Theodor Kocher, Oskar Hirsch, and Norman Dott. J Neurosurg 2001;95:1097–1103
6. Hirsch O. Endonasal method of removal of hypophyseal tumors. With report of two successful cases. JAMA 1910;55:772–774
7. Lanzino G, Laws ER Jr. Key personalities in the development and popularization of the transsphenoidal approach to pituitary tumors: an historical overview. Neurosurg Clin N Am 2003;14:1–10
8. Liu JK, Das K, Weiss MH, Laws ER Jr, Couldwell WT. The history and evolution of transsphenoidal surgery. J Neurosurg 2001;95:1083–1096
9. Cohen-Gadol AA, Liu JK, Laws ER Jr. Cushing's first case of transsphenoidal surgery: the launch of the pituitary surgery era. J Neurosurg 2005;103:570–574

10. Halstead AE. Remarks on the operative treatment of tumors of the hypophysis. With the report of two cases operated on by an oronasal method. Surg Gynecol Obstet 1910;10:494–502
11. Cushing H. Disorders of the pituitary gland. Retrospective and prophetic. JAMA 1921;76:1721–1726
12. Apuzzo ML, Heifetz MD, Weiss MH, Kurze T. Neurosurgical endoscopy using the side-viewing telescope. J Neurosurg 1977;46:398–400
13. Bushe KA, Halves E. [Modified technique in transsphenoidal operations of pituitary adenomas. Technical note (author's transl)]. Acta Neurochir (Wien) 1978;41:163–175
14. Jankowski R, Auque J, Simon C, Marchal JC, Hepner H, Wayoff M. Endoscopic pituitary tumor surgery. Laryngoscope 1992;102:198–202
15. Prevedello DM, Doglietto F, Jane JA Jr, Jagannathan J, Han J, Laws ER Jr. History of endoscopic skull base surgery: its evolution and current reality. J Neurosurg 2007;107:206–213
16. Jho HD. Endoscopic pituitary surgery. Pituitary 1999;2:139–154
17. Couldwell WT. Transsphenoidal and transcranial surgery for pituitary adenomas. J Neurooncol 2004;69:237–256
18. de Divitiis E, Cappabianca P. Microscopic and endoscopic transsphenoidal surgery. Neurosurgery 2002;51:1527–1529, author reply 1529–1530
19. Jane JA Jr, Thapar K, Kaptain GJ, Maartens N, Laws ER Jr. Pituitary surgery: transsphenoidal approach. Neurosurgery 2002;51:435–442, discussion 442–444
20. Griffith HB, Veerapen R. A direct transnasal approach to the sphenoid sinus. Technical note. J Neurosurg 1987;66:140–142
21. Laws ER, Jane JA Jr. Neurosurgical approach to treating pituitary adenomas. Growth Horm IGF Res 2005;15(Suppl A):S36–S41
22. Laws ER, Kanter AS, Jane JA Jr, Dumont AS. Extended transsphenoidal approach. J Neurosurg 2005;102:825–827, discussion 827–828
23. Kouri JG, Chen MY, Watson JC, Oldfield EH. Resection of suprasellar tumors by using a modified transsphenoidal approach. Report of four cases. J Neurosurg 2000;92:1028–1035
24. Jane JA Jr, Han J, Prevedello DM, Jagannathan J, Dumont AS, Laws ER Jr. Perspectives on endoscopic transsphenoidal surgery. Neurosurg Focus 2005;19:E2
25. de Divitiis E, Cappabianca P, Cavallo LM. Endoscopic transsphenoidal approach: adaptability of the procedure to different sellar lesions. Neurosurgery 2002;51:699–705, discussion 705–707
26. Kassam AB, Gardner P, Snyderman C, Mintz A, Carrau R. Expanded endonasal approach: fully endoscopic, completely transnasal approach to the middle third of the clivus, petrous bone, middle cranial fossa, and infratemporal fossa. Neurosurg Focus 2005; 19:E6
27. Prevedello DM, Thomas A, Gardner P, Snyderman CH, Carrau RL, Kassam AB. Endoscopic endonasal resection of a synchronous pituitary adenoma and a tuberculum sellae meningioma: technical case report. Neurosurgery 2007;60(4, Suppl 2):E401, discussion E401
28. Schwartz M, Swearingen B, Black P. Transsphenoidal surgery for pituitary tumors. In: Kaye AH, Black P, eds. Operative Neurosurgery. London: Churchill Livingstone; 2000:672–683
29. Cappabianca P, Cavallo LM, de Divitiis E. Endoscopic endonasal transsphenoidal surgery. Neurosurgery 2004;55:933–940, discussion 940–941
30. Tyrrell JB, Lamborn KR, Hannegan LT, Applebury CB, Wilson CB. Transsphenoidal microsurgical therapy of prolactinomas: initial outcomes and long-term results. Neurosurgery 1999;44:254–261, discussion 261–263
31. Pouratian N, Prevedello DM, Jagannathan J, Lopes MB, Vance ML, Laws ER Jr. Outcomes and management of patients with Cushing's disease without pathological confirmation of tumor resection after transsphenoidal surgery. J Clin Endocrinol Metab 2007;92:3383–3388
32. Meij BP, Lopes MB, Ellegala DB, Alden TD, Laws ER Jr. The long-term significance of microscopic dural invasion in 354 patients with pituitary adenomas treated with transsphenoidal surgery. J Neurosurg 2002;96:195–208
33. Weiss MH. Transnasal transsphenoidal approach. In: Apuzzo ML, ed. Surgery of the Third Ventricle. Baltimore: Williams & Wilkins; 1987:476–494
34. Cappabianca P, Alfieri A, Thermes S, Buonamassa S, de Divitiis E. Instruments for endoscopic endonasal transsphenoidal surgery. Neurosurgery 1999;45:392–395, discussion 395–396
35. Cappabianca P, Cavallo LM, Esposito F, de Divitiis E. Endoscopic endonasal transsphenoidal surgery: procedure, endoscopic equipment and instrumentation. Childs Nerv Syst 2004;20:796–801
36. Cavallo LM, de Divitiis O, Aydin S, et al. Extended endoscopic endonasal transsphenoidal approach to the suprasellar area: anatomic considerations—part 1. Neurosurgery 2007;61(3, Suppl):24–33, discussion 33–34
37. Magro F, Solari D, Cavallo LM, et al. The endoscopic endonasal approach to the lateral recess of the sphenoid sinus via the pterygopalatine fossa: comparison of endoscopic and radiological landmarks. Neurosurgery 2006;59(4, Suppl 2):ONS237–ONS242, discussion ONS242–ONS243
38. Kabil MS, Eby JB, Shahinian HK. Fully endoscopic endonasal vs. transseptal transsphenoidal pituitary surgery. Minim Invasive Neurosurg 2005;48:348–354
39. Ciric I, Ragin A, Baumgartner C, Pierce D. Complications of transsphenoidal surgery: results of a national survey, review of the literature, and personal experience. Neurosurgery 1997;40:225–236, discussion 236–237
40. Frank G, Pasquini E, Farneti G, et al. The endoscopic versus the traditional approach in pituitary surgery. Neuroendocrinology 2006;83:240–248
41. Zada G, Kelly DF, Cohan P, Wang C, Swerdloff R. Endonasal transsphenoidal approach for pituitary adenomas and other sellar lesions: an assessment of efficacy, safety, and patient impressions. J Neurosurg 2003;98:350–358

23 Microscopic and Endoscopic Transsphenoidal Pituitary Surgery: A Reasoned and Balanced Dialectic

Nathan C. Rowland, Ammara Abbasi, David V. LaBorde, and Nelson M. Oyesiku

The transnasal or endonasal transsphenoidal approach to the sella, developed in the early 20th century, was a remarkably elegant solution to the problems that early surgeons faced with intracranial access to the pituitary gland.[1–12] This approach has evolved over the last century, resulting in the application of radiofluoroscopy,[13] the operative binocular microscope[14] (by which most pituitary surgery is performed today), ultrasound, magnetic resonance imaging (MRI)-based image guidance, and intraoperative MRI. More recently pituitary neurosurgeons have rediscovered the endoscope, deploying it in endoscopic-assisted and endoscopic-based transsphenoidal operations to refine illumination and visualization of the sella and parasellar regions during pituitary procedures.[15,16] Endoscopic surgery of the pituitary was an extension of the use of endoscopy for sinus disease. As experience with endoscopic sinus surgery increased, endoscopic endonasal techniques were adapted and expanded for use in other conditions affecting the paranasal sinuses and skull base. Initially this was directed toward nonneoplastic conditions. Endoscopic treatment of cerebrospinal fluid (CSF) leaks was reported in the early 1980s, and then endoscopic repairs of encephaloceles and mucoceles were reported.[17–19] Pituitary tumors were soon managed by endoscopic removal, and there followed debate as to the relative merits and demerits of each instrument—microscope or endoscope. Evangelism and proselytism now compete with cautious clinicians and careful analysis. Opinion and bias now rival balanced consensus and equanimity.

The arguments are by now familiar: "minimally invasive" (yet both are endonasal—endonasal microscopic or endonasal endoscopic); shorter length of stay (length of stay has nothing to do with a microscope or an endoscope); nasal packing (packing has nothing to do with a microscope or an endoscope); the view is three-dimensional (3D) and stereoscopic versus two-dimensional (2D) and somewhat distorted (yes, but 3D endoscopes are now being developed); panoramic visibility and ability to see around corners (yes, but this provides little added advantage in cases where the lesion is small and straight ahead at 0 degrees). Both hands are free to handle instruments (yes, bimanual surgery is safer and more effective, but get an endoscope driver or holder and you can free up the neurosurgeon to use both hands); enhanced illumination at the source versus loss of illumination with depth (fine, just as long as the lens is clean and free of blood); enhanced resection (yes, if it is safe without added complications, and the enhancement results in 100% removal and disease remission or cure; otherwise little additional benefit has been achieved if adjuvant therapy is still needed); operating times are shorter or longer (that depends on whom one reads and his or her veracity). The litany of claims and counterclaims goes on and on as protagonists are swept up in the tide and emotion.

A careful consideration of the advantages and disadvantages of both techniques allows the rational surgeon to individualize the approach to each patient's lesion. Not every patient is best served by the exclusive use of either a microscopic or an endoscopic approach. In fact, in certain situations, a combination of microscopic and endoscopic techniques may provide the best combination of safety and efficacy. Surgeons need to be comfortable with all the available technology to address a patient's pathology, or they may fall into the trap of seeing everything as a nail when all they have is a hammer. Conversely, any tool in the hands of surgeons must be carefully deployed; "a fool with a tool is still a fool, only a more dangerous fool."

No instrument or equipment can make one a surgeon. Surgeons achieve expertise by years of training and the acquisition of experience. Good judgment comes from experience, whereas experience comes from bad judgment (Jim Horning). The critical question facing pituitary neurosurgeons today becomes when and how to deploy endoscopic and microscopic techniques, based on available data and experience. In this chapter, we present clinical decision-making factors that should guide the discerning and discriminating neurosurgeon as to whether microscopy-based, endoscopy-based, or a hybrid of the two techniques represents the optimal procedure for successfully resolving pituitary lesions.

A Comparison of Microscopic Versus Endoscopic Transsphenoidal Methods

The state of the literature surrounding this debate is at present polarized between traditional microscopists and evangelical endoscopists, both arguing in favor of their procedural biases. To be sure, there is a middle ground. Most descriptions of these techniques occur with little attempt to appreciate their common features, which are many.

Planning and Positioning

The differential diagnosis of pathologies that may occupy the sella turcica includes tumors and nonneoplasms and is extensive.[20] Even the most common lesion, pituitary adenomas, frequently have parasellar extensions (**Fig. 23.1**). Thus, the strategy of how microscopic and endoscopic techniques are applied must begin at the planning stage, which should be given considerable thought.

Assistant surgeons, most commonly otorhinolaryngologists, may be included if an endoscopic approach is under consideration. This multidisciplinary approach, although still institution-dependent, is a very common and reasonable practice, especially when planning for complex lesions. In this scenario, the operating room should be accommodated to facilitate both teams. If a pure microscopic approach is planned, the use of fluoroscopy or MRI/computed tomography image guidance, depending on the neurosurgeon's preference, may be included at the beginning of the procedure without requirements for an endoscopic setup. If fluoroscopy is anticipated, care should be taken to make sure the head pin position does not obstruct the sella and sphenoid on a lateral view. With both procedures, induction of general anesthesia and placement of a lumbar drain (if needed) are identical. Positioning of the head should be fixed approximately 10 degrees toward the surgeon. For sellar lesions, the head is generally flexed approximately 20 degrees and even more so if the disease is clival in origin. The head should be extended if the lesion is suprasellar. That being said, some surgeons do not use a Mayfield head holder in endoscopic approaches. If an endoscope will be used, typically the endoscope monitor is positioned behind the patient; the surgeon stands on the right, the assistant stands on the left, and anesthesia is situated on the side opposite the surgeon behind the assistant. If a microscope will be used, this is an appropriate time to balance and drape it. Also, intraoperative guidance systems, if any, should be readied. Next, the nasal mucosa is prepared with a vasoconstrictive agent, for example, 4% cocaine or oxymetazoline. In the endonasal transseptal microscopic-based procedure, the nasal mucosa may be injected with local anesthetic to aid in the dissection of the rhinoseptal mucosa. In the direct endonasal microscopic approach there is no septal mucosal dissection.[21]

Approach and Exposure

In practical terms, the ergonomics of the operation are dependent on the hardware used, whether a microscope or endoscopic instrumentation. When the microscope is used, the entire procedure is usually performed indepen-

A

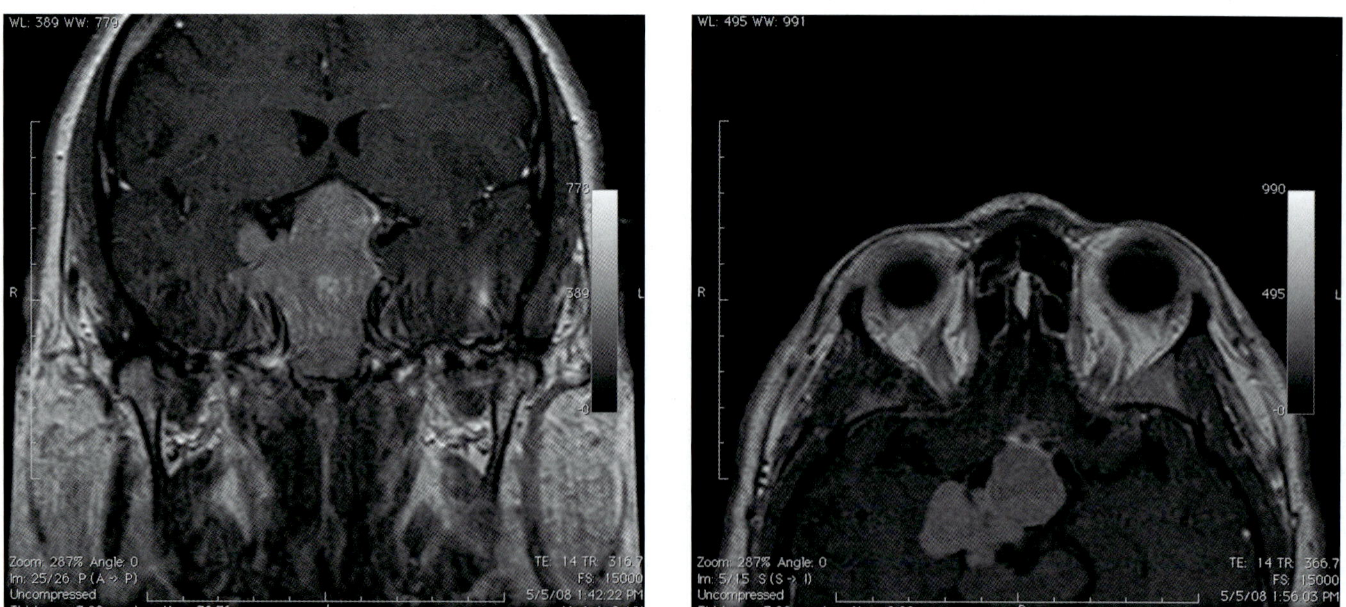

B

Fig. 23.1 **(A,B)** A pituitary lesion with asymmetric parasellar extension suitable for hybrid or pure endoscopic resection, permitting the surgeon to look "around the corner."

dently by a neurosurgeon, with the assistant observing through the observer scope. An array of nasosphenoidal routes exist, including sublabial-paraseptal, endonasal-unilateral-septal,[22] and direct endonasal.[21,23] The sublabial route is presently the least used. If a septal mucosal dissection is done, it is usually necessary to insert a nasal speculum to hold the nasal mucosa out of the line of sight and to push the middle turbinate laterally. If a direct endonasal approach is performed, there is no septal dissection and the nasal speculum is inserted into the nostril and opened at the face of the sphenoid between the ostium and the septum, subluxing the septum and exposing the face of the sphenoid.[21] The operation usually takes place through the nostril containing the nasal speculum. As mentioned, in endoscopic-based procedures, the procedure is typically multidisciplinary, with the otolaryngologist completing the endoscopic endonasal approach to the sphenoid sinus and the neurosurgeon opening the sella and resecting the tumor. However, many neurosurgeons perform the approach without an otolaryngologist. A unilateral or bilateral nostril approach may be used, and the assistant usually drives the camera. The use of a speculum is not necessary, as there is no need for mucosal retraction and no "line-of-sight" vision requirements. Moreover, a speculum would limit the space available for the endoscope and surgical instruments. However, because no speculum is present, the endoscope and instruments can abrade the mucosa and cause bleeding that can obstruct the endoscope lens. Because of this, and due to the proximity of the lens to the operative field, during endoscopic-based procedures frequent and repeated cleansing of the endoscope is often required. In contrast, the microscope, at a fixed distance away from the field, does not usually get soiled with blood and does not require frequent cleaning, if at all.

As the endoscopic procedure commences, the camera and instruments are introduced parallel to one another through one or both nostrils. It is important not to lose sight of the instruments in front of the endoscope to prevent trauma to the mucosa or important neurovascular structures. The surgeon is offered a wide viewing angle with the endoscope that provides a panoramic view of the sphenoid sinus, the face of the pituitary gland, and the interior of the tumor cavity in trajectories unavailable to the microscope. In a combined approach, the bulk of the tumor is resected using the microscope, and the endoscope then provides illumination and magnification of regions of interest outside the view of the microscope, including the cavernous, suprasellar, anterosellar, parasellar (**Fig. 23.1**), and retrosellar regions. In a study of cadaver sellae, Spencer et al[24] quantified the volume of space accessible under both microscopic and endoscopic guidance. In this study, a significantly greater volume of 3D space was visualized using the endoscope versus the microscope in both the endonasal-transsphenoidal (225 mm^3 versus 75 mm^3, p <.0001) and sublabial-transsphenoidal (350 mm^3 versus 200 mm^3, p <.0001) approaches.

Apart from differences in optical properties, another difference between the procedures is in the exposure of the nasal passage and sphenoid sinus. In the microscope-based transseptal (but not the direct endonasal procedure), a small vertical buried incision is made within the nasal mucosa in either nare but usually ipsilateral to the operating surgeon. A complete dissection of the rhinoseptal mucosa from the nasal septum is performed following the initial incision. A handheld nasal speculum is inserted medial to the septum and lateral to the rhinoseptal mucosa, taking care not to tear the mucosa. Any remaining attachment of mucosa to the septum is freed at this time. The perpendicular plate of the ethmoid and the vomer between the surgeon and the sella are removed. The nasal speculum is then arranged in the newly formed submucosal cavity with the tips of the blades nearly at the base of the sphenoid sinus. Once the speculum is in good position, the blades are gently opened to keep the mucosa out of the operative field.

The endoscopic procedure and the direct endonasal microscopic procedure both obviate an initial nasal mucosal incision.[21] However, in the endoscopic approach, in lieu of the nasal mucosal incision, a large bilateral sphenoidectomy and posterior one-third septectomy are created to provide for entry of the instruments and the endoscope into the sphenoid sinus. This opening is invasive and indeed quite so in that the mucosa and bone over the sphenoid sinus wall are extensively debrided and approximately one third of the posterior septum is removed (fortunately this is not externally visible).

In contrast to the microscopic approach, with the endoscopic approach, one of the nuances that must be mastered is driving the camera. Upon entry of the endoscope into the nare, the camera is oriented with the following important landmarks identified: (1) the inferior turbinate and eustachian tube in the lateral field, (2) the nasal septum in the medial field, (3) the nasal cavity floor in the inferior field, and (4) the middle turbinate head in the superior field. It may sometimes be necessary to decongest and perhaps laterally dislocate the middle turbinate head, which usually closely approximates the nasal septum.

Next, in both the microscopic and endoscopic procedures, the sphenoid ostia are identified. These are normally located approximately 1.5 cm above the roof of the choana and are of variable shape and size. The ostia initially may not be visible, as the view can be obstructed by the superior turbinate. Again, it may be necessary to lateralize or partially remove this structure. The surgeon should note, however, that the lateral lamella of the cribriform plate is thin, which poses a risk of ethmoid CSF leak. Starting 0.5 cm from the top of the choana while taking care to avoid the sphenopalatine artery branches, the sphenoethmoid recess and sphenoid ostia are carefully coagulated. At this point, the nasal septum may be detached from the sphenoid rostrum and the bone of the vomer between the ostia can be removed. In both procedures, the sphenoid ostia are opened using a bone punch or microdrill. Once the sphenoid sinus is opened, the midline is identified. Surgeons should note the location of the septum in relation to the midline on preoperative imaging as the midline can be markedly asymmetric.[25] Next, the mucosa over the face of the sella is removed or cauterized and the sella itself is opened.

Optical Properties

Once in the sphenoid sinus and the sella, the differences in optical properties between the microscope and endoscope are best appreciated. However, it is imperative to note that these differences are not mutually exclusive but complementary. Within the sphenoid sinus, the endoscope allows direct visualization of the carotid and optic nerve prominences before proceeding with opening the sella turcica. The microscope, conversely, does not offer this ability to look "around the corner" and panoramically inspect the sella widely to identify these landmarks. However, this is neither necessary nor essential if the operation is for retrieval of a small or wholly intrasellar lesion. The microscope, however, does offer depth perception, which the endoscope lacks. Currently, endoscopes provide only 2D (monocular) images that by definition lack depth, and thus restrict the surgeon's perspective, which can limit the ability to perform critical aspects of some surgeries. To be sure, part of this limitation can be obviated by movement of the endoscope to allow perception of relative positional anatomy. Stereoscopic vision better facilitates understanding of the anatomy, hand–eye coordination, and the use of surgical instruments. Technological refinements from industry (Visionsense, Orangeburg, NY) have led to the development of proprietary miniature sensors that offer natural stereoscopic vision. The technology is based on a single stereoscopic (3D) sensor that imitates an insect's compound eye[26] and offers the ability to surpass the 2D limitation of the endoscope. However, the market penetration and adaptation of this technology are in their infancy, and the ultimate impact it will have on pituitary surgery remains to be seen. Thus, at present, the optical properties of the endoscope present a learning curve for neurosurgeons trained solely using microscopic techniques, a deficiency that can be overcome with preoperative practice in the anatomy laboratory, practical courses, and increasing exposure and experience.[25] Furthermore, with the current rediscovery of the endoscope, more neurosurgeons are gaining familiarity with use of the endoscope, particularly in centers with endoscopic surgeons, those with multidisciplinary teams of otolaryngologists and neurosurgeons, and those with neurosurgery faculty trained in both techniques. As a result, increasing numbers of neurosurgeons in training and neurosurgeons recently out of training have gained exposure to endoscopic techniques. This trend is overall positive and likely will facilitate the appropriate and judicious use of one or both techniques dictated by the anatomy of each patient's tumor rather than by the surgeon's comfort with one particular technology over the other.

Tumor Removal

Using bayoneted instruments in the microscopic approach, the tumor is resected from normal pituitary glandular tissue under direct visualization.[23] Bayoneted instruments may be used in the endoscopic approach as well but are not usually necessary, and straight shafts are preferable.[25] As a general principle, in both approaches, the inferior and lateral fragments of the lesion are removed before the superior aspect to prevent redundant diaphragm or arachnoid from entering the field. A Valsalva maneuver can be performed if descent of the suprasellar portion does not occur spontaneously or saline can be infused into the lumbar drain if one was placed preoperatively. Following tumor removal, the tumor cavity should be thoroughly inspected. In a hybrid approach, the lesion may be resected mainly using the microscopic approach with angled endoscopes used to inspect for residual tumor. The 30- and 45-degree angled scopes are useful for this maneuver. Tumor fragments may be discovered in the medial cavernous sinus wall or elsewhere out of the line of sight of the microscope (**Fig. 23.1**).

Closing

As the procedure nears its end, the pseudocapsule (if present) is dissected away from the wall of the sella, and any sellar reconstruction to be done is completed, which varies by surgeon. Hemostasis is meticulously pursued. In the microscopic approach, the final stages involve removing the speculum, positioning the nasal septum back to midline, closing and reapproximating the mucosal incision just inside the nare, inspecting the mucosa, placing a nasal airway (if necessary), and occasional nasal packing with a Gelfoam tampon if mucosal injury is present. In the endoscopic approach, the endoscope is simply removed to finish the procedure, most often without the need for nasal packing, although most surgeons place Gelfoam or a similar material over the sellar opening.

Summary of Advantages and Disadvantages of Microscopic and Endoscopic Transsphenoidal Approaches

A body of evidence of varying levels now exists regarding the efficacy of endoscopic transsphenoidal procedures from several groups using endoscopic transsphenoidal techniques. Most groups acknowledge the superior viewing angles provided by the endoscope when dealing with tumors that have retrosellar, parasellar (**Fig. 23.1**), and subfrontal configurations. However, there are other significant advantages as well. The endoscopic technique generally causes less trauma to the nasal septal mucosa (though it does involve extensive trauma to the nasal mucosa over the sphenoid sinus). Thus, during the procedure, there is little or no need for vasoconstrictors, and often no nasal packing is needed postoperatively (this is an often-touted advantage; however, nasal packing is not necessary in the unilateral septal or direct endonasal microscopic approaches either). A nasal speculum is not needed in purely endoscopic procedures as it is in microscopic procedures. Microscopic transsphenoidal techniques benefit from the stereoscopic view of the microscope, providing the surgeon with excellent 3D depth perception and proper comprehension of the critical surgical anatomy without the optical distortion that may lead to disorientation, misdirection, and possibly technical errors. Microsurgeons rightly routinely cite the ability to operate with both hands in the surgical field with the microscope a fixed distance away as a major benefit during these procedures. In contrast, the endoscope, although accommodating exceptional views of sellar blind angles, provides only a 2D visual image on the screen (that frequently is obscured by blood) and may be limited even more so by the "barrel"-type spatial distortion of the peripheral view emanating from the camera.[25] Moreover, the endoscopic instrumentation occupies a portion of the surgical field, which can preclude its use in patients with especially narrow nasal passages.

Reported Outcomes of Microscopic Versus Endoscopic Transsphenoidal Procedures

To date, no large, prospective, randomized study directly comparing microscopic and endoscopic transsphenoidal approaches to the pituitary adenectomy has been performed. Nevertheless, the safety and effectiveness of endoscopic transsphenoidal surgery have been demonstrated in recent reviews of the endoscopic and microscopic literature covering this topic.[27] Unfortunately, many of these reports offer spurious comparisons and reflect the bias of the authors. For example, many reports use a sublabial incision as a proxy for microscopic techniques even though it is not, as most microsurgeons use a direct endonasal transseptal approach. It is essential to evaluate these techniques using objective measures of efficacy and by asking the right questions.

Tumor Resection

The improved visualization of sellar blind angles with the endoscope has been offered as a basis for predicting superior tumor resection during endoscopic approaches as compared with microscopic approaches. This is quite true, to a point. For example, there are many tumors that have extension into areas where they are visible with the endoscope, but they are not resectable because of unacceptable risk (**Fig. 23.2**).

A

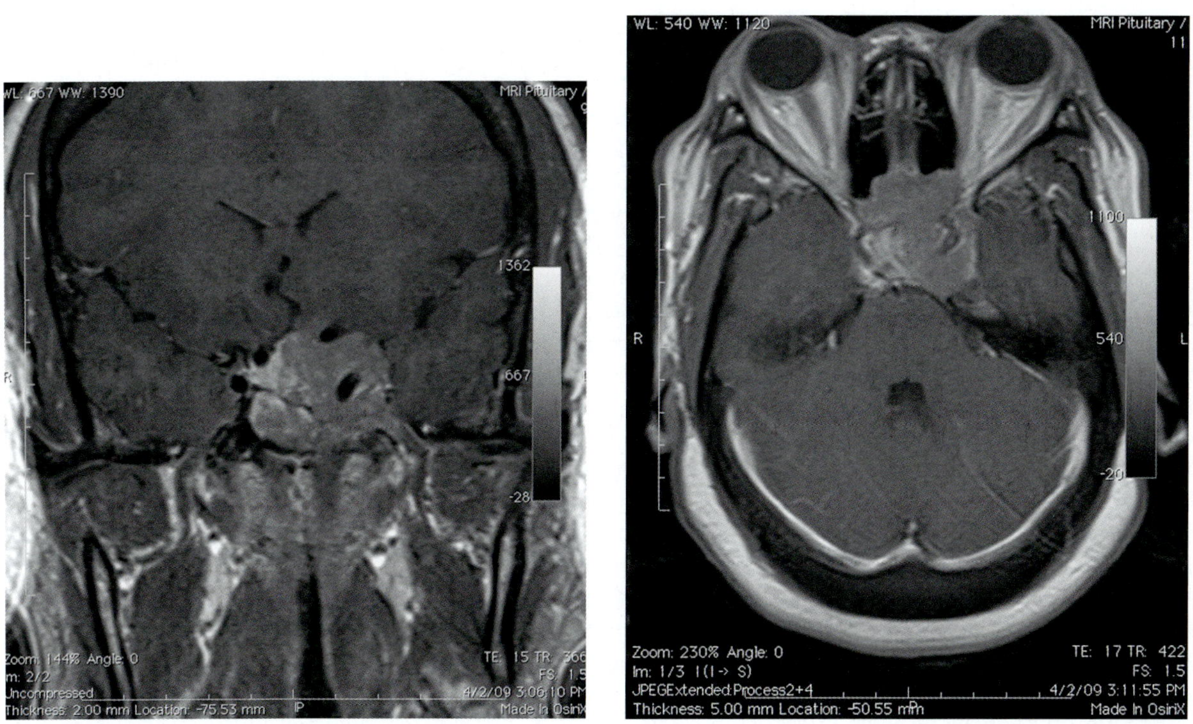

B

Fig. 23.2 **(A,B)** An invasive growth hormone adenoma, for which complete resection or remission is highly unlikely by endoscope or microscope.

Nevertheless, in one study of 37 patients, Helal[28] removed sellar lesions with a microscope followed by inspection of the sellar regions with a rigid 30-degree endoscope. Tumor residues were ultimately detected in 40.5% of patients undergoing the procedure, and hidden areas could be visualized in 84% of patients. Helal concluded that endoscopy improves tumor resection by allowing a more complete visualization of the operating field. However, one might argue that the percentage of cases that were likely to have residual tumor after microscopic resection could have been predicted to some degree based on the preoperative imaging. Jarrahy et al[29] employed the endoscope as an adjunctive imaging modality following microscopic tumor resection and report results in nine patients in whom gross tumor resection was achieved. In their series, tumor remnants not visualized by the microscope were identified and extracted (by using an endoscope after the microscopic resection) in three of the nine patients. Other groups using a hybrid microscopy-endoscopy approach have also reported their findings. Operating through a widened nasal cavity to enable conversion between microscopic and endoscopic approaches, Kim et al[30] noted residual tumor in two of five patients using the hybrid microscopic-endoscopic technique. Kawamata et al[31] found a flexible endoscope useful in resecting residual tumor inaccessible by both microscope and rigid endoscope in five of 34 patients. Finally, residual tumor was discovered and removed in seven of 13 patients operated on by Baussart et al.[32] These studies support the fact that using the endoscope to inspect the sellar cavity following resection under microscopic guidance can allow for a greater degree of tumor resection in cases where the tumor extends outside of the line of sight of the microscope. Nevertheless, in cases where there is extension into the suprasellar (**Fig. 23.3**) and cavernous regions, it can still be inherently difficult to access the entire tumor, be it with the microscope or the endoscope.

Moreover, few reports, if any, exist on tumor recurrence and long-term cure rates comparing the two techniques.

Cost Analysis

The enhanced minimal invasiveness in approaching pituitary lesions using endoscopic techniques has been proffered as a basis for reducing costs associated with these procedures. In one series of 160 patients undergoing purely endoscopic pituitary resection, 111 patients stayed in the hospital only overnight.[33] This constitutes one of the most unscholarly contentions because it is apparent to most clinicians caring for patients following pituitary surgery that the length of hospital stay is not determined by a microscope or endoscope but by the dictates of the disease and its management. Cappabianca et al[34] reported the outcomes from their series of 100 patients using the endoscopic procedure. They found that 40 of these patients had postoperative hospital stays of 2 days or less. Hospital stay was also shorter by 2.1 days in Cho and Liau's[35] series, which compared the endoscopic and sublabial transsphenoidal approaches ($p < .05$). White et al[36] also noted significantly reduced hospital stay in their series of 100 patients. However, these case studies represent spurious comparisons because the wrong question is being asked—comparing a sublabial approach using the microscope to a direct endonasal approach using the endoscope. A more relevant and useful investigation would be to determine whether there is any difference in length of stay when using the microscope as compared with endoscope through a similar channel—the direct endonasal approach. That question was not asked. Collectively, these studies provide a nonevidentiary argument in favor of adopting endoscopic techniques from the viewpoint of reducing patient hospital length of stay, primarily because the question was asked incorrectly and the comparisons made were inappropriate.

Hormonal Homeostasis

Successful treatment of hormonal hypersecretion should also be considered an endpoint in the comparison of outcomes between endoscopic and microscopic transsphenoidal pituitary surgery in patients with functional tumors. Tabaee et al[27] reported in a recent meta-analysis that the overall hormonal remission rate from six pooled studies using endoscopic pituitary removal was 79%. These authors calculated an overall hormonal remission rate of 81% for adrenocorticotropic hormone–secreting tumors, 84% for growth hormone–secreting tumors, and 82% for prolactin-secreting tumors.[27] Cho and Liau[35] directly compared the traditional sublabial microscopic (22 patients) and purely endoscopic (22 patients) approaches for removal of prolactinomas, and no overall differences in prolactin homeostasis or visual improvement could be demonstrated using these techniques. At present, no studies have challenged the view that the effectiveness of the procedures is essentially the same with regard to these outcome measures. As mentioned, randomized prospective studies with sufficient power are needed to differentiate any inherent differences between these approaches.

Complications

Along with efficacy, safety is of primary importance to neurosurgeons contemplating the adoption of endoscopic techniques. Anecdotally, endoscopic transsphenoidal pituitary surgery has been reported to be a safe procedure from the perspective of those familiar with the instrumentation and methods.[37] Tabaee et al's[27] meta-analysis reported pooled complication rates of 2% for CSF leak and 1% for permanent diabetes insipidus in exclusively endoscopic pituitary operations.[27] Two deaths were reported in this study caused by vascular injury, resulting in an overall mortality rate of 0.24%.

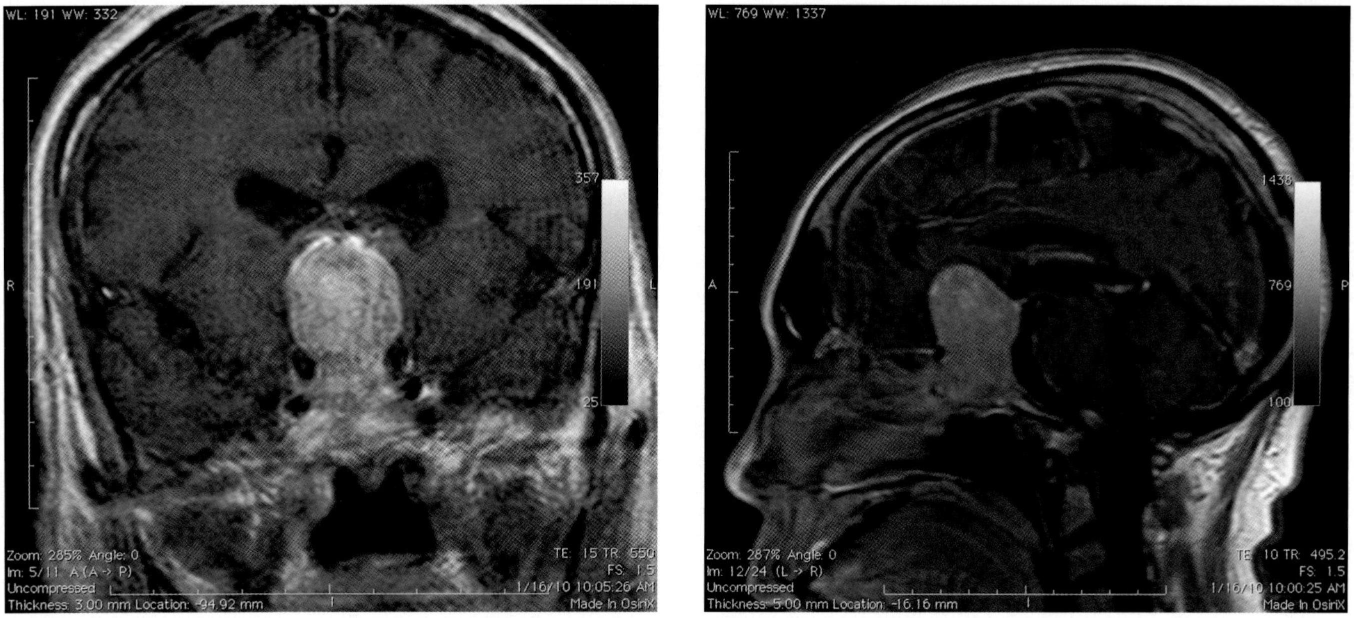

A B

Fig. 23.3 (A,B) A pituitary lesion with suprasellar extension in the setting of a narrow diaphragmatic hiatus. Here, endoscopic assistance would be helpful.

These rates are similar to those reported in the literature for traditional microscopic transsphenoidal surgery.[38–45]

Cho and Liau[35] found a significant (*p* <.05) reduction in complication rates when an endonasal endoscopic approach was used (22 patients) versus a sublabial microscopic technique (22 patients), which was attributed to less mucosal trauma in the more minimally invasive approach. However, again the wrong question was framed. The appropriate and more relevant investigation would be to compare the use of the microscope versus the use of the endoscope through the same endonasal aperture. Casler et al[46] compared an endoscopic transsphenoidal approach (15 patients) with an open transsphenoidal approach (15 patients) for pituitary tumor resection. They reported no statistically significant difference in operative time, gross complete resection, blood loss, intensive care unit stay, CSF leak, or diabetes insipidus. They did, however, discover a significant decrease in hospital length of stay (4.4 days versus 5.73 days for the endoscopic and open approaches, respectively; *p* <.03) and in the number of patients who were pain free on postoperative day 1 (10/15 versus 2/15 patients for the endoscopic and open approaches, respectively; *p* <.003). White et al[36] retrospectively reviewed 50 cases of sublabial, transseptal procedures along with 50 cases of endoscopic, minimally invasive pituitary surgery at the same institution to compare complication rates. The sublabial, transseptal group experienced significantly higher total complications per patient, including postoperative epistaxis, lip anesthesia, and deviated septum (*p* <.05). Additionally, the endoscopic group experienced significantly reduced hospital length of stay, lumbar drain use, and nasal packing (*p* <.05). However, no statistically significant differences were found in CSF leakage, meningitis, ophthalmoplegia, visual acuity loss, diabetes insipidus, intracranial hemorrhage, or death. This is all correct, which is why most microscope pituitary surgeons have long ago abandoned the sublabial approach. The direct endonasal microscope approach was described in 1987.

The reader may wonder why again and again the wrong question has been framed. The answer, of course, lies in the observation that surgeons on each side in the debate have endeavored to frame the argument in ways that would favor the point they wish to address or prove. The appropriate question again is the use of the microscope versus the use of the endoscope through the same endonasal aperture. In 2009, Charalampaki et al[47] reported on their retrospective analysis of complication rates for a group of patients treated endoscopically versus a historical control group of patients treated microscopically. In the endoscopically treated group, they report a 0.7% rate of sphenopalatine artery bleeding, a 2% rate of postoperative sinusitis, and a 3.3% rate of postoperative CSF leak. One patient in the endoscopic group died during surgery secondary to a lacerated posterior cerebral artery, and another suffered rupture of a carotid artery aneurysm within the cavernous sinus. The authors contended that most of their major complications occurred early on in their technical experience with the endoscope and that as their skills improved, the complication rate concomitantly decreased. Still, complications from the endoscopic-based procedures were noted to be less frequent than those from the transseptal-, paraseptal-, and sublabial-transsphenoidal microscopic pituitary procedures, and this reduced morbidity was ascribed to better visualization provided by the endoscope and the avoidance of using a nasal speculum and transsphenoidal retractor. However, these results, like others discussed, are again confounded by the comparison of differing operative apertures, which severely limits the actual relevance of the conclusions to the respective technologies. Moreover, the bias inherent in this comparison of lumped historical "controls" versus a current series is self-evident.

Clinical Decision-Making Factors in Selecting Microscopic and Endoscopic Approaches

Determining whether the microscope or the endoscope will be most beneficial should not be viewed as binary, as the factors that frame this decision-making process certainly are not. Although the indications are almost identical for microscopic and endoscopic pituitary surgery, certain situations may be better suited for a particular approach. As de Divitiis and Cappabianca point out,[48] a relatively smaller sella may be better approached via a microscope. This is because the constraints of a small sella force the endoscope and surgical instruments to converge near the same target, resulting in a difficult operating field in which to maneuver. If the nasal aperture is wide and the tumor is small to medium and central (**Fig. 23.4**), it is easily managed by rapid direct endonasal microscopic resection.

The appeal of a panoramic view provided by the endoscope is lost in the confines of a smaller space and may not be necessary in such a case. In contrast, the microscope's ability to zoom into the surgical area without significant interference with surgical instruments makes it a stronger candidate in such cases.[48] Furthermore, endoscopic instrumentation can be particularly difficult when two surgeons are working together in the same surgical field.[49] Conch-type sphenoid sinuses also present a unique obstacle for endoscopes, requiring removal of the posterior aspect of the nasal septum to have sufficient ability to maneuver within the nasal passage,[48] and poor pneumatization can impede recognition of important landmarks within the sinus.[25] Other factors that may affect visualization of the sinus are narrow passages and tissue hypertrophy from glandular hypersecretion.

Alternatively, the endoscopic approach is advantageous for surgical patients who have previously undergone surgery via the transsphenoidal approach. This is because the sphenoid ostium is already enlarged and contains scars and surgical adhesions in the visual field that are better explored with the panoramic views provided by endoscopes.[48] Additionally, for resection, large pituitary adenomas, particularly those with less accessible antero-, supra-, para-, and retrosellar extensions, are better suited for visualization through angled views provided by the endoscope.[50,51] Cavallo et al[25] suggest that the patients who represent the optimal candidates for the neurosurgeon initially learning the endoscopic method are elderly patients, who generally have spacious nasal passages; those with nonfunctioning adenomas; and those with well-pneumatized sinuses.[25] As mentioned above, patients with presellar or conchal sphenoid sinus types and also patients with functional adenomas should be reserved until more advanced skills have been acquired.

The Future of Pituitary Surgery

The microscope is still appropriate for resection of most pituitary neoplasms and should not be considered outdated. Neurosurgeons are already able to work quickly, safely, and with familiarity using the microscope. This fact in itself is beneficial for the patient, and the microscope is adequate for many pituitary neoplasms, particularly those that are isolated within the sella.

Additionally, most neurosurgeons will overcome their hesitation to transcend the learning curve of endoscopy. Incorporating endoscopes by using them as supplementary visual tools for tumor remnants after typical microscopic resection is one pathway toward gaining endoscopic skills. Ultimately, facility with both modalities is most advantageous for the patient as it allows the neurosurgeon to select the method most appropriate for the patient and pathology at hand rather than fitting the patient into a procedure solely because it is the only one in the surgeon's repertoire.

The learning curve for endoscopic surgery can also be overcome with collaborative efforts that bring together otorhinolaryngologists and neurologic surgeons. "Four-handed" approaches in which the otorhinolaryngologist provides access into the sella with tumor resection by the neurosurgeon are efficient. Though eventually the neurosurgeon may learn to perform the entire procedure alone, the advantage of the otorhinolaryngologist's oversight can be beneficial and instructive when initially learning to enter the sphenoid sinus with the endoscope. Neurosurgeons can also help otorhinolaryngologists become more comfortable with working in the proximity of intracranial contents at the base of the skull.[52] As Harvey Cushing himself succinctly stated when discussing transsphenoidal surgery at its very beginning, "The performance becomes progressively simplified by the combined suggestion and experience of many."[53]

Conclusion

Since its inception in 1907, transsphenoidal surgery of the pituitary gland has undergone several developments to

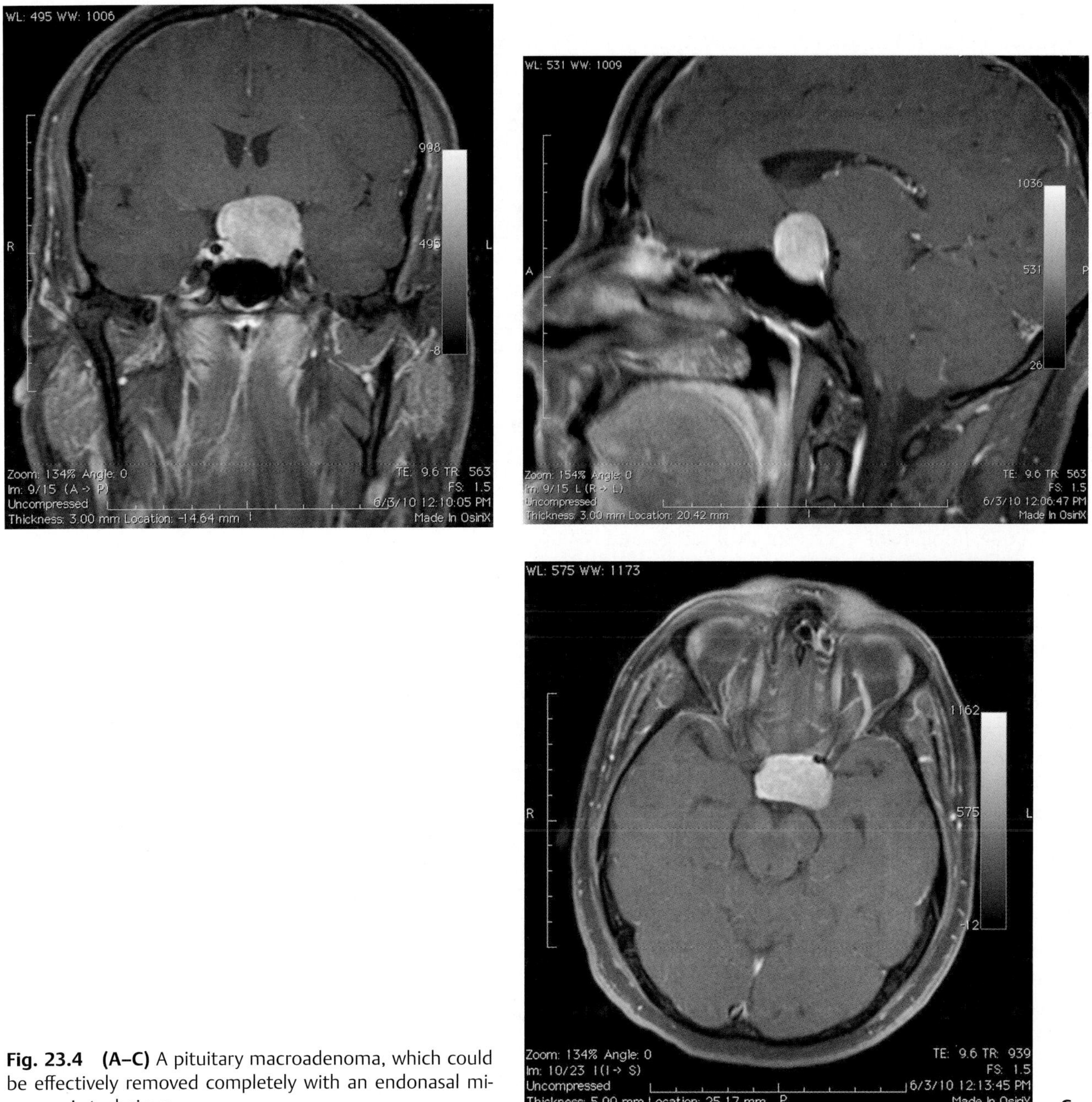

Fig. 23.4 **(A–C)** A pituitary macroadenoma, which could be effectively removed completely with an endonasal microscopic technique.

become a minimally invasive and highly effective treatment for pituitary lesions. The introduction of the surgical microscope in the 1960s coinciding with the wide use of hormonal replacements enabled the microscopic transsphenoidal approach to gain popularity and become the procedure of choice for treating pituitary neoplasms.[54]

The past decade has seen renewed interest in the use of endoscopes in performing transsphenoidal surgeries, particularly among otorhinolaryngologists. The panoramic views of the endoscope have piqued the interest of neurosurgeons. These advantages in the hands of experienced surgeons have warranted further use and investigation of endoscopic transnasal resections of pituitary lesions.[55]

However, the potential of endoscopic-based transsphenoidal surgery has not been fully realized. This is in part due to the reluctance of neurosurgeons to incorporate endoscopic techniques into their armamentarium because of unfamiliarity with the use of the scope and in part because of the inherent disadvantages and limitations of the endoscope such as optical distortion (2D not 3D), frequent lens obscurations, and lengthier procedures. So far, it has been demonstrated to be reliable and as safe as the traditional microscopic approach in experienced hands. However, long-term objective measures, such as tumor recurrence and cure rates, are not known.

Advances in medicine and surgery share many features; however, they also exhibit some sharp contrasts. In common, they can experience bold paradigm shifts led by pioneering investigators or teams motivated by solving difficult problems. Witness the changes wrought by antibiotics, antihypertensives, and cancer chemotherapies in medicine or laparoscopic surgery, coronary artery bypass grafting, or endovascular coiling of aneurysms in surgery.

But there are also sharp contrasts. Although medical advances are typically characterized by the rigid protocols of phased clinical trials and diligent reporting monitored by many skeptical eyes of the medical profession, competitors in the pharmaceutical industry, and the government, these protocols infrequently occur in surgery. Rarely is there a clear path from conception to implementation. Oftentimes a lone figure or small core team will formulate a new operation or technique, implement it, present its findings, and tutor others, and then surgeon-to-surgeon, institution-by-institution propagation takes place until it becomes the standard of care.

Phased trials are rarely performed, required, or reported, let alone randomized controlled trials. Few surgeons even rigorously compare data with established or proven techniques until compelled to do so. The profession is thus almost always at the mercy of the skills, transparency, and reporting of those initiating the advance. Even with properly executed, evidence-based investigation, there would still be the matter of surgical judgment and patient selection as key elements in the application of surgical therapies, new or old. Tools, no matter how advanced, cannot interpret anatomy, select patients, or make surgical judgments—that is the work of trained, experienced surgeons.

To make matters more imprecise, the world is smaller today than it ever was thanks to the Internet, globalization, wireless communication, and the unfettered access to information and disinformation, so that it is just as easy to spread good data as it is to spread bad data. This may leave some practitioners partially educated or vulnerable to self-claims of evangelists not vetted by scientific tribunals or other more trusted discourse. Unaudited feats of glory and uncomplicated rewards pressure other "forty-niners" unprepared for the hazards of exploration. In spite of this, surgical innovation, has survived and will continue to survive, bypassing amber-entombed fossils and entrenched postures.

We must foster and breed bold shifts and advances in our surgical portfolio, and change must occur for the field to evolve and improve. This demands courage, skill, contrariness, a pioneering spirit, and a will to accept challenges or even defeat, should it come. But in doing so we must never shed our willingness and readiness to query, assess, and report the gains or cost of such advances so that those who depend on us—patients (most importantly), our profession (later adopters), and our trainees (our future)—will have access to the truth and objectivity.

Such assessment will include answers to the following questions: What problems beg for a solution? What advantages does this advance bring to the table? What gains accrue as a result? At what cost? When and how should it be deployed? In doing so, we will have fulfilled our mission.

In closing, we are reminded of the words of Czesław Miłosz, the Polish-American poet, prose writer, and Nobel Laureate in Literature: "In a room where people unanimously maintain a conspiracy of silence, one word of truth sounds like a pistol shot."

References

1. Caton R, Paul FT. Notes of a case of acromegaly treated by operation. BMJ 1893;2:1421–1423
2. Horsley V. On the technique of operations on the central nervous system. BMJ 1906;2:411–423
3. Schloffer H. Zur frage der operationen an der hypophyse. Beitr Klin Chir. 1906;50:767–817
4. Schloffer H. Erfolgreiche operation eines hypophysentumor auf nasalem wege. Wien Klin Wochenschr 1907;20:621–624
5. Schloffer H. Weiterer bericht uber den fall von operiertem hypophysen-tumor. Wien Klin Wochenschr 1907;20:1075–1078
6. Cushing H. III. Partial hypophysectomy for acromegaly: with remarks on the function of the hypophysis. Ann Surg 1909;50:1002–1017
7. Halstead AE. Remarks on the operative treatment of tumors of the hypophysis: with report of two cases operated on by an oronasal method. Surg Gynecol Obstet 1910;10:494–502
8. Hirsch O. Endonasal method of removal of hypophyseal tumors with a report of two successful cases. JAMA 1910;55:772–774
9. Biggart JH, Dott NM. Pituitary tumours: their classification and treatment. BMJ 1936;2:1206–1208
10. Guiot G, Thibaut B. [Excision of pituitary adenomas by trans-sphenoidal route.]. Neurochirurgia (Stuttg) 1959;1:133–150
11. Tindall GT, Tindall SC. Surgery of the pituitary gland. Curr Probl Surg 1981;18:609–679
12. Couldwell WT. Transsphenoidal and transcranial surgery for pituitary adenomas. J Neurooncol 2004;69:237–256
13. Hardy J, Wigser SM. Trans-sphenoidal surgery of pituitary fossa tumors with televised radiofluoroscopic control. J Neurosurg 1965;23:612–619
14. Hardy J. [Surgery of the pituitary gland, using the trans-sphenoidal approach. Comparative study of 2 technical methods]. Union Med Can 1967;96:702–712
15. Bushe KA, Halves E. [Modified technique in transsphenoidal operations of pituitary adenomas. Technical note (author's transl)]. Acta Neurochir (Wien) 1978;41:163–175
16. Jho HD, Carrau RL. Endoscopic endonasal transsphenoidal surgery: experience with 50 patients. J Neurosurg 1997;87:44–51
17. Wigand ME. Transnasal ethmoidectomy under endoscopical control. Rhinology 1981;19:7–15
18. Lanza DC, O'Brien DA, Kennedy DW. Endoscopic repair of cerebrospinal fluid fistulae and encephaloceles. Laryngoscope 1996;106 (9 Pt 1):1119–1125

19. Har-El G. Endoscopic management of 108 sinus mucoceles. Laryngoscope 2001;111:2131–2134
20. Freda PU, Post KD. Differential diagnosis of sellar masses. Endocrinol Metab Clin North Am 1999;28:81–117
21. Griffith HB, Veerapen R. A direct transnasal approach to the sphenoid sinus. Technical note. J Neurosurg 1987;66:140–142
22. Tindall GT, Collins WF Jr, Kirchner JA. Unilateral septal technique for transsphenoidal microsurgical approach to the sella turcica. Technical note. J Neurosurg 1978;49:138–142
23. Buchfelder M, Fahlbusch R. The "classic" transsphenoidal approach for resection of pituitary tumors. Operative Techniques in Neurosurgery. 2002;5:210–217
24. Spencer WR, Das K, Nwagu C, et al. Approaches to the sellar and parasellar region: anatomic comparison of the microscope versus endoscope. Laryngoscope 1999;109:791–794
25. Cavallo LM, Dal Fabbro M, Jalalod'din H, et al. Endoscopic endonasal transsphenoidal surgery. Before scrubbing in: tips and tricks. Surg Neurol 2007;67:342–347
26. Visionsense, Inc. Orangeburg, NY. http://www.visionsense.com/index.htm
27. Tabaee A, Anand VK, Barrón Y, et al. Endoscopic pituitary surgery: a systematic review and meta-analysis. J Neurosurg 2009;111:545–554
28. Helal MZ. Combined micro-endoscopic trans-sphenoid excisions of pituitary macroadenomas. Eur Arch Otorhinolaryngol 1995;252:186–189
29. Jarrahy R, Berci G, Shahinian HK. Assessment of the efficacy of endoscopy in pituitary adenoma resection. Arch Otolaryngol Head Neck Surg 2000;126:1487–1490
30. Kim EY, Park HS, Kim JJ, et al. Endoscopic transsphenoidal approach through a widened nasal cavity for pituitary lesions. J Clin Neurosci 2001;8:437–441
31. Kawamata T, Kamikawa S, Iseki H, Hori T. Flexible endoscope-assisted endonasal transsphenoidal surgery for pituitary tumors. Minim Invasive Neurosurg 2002;45:208–210
32. Baussart B, Aghakhani N, Portier F, Chanson P, Tadié M, Parker F. [Endoscope-assisted microsurgery for invasive endo- and suprasellar pituitary macroadenomas: a consecutive retrospective study with 13 patients]. Neurochirurgie 2005;51:455–463
33. Jho HD. Endoscopic transsphenoidal surgery. J Neurooncol 2001;54:187–195
34. Cappabianca P, Cavallo LM, Colao A, et al. Endoscopic endonasal transsphenoidal approach: outcome analysis of 100 consecutive procedures. Minim Invasive Neurosurg 2002;45:193–200
35. Cho DY, Liau WR. Comparison of endonasal endoscopic surgery and sublabial microsurgery for prolactinomas. Surg Neurol 2002;58:371–375, discussion 375–376
36. White DR, Sonnenburg RE, Ewend MG, Senior BA. Safety of minimally invasive pituitary surgery (MIPS) compared with a traditional approach. Laryngoscope 2004;114:1945–1948
37. Koren I, Hadar T, Rappaport ZH, Yaniv E. Endoscopic transnasal transsphenoidal microsurgery versus the sublabial approach for the treatment of pituitary tumors: endonasal complications. Laryngoscope 1999;109:1838–1840
38. Ciric I, Mikhael M, Stafford T, Lawson L, Garces R. Transsphenoidal microsurgery of pituitary macroadenomas with long-term follow-up results. J Neurosurg 1983;59:395–401
39. Fahlbusch R, Buchfelder M. Present status of neurosurgery in the treatment of prolactinomas. Neurosurg Rev 1985;8:195–205
40. Fahlbusch R, Buchfelder M, Müller OA. Transsphenoidal surgery for Cushing's disease. J R Soc Med 1986;79:262–269
41. Black PM, Zervas NT, Candia GL. Incidence and management of complications of transsphenoidal operation for pituitary adenomas. Neurosurgery 1987;20:920–924
42. Ciric I, Ragin A, Baumgartner C, Pierce D. Complications of transsphenoidal surgery: results of a national survey, review of the literature, and personal experience. Neurosurgery 1997;40:225–236; discussion 236–227
43. Semple PL, Laws ER Jr. Complications in a contemporary series of patients who underwent transsphenoidal surgery for Cushing's disease. J Neurosurg 1999;91:175–179
44. Jane JA Jr, Laws ER Jr. The surgical management of pituitary adenomas in a series of 3,093 patients. J Am Coll Surg 2001;193:651–659
45. Barker FG II, Klibanski A, Swearingen B. Transsphenoidal surgery for pituitary tumors in the United States, 1996–2000: mortality, morbidity, and the effects of hospital and surgeon volume. J Clin Endocrinol Metab 2003;88:4709–4719
46. Casler JD, Doolittle AM, Mair EA. Endoscopic surgery of the anterior skull base. Laryngoscope 2005;115:16–24
47. Charalampaki P, Ayyad A, Kockro RA, Perneczky A. Surgical complications after endoscopic transsphenoidal pituitary surgery. J Clin Neurosci 2009;16:786–789
48. de Divitiis E, Cappabianca P. Microscopic and endoscopic transsphenoidal surgery. Neurosurgery 2002;51:1527–1529, author reply 1529–1530
49. Sethi DS, Leong JL. Endoscopic pituitary surgery. Otolaryngol Clin North Am 2006;39:563–583
50. Gamea A, Fathi M, el-Guindy A. The use of the rigid endoscope in trans-sphenoidal pituitary surgery. J Laryngol Otol 1994;108:19–22
51. Fatemi N, Dusick JR, de Paiva Neto MA, Kelly DF. The endonasal microscopic approach for pituitary adenomas and other parasellar tumors: a 10-year experience. Neurosurgery 2008;63(4, Suppl 2):244–256, discussion 256
52. Snyderman CH, Carrau RL, Kassam AB, et al. Endoscopic skull base surgery: principles of endonasal oncological surgery. J Surg Oncol 2008;97:658–664
53. Doglietto F, Prevedello DM, Jane JA Jr, Han J, Laws ER Jr. Brief history of endoscopic transsphenoidal surgery—from Philipp Bozzini to the First World Congress of Endoscopic Skull Base Surgery. Neurosurg Focus 2005;19:E3
54. Bassim MK, Senior BA. Minimally invasive pituitary surgery. Operative Techniques in Otolaryngology. 2006;17:31–36
55. Jankowski R, Auque J, Simon C, Marchal JC, Hepner H, Wayoff M. Endoscopic pituitary tumor surgery. Laryngoscope 1992;102:198–202

24 Extended Endonasal, Endoscopic Transsphenoidal Approach versus Craniotomy for Giant Pituitary Macroadenomas

Christoph P. Hofstetter, Yaron Moshel, Michael Nanaszko, Vijay K. Anand, and Theodore H. Schwartz

With the exception of medically treatable prolactinomas, surgery is the first-line treatment for symptomatic giant pituitary adenomas. The surgical treatment for giant pituitary macroadenomas has evolved considerably over the past 100 years including the development of the transsphenoidal approach, extended transsphenoidal approach, endoscopic endonasal skull base techniques, and advances in transcranial and open skull base techniques. Either transcranial or transsphenoidal techniques can be employed for the treatment of giant pituitary macroadenomas; sometimes both approaches have been used either simultaneously or in a staged fashion.[1–7] The goals of surgical treatment include improvement of visual function, endocrinologic function, and neurologic symptoms. Maximizing the extent of resection in the setting of a low morbidity and mortality rate is also a goal of surgery.

The surgical outcome in cases with giant pituitary adenoma have generally been reported to be poor because of a high rate of surgical morbidity secondary to small vessel ischemia of the hypothalamic walls and brainstem.[8–10] A partial or subtotal resection can lead to infarction and edema of the residual tumor, in turn leading to postoperative neurologic deterioration.[5,11] The high mortality rate during the early macrosurgical experience with transcranial surgery for pituitary tumors in general led to development of extracranial approaches to the sella.[12,13] The transsphenoidal approach quickly became the most widely adopted technique, and the transcranial approaches were often reserved for giant pituitary macroadenomas with complex extensions into the retrochiasmatic region, ventricular system, and anterior or middle fossa.[10,14,15] However, with recent introduction of endoscopic endonasal techniques for access to the ventral skull base and the suprasellar cisterns, the indications for transcranial and transsphenoidal surgery are once again being redefined.[16–20]

Definition of Giant Macroadenomas

The definition of a giant pituitary macroadenoma has been somewhat arbitrary. Using pneumoencephalography Hardy classified tumors as follows: type A, tumor that is bulging into the chiasmatic cisterns; type B, tumor that reaches the floor of the third ventricle; type C, large suprasellar tumor growth into the third ventricle up to the foramen of Monro; and type D, tumors that extend into the anterior or middle cranial fossa.[21] This classification was then modified to incorporate modern computed tomography (CT) and magnetic resonance imaging (MRI). The suprasellar extensions of macroadenomas were graded, and the giant tumors were considered to be grades C and D. Grade C included tumors with large suprasellar extensions up to 3 cm filling the anterior third ventricle, and grade D were either huge tumors with >3 cm suprasellar extension above the foramen of Monro or a grade C tumor with asymmetrical or multiple lateral extensions.[9] The critical threshold was a superior tumor margin greater than 2 cm above the jugum sphenoidale.[9] However, these classifications consider the tumor from the transsphenoidal approach.

Symon et al[15,22] defined giant pituitary tumors as those with suprasellar extensions over 4 cm above the jugum sphenoidale and that had less than 6 mm from the highest point of the tumor to the foramen of Monro. Not all giant pituitary adenomas extend into the third ventricle, and other studies have limited them to tumors over 3 or 4 cm in diameter regardless of the direction of growth.[23,24] In general, the extrasellar extension of a giant pituitary adenoma can occur in any direction.[10] Yasargil[25] incorporated elements of these classification schemes and classified giant pituitary adenomas as tumors that extend out of the sella in any direction and divided them into four subgroups: (1) suprasellar-suprachiasmatic: tumors that grow in front of the chiasm with greater than 2 cm above the planum sphenoidale; (2) suprasellar-retrosellar: tumor growth behind the chiasm filling the interpeduncular cistern and into the third ventricle or the prepontine cistern; (3) parasellar-cavernous: tumor growth laterally into the cavernous sinus or into the middle fossa; and (4) paninvasive: tumor invading in all directions retrochiasmatic, epidurally into the middle fossa and prepontine cistern.

Transcranial Surgery for Giant Macroadenomas

Horsley[26] is credited with performing the first successful resection of a pituitary tumor in 1889. He then used a subfrontal and middle fossa approach with a mortality rate of 20% in 10 patients between 1904 and 1906. At the same time Krause[27,28] removed a pituitary tumor using a mostly extradural subfrontal approach in 1905. McArthur[29] incorporated removal of the supraorbital ridge and orbital roof to expose a pituitary tumor in 1908. Frazier[30,31] shifted to an intradural frontobasal approach and considered it superior to the transsphenoidal approach in patients with visual disturbances. These techniques were later modified by Cushing,[32] Dandy,[3] and Heuer,[33] and a large experience with transcranial surgery for pituitary tumors was developed.[34–36] With development of microsurgical techniques to open the sylvian fissure and refinement of the pterional approach with sphenoid wing removal, Yasargil et al[37] described an unobstructed direct view to the parasellar structures. The shift from macrosurgical approaches to microsurgical approaches in the 1970s dramatically reduced the morbidity and mortality of transcranial surgery for giant pituitary adenomas.[10,15,38] Variations of these approaches were then introduced depending on the extension of the tumor laterally, into the suprasellar space, into the third ventricle, and to minimize brain retraction (orbitozygomatic, interhemispheric transcallosal, and frontobasal interhemispheric approaches).[25,37,39–45]

As the transsphenoidal approach gained in popularity, these transcranial approaches were eventually reserved for (1) pituitary tumors with extension into the anterior, middle, or posterior fossa; (2) hourglass-shaped tumors presumably with a small diaphragmatic hiatus; (3) presence of a suprasellar tumor in the setting of a small sella; and (4) fibrous tumors that proved too difficult to remove from a transsphenoidal approach.[5,38,46] Other indications for a transcranial approach include an active sinus infection in a patient for whom surgical delay poses the threat of acute neurologic deterioration; the presence of dolichoectatic internal carotid arteries that meet in the sella, that is, "kissing" carotid arteries; persistent visual loss after incomplete resection via the transsphenoidal route; and loss of occulomotor function.[45,47]

The operative mortality after transcranial surgery for giant pituitary adenomas was unacceptably high in the macrosurgical era, ranging from 18 to 33% in the acute postoperative period.[34,48–51] In one retrospective review with 16 cases of giant pituitary macroadenomas there was an 18% acute operative mortality rate associated with a 61% rate of radical excision, with one patient having a transient postoperative visual deterioration.[15] Microsurgery and experience dramatically lowered the operative mortality rate, which trended from 30% in 1953–1972 to 10% in 1973–1977 and to 6% in 1978–1983.[10] Unfortunately, the literature regarding transcranial approaches to giant pituitary macroadenomas is heterogeneous without clear selection criteria for a surgical approach and with variable data regarding the extent of resection.

The use of the microsurgical technique in combination with traditional transfrontal or transtemporal approaches to giant pituitary adenomas led to a substantial reduction in operative mortality. In one surgical series of 21 patients with giant pituitary adenomas measuring >4 cm in diameter, there was only one postoperative mortality secondary to renal failure and no postoperative cerebrospinal fluid (CSF) leak, worsening of vision, or reported diabetes insipidus (DI). Six patients had prolactinomas and 10 patients had evidence of hypopituitarism before surgery. Postoperatively, seven patients had improvement in their endocrinologic and ophthalmologic symptoms, and the rest were unchanged. However, a radical excision was not achieved in any of the 21 patients[52] (**Table 24.1**). In contrast, in a series of 319 patients with pituitary adenomas, there were 21 patients with giant adenomas (the authors define giant adenomas vaguely as adenomas with massive suprasellar extension) who underwent transcranial tumor resection with a subfrontal pterional approach.[53] The increased gross total resection rate that was achieved in eight patients (38%) was associated with a 10% (two patients) operative mortality. Postoperative worsening of visual function occurred in two (9.5%) patients, and none of the patients had evidence of CSF leak. Postoperative DI occurred in four patients (19%). All 21 patients had marked hypopituitarism on presentation, and 10 (48%) demonstrated improvements in anterior pituitary function after surgery (**Table 24.1**). It is unclear to what degree the growth hormone/insulin-like growth factor (GH/IGF) levels were normalized in the three patients with GH-secreting giant adenomas.[53]

In a separate series of 26 patients who underwent transcranial surgery and 85 patients who underwent transsphenoidal surgery for giant pituitary adenomas (>4 cm diameter), the pterional transsylvian approach was used in 12 patients earlier in the series, and either the fronto-orbito-zygomatic approach (seven patients) or the extended subfrontal approach incorporating a bilateral frontonasal-orbital craniotomy (seven patients) was used later in the series. Following transcranial surgery there was one perioperative mortality secondary to a pulmonary embolism 2 months after surgery. The rate of CSF leak requiring lumbar drainage was 7.7% (two patients), and the rate of permanent visual worsening was 15.4% (four patients) after transcranial surgery.[24] The rate of visual worsening was lower in the patients who underwent cranial base operations (7.8%); however, this was not statistically significant. Postoperative hypopituitarism occurred in six patients (23%), and permanent DI occurred in four patients (15%) after transcranial surgery. These complications were greater in the transcranial

Table 24.1 Microsurgical Technique in Combination with Traditional Transfrontal or Transtemporal Approaches to Giant Pituitary Adenomas

First Author	*N*	GTR	CSF Leak	Permanent DI	Decreased Vision	Mortality
		n (%)	*n* (%)	*n* (%)	*n* (%)	*n* (%)
Transcranial						
Dolenc[18]						
Group I	120	81 (68)	10 (8)	n/a	21 (18)	0
Group II	90	83 (92)	1 (1)	n/a	1 (1)	0
Symon[72]	16	11 (69)	n/a	n/a	1 (6)	3 (19)
Pia[64]	54	n/a	5 (9)	0	4 (7)	4 (7)
Grote[32]	21	0	0	0	0	1 (5)
Guidetti[33]	21	8 (38)	0	4 (19)	2 (10)	2 (10)
Mortini[60]	26	1 (4)	2 (8)	4 (15)	4 (15)	1 (4)
Total	348	184 (53)	18 (5)	8 (2)	33 (9)	11 (3)
Microscopic Transsphenoidal						
Henderson[41]	231	n/a	n/a	n/a	6 (3)	13 (6)
Ciric[8]	117	17 (15)	4 (3)	0	0	0
Black[4]	144	n/a	6 (4)	1 (1)	0	0
Bohinski[5]	30	10 (33)	1 (3)	0	1 (3)	0
Kitano[49]	*36	26 (72)	13 (4)	3 (9)	0	0
Total	558	53 (9)	24 (4)	4 (1)	7 (1)	13 (2)
Combined Transcranial/Microscopic Transsphenoidal						
D'Ambrosio[12]	11	6 (55)	2 (18)	3 (27)	0	0
Takakara[73]						
Cranial alone	40	n/a	n/a	n/a	3 (8)	10 (25)
Combined	17	n/a	n/a	n/a	0	0
Alleyne[1]	10	4 (40)	0	1 (10)	0	0
Total	78	10 (13)	2 (3)	4 (4)	3 (4)	10 (13)
Endonasal Endoscopic Transsphenoidal						
Dehdashti[17]	3	3 (100)	0	0	0	0
Cornell	62	45 (73)	1 (2)	9 (15)	0	1 (2)
Total	65	48 (74)	1 (2)	9 (14)	0	1 (2)

Abbreviations: CSF, cerebrospinal fluid; DI, diabetes insipidus; GTR, gross total resection; n/a, not applicable.
*Although microsurgical technique was used for exposure and resection of the lesion, a 70-degree endoscope was intermittently used to inspect the cavernous sinus for residual disease.

group compared with the transsphenoidal group. Only one patient (3.8%) in the transcranial group had complete tumor resection[24] (**Table 24.1**).

Other surgeons shifted to a combined transsphenoidal and pterional craniotomy approach to giant pituitary adenomas. In one series of 40 patients with giant pituitary adenomas (>5 cm in diameter) the older strategy of transcranial surgery alone was compared with a newer staged transsphenoidal and transcranial approach.[7] In the older subgroup managed by transcranial surgery alone, a 25% mortality rate was reported, with the highest mortality rate, 57%, seen in the group who underwent radical surgical removal. This decreased to 26% in the partial-removal group. Worsening postoperative vision was noted in 10% after transcranial surgery, and the authors did not specifically report on endocrinologic outcomes[7] (**Table 24.1**). The high mortality rate led them to shift to an initial transsphenoidal removal of the intrasellar component of the tumor and decompression of the suprasellar component if it descends during the operation. The patients were then followed by repeat MRI scans for up to 3 months. At that time, suprasellar components descended into the vacant sella space and a second transsphenoidal or transcranial operation was performed. With this approach in 17 patients no operative mortality or major complications were reported; however, specific endocrine outcomes were not reported.[7]

The staged combined approach was also attempted as a simultaneous combined transsphenoidal and pterional approach.[1,2] In a series of 10 patients who underwent the simultaneous combined surgical approach, six had gross total or near total removal of the tumor. All nine patients who presented with visual loss had postoperative resolution, and there was no operative mortality or postoperative CSF leak. Postoperative DI occurred in one patient, and hypopituitarism persisted in all five patients who presented with DI preoperatively[1] (**Table 24.1**).

Improved visualization of the surgical anatomy with use of skull base techniques substantially decreased the operative morbidity and mortality of giant pituitary adenomas. In a series of 210 patients with large or giant pituitary adenomas with suprasellar and parasellar extension, a classic frontotemporal transcranial approach was used for the first 120 patients and an extradural transcavernous skull base approach was used for the next 90 patients.[41] The skull base approach incorporated extradural anterior clinoidectomy, orbitotomy, optic canal unroofing, and intradural exposure of the cavernous sinus, and it combined intradural and extradural transcavernous tumor resection. Although the author's exact definition of giant adenoma was unclear, these tumors required transcranial surgery for removal of their various suprasellar and parasellar extensions. With the classic approach in patients undergoing their first operation, complete resection was achieved in 63% of patients. New visual field deficits were observed in 29% of patients, and CSF leak occurred in 6% of patients. In contrast, with the extradural skull base approach, complete resection was achieved in 93% of patients. None of the patients who underwent the skull base approach had postoperative visual field deterioration or CSF leak.[41] In both groups of patients, almost all had significant endocrinologic deficits present preoperatively, and they did not change after surgery. Specific anterior or posterior pituitary endocrine deficits were not reported. No perioperative mortalities were described with either approach (**Table 24.1**).

Transsphenoidal Surgery for Giant Macroadenomas

The transsphenoidal approach for the resection of a pituitary tumor was first described by Herman Schloffer[54] at the University Clinic in Innsbruck, Austria. He performed a superior nasal transsphenoidal approach on a 30-year-old man with a 6-year history of severe headaches and declining vision who was found to have an enlarged sella on a lateral skull x-ray. Although the surgery proceeded without serious complications, the patient died postoperatively from obstructive hydrocephalus. During the following years the transsphenoidal approach was modified, and Harvey Cushing was the first to present a large clinical series of 231 transsphenoidal pituitary adenoma resections in 1939.[55] Cushing compared the clinical outcome between the transsphenoidal and transcranial approaches for resection of pituitary adenomas. In his series the perioperative mortality rate following transsphenoidal and transcranial pituitary adenoma resection was similarly low (5.2% versus 4.5%). However, the cause of death was different depending on the approach. Mortality following a transsphenoidal approach was due to infections, swelling of residual tumor tissue, and in one case uncontrollable intraoperative hemorrhage. Mortality following a transcranial pituitary adenoma resection was caused by postoperative blood clots in the majority of cases. Clinical follow-up data were available for almost all patients. Ten years after the operation half of the patients were still alive. Preoperative impaired vision improved in approximately two thirds of patients. Two major disadvantages of the transsphenoidal approach prompted Cushing to abandon the transsphenoidal approach. First, given the lack of preoperative imaging, possible suprasellar extension of a pituitary adenoma was unknown and the transsphenoidal approach was not suitable for intraoperative exploration. Consequently, tumor was left behind and caused half of the perioperative mortality associated with the transsphenoidal approach. Second, high-power illumination or magnification was not available, which severely limited access and visibility. Hence, in the late 1920s Cushing preferentially used the transfrontal approach, as it allowed for intraoperative visualization of suprasellar tumor extension and better decompression of the optic chiasm.

For the next decades the use of transsphenoidal operations diminished greatly. Two technologic milestones paved the way for the revival of the transsphenoidal technique. First, the intraoperative use of the operating microscope improved intraoperative illumination and visualization.[56] Second, preoperative CT provided information about the size and location of the lesion and facilitated patient selection and choice of appropriate surgical access. Using these technologic tools, a high incidence of complete tumor removal and low complication rate was reported for the transsphenoidal resection of pituitary microadenomas.[57,58] Rapidly, transsphenoidal surgery was also adopted for pituitary macroadenomas.

In 1983, Ciric and colleagues[59] reported transsphenoidal resection of pituitary macroadenomas (diameter >2 cm) in 108 patients. No perioperative mortality was encountered. Preoperative visual field impairment improved in 90% of patients. Normalization of prolactin- and GH-secreting tumors was achieved in approximately one third of the patients. Specific anterior or posterior pituitary endocrine deficits were not reported, and no case with DI lasting longer than 3 months was seen. Postoperative CT imaging revealed gross total tumor resection in 59% of patients; however, this number might be optimistic, given that CT imaging was used. The main complication in this series was CSF rhinorrhea, which complicated the postoperative course of 3.5% of patients, and one of these patients developed meningitis (**Table 24.1**).

Black and colleagues[60] described their experience with transsphenoidal procedures for pituitary adenomas in 255 patients. Of these lesions, 44% had suprasellar extension and 15% were intrasellar macroadenomas. In this series there was no perioperative death. Importantly, Black and colleagues correlated complications with tumor size. CSF leaks were the major complication encountered. Although only 1% of microadenomas were complicated by CSF leaks, this complication was seen in 3% of tumors with suprasellar extension and 9.5% of macroadenomas (>1 cm in diameter). A similar increase of adverse outcome was seen with regard to the rate of DI following removal of microadendomas (1%) and macroadenomas (9.5%). In all but one patient (0.4%), DI resolved within 1 year (**Table 24.1**). This study was limited to perioperative complications and did not address the radiographic extent of resection and clinical outcome.

Bohinski and colleagues[61] used intraoperative MRI to study the extent of resection in 30 patients who underwent transsphenoidal resection of pituitary macroadenomas (measuring ≥1 cm). In this series, a gross total resection was achieved in 34% of patients (**Table 24.1**). One transsphenoidal approach was converted to a craniotomy due to laceration of the anterior cerebral artery.

Han and colleagues[62] analyzed factors associated with CSF leaks in a series of 592 patients who underwent a transsphenoidal approach for pituitary macroadenomas. They found that transsphenoidal resection of macroadenomas (diameter ranging from >1 cm to <4 cm) was associated with a 2.7% risk of postoperative CSF leak compared with 9.1% in patients after resection of a giant adenoma (diameter 4 cm or larger). Indistinct tumor borders and tenacious tumor consistency were other factors increasing the risk of postoperative CSF leaks (**Table 24.1**).

Extended Endoscopic Approaches for Pituitary Macroadenomas

Endoscope-assisted transsphenoidal surgery has gained widespread use during the last decade. Several authors propose that visualization of endoscope-assisted surgery is superior compared with that of microsurgery. In particular, the endoscope enables distinct resolution of anatomical details and better demarcation of tumor tissue from surrounding structures compared with microsurgery. Moreover, the use of angled endoscopes enables the surgeon to look around corners and expands the traditional indications of transsphenoidal surgery with regard to the lesion location and size.[63–69] This appears to be a particular advantage when dealing with tumors that extend beyond the sella. The microscope-based approach, which requires a speculum to maintain an adequately large corridor for visualization, also limits the field of view and maneuverability of the instruments. The endonasal endoscopic approach avoids the use of retractors and moves the lens and light source into the sphenoid sinus and intracranial cavity, which increases visualization.[69–71] The other main advantage of the endonasal approach is the development of expanded approaches, in which large areas of bone of the anterior skull base are removed to increase visualization.[17,18,72] For giant macroadenomas, removal of the tuberculum sellae and planum sphenoidale permits direct visualization of the suprasellar extent of macroadenomas, previously invisible to the microscope-based transsphenoidal approaches.[69,72] Likewise, the transcavernous approach allows the removal of tumor in the cavernous sinus, and the transclival approach allows the surgeon to remove tumor extending through the back wall of the sphenoid sinus into the posterior fossa.[67,72–74] These areas were previously accessible only with a craniotomy. By using a transsphenoidal approach, the surgeon can stay within the capsule of the tumor, which also decreases the risk of surrounding critical structures such as the optic nerves and carotid arteries and its branches. Critical to these novel expanded approaches is the ability to reconstruct the floor of the skull base in a watertight fashion to prevent postoperative CSF leak and meningitis. The use of novel multilayer closures, such as the gasket seal[75] and nasoseptal flap,[76] increases the surgeon's confidence that any size opening can be adequately secured with a postoperative CSF leak of under 5 to 10%.

Only a few studies have explored expanded endoscope-assisted transsphenoidal approaches for resection of pituitary macroadenomas. Kitano and colleagues[77] reported an extended endoscope-assisted transsphenoidal approach for pituitary adenomas invading the cavernous sinus. The authors used microsurgical technique for exposure and tumor resection. Intermittently, a 70-degree rigid endoscope was used to assist with resection of tumor in the cavernous sinus. This series included 36 patients with pituitary adenomas ranging from 0.5 to 114.6 mm.[34] Access to the cavernous sinus was gained medial to the intracavernous internal carotid artery for the resection of smaller lesions and lateral to the internal carotid artery for the resection of larger adenomas. The extent of resection was similar between these two approaches, and a gross total tumor resection was achieved in 72% of patients. Patients with larger tumors who required a lateral approach had a greater blood loss compared with patients who underwent the medial approach. The most common complications were transient double vision, which was found in 42% of patients after a lateral approach and in 14% of patients after a medial approach (**Table 24.1**). Of 12 patients with acromegaly treated with the expanded transsphenoidal approach, eight patients had normalization of their GH levels. No cases of postoperative hypopituitarism were reported.

Dehdashti and colleagues[78] included three patients with pituitary macroadenoma in their series of 22 patients using a pure endoscopic expanded transsphenoidal approach. They were able to achieve a gross total resection and noticed a marked improvement of vision. The operation did not alter the existing hypopituitarism in two patients (**Table 24.1**).

Extended Endoscopic Transsphenoidal Approach: Surgical Technique

At our institution we perform an expanded endonasal transsphenoidal approach as the initial surgery for essentially every macroadenoma, regardless of size or extension. If significant residual tumor remains, a craniotomy could be a second procedure, but this has rarely, if ever, been required. The technique can be divided into the approach, the resection, and the closure, each of which is tailored to the size and compartments involved by the tumor.

Setup

The patient is placed under general anesthesia and administered antibiotics and glucocorticoids. We routinely use cephazolin (2 g intravenous [IV]) and dexamethasone (10 mg IV). Many patients already have a decreased ability to produce a steroid stress response given the size of the tumor, and this number increases postoperatively. For this reason we do not generally test the adrenal axis prior to surgery and just assume stress steroids will be needed in large macroadenomas. Postoperative cortisol levels are established prior to discharging patients. We also administer steroids to decrease the potential inflammatory response from the administration of intrathecal fluorescein and additionally administer diphenhydramine (50 mg IV). A lumbar puncture is performed, and 0.2 mL of 10% fluorescein is injected in 10 mL of CSF to help visualize CSF leaks. If a large CSF leak is expected (such as in tumors extending >2 cm above the jugum), we often place a lumbar drain for prophylactic drainage. The drain is left in place for 1 to 2 days and drained at a rate of no more than 5 mL/h. Cottonoids soaked in 4 mL of 4% cocaine (topical) are placed over the nasal mucosa for vasoconstriction. The patient's head is placed in three-point fixation and elevated above the heart to facilitate venous drainage and positioned in slight extension and turned slightly to the right. We generally use the Brainlab neuronavigation system (Brainlab Inc., Westchester, IL), and the patient is registered with a preoperative CT or MRI scan. The lateral thigh is prepared for autologous fat grafts. The mucosa of the middle turbinates is injected with a mixture of lidocaine 1% and epinephrine (1:100,000).

Approach

Under endoscopic view, the inferior, middle, and superior turbinates are identified. The middle and superior turbinates are retracted laterally, and the sphenoid ostia are identified bilaterally. If a nasoseptal flap is indicated, it is harvested by making cuts in the septal mucosa 1 mm above the palate and 2 to 3 mm below the cribriform plate until they meet anteriorly (**Fig. 24.1**). The mucosa is elevated off the septum, with care taken to preserve the vascular supply

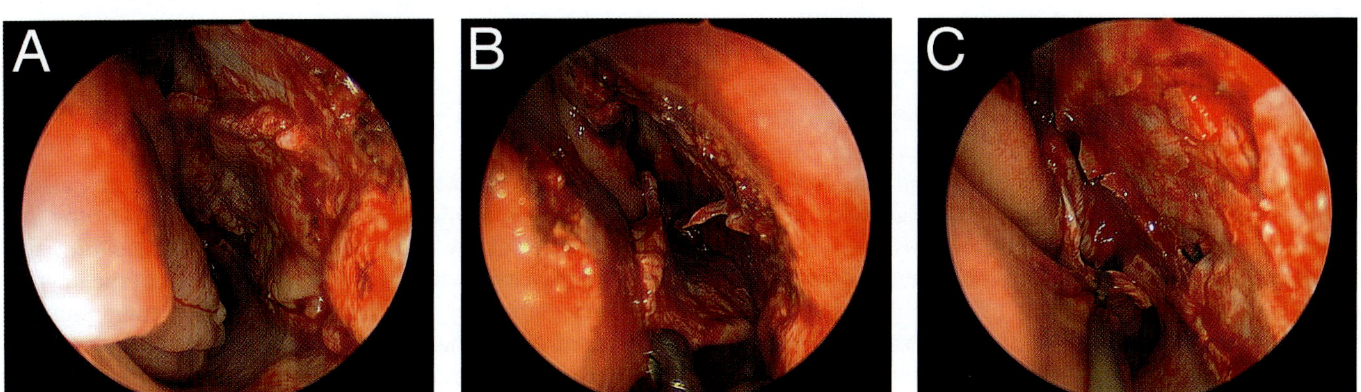

Fig. 24.1 Harvesting of the nasoseptal flap. The flap constitutes a mucoperichondrial pedicled flap based on the nasoseptal artery. **(A)** With the help of a needle-point electrocautery, the septal mucosa is incised just above the palate and below the cribriform plate. These cuts meet anteriorly. **(B)** The mucosa is elevated off the septum and then **(C)** stored in the choana until the end of the operation.

from the sphenopalatine artery. The flap is dissected off the face of the sphenoid sinus and retracted into the choana, where it is stored until the end of the operation (**Fig. 24.1**). We do not place a flap in all pituitary tumors, but only those macroadenomas with a significant suprasellar extension for which we expect a large CSF leak. However, one cannot harvest the flap at the end of the procedure after the septal mucosa has been removed. Therefore, if one feels that it might be needed, it is worth the time to harvest it even in questionable cases.

The sphenoid ostia lie just above the sphenoethmoid recess, approximately 1.5 cm above the choana. In some circumstances, the ostium is covered by a supreme turbinate, which can be gently retracted laterally or resected if necessary. The mucosa around the ostium is cauterized and enlarged with a mushroom punch and Kerrison rongeur. Care is taken not to wander inferolaterally into the territory of the sphenopalatine artery. The posterior third of the nasal septum adjacent to the vomeric bone and maxillary crest is resected with a tissue shaver. This step permits a panoramic view of the sphenoid sinus rostrum and the ostia bilaterally and provides the ability to use four separate instruments, two through each nostril, for the remainder of the procedure. A graft of vomer or cartilage can be harvested to reconstruct the floor of the sella at the end of the operation. Alternatively, synthetic material can be used. The mucosa of the sphenoid sinus rostrum is retracted laterally and inferiorly, and the rostrum is removed and the floor and lateral wall of the sphenoid sinus are drilled down to facilitate placement of the nasoseptal flap at the end of the operation. If the floor of the sinus is not flattened, the flap will extend over a large lip of sphenoid sinus and subsequently hang off the posterior wall of the sinus and not adequately cover the defect. It is important to remove the entire anterior wall of the sphenoid sinus to provide enough room for the endoscope and instruments to sit within the sphenoid during the procedure. Care must be taken to avoid fracturing the cribriform plate superiorly, a common site of iatrogenic CSF leak after surgery.

All sphenoid septa are removed with a drill, and the mucosa of the sphenoid sinus is completely removed so that a mucocele does not form under the nasoseptal flap. Bleeding is stopped either with warm saline irrigation or Gelfoam. It is important to examine the preoperative MRI or CT to determine the location of the carotid arteries with respect to the intersphenoidal septations. Septations overlying the carotids can be left in place if there is no intercavernous extent of the tumor. A diamond drill is useful to remove these septations if necessary to avoid iatrogenic carotid injury. The middle turbinate on one side can be removed to increase the exposure, although we try to preserve the middle turbinate if possible. Often, the posterior ethmoids must be completely removed to visualize the tuberculum sellae and planum sphenoidale if an extended transtuberculum, transplanum approach is being used. Care must be taken to avoid injuring the posterior ethmoidal arteries or to identify and coagulate them upfront. Thus, the posterior wall of the sphenoid sinus is brought into full view.

A 0-degree, 30-cm long, 4-mm diameter rigid endoscope (Karl Storz, Tuttlingen, Germany) is introduced through the left nostril and held in place with a flexible scope holder. The carotid protuberance, optic protuberance, and opticocarotid recesses are identified. Although the extent of bone removal varies depending on the location of the pathology, we generally start by thinning the tuberculum sellae with a high-speed diamond drill under constant irrigation. The opening extends between the middle clinoids, also called the "medial opticocarotid recess." The inferior extent of the bone opening extends down to roughly 1 mm above the floor of the sella. We usually leave a lip of the sella floor to hold the fat graft in place in cases where there is a CSF leak but not so much as to prevent complete resection of the inferior portion of the tumor. The thinned bone is removed with a curette and Kerrison rongeur. Care is taken when opening over the intercavernous sinus to coagulate the dura and sinus with a bipolar. The opening is extended above the level of the diaphragma, and the planum sphenoidale is removed. The anterior extent of removal of the planum is determined with image guidance to ensure adequate exposure of the tumor and that the top of the tumor will be seen, to maximize the possibility of a complete removal of the suprasellar component (**Fig. 24.2**). Often, this portion of the procedure requires a 30-degree, 30-cm long, 4-mm diameter rigid endoscope to achieve adequate upward visualization. If the tumor extends into the cavernous sinus, then the bone over the cavernous sinus is removed (**Fig. 24.3**). This maneuver can be done safely with a 1-mm Kerrison rongeur if the footplate is in the correct plane. Venous bleeding is stopped with Gelfoam soaked in thrombin and gentle pressure. The course of the carotid artery is identified with navigation and a Doppler. Tumors that extend into the clivus require additional removal of clival bone below the sphenoid sinus between the vertical segments of the internal carotid artery.

Resection

First the dura is opened over the sella in a cruciate pattern and the leaves of the dura are dissected free from the anterior border of the tumor. It is important to examine the preoperative MRI scan to identify the location of the normal pituitary gland and stalk because these structures must be preserved. Often the normal pituitary gland is draped over the top of the tumor (**Fig. 24.3**). However, the gland can be pushed laterally or, less commonly, anteriorly, and one must be careful to avoid resecting normal pituitary during this procedure. If the normal gland is anterior, a vertical cut can be made in the gland to enter the tumor, and the gland

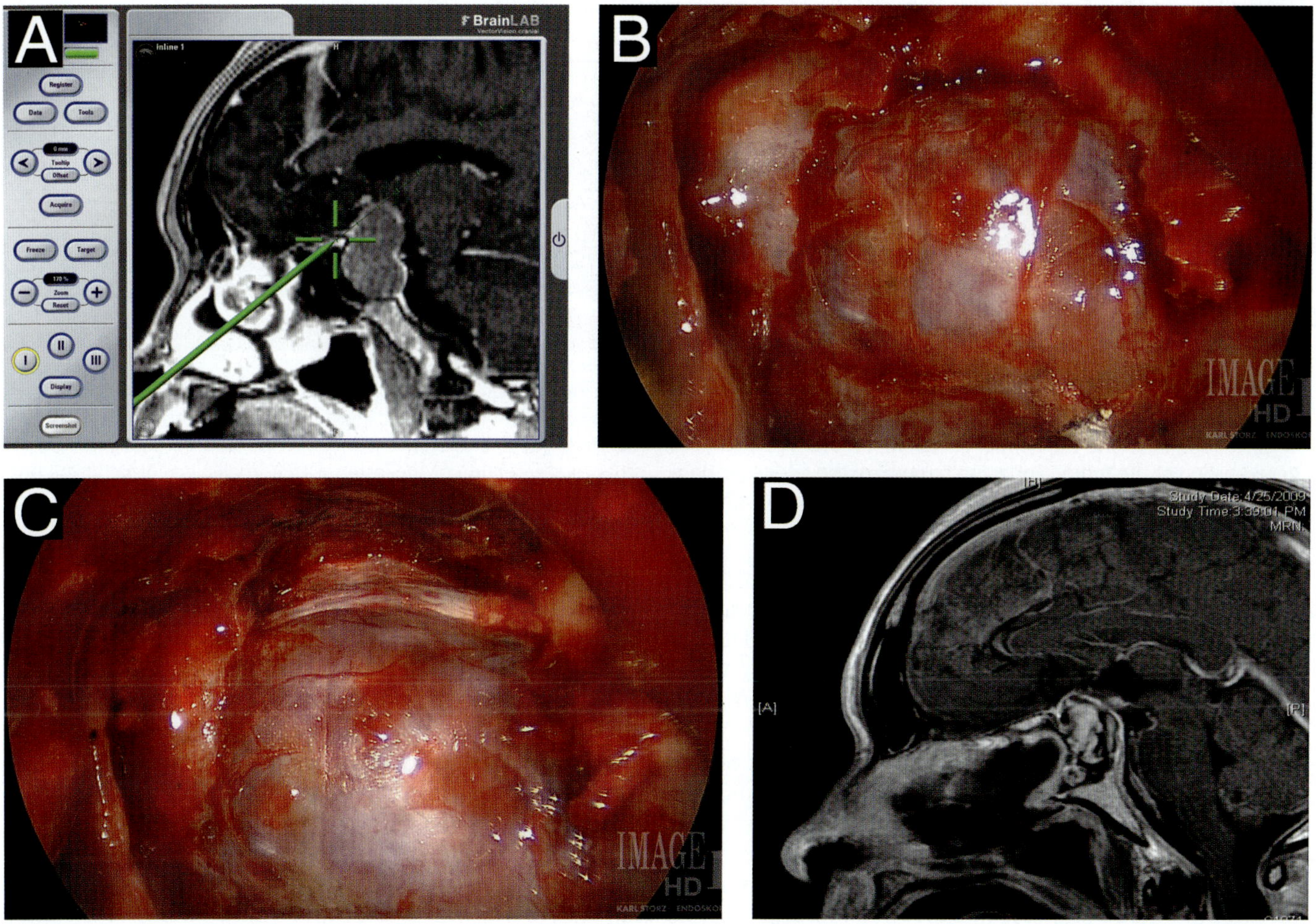

Fig. 24.2 Removal of tuberculum sellae and planum sphenoidale to facilitate the resection of the suprasellar portion of the tumor. **(A)** Sagittal preoperative contrast-enhanced magnetic resonance imaging (MRI) reveals suprasellar extension of a pituitary macroadenoma. The *green line*, derived from the stereotactic navigation software, indicates the trajectory necessary to access the superior extend of the lesion and the amount of bone required to see over the top of the tumor. **(B)** Intraoperative image following the removal of the posterior wall of the sphenoid sinus depicts the bulging dura over the floor and anterior face of the sella behind which lies the tumor. **(C)** Removal of the tuberculum sellae and part of the planum sphenoidale prepares the surgical corridor for removal of the suprasellar part of the lesion. Note the change in consistency of the dura over the floor of the sella and the dura behind the tuberculum sellae and planum sphenoidale. **(D)** Postoperative sagittal MRI demonstrates a complete resection of the tumor, the extent of the resected bone, and the nasoseptal flap holding the fat graft in place. Note how the lip of bone at the floor of the sphenoid sinus and top of clivus can hinder the flap from draping onto the posterior wall of the sinus.

can be pushed to either side to create a corridor for surgery. Care must be taken to avoid disconnecting the gland from the stalk.

Although it is important to try to find a plane of dissection between the normal pituitary gland and the tumor, with giant macroadenomas this is often quite difficult at the start of the operation. For this reason, we often start with internal decompression. If the tumor is soft, this can be done with one or two suctions as well as ring curettes. Frozen and permanent sections are sent to the pathology lab. If the tumor is firm, we have used a Cavitron ultrasonic surgical aspirator (Valleylab, Boulder, CO) or Elliquence monopolar (Elliquence, Oceanside, NY). Another very useful device is called the Myriad (NICO Corp., Indianapolis, IN), which side-cuts and aspirates simultaneously. Visualization is obtained with a 30-degree, 30-cm long, 4-mm diameter rigid endoscope. It is important to remove the inferior portion of the tumor and then the lateral portions to prevent the suprasellar arachnoid from herniating down into the sella and obstructing the view. Tumor is dissected off the medial wall of the cavernous sinus. If there is cavernous invasion, the carotid is often pushed laterally and the dura can be opened over the cavernous sinus medially and removed through the defect in the medial wall of the cavernous sinus (**Fig. 24.3**).

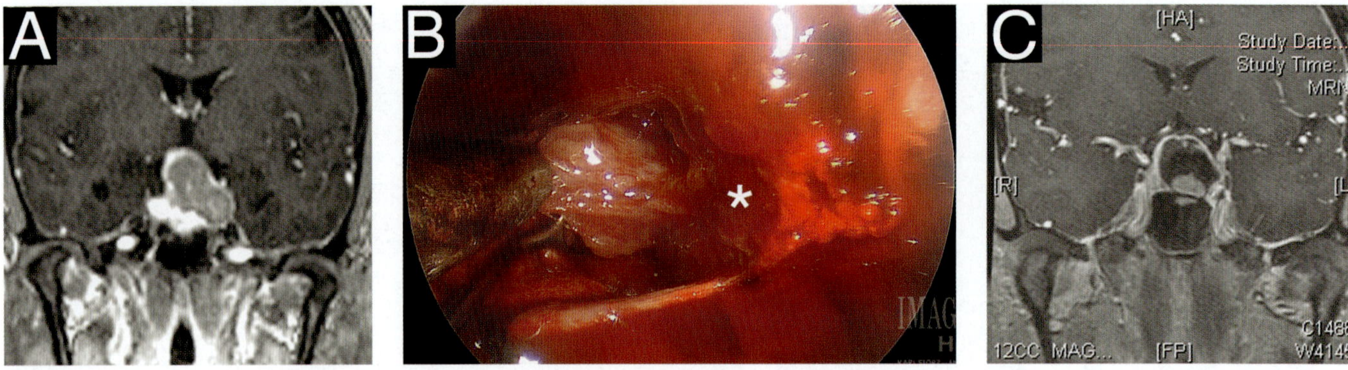

Fig. 24.3 Removal of tumor extending into the cavernous sinus. **(A)** Preoperative contrast-enhanced coronal MRI reveals invasion of the left cavernous sinus and the normal gland draped over the superior-lateral portion of the tumor. Following removal of the lateral portion of the sella floor, the inferior wall of the cavernous sinus is exposed. **(B)** Using an angled endoscope the medial cavernous sinus can be visualized and tumor removed from behind the internal carotid artery (*asterisk*). **(C)** Postoperative contrast-enhanced coronal MRI reveals gross total resection of the lesion with a small piece of fat at the bottom of the sella.

Although it is also possible to open the cavernous sinus lateral to the carotid, one must carefully weigh the safety of this maneuver with the increased extent of resection that it will facilitate and how this will affect the long-term outcome of the patient versus treatment with stereotactic radiosurgery.

Attention is then turned to the suprasellar extent of the tumor. Using a 30-degree scope and removing the tuberculum sella and planum sphenoidale will facilitate direct visualization of this component of the tumor (**Fig. 24.2**). Initially, we try to stay within the tumor and dissect the tumor off the pituitary gland and arachnoid. The diaphragm sella is usually enlarged and not visualized. If the diaphragma is intact, in the case of a dumbbell tumor, then the anterior intercavernous sinus can be cauterized and cut and the diaphragm opened. Tears in the arachnoid are common with giant macroadenomas and should not be cause for concern as long as one has prepared for the closure. Tumor that extends into the third ventricle or between the optic nerves must be carefully dissected free of these structures under direct vision. Aggressive internal decompression usually facilitates descent of the tumor into the sella. However, if the tumor is firm or the capsule adherent, the suprasellar tumor may remain in place. With the removal of the bone of the tuberculum sella and planum sphenoidale, the surgeon can dissect over the top of the capsule and push the tumor down off the optic chiasm and out of the third ventricle so complete removal can be obtained (**Fig. 24.4**). In some

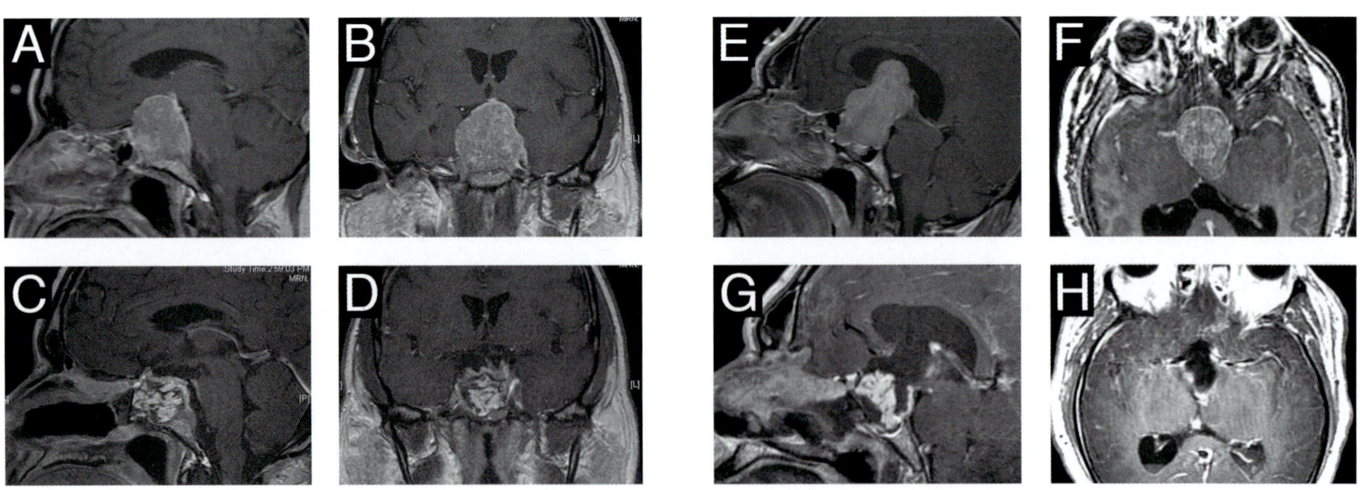

Fig. 24.4 Examples for pre- and postoperative contrast-enhanced MRI studies. Sagittal **(A)** and coronal **(B)** images reveal a homogeneously enhancing mass with a suprasellar extension reaching the floor of the third ventricle and clival and bilateral cavernous sinus invasion. Postoperative sagittal **(C)** and coronal **(D)** images show complete resection of the lesion with a fat graft in the resection cavity. Preoperative contrast-enhanced sagittal **(E)** and axial **(F)** images depict a lesion with suprasellar extension through the third ventricle and into the lateral ventricle. Postoperative contrast-enhanced sagittal **(G)** and axial **(H)** images depict interval complete removal of the lesion.

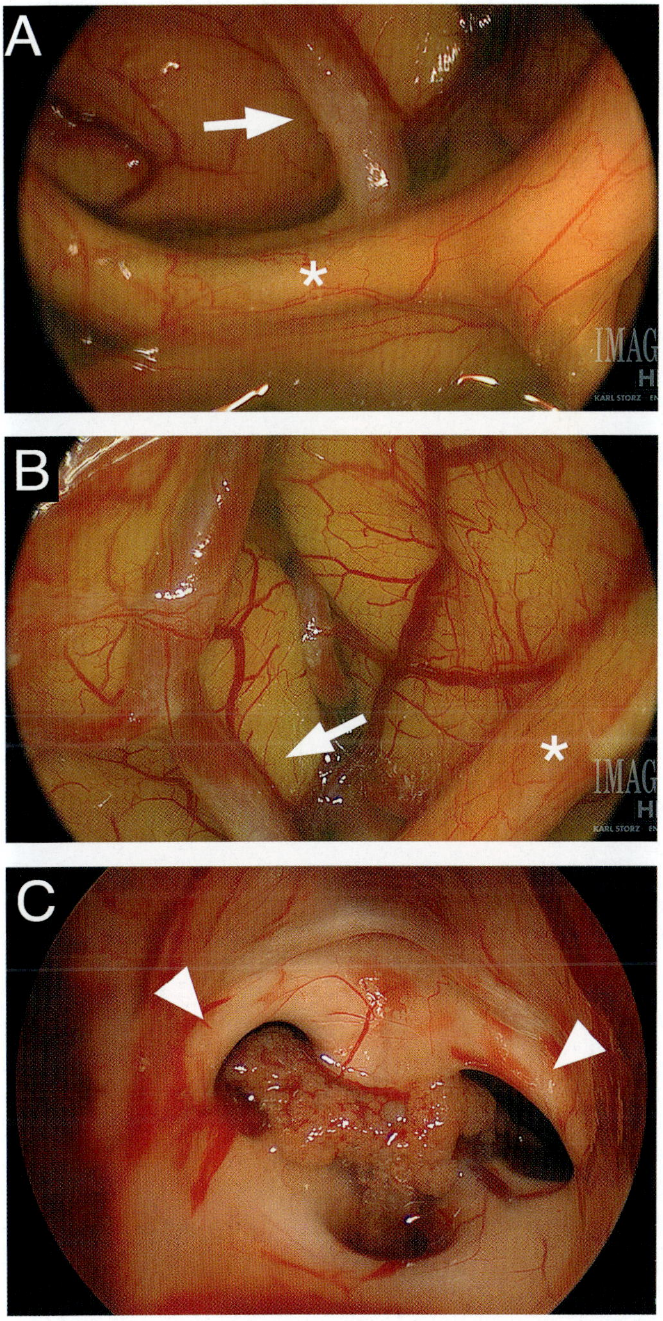

Fig. 24.5 Final inspection of the surgical site. **(A)** Using a 45-degree rigid scope the splayed optic nerve (*asterisk*) and the second segment of the anterior cerebral artery (A2 segment, *arrow*) are visualized. **(B)** The A2 segment (*arrow*) is followed to the interhemispheric fissure, and the thinned optic nerve (*asterisk*) is seen as well. **(C)** Resection of a lesion extending in the third ventricle allows for the inspection of the roof of the third ventricle including the foramina of Monro (*arrowheads*) and choroid plexus.

circumstances, if the nerves or vessels are encased in fibrous tumor, complete resection may not be possible. At the end of the resection, a 45-degree, 18-cm long, 4-mm diameter rigid endoscope is advanced into the cavity to ensure the absence of any residual tumor (**Fig. 24.5**). Curved suctions, angled micropituitary rongeurs, and dissectors can be used to reach residual pieces of tumor.

Closure

The use of intrathecal fluorescein helps to ensure adequate closure at each stage (**Fig. 24.6**). Intraoperative CSF leakage is very common after transsphenoidal resection of giant macroadenomas and is not of concern if one is well prepared. However, residual CSF leak is unacceptable at the end of the closure, and fluorescein is useful to ensure a watertight closure at the end of the procedure. Closure is performed in a multilayer fashion. The first step is to fill any dead space with autologous fat graft. Care must be taken to avoid placing too much fat that might compress the optic nerves. Although macroadenomas may have a large intracranial extension, they are still predominantly extra–arachnoidal tumors. Depending on the size of the arachnoid defect, the amount of CSF leak, and the degree of removal of the planum sphenoidale, the closure can be tailored. If the arachnoid is somewhat preserved and only a small amount of the planum sphenoidale has been removed, then the fat is held in place with Medpor (Porex, Newnan, GA) or vomer and covered with a nasoseptal flap (**Fig. 24.6**). If, however, there is a very large rent in the arachnoid and a significant amount of the planum has been removed, we place an onlay of fascia lata that is countersunk into the cavity with Medpor or vomer, the so-called gasket-seal closure.[75] This is covered with the nasoseptal flap. In both circumstances, after the flap is placed, a layer of DuraSeal (Confluent Surgical, Waltham, MA) is used to keep the flap in position and provide a temporary watertight seal. Although we do not use an inflated Foley to keep the flap in position, other institutions find this helpful.[76] It is critical to ensure that the nasoseptal flap is positioned over the entire defect, making sure that it is not doubled over on itself and that the mucosal surface is facing the nasal cavity (**Fig. 24.6**). If fascia lata is used, it is critical that the nasoseptal flap lies beyond the edges of the fascia lata so that the flap is in contact with the sphenoid bone to fully cover the defect. The nasal cavity is then filled with FloSeal (Baxter, Deerfield, IL). A small piece of Telfa (Kendall, Mansfield, MA) is placed in each nostril overnight to absorb any drainage and is removed in the morning. The lumbar drain is left open at 5 mL/h for 1 to 2 days depending on the size of the leak and the adequacy of the closure. Patients are placed on low doses of heparin to prevent deep venous thrombosis.

■ Our Series

In our experience, approximately one third of patients with pituitary macroadenomas (maximal diameter >1 cm)

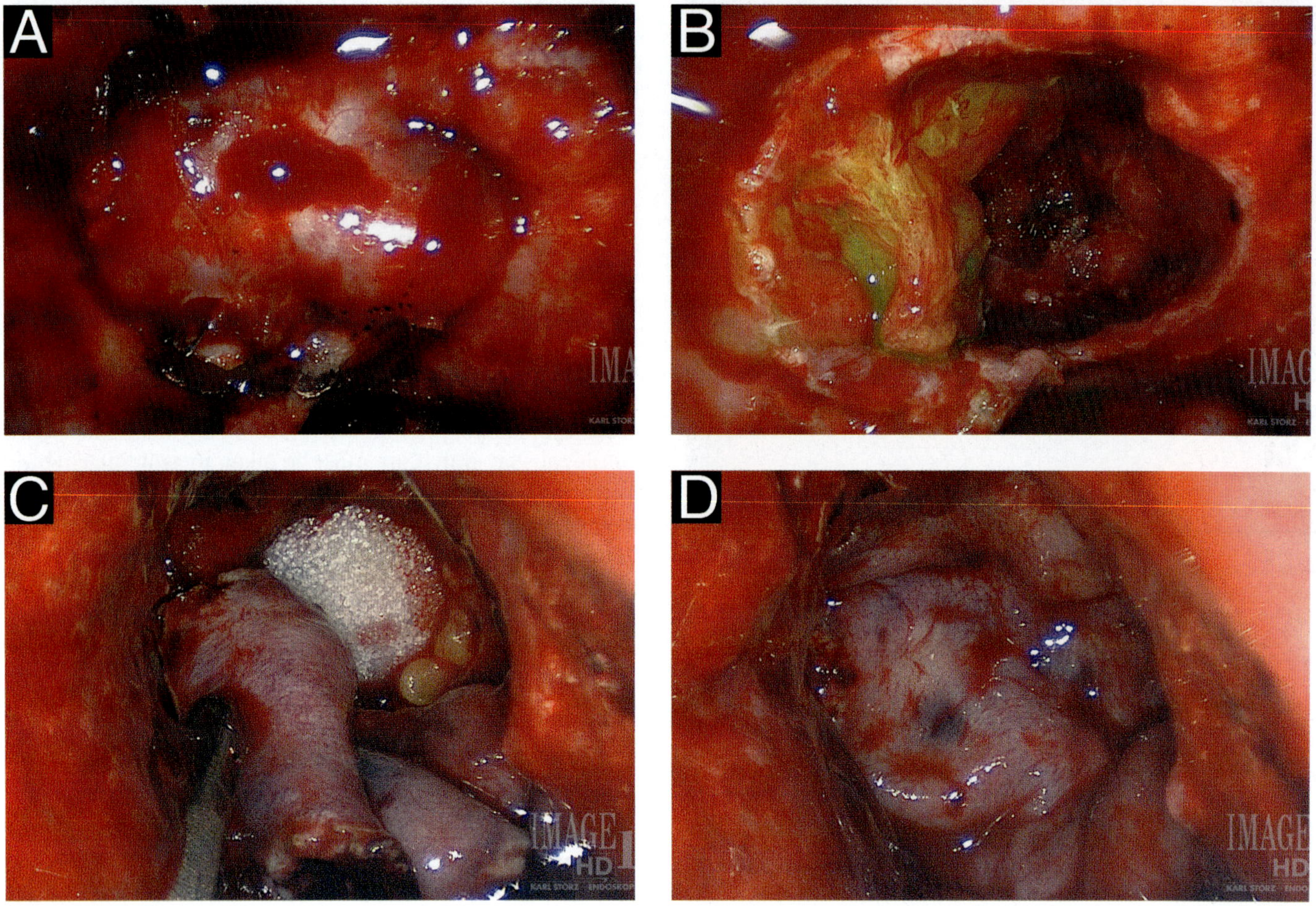

Fig. 24.6 Multilayer closure. **(A)** Prior to resection of the lesion, the bulging dura containing the lesion is seen. The bone over the cavernous sinus containing the internal carotid artery has been completely exposed on the far right of the image. **(B)** Downward herniation of arachnoid and minimal fluorescein-marked cerebrospinal fluid leakage is noted around the thinned normal pituitary gland. **(C)** The bony defect is repaired first with a fat graft that is held in place with a piece of Medpor. The nasoseptal flap is being moved into place and can be seen just below the Medpor. **(D)** The flap is placed over the entire closure with its vascular pedicle intact below.

present with visual field defects, whereas other patients commonly present with complaints of headaches, amenorrhea, or decreased libido. Analysis of contrast-enhanced postoperative MRI studies revealed that the extent of resection depends mainly on whether or not the invasion of the cavernous sinus has occurred. Thus, a gross total resection is accomplished in 93% of macroadenomas without invasion of the cavernous sinus. Once invasion of the cavernous sinus has occurred, a gross total resection is achieved in only 29% of patients. Although some tumor tissue is left behind in the cavernous sinus, we can still achieve a 93% average amount of resection. We routinely follow residual tumor in the cavernous sinus with serial MRI, and eventually half of these patients undergo radiosurgery. Tumor size is positively correlated with invasion of the cavernous sinus. Tumor size does not appear to be an independent predictor for complete resectability of pituitary macroadenomas. Besides the cavernous sinus, residual tumor was most often detected in the suprasellar compartment, frontal lobe, and the most posterosuperior extent of the lesion. We find that endoscopic resection of pituitary macroadenomas via an extended transsphenoidal approach yields an 80% rate of improvement in preoperative visual field defects, whereas the remaining patients experience stabilization of their visual field defect. In two thirds of hormone-producing adenomas, a normalization of the endocrine panel is observed, and patients may discontinue medical therapy. In our series, we encountered one perioperative mortality. A 59-year-old man died 7 days after the procedure of cardiopulmonary arrest due to dilated cardiomyopathy. Our main complications are postoperative panhypopituitarism and DI, which are encountered in approximately 6%

of patients who had an intact hypothalamic-pituitary axis prior to the resection of their macroadenoma. Notably, all of the patients who suffered from postoperative panhypopituitarism had lesions with diameters greater than 4 cm. CSF leaks were encountered in 1.6% of our patients. Intraoperative hemorrhage due to laceration of the ophthalmic artery, bilateral subdural hematomas due to CSF leakage from the lumbar drain site, and postoperative hydrocephalus requiring placement of a ventriculoperitoneal shunt are other complications that we have experienced with this intervention.

Discussion

With the advance of preoperative imaging, constant modification, and improvement of endoscopic equipment and surgical tools, pituitary macroadenomas, even giant ones with significant suprasellar and cavernous sinus extension, are increasingly amenable to resection via an extended endonasal endoscopic transsphenoidal approach. In our institution, there is almost no role for craniotomy in the management of these tumors, and it is likely that the introduction of endoscopic skull base techniques will gradually decrease the numbers of craniotomies required for these tumors in other centers as well. As we have shown in our series, the use of multilayer closures with a nasoseptal flap has decreased the rate of CSF leak in giant macroadenomas to very low levels. The advantages of the endonasal endoscopic approach are multiple, including the absence of brain retraction, the position of the cranial nerves and arteries outside the central trajectory of the surgery, and the potential ability to stay within the pseudocapsule of the tumor and arachnoid to minimize trauma to neurovascular structures. With extended bone openings and angled endoscopes, visualization is not as limited as with the microscope and the Hardy retractor.

Although gross-total resection is generally the surgical goal, in elderly patients or if the tumor densely adherent to neurovascular structures, a subtotal resection with subsequent radiation therapy may be a more appropriate treatment plan once decompression of mass effect is achieved. For hormone-secreting tumors, however, complete resection is more critical to eliminate hormone overproduction. Although traditional teaching demands a craniotomy for radical resection of lesions invading the cavernous sinus, a gross total resection may be accomplished using a transcavernous approach, or tumor may be left in the cavernous sinus and treated with radiosurgery.[73] In spite of the advances in endoscopic skull base surgery, certain situations still require a craniotomy for adequate resection of the tumor, the indications for which will vary based on the individual needs of the patient and the judgment and training of the treating physician.

References

1. Alleyne CH Jr, Barrow DL, Oyesiku NM. Combined transsphenoidal and pterional craniotomy approach to giant pituitary tumors. Surg Neurol 2002;57:380–390, discussion 390
2. D'Ambrosio AL, Syed ON, Grobelny BT, Freda PU, Wardlaw S, Bruce JN. Simultaneous above and below approach to giant pituitary adenomas: surgical strategies and long-term follow-up. Pituitary 2009;12:217–225
3. Dandy W. A new hypophysis operation. Bull Johns Hopkins Hosp 1918;29:154–155
4. Loyo M, Kleriga E, Mateos H, de Leo R, Delgado A. Combined supra-infrasellar approach for large pituitary tumors. Neurosurgery 1984;14:485–488
5. Maartens NF, Kaye AH. Role of transcranial approaches in the treatment of sellar and suprasellar lesions. Front Horm Res 2006;34:1–28
6. Saito K, Kuwayama A, Yamamoto N, Sugita K. The transsphenoidal removal of nonfunctioning pituitary adenomas with suprasellar extensions: the open sella method and intentionally staged operation. Neurosurgery 1995;36:668–675, discussion 675–676
7. Takakura K, Teramoto A. Management of huge pituitary adenomas. Acta Neurochir Suppl (Wien) 1996;65:13–15
8. Hashimoto N, Handa H, Yamashita J, Yamagami T. Long-term follow-up of large or invasive pituitary adenomas. Surg Neurol 1986;25:49–54
9. Mohr G, Hardy J, Comtois R, Beauregard H. Surgical management of giant pituitary adenomas. Can J Neurol Sci 1990;17:62–66
10. Pia HW, Grote E, Hildebrandt G. Giant pituitary adenomas. Neurosurg Rev 1985;8:207–220
11. Goel A, Deogaonkar M, Desai K. Fatal postoperative "pituitary apoplexy": its cause and management. Br J Neurosurg 1995;9:37–40
12. Buchfelder M, Kreutzer J. Transcranial surgery for pituitary adenomas. Pituitary 2008;11:375–384
13. Grosvenor AE, Laws ER. The evolution of extracranial approaches to the pituitary and anterior skull base. Pituitary 2008;11:337–345
14. Couldwell WT. Transsphenoidal and transcranial surgery for pituitary adenomas. J Neurooncol 2004;69:237–256
15. Symon L, Jakubowski J, Kendall B. Surgical treatment of giant pituitary adenomas. J Neurol Neurosurg Psychiatry 1979;42:973–982
16. de Divitiis E, Cavallo LM, Cappabianca P, Esposito F. Extended endoscopic endonasal transsphenoidal approach for the removal of suprasellar tumors: Part 2. Neurosurgery 2007;60:46–58, discussion 58–59
17. Kassam A, Snyderman CH, Mintz A, Gardner P, Carrau RL. Expanded endonasal approach: the rostrocaudal axis. Part I. Crista galli to the sella turcica. Neurosurg Focus 2005;19:E3
18. Kassam A, Snyderman CH, Mintz A, Gardner P, Carrau RL. Expanded endonasal approach: the rostrocaudal axis. Part II. Posterior clinoids to the foramen magnum. Neurosurg Focus 2005;19:E4
19. Schwartz TH, Anand VK. The endoscopic endonasal transsphenoidal approach to the suprasellar cistern. Clin Neurosurg 2007;54:226–235
20. Schwartz TH, Stieg PE, Anand VK. Endoscopic transsphenoidal pituitary surgery with intraoperative magnetic resonance imaging. Neurosurgery 2006;58(1, Suppl):ONS44–ONS51, discussion ONS44–ONS51
21. Hardy J, Vezina JL. Transsphenoidal neurosurgery of intracranial neoplasm. Adv Neurol 1976;15:261–273

22. Symon L, Jakubowski J. Transcranial management of pituitary tumours with suprasellar extension. J Neurol Neurosurg Psychiatry 1979;42:123–133
23. Garibi J, Pomposo I, Villar G, Gaztambide S. Giant pituitary adenomas: clinical characteristics and surgical results. Br J Neurosurg 2002;16:133–139
24. Mortini P, Barzaghi R, Losa M, Boari N, Giovanelli M. Surgical treatment of giant pituitary adenomas: strategies and results in a series of 95 consecutive patients. Neurosurgery 2007;60:993–1002, discussion 1003–1004
25. Yasargil MG. Microneurosurgery, Volume 4b: Microneurosurgery of CNS Tumors. New York: Thieme Medical Publishers; 1996
26. Horsley V. On the technique of operations on the central nervous system. BMJ 1906;2:411–423
27. Krause F. Bemerkungen zur Operation der Hypophysen Geschwulste. Dtsch Med Wochenschr 1927;53:691–694
28. Krause F. Hirnchirurgie (freilegung do hypophyse). Deutsche Klin 1905;8:953–1024
29. McArthur L. An aseptic surgical access to the pituitary body and its neighborhood. JAMA 1912;58:2009–2011
30. Frazier C. Choice of method in operations upon the pituitary body. Surg Gynecol Obstet 1919;29:9–16
31. Frazier C. Lesions of the hypophysis from the viewpoint of the surgeon. Surg Gynecol Obstet 1913;17:724–736
32. Cushing H. The Pituitary Body and Its Disorders. Philadelphia: JB Lippincott; 1912
33. Heuer G. The surgical approach and the therapy of tumors and other lesions about the optic chiasm. Surg Gynecol Obstet 1931;53:489–518
34. Bakay L. The results of 300 pituitary adenoma operations (Prof. Herbert Olivecrona's series). J Neurosurg 1950;7:240–255
35. Luft R, Olivecrona H. Experiences with hypophysectomy in man. J Neurosurg 1953;10:301–316
36. Pearson OH, Ray BS. Hypophysectomy in the treatment of advanced cancer of breast. Ann Surg 1956;144:394–406
37. Yasargil MG, Kasdaglis K, Jain KK, Weber HP. Anatomical observations of the subarachnoid cisterns of the brain during surgery. J Neurosurg 1976;44:298–302
38. Patterson RH. The role of transcranial surgery in the management of pituitary adenoma. Acta Neurochir Suppl (Wien) 1996;65:16–17
39. Aziz KM, Froelich SC, Cohen PL, Sanan A, Keller JT, van Loveren HR. The one-piece orbitozygomatic approach: the MacCarty burr hole and the inferior orbital fissure as keys to technique and application. Acta Neurochir (Wien) 2002;144:15–24
40. Dehdashti AR, de Tribolet N. Frontobasal interhemispheric trans-lamina terminalis approach for suprasellar lesions. Neurosurgery 2008;62(6, Suppl 3):1233–1239
41. Dolenc VV. Transcranial epidural approach to pituitary tumors extending beyond the sella. Neurosurgery 1997;41:542–550, discussion 551–552
42. Fahlbusch R, Honegger J, Paulus W, Huk W, Buchfelder M. Surgical treatment of craniopharyngiomas: experience with 168 patients. J Neurosurg 1999;90:237–250
43. Hakuba A, Liu S, Nishimura S. The orbitozygomatic infratemporal approach: a new surgical technique. Surg Neurol 1986;26:271–276
44. Patterson RH Jr, Danylevich A. Surgical removal of craniopharyngiomas by the transcranial approach through the lamina terminalis and sphenoid sinus. Neurosurgery 1980;7:111–117
45. Youssef AS, Agazzi S, van Loveren HR. Transcranial surgery for pituitary adenomas. Neurosurgery 2005;57(1, Suppl)168–175, discussion 168–175
46. Snow RB, Lavyne MH, Lee BC, Morgello S, Patterson RH Jr. Craniotomy versus transsphenoidal excision of large pituitary tumors: the usefulness of magnetic resonance imaging in guiding the operative approach. Neurosurgery 1986;19:59–64
47. Wilson CB. Surgical management of pituitary tumors. J Clin Endocrinol Metab 1997;82:2381–2385
48. Elkington SG, McKissock W. Pituitary adenoma: results of combined surgical and radiotherapeutic treatment of 260 patients. BMJ 1967;1:263–266
49. Heimbach SB. Follow-up studies on 105 cases of verified chromophobe and acidophile pituitary adenomata after treatment by transfrontal operation and x-ray irradiation. Acta Neurochir (Wien) 1959;7:101–155
50. Jefferson G. Extrasellar extensions of pituitary adenomas: (section of neurology). Proc R Soc Med 1940;33:433–458
51. Wirth FP, Schwartz HG, Schwetschenau PR. Pituitary adenomas: factors in treatment. Clin Neurosurg 1974;21:8–25
52. Grote E. Characteristics of giant pituitary adenomas. Acta Neurochir (Wien) 1982;60:141–153
53. Guidetti B, Fraioli B, Cantore GP. Results of surgical management of 319 pituitary adenomas. Acta Neurochir (Wien) 1987;85:117–124
54. Schloffer H. Erfolgreiche Operation eines Hypophysen-tumors of nasalem Wege. Wiener Klinische Wochenzeitschrift 1907;20:621–624
55. Henderson WR. The pituitary adenomata. A follow-up study of the surgical results in 338 cases (Dr. Harvey Cushing's series). Br J Surg 1939;26:811–921
56. Hardy J. Transsphenoidal hypophysectomy. J Neurosurg 1971;34:582–594
57. Faria MA Jr, Tindall GT. Transsphenoidal microsurgery for prolactin-secreting pituitary adenomas. J Neurosurg 1982;56:33–43
58. Laws ER, Ebersold MJ, Piegras DG. The results of transsphenoidal surgery in specific clinical entities. In: Laws ER, ed. Management of Pituitary Adenomas and Related Lesions with Emphasis on Transsphenoidal Microsurgery: New York: Appleton-Century-Crofts; 1982:277–306
59. Ciric I, Mikhael M, Stafford T, Lawson L, Garces R. Transsphenoidal microsurgery of pituitary macroadenomas with long-term follow-up results. J Neurosurg 1983;59:395–401
60. Black PM, Zervas NT, Candia GL. Incidence and management of complications of transsphenoidal operation for pituitary adenomas. Neurosurgery 1987;20:920–924
61. Bohinski RJ, Warnick RE, Gaskill-Shipley MF, et al. Intraoperative magnetic resonance imaging to determine the extent of resection of pituitary macroadenomas during transsphenoidal microsurgery. Neurosurgery 2001;49:1133–1143, discussion 1143–1144
62. Han ZL, He DS, Mao ZG, Wang HJ. Cerebrospinal fluid rhinorrhea following trans-sphenoidal pituitary macroadenoma surgery: experience from 592 patients. Clin Neurol Neurosurg 2008;110:570–579
63. Catapano D, Sloffer CA, Frank G, Pasquini E, D'Angelo VA, Lanzino G. Comparison between the microscope and endoscope in the direct endonasal extended transsphenoidal approach: anatomical study. J Neurosurg 2006;104:419–425
64. Couldwell WT, Weiss MH, Rabb C, Liu JK, Apfelbaum RI, Fukushima T. Variations on the standard transsphenoidal approach to the sellar region, with emphasis on the extended approaches and parasellar

approaches: surgical experience in 105 cases. Neurosurgery 2004; 55:539–547, discussion 547–550

65. de Divitiis E, Cappabianca P. Microscopic and endoscopic transsphenoidal surgery. Neurosurgery 2002;51:1527–1529, author reply 1529–1530
66. Dusick JR, Esposito F, Kelly DF, et al. The extended direct endonasal transsphenoidal approach for nonadenomatous suprasellar tumors. J Neurosurg 2005;102:832–841
67. Frank G, Pasquini E, Mazzatenta D. Extended transsphenoidal approach. J Neurosurg 2001;95:917–918
68. Frank G, Sciarretta V, Calbucci F, Farneti G, Mazzatenta D, Pasquini E. The endoscopic transnasal transsphenoidal approach for the treatment of cranial base chordomas and chondrosarcomas. Neurosurgery 2006;59(1, Suppl 1):ONS50–ONS57, discussion ONS50–ONS57
69. Laufer I, Anand VK, Schwartz TH. Endoscopic, endonasal extended transsphenoidal, transplanum transtuberculum approach for resection of suprasellar lesions. J Neurosurg 2007;106:400–406
70. Jho HD, Carrau RL. Endoscopic endonasal transsphenoidal surgery: experience with 50 patients. J Neurosurg 1997;87:44–51
71. Jho HD, Carrau RL, Ko Y, Daly MA. Endoscopic pituitary surgery: an early experience. Surg Neurol 1997;47:213–222, discussion 222–223
72. Schwartz TH, Fraser JF, Brown S, Tabaee A, Kacker A, Anand VK. Endoscopic cranial base surgery: classification of operative approaches. Neurosurgery 2008;62:991–1002, discussion 1002–1005
73. Fraser JF, Mass AY, Brown S, Anand VK, Schwartz TH. Transnasal endoscopic resection of a cavernous sinus hemangioma: technical note and review of the literature. Skull Base 2008;18:309–315
74. Fraser JF, Nyquist GG, Moore N, Anand VK, Schwartz TH. Endoscopic endonasal transclival resection of chordomas: operative technique, clinical outcome, and review of the literature. J Neurosurg 2010; 112:1061–1069
75. Leng LZ, Brown S, Anand VK, Schwartz TH. "Gasket-seal" watertight closure in minimal-access endoscopic cranial base surgery. Neurosurgery 2008;62(5, Suppl 2):E342–E343, discussion E343
76. Hadad G, Bassagasteguy L, Carrau RL, et al. A novel reconstructive technique after endoscopic expanded endonasal approaches: vascular pedicle nasoseptal flap. Laryngoscope 2006;116:1882–1886
77. Kitano M, Taneda M, Shimono T, Nakao Y. Extended transsphenoidal approach for surgical management of pituitary adenomas invading the cavernous sinus. J Neurosurg 2008;108:26–36
78. Dehdashti AR, Ganna A, Witterick I, Gentili F. Expanded endoscopic endonasal approach for anterior cranial base and suprasellar lesions: indications and limitations. Neurosurgery 2009;64:677–687, discussion 687–689

25 Stereotactic Radiosurgery and Fractionated Radiation for Pituitary Tumors

Bruce E. Pollock and Paul D. Brown

The use of radiation for scientific and medical purposes dates back over 100 years with the discovery of the x-ray by Conrad Roentgen in 1895[1] and the isolation of radium by Madame and Pierre Curie in 1898.[2] Early external-beam techniques were developed for clinical use, but these devices produced very low-energy x-rays resulting in poor tissue penetration and severe skin damage. In the 1920s, Coutard and Regaud showed that by dividing the total dose into many smaller treatments, delivered over several weeks, tumors could be cured without severe normal tissue damage.[3] This method was quickly adopted by others and ushered in as the concept of dose fractionation. The start of the modern era of external-beam radiation therapy began with the appearance of the cobalt-60 machines in the mid-1950s. Cobalt machines were less complex and delivered high-energy rays in the megavoltage (MV) range. Throughout the 1960s and 1970s, cobalt machines gave way to linear accelerators. In addition to photons, linear accelerators are able to produce electrons, which have a finite range in tissue that allows tailoring the depth of penetration to the exact clinical situation. Other advantages of linear accelerators include increased precision and variable dose rates. The technology of radiation delivery continues to undergo rapid development and change.

Physical Properties of Radiation

Ionizing radiation is composed of particulate radiation and electromagnetic radiation. Although some radiation treatments use electrons, protons, or neutrons (particulate radiation), the vast majority of radiation treatments are delivered via photons (electromagnetic radiation). Electromagnetic radiation is part of a continuum of waveform energy known as the electromagnetic spectrum. Near the high-energy (short wavelength) end of this spectrum lie the electromagnetic waves used therapeutically (x-rays, gamma rays) to treat patients. Gamma rays and x-rays are essentially identical, with the only difference being their origin. X-rays are obtained from an extranuclear process when an accelerated electron strikes a target with a high atomic number, causing deceleration of the electron with the production of polyenergetic x-rays through the process of "bremsstrahlung" (braking radiation). In contrast, gamma rays are emitted from the nucleus during nuclear decay.

High-energy electromagnetic radiation interacts with matter, removing electrons from their orbits, resulting in ionization and the release of energy. In this process the photon interacts with an outer shell electron, resulting in the release of the electron and a photon of lower energy deflected from its original course (Compton effect). These interactions are not dependent on the atomic number of the substance with which the x-ray is interacting, but only on the density of the absorbing material. The amount of radiation absorbed is roughly equal, gram for gram, whether the material is soft tissue or bone. This explains why body lead is protective in the energies typically used for diagnostic radiology but is ineffective with the higher energies typically used in radiosurgery and radiation therapy.

Electrons are the most commonly used particulate radiation in general radiotherapy practice. However, due to the lack of penetration of electrons, they are rarely used in the treatment of intracranial diseases. In contrast, other forms of particulate radiation, such as protons and neutrons, are utilized in the treatment of intracranial diseases. Neutrons interact with the nuclei of atoms and produce much heavier particles, such as protons, α-particles (nuclei of helium atoms), and even heavier nuclear fragments. The density of ionizations along the pathway of these particles is much greater than that of x-rays. In contrast to neutrons, the advantage of protons is in their dose distribution.[4] Protons deposit most of their energy at the end of their track range in tissue, called the Bragg peak. The energy delivered to tissue proximal to the peak is minimal. The energy delivered at the peak is high, and essentially none passes beyond the peak. This allows energy to be deposited in large amounts in a region while sparing the adjacent tissues. However, due to the complexity of particle beam treatment planning, the need for a cyclotron to generate the protons, and the expense of these units, there are only a limited number of facilities around the world.

Biologic Properties of Radiation

When photon radiation hits a cell it will most likely interact with water because cells are primarily composed of water. This creates unstable molecules called free radicals that may interact with DNA. Free radicals damage DNA and can result in permanent cell injury or death. This is called the indirect effect of radiation. Less commonly, photon radiation may interact directly with DNA, or other cellular molecules, leading to damage and possibly cell death. This direct effect is the predominant process in heavy particle radiation.

Cell Death from Radiation

Radiation of the cell leads to damage of the DNA, but not all of the damage is equally capable of producing biologic injury. DNA–protein cross-links, direct base damage, and single-strand breaks seem to play a relatively minor role in the lethality of ionizing radiation compared with double-strand breaks.[5] Provided the opposite strand is intact, cells remain capable of repairing single-strand breaks with great efficiency. Therefore, the critical lesions caused by radiation are double-strand breaks. The most common types of cell death after radiotherapy are mitotic cell death and apoptosis. If a cell accumulates sufficient radiation damage, its later progeny may be unable to go through mitosis successfully and will die. Several cell divisions may occur before the lethal effects of radiation are expressed. Consequently, rapidly dividing normal tissues (i.e., oral mucosa) or malignant tumors express radiation damage sooner than slower dividing normal tissues (i.e., brain) or benign tumors such as pituitary adenomas. Some cells do not have to go through mitosis to succumb to radiation but instead die from programmed cell death or apoptosis.[6] An apoptotic event is irreversible, and there is no capability for repair of radiation damage, which characterizes cells dying from mitotically expressed DNA damage.

Therapeutic Ratio

To have a therapeutic effect, radiation must differentially damage a tumor more than the adjacent normal tissues. This is accomplished physically by designing radiation treatments that deliver high doses of radiation to the tumor with less radiation going to nearby structures. The therapeutic ratio can also be improved biologically by utilizing the advantages of differential radiosensitivity of normal tissues and tumors with dose fractionation. In general, normal tissues are better able to repair DNA damage than tumors because of the aberrant cell cycle control mechanisms in tumors. However, at the doses typically used for radiosurgery the repair mechanisms of even normal tissues can be overwhelmed, and radiation damage can occur along with the desired effect on the tumor.[7] Therefore, unless the radiation dose delivery is highly conformal, it is advantageous to deliver multiple small doses of radiation because of the normal cells' inherent superiority in repairing sublethal damage compared with tumor cells.

Fractionated Radiation Therapy

Proper immobilization and consistent reproducibility of the treatment position are essential for patients undergoing radiotherapy. Therefore, a device is needed to accurately reposition the patient on a day-to-day basis. Most radiation therapy centers fabricate a thermoplastic mask for each patient to prevent the head from moving during treatment. To provide consistent references points, fiducial markers are placed on the mask. Each day during treatment setup, these markers are aligned with lasers in the linear accelerator treatment room, allowing precise alignment of patients on a daily basis. Because the treatment may last several weeks, a repeatable head fixation device is an absolute requirement for any facility performing stereotactic radiation therapy (SRT). These devices often include a relocatable head frame stabilized by a mouth-guard–type bite block. These "pinless" stereotactic systems can achieve an accuracy of better than 2 mm.

Once an immobilization device has been constructed, the patient undergoes a treatment simulation and planning session in the treatment position. Historically, this was performed using conventional fluoroscopic units to visualize bony anatomical landmarks. More recently, simulators using computed tomography (CT) to image the region of interest are obtained to plan the radiation treatments. The planning CT scanners are similar to diagnostic scanners, except that planning scans are conducted under the same conditions (on a flat table with custom immobilization devices) used for treatment of the patient on the linear accelerator. The CT simulators incorporate workstations allowing efficient target contouring, image manipulation, and simulation of beam arrangements. Image fusion between CT and other imaging modalities, such as magnetic resonance imaging (MRI), can also be performed on these workstations.

Once the planning CT images are in the treatment planning computer, the radiation oncologist defines the gross tumor volume, volumes at risk for tumor spread (clinical target volume [CTV]) without obvious gross disease on imaging, and critical normal structures. A planning target volume (PTV) is then generated by enlarging the CTV with a margin of approximately 2 to 4 mm to account for patient setup error and inaccuracies in imaging. A treatment plan is then a constructed plan to deliver a homogeneous radiation dose to cover the PTV while minimizing the dose to critical structures outside the PTV. By achieving a homogeneous dose distribution, areas of excessive dose are avoided, thereby decreasing the risk of radiation damage. The radiation oncologist reviews the computerized dose distributions (isodose lines) displayed and determines whether the plan is acceptable or in need of modification.

With the advent of sophisticated computerized planning systems and advances in neuroimaging, it is now possible to deliver high does of radiation to the sellar region while sparing the surrounding normal structures from these high doses of radiation. Methods to accomplish this dosimetric goal include the use of multiple, nonoverlapping, conformal radiation beams shaped by custom-made blocks to the configuration of the tumor volume, also called three-dimensional (3D) conformal radiotherapy. Computer-controlled tungsten leaves, or multileaf collimators, are individual leaves that shift to form specific patterns, conforming the radiation beam to the target. In addition to blocks, wedges are often added to alter the radiation beam dose distribution to allow more uniform dose distribution within the treatment volume.

Another recent innovation, intensity modulated radiation therapy (IMRT), provides a completely different approach to treatment planning. Instead of clinicians defining beam directions, beam weights, wedges, blocks, and margins, and then computing and displaying dose distributions to assess whether the treatment plan will lead to an acceptable outcome, they do the opposite or "inverse" treatment planning. The radiation oncologist specifies the prescribed target dose and the dose constraints for normal structures. Sophisticated algorithms of the inverse treatment planning system enable the evaluation of millions of possible beam arrangements and determine the clinically optimized treatment plan, maximizing the dose to the tumor while minimizing exposure to surrounding healthy tissue. Hundreds to thousands of small, modulated radiation beams strike a tumor site with varying intensities, and from many angles, to attack the target in a complete 3D manner. A comparison of linear accelerator–based radiosurgery, fixed noncoplanar 3D custom blocked fields, and IMRT did find improved dose conformity and decreased dose to nontarget brain in high and low isodose regions for the IMRT plans for the irregular tumor targets.[8]

Typically, the patient receives five treatments a week, one a day, Monday through Friday. Along with these daily treatments, most centers utilizing stereotactic radiotherapy also utilize image-guided radiation therapy (IGRT), which involves two-dimensional (2D) or 3D imaging that is obtained before treatment to direct the radiation therapy to the correct location with high precision. An example of 3D IGRT is cone-beam computed tomography, which acquires many 2D projections over the entire volume of interest in each projection. These projections are then reconstructed into a 3D volume analogous to the CT planning data set and then used to align the patient into the correct position.

An example of 2D IGRT is obtaining an orthogonal pair of kilovoltage radiographs before treatment, then using an automated matching system, the patient is moved robotically to correct patient setup errors and to track any patient movement throughout the treatment.

Most conventional fractionation schedules are delivered with 1.8 to 2 Gy fractions daily. Smaller doses per fraction allow more healing of sublethal damage between treatments. Hypofractionation, using fewer fractions but larger doses per fraction (3 to 7 Gy) to achieve a lower total dose (20 to 30 Gy), has also been employed by some centers. Despite the theoretical radiobiologic equivalence of such hypofractionated schedules with either conventional dose fractionation or high-dose, single-fraction techniques, there are no long-term studies on tumor control or toxicities.

Stereotactic Radiosurgery

Stereotactic radiosurgery is a surgical procedure that combines the principles of stereotactic localization with the precise delivery of radiation to an imaging-defined target. Lars Leksell,[9] neurosurgeon at the Karolinska Institute in Stockholm, Sweden, conceived the concept of stereotactic radiosurgery in 1951. His goal was to develop a method for the noninvasive destruction of intracranial lesions that were at high risk for surgical resection. To accomplish this goal, Leksell[10] coupled stereotactic localization with the delivery of a large, single-fraction dose of ionizing radiation. In 1968 Leksell and Börje Larsson developed the first cobalt-60 gamma unit (the Gamma Knife, Elekta Instruments, Norcross, GA). Over the past two decades radiosurgery has gained acceptance and has become an integral part of both neurosurgery and radiation oncology. Advances in neuroimaging and improved computer software have made radiosurgery safer and more effective in the management of a wide range of disorders affecting the nervous system. Today, radiosurgery is available to patients at the majority of large medical centers.

The goal of radiosurgery is to deliver a high radiation dose to an imaging-defined target. In contrast to conventional fractionated radiation therapy, radiosurgery does not rely on the increased radiation sensitivity of the target compared with the normal brain. Instead, radiosurgery spares normal structures using conformal dose plans that deposit large radiation doses into the target with a rapid fall-off of radiation at the edges of the dose plan (**Fig. 25.1**). Different radiosurgical systems satisfy these essential criteria by using various technical solutions.

Leksell Gamma Knife

Several versions of the Leksell gamma knife have been developed over time with the goals of increased precision and accuracy of radiation delivery. Recently the Perfexion (Elekta Instruments, Norcross, GA) was introduced as the latest version of this device. It contains 192 individual cobalt-60 sources that naturally decay to nickel (^{60}Ni). During this process gamma photons are released with energies of 1.17 and 1.33 MeV. The emitted photons are precisely directed

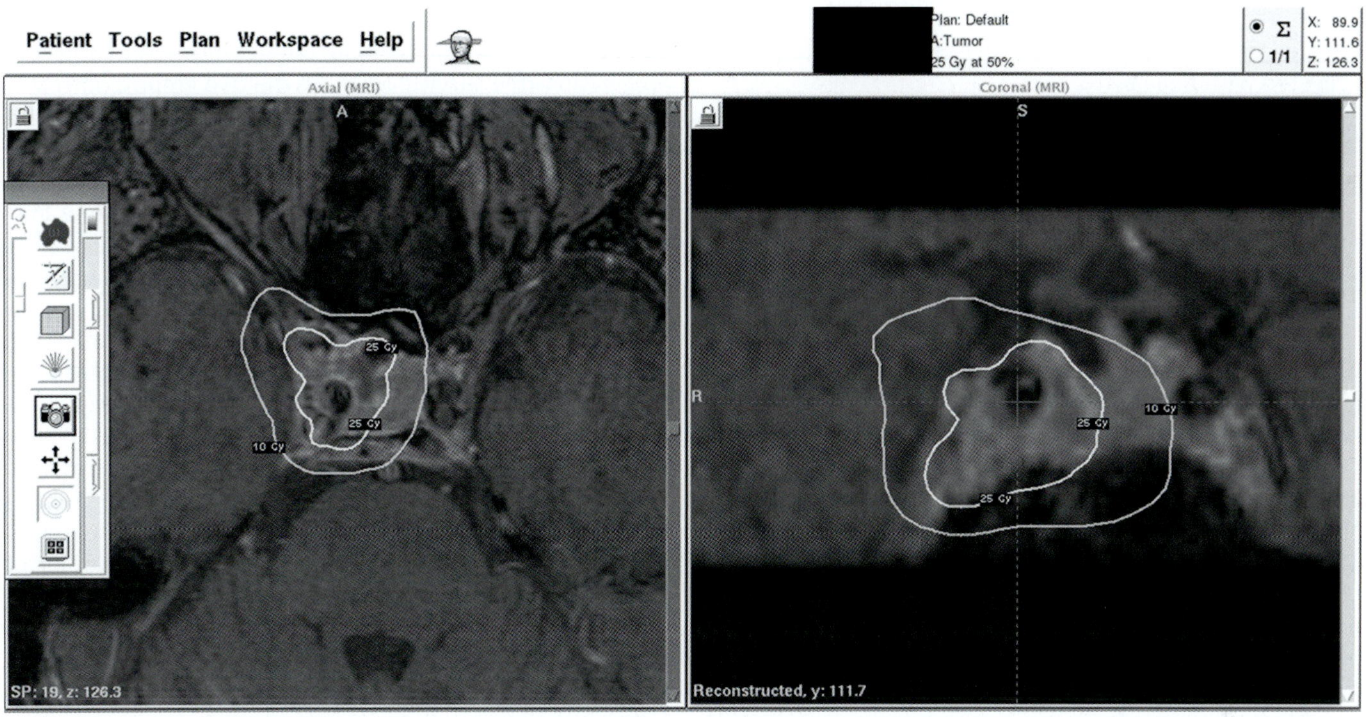

Fig. 25.1 Dose plan of a 50-year-old man with recurrent Cushing's disease after prior transsphenoidal resection. A total of 17 isocenters of radiation were used to cover a volume of 3.8 cm^3. The tumor margin dose was 25 Gy and the maximum radiation dose was 50 Gy. The maximum dose received by the right optic nerve was 10.1 Gy.

through circular channels drilled into a high-density metal helmet. Secondary collimation is accomplished through eight sectors containing 4-, 8-, and 16-mm openings, as well as a closed position. Isocenter shaping is achieved by arranging the size of the different sector openings; one or more of the sectors may be blocked to eliminate radiation from that direction. Isocenter coordinates, beam openings, and relative weighting of each isocenter are entered into the treatment-planning computer. Because the gamma knife employs fixed sources with a constant relation to the collimator helmet and stereotactic frame, isocenter verification films or port films are unnecessary. Patient positioning is robotically controlled, repositioning the patient at each isocenter by digitally transferred information from the operator's console.

Linear Accelerator (LINAC)-Based Radiosurgery

The development of LINAC-based radiosurgical systems began in the 1980s.[11–13] These systems generally consist of a stereotactic head frame, floor stand, and a 6-MV linear accelerator. Multiple (often four or more) sagittally oriented irradiation arcs are delivered using a wide range of circular collimators. Detection of mechanical inaccuracy is performed by a phantom-target film technique for every treatment arc. Friedman and Bova[12] further refined LINAC-based radiosurgery by adding a high-precision attachment to control movements of the patient's head and the tertiary collimators (5 to 35 mm diameter) independent of potential variations in gantry or treatment couch alignment. The majority of targets are treated at the 70 to 80% isodose line.

CyberKnife

John Adler and colleagues[14] at Stanford University have developed a new radiosurgical device called the CyberKnife (Accuray, Sunnyvale, CA) that incorporates recent advances in robotics and computerized image recognition. The CyberKnife has a compact, lightweight linear accelerator mounted on a robotic arm. For intracranial targets, patients are fitted with a noninvasive flexible mesh mask to limit large movements. Because skeletal landmarks are used to define stereotactic space, fixation using a stereotactic head frame is not required. Radiographs of the treatment site are taken and image registration performed to determine the target's coordinates with respect to the linear accelerator. The target coordinates are transferred to the robot, which directs the beam to the treatment site. The system has dynamic tracking software that can follow lesions in six dimensions (three translational and three rotational axes) to account and compensate for any patient movement. If any movement of the target during treatment is detected, the LINAC is repositioned to the new target location. The majority of targets are treated at the 70 to 80% isodose line. Hypofractionated treatments over three to five sessions are frequently delivered with this device.

Radiation Management of Patients with Pituitary Adenomas

Patient Selection

A complete patient evaluation is essential before initiating radiation therapy or stereotactic radiosurgery for patients with pituitary adenomas. This assessment must include a review of prior surgical procedures, the pathology, the history of previous radiation exposure, the status of anterior and posterior pituitary function, visual acuity and fields, and other patient comorbidities. Critical in the decision-making process are the size and location of the tumor, especially in relationship to the optic nerves and chiasm, as determined by high-quality MRI. In our practice, patients with a clearly defined tumor that does not directly involve the optic apparatus typically undergo radiosurgery, whereas patients with poorly defined tumors, or those with compression of the optic structures, are generally considered better suited to stereotactic radiotherapy. Moreover, patients with new or progressive visual field deficits in the setting of an enlarging tumor are referred for surgical resection to reduce mass effect and improve neurologic function.

Radiation Therapy of Nonfunctioning Pituitary Adenomas

Nonfunctioning pituitary adenomas (NFAs) constitute approximately 30% of diagnosed pituitary tumors. Most patients with NFA have macroadenomas, and surgical resection is indicated to decompress the optic apparatus as well as the remaining functioning pituitary gland. Improved surgical techniques utilizing endoscopy and intraoperative MRI permit more complete tumor removal in the sellar and suprasellar regions. Nonetheless, complete resection is not possible for patients with tumors extending into the cavernous sinuses with acceptable morbidity.

The management of patients with NFA who have residual tumor after initial surgery remains controversial. Observation after subtotal resection is frequently recommended by neurosurgeons to minimize the number of patients being exposed to the risks, primarily hypopituitarism, associated with radiotherapy. Neurosurgeons believe that tumor progression or recurrence can be detected early on postoperative MRI before it becomes symptomatic. Park et al[15] reviewed 176 NFA patients having surgery between 1979 and 1999. The actuarial tumor progression rate at 10 years was 2.3% for patients receiving early radiation compared with 50.5% for patients not receiving planned postoperative radiotherapy. Despite the significant differences in progression-free survival (PFS) for the two groups, outcomes at last follow-up were similar. The authors concluded that using radiation only for patients with proven tumor recurrence is safe for patients with complete or near-complete resection of NFA, if they agree to ongoing follow-up for a long period after surgery. Conversely, most radiation oncologists recommend upfront radiation therapy for patients with residual NFA after resection. Van den Bergh and colleagues[16] analyzed 122 NFA patients operated between 1979 and 1998. Group 1 patients ($n = 76$) underwent immediate postoperative radiotherapy, whereas group 2 ($n = 28$) patients were followed with serial imaging following surgery. The 10-year PFS was 95% for group 1 compared with 22% for group 2. There was no difference in the percentage of patients requiring hormone substitution at last follow-up, and life expectancy for the two groups did not differ from each other or from that for the general population. The authors concluded that immediate postoperative radiation therapy provides a marked improvement in tumor control without additional negative effect on pituitary function. In the absence of class 1 data, either approach can be supported based on the available information. Nonetheless, it is reasonable to state that patients who have a clearly definable tumor mass following surgery and who have a life expectancy greater than 10 years will likely require additional tumor-directed therapy.

One of the primary concerns of radiotherapy for patients with pituitary adenomas relates to the long-term cognitive effects secondary to radiation exposure.[17,18] In an effort to reduce the radiation exposure of these adjacent structures, many centers have incorporated more complex dose planning to improve dose conformality. Paek et al[19] analyzed the clinical records of 68 patients with NFA undergoing fractionated SRT. At a median follow-up of 30 months, 67 patients (99%) had stable ($n = 41$) or decreased ($n = 26$) tumor volumes. Two patients (3%) developed radiation-related optic neuropathy and four patients (6%) had new pituitary deficits. Minniti et al[20] reviewed 92 patients with secreting adenoma ($n = 25$) or NFA ($n = 67$) having fractionated SRT between 1995 and 2003. At a median follow-up of 32 months, one patient (1%) suffered a unilateral quadrantopia without tumor progression, and 22% of patients developed hypopituitarism. Intensity modulated radiotherapy is also being increasingly used to treat patients with pituitary adenomas. Mackley et al[21] analyzed 34 patients with pituitary adenomas having IMRT from 1998 to 2003. With a median follow-up of 43 months, new hormonal supplementation was required in 40% of patients. So although these series show that both fractionated SRT and IMRT are safe in the treatment of patients with pituitary adenomas, the theoretical advantage of these more complex fractionated radiation techniques on preserving cognitive function has yet to be demonstrated.

Another drawback of radiation therapy for patients with NFA is the risk of developing a radiation-induced neoplasm. Breen et al[22] evaluated 120 patients with NFA who underwent external-beam radiotherapy (median dose, 46.7 Gy) between 1960 and 1991. Two radiation-induced tumors were noted (meningioma and glioblastoma multiforme); the 10- and 30-year actuarial risk was 2.7%. Minniti et al[23] assessed the risk of secondary brain tumor formation on 426 pituitary adenoma patients who received radiotherapy from 1962 to 1994. Overall, 11 patients developed radiation-induced brain tumors in 5749 patient-years of follow-up. The tumors included meningiomas (n = 5), high-grade astrocytomas (n = 4), meningeal sarcoma (n = 1), and primitive neuroectodermal tumor (n = 1). The cumulative risk was 2.0% at 10 years and 2.4% at 20 years.

Radiosurgery of Nonfunctioning Pituitary Adenomas

As an alternative to radiation therapy, radiosurgery is increasingly used to manage patients with residual or recurrent NFA after surgical resection.[24–27] Radiosurgery is more convenient (1 day versus 6 weeks); has less radiation exposure to adjacent structures, thereby potentially reducing the chance of cognitive decline; and has a lower risk of radiation-induced tumors.[28]

We recently performed a retrospective review of 62 patients with NFA having radiosurgery between 1992 and 2004.[27] Fifty-nine patients (95%) underwent prior tumor resection. The median treatment dose to the tumor margin was 16 Gy. At a median follow-up interval of 64 months, tumor size decreased for 37 patients (60%) and remained unchanged for 23 patients (37%) (**Fig. 25.2**). Two patients (3%) had tumor growth outside the prescribed treatment volume and required additional treatment. Tumor growth control was 95% at 3 and 7 years after radiosurgery. The risk of developing new anterior pituitary deficits at 5 years was 32%. No patient had a decline in visual function.

Other centers have also reported high tumor control rates (87 to 98%) after radiosurgery for patients with NFA.[24–26] Interestingly, Losa et al[25] noted out-of-field tumor growth on the contralateral side of the sella turcica in two of the 52 patients (4%) they reported after NFA radiosurgery. The primary complication in these other series was also the development of new anterior pituitary deficits, ranging from 7 to 25%. The wide range noted in new anterior pituitary deficits likely relates to length of follow-up and completeness of the patients' endocrine evaluation. Feigl et al[28] reported 92 patients (61 with NFA) having radiosurgery for pituitary adenomas. The mean follow-up was of 4.6 years. Overall, 41% of patients developed pituitary deficits of one or more hormonal axes.

A clear benefit of radiosurgery compared with radiation therapy is a significant reduction in the risk of radiation-induced tumors. Whereas the risk of second tumor formation is between 2 and 3% following fractionated radiation therapy,[22,23] the risk of radiation-induced tumors after radiosurgery has been estimated to be 0.01%. Rowe and colleagues[29]

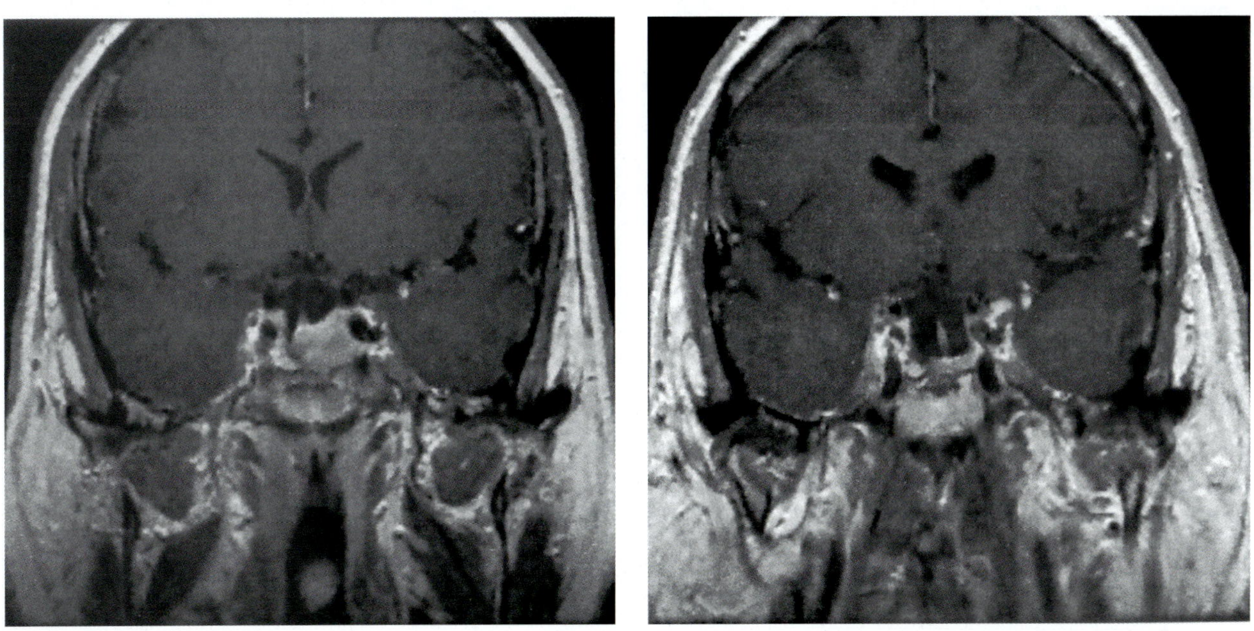

A B

Fig. 25.2 Coronal postgadolinium magnetic resonance imaging (MRI) scans of a 59-year-old man with an enlarging nonfunctioning pituitary adenoma after transsphenoidal resection 3 years earlier. **(A)** MRI before radiosurgery. **(B)** MRI performed 52 months after radiosurgery shows a significant reduction in tumor size.

from the National Centre for Stereotactic Radiosurgery in Sheffield, England, reviewed one of the world's largest radiosurgical experiences and compared the incidence of new central nervous system malignancies in their patient population with the national incidence in the United Kingdom over the same time frame. Based on almost 5000 patients and over 30,000 patient-years of follow-up, they did not find an increased incidence in their radiosurgical patients compared with the age- and sex-adjusted national cohort. The primary weakness of this study is the relative short mean follow-up interval (6.1 years) after radiosurgery, relative to the life expectancy of patients having radiosurgery for benign conditions.

Radiation Therapy of Hormone-Secreting Pituitary Adenomas

The goals of treatment for patients with hormone-secreting pituitary adenomas are tumor control, endocrine normalization, preservation of anterior pituitary function, and minimizing the risk of damage to the optic apparatus and cavernous sinuses. Medical therapy and surgical resection are the primary methods to normalize hormonal overproduction syndromes. However, not all patients respond to or tolerate medical treatment, and not all tumors are amenable to complete resection. For these patients, radiation is generally considered as a salvage technique to stop tumor growth and produce biochemical remission.

Conventional dose-fractionation schedules and maximum radiation doses from 45 to 50 Gy are most commonly used to manage patients with hormone-secreting pituitary adenomas. Radiotherapy has been shown to normalize insulin-like growth factor-1 (IGF-1) levels in approximately 40 to 55% of patients with acromegaly.[30,31] Epaminonda et al[30] reviewed 67 patients having radiotherapy for persistent acromegaly after resection. Thirty-seven patients (55%) had normal or low IGF-1 levels documented at a mean of 12 years after radiation therapy. Powell et al[31] noted normal IGF-1 levels in 17 of 47 patients followed for an average of 5.2 years after radiotherapy. Notably, 27% of patients followed for less than 6 years were considered in remission compared with 69% of patients who were followed for intervals longer than 6 years. Minniti and colleagues[32] recently reviewed the outcomes of 40 patients with Cushing's disease who underwent radiation therapy with doses of 45 to 50 Gy. Normalization of cortisol production was seen in 28% of patients at 1 year, 73% at 3 years, and 84% at 10 years. The mean time to remission was 24 months. Hypopituitarism was detected in 62% of patients 5 years after radiotherapy and 76% at 10 years after radiotherapy. The endocrine results available for radiation therapy of patients with prolactin-secreting tumors are limited. This is no doubt directly related to the success of dopamine agonist therapy in treating these patients. Consequently, patients undergoing either surgical resection or radiotherapy commonly have large tumors that often extend into either one or both cavernous sinuses. For such patients, tumor control, rather than biochemical remission, is the most important consideration. Sasaki et al[33] had a 10-year tumor control rate of 83% for patients with prolactin-secreting tumors. Symptoms related to mass effect improved in almost 80% of these patients.

Radiosurgery of Hormone-Secreting Pituitary Adenomas

Stereotactic radiosurgery has emerged as a safe and effective treatment for patients with hormone-secreting pituitary adenomas (**Fig. 25.3**). However, a wide range of biochemical remission rates have been reported (17–54%),[34–44] making direct comparison of these studies difficult. It is critical that studies apply standardized criteria for biochemical remission and have adequate follow-up. Moreover, it remains controversial whether pituitary suppressive medications taken at the time of radiosurgery negatively impact the chance of

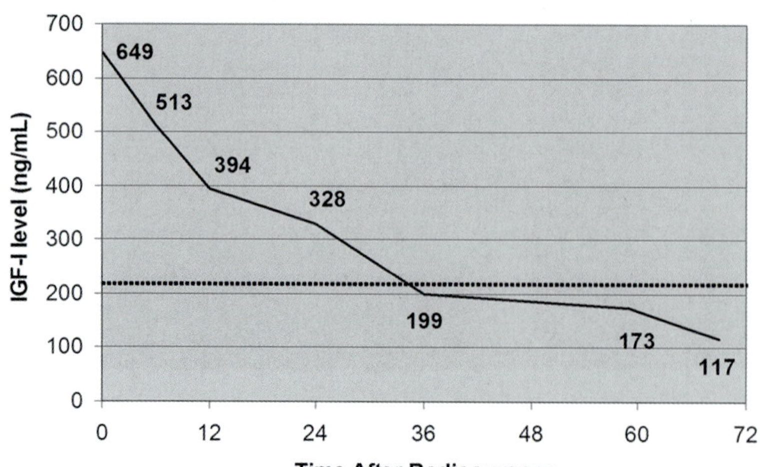

Fig. 25.3 Graph showing serum insulin-like growth factor-1 (IGF-1) after radiosurgery of a patient with persistent acromegaly after transsphenoidal resection. Dotted line shows the age- and sex-adjusted upper limit of normal (212 ng/mL).

biochemical remission. Landolt and colleagues[38,39] originally noted that patients using either somatostatin or dopamine agonists at the time of radiosurgery for their growth hormone (GH)- and prolactin (PRL)-secreting tumors achieved biochemical remission less frequently. Our center and others have confirmed that pituitary suppressive medications adversely affect endocrine outcomes.[41,42,44] Pouratian and colleagues,[44] in a study of 23 patients with PRL-secreting tumors, found remission was significantly associated with not taking a dopamine agonist at the time of radiosurgery. We recently reviewed our experience with 46 acromegalic patients having radiosurgery and found that patients not receiving pituitary suppressive medications were more than four times more likely to reach normal GH and IGF-1 levels off medications than if they were receiving octreotide or a dopamine agonist at the time of radiosurgery.[41] Conversely, two studies failed to find any association between biochemical remission rates for acromegalic patients who received somatostatin agonists at the time of radiosurgery and those who did not.[34,36] Possible explanations for this discrepancy may relate to the duration of follow-up after radiosurgery and the completeness of tumor coverage during radiosurgery. Despite the conflicting results, most authors recommend that patients be off pituitary suppressive medications for several months to maximize the chance of biochemical remission after radiosurgery.

A clear benefit of radiosurgery compared with radiation therapy for patients with hormone-secreting tumors is the time required to achieve biochemical remission.[45,46] Landolt et al[46] compared 16 patients having radiosurgery with 50 patients undergoing radiotherapy for persistent acromegaly. Despite the number of patients cured being similar after radiosurgery or radiotherapy, the mean interval to remission was significantly shorter for the radiosurgery group (1.4 years versus 7.1 years). In a similar study, Kong et al[45] reviewed 54 patients with a variety of hormone-secreting pituitary adenomas having radiation therapy or radiosurgery from 1995 to 2006. No difference was noted in endocrine outcomes: complete remission was documented in 44% of patients having radiosurgery and 36% of patients having radiotherapy. Median times to remission, however, were significantly shorter in the radiosurgery group (26 months) compared with the radiotherapy group (63 months). The ability to normalize hormone levels more rapidly makes radiosurgery the preferred radiation management for patients with either acromegaly or Cushing's disease to minimize the metabolic consequences of these conditions.

Dose Selection in Radiosurgery of Pituitary Adenomas

As mentioned earlier, the goals of pituitary adenoma radiosurgery are tumor control, biochemical remission for patients with hormone-secreting tumors, and avoidance of damage to adjacent optic apparatus and functioning pituitary tissue. Appropriate dose selection is critical to achieve these objectives and must take into account the type of tumor being treated, any history of prior radiation treatment, and the tumor's size and shape. In general, the dose required for tumor control is far less than the dose required for hormonal normalization in patients with secreting tumors. Whereas a tumor margin dose of 12 to 15 Gy appears to provide growth control rates exceeding 90% in patients with NFAs,[24–27] the tumor margin doses prescribed for secreting adenomas typically exceed 20 Gy, and many authors believe doses of 25 to 30 Gy are optimal.[34–37,41,42,44] Recently we reviewed 46 patients with hormone-secreting tumors having radiosurgery from 1991 to 2003.[47] All received a tumor margin dose of 18 Gy or more and were off pituitary suppressive medications for at least 1 month before radiosurgery. The groups were similar with regard to irradiated volume, radiation dose, and follow-up. At a median endocrinologic follow-up of 54 months after radiosurgery, 4-year remission rates were 87% for patients with Cushing's disease, 67% for patients with acromegaly, and 18% for patients with prolactinomas. Patients with oversecretion of adrenocorticotropic hormone or GH were more than four times more likely to achieve remission after radiosurgery compared with patients with prolactinomas. Such a differential sensitivity suggests that higher doses should be prescribed for patients with prolactinomas compared with patients with Cushing's disease and acromegaly, but further study is needed to validate these findings.

However, increasing the radiation dose to the tumor also increases the radiation dose to the optic nerves/chiasm and the adjacent functioning pituitary gland. Despite early concerns that 8 Gy was the radiation tolerance of the anterior optic pathways, more recent studies have shown that doses between 10 and 12 Gy to small volumes are associated with less than a 2% chance of new visual deficits.[48,49] It has also been recognized that the chance of new hormonal deficits after radiosurgery correlate with the radiation dose received by the anterior pituitary gland. Vladyka et al[50] performed detailed dosimetric analysis of pituitary adenoma patients having radiosurgery at the Hospital Na Homolce, Prague, Czech Republic. Using dose-volume determinations, they concluded that the primary factor associated with new anterior pituitary deficits was the mean radiation dose to the pituitary gland. In their study, the safe mean pituitary dose was 15 Gy to maintain gonadotropic and thyrotropic function, and 18 Gy to maintain adrenocorticotropic function. Leenstra et al[51] analyzed the dose plans of the 82 patients (secreting tumors, $n = 53$; nonsecreting tumors, $n = 29$) and created dose-volume histograms of the identifiable pituitary tissue. The risk of developing new anterior pituitary deficits was 16% and 45% at 2 and 5 years, respectively. Dosimetric analysis of 60 patients whose pituitary gland could be clearly identified showed that increasing mean pituitary gland radiation dose correlated with new anterior pituitary deficits. New anterior pituitary deficits stratified by mean pituitary gland radiation dose were as follows: ≤7.5 Gy, 0% (0/7); 7.6 to 13.2 Gy, 29% (7/24); 13.3 to 19.1 Gy, 39% (9/23); >19.1 Gy, 83% (5/6). Consequently, methods that limit the radiation dose to the pituitary gland during radiosurgery should be used whenever possible to increase the probability of preserving pituitary function.

References

1. Rossi HH, Kellerer AM. Roentgen. Radiat Res 1995;144:124–128
2. Sherman AA. Translation of an historic paper. On a new, strongly radioactive substance, contained in pitchblende: by M.P. Curie, Mme P. Curie and M.G. Bémont; presented by M. Becquerel. J Nucl Med 1970;11:269–270
3. del Regato JA. Fractionation: a panoramic view. Int J Radiat Oncol Biol Phys 1990;19:1329–1331
4. Miller DW. A review of proton beam radiation therapy. Med Phys 1995;22(11 Pt 2):1943–1954
5. Frankenberg-Schwager M. Review of repair kinetics for DNA damage induced in eukaryotic cells in vitro by ionizing radiation. Radiother Oncol 1989;14:307–320
6. McCarthy NJ, Hazlewood SA, Huen DS, Rickinson AB, Williams GT. The Epstein-Barr virus gene BHRF1, a homologue of the cellular oncogene Bcl-2, inhibits apoptosis induced by gamma radiation and chemotherapeutic drugs. Adv Exp Med Biol 1996;406:83–97
7. Hall EJ, Brenner DJ. The radiobiology of radiosurgery: rationale for different treatment regimes for AVMs and malignancies. Int J Radiat Oncol Biol Phys 1993;25:381–385
8. Cardinale RM, Benedict SH, Wu Q, Zwicker RD, Gaballa HE, Mohan R. A comparison of three stereotactic radiotherapy techniques; ARCS vs. noncoplanar fixed fields vs. intensity modulation. Int J Radiat Oncol Biol Phys 1998;42:431–436
9. Leksell L. The stereotaxic method and radiosurgery of the brain. Acta Chir Scand 1951;102:316–319
10. Leksell L. Stereotactic radiosurgery. J Neurol Neurosurg Psychiatry 1983;46:797–803
11. Colombo F, Benedetti A, Pozza F, et al. Stereotactic radiosurgery utilizing a linear accelerator. Appl Neurophysiol 1985;48:133–145
12. Friedman WA, Bova FJ. The University of Florida radiosurgery system. Surg Neurol 1989;32:334–342
13. Winston KR, Lutz W. Linear accelerator as a neurosurgical tool for stereotactic radiosurgery. Neurosurgery 1988;22:454–464
14. Adler JR Jr, Chang SD, Murphy MJ, Doty J, Geis P, Hancock SL. The Cyberknife: a frameless robotic system for radiosurgery. Stereotact Funct Neurosurg 1997;69(1-4 Pt 2):124–128
15. Park P, Chandler WF, Barkan AL, et al. The role of radiation therapy after surgical resection of nonfunctional pituitary macroadenomas. Neurosurgery 2004;55:100–106, discussion 106–107
16. van den Bergh AC, van den Berg G, Schoorl MA, et al. Immediate postoperative radiotherapy in residual nonfunctioning pituitary adenoma: beneficial effect on local control without additional negative impact on pituitary function and life expectancy. Int J Radiat Oncol Biol Phys 2007;67:863–869
17. Guinan EM, Lowy C, Stanhope N, Lewis PD, Kopelman MD. Cognitive effects of pituitary tumours and their treatments: two case studies and an investigation of 90 patients. J Neurol Neurosurg Psychiatry 1998;65:870–876
18. Noad R, Narayanan KR, Howlett T, Lincoln NB, Page RC. Evaluation of the effect of radiotherapy for pituitary tumours on cognitive function and quality of life. Clin Oncol (R Coll Radiol) 2004; 16:233–237
19. Paek SH, Downes MB, Bednarz G, et al. Integration of surgery with fractionated stereotactic radiotherapy for treatment of nonfunctioning pituitary macroadenomas. Int J Radiat Oncol Biol Phys 2005;61:795–808
20. Minniti G, Traish D, Ashley S, Gonsalves A, Brada M. Fractionated stereotactic conformal radiotherapy for secreting and nonsecreting pituitary adenomas. Clin Endocrinol (Oxf) 2006;64:542–548
21. Mackley HB, Reddy CA, Lee SY, et al. Intensity-modulated radiotherapy for pituitary adenomas: the preliminary report of the Cleveland Clinic experience. Int J Radiat Oncol Biol Phys 2007;67:232–239
22. Breen P, Flickinger JC, Kondziolka D, Martinez AJ. Radiotherapy for nonfunctional pituitary adenoma: analysis of long-term tumor control. J Neurosurg 1998;89:933–938
23. Minniti G, Traish D, Ashley S, Gonsalves A, Brada M. Risk of second brain tumor after conservative surgery and radiotherapy for pituitary adenoma: update after an additional 10 years. J Clin Endocrinol Metab 2005;90:800–804
24. Iwai Y, Yamanaka K, Yoshioka K. Radiosurgery for nonfunctioning pituitary adenomas. Neurosurgery 2005;56:699–705, discussion 699–705
25. Losa M, Valle M, Mortini P, et al. Gamma knife surgery for treatment of residual nonfunctioning pituitary adenomas after surgical debulking. J Neurosurg 2004;100:438–444
26. Mingione V, Yen CP, Vance ML, et al. Gamma surgery in the treatment of nonsecretory pituitary macroadenoma. J Neurosurg 2006;104:876–883
27. Pollock BE, Cochran J, Natt N, et al. Gamma knife radiosurgery for patients with nonfunctioning pituitary adenomas: results from a 15-year experience. Int J Radiat Oncol Biol Phys 2008;70: 1325–1329
28. Feigl GC, Bonelli CM, Berghold A, Mokry M. Effects of gamma knife radiosurgery of pituitary adenomas on pituitary function. J Neurosurg 2002;97(5, Suppl):415–421
29. Rowe J, Grainger A, Walton L, Silcocks P, Radatz M, Kemeny A. Risk of malignancy after gamma knife stereotactic radiosurgery. Neurosurgery 2007;60:60–65, discussion 65–66
30. Epaminonda P, Porretti S, Cappiello V, Beck-Peccoz P, Faglia G, Arosio M. Efficacy of radiotherapy in normalizing serum IGF-I, acid-labile subunit (ALS) and IGFBP-3 levels in acromegaly. Clin Endocrinol (Oxf) 2001;55:183–189
31. Powell JS, Wardlow SL, Post KD, Freda PU. Outcome of radiotherapy for acromegaly using normalization of insulin-like growth factor I to define cure. J Clin Endocrinol Metab 2000;82:3187–3191
32. Minniti G, Osti M, Jaffrain-Rea ML, Esposito V, Cantore G, Maurizi Enrici R. Long-term follow-up results of postoperative radiation therapy for Cushing's disease. J Neurooncol 2007;84:79–84
33. Sasaki R, Murakami M, Okamoto Y, et al. The efficacy of conventional radiation therapy in the management of pituitary adenoma. Int J Radiat Oncol Biol Phys 2000;47:1337–1345
34. Attanasio R, Epaminonda P, Motti E, et al. Gamma-knife radiosurgery in acromegaly: a 4-year follow-up study. J Clin Endocrinol Metab 2003;88:3105–3112
35. Castinetti F, Nagai M, Dufour H, et al. Gamma knife radiosurgery is a successful adjunctive treatment in Cushing's disease. Eur J Endocrinol 2007;156:91–98

36. Castinetti F, Taieb D, Kuhn JM, et al. Outcome of gamma knife radiosurgery in 82 patients with acromegaly: correlation with initial hypersecretion. J Clin Endocrinol Metab 2005;90:4483–4488
37. Jagannathan J, Sheehan JP, Pouratian N, Laws ER, Steiner L, Vance ML. Gamma Knife surgery for Cushing's disease. J Neurosurg 2007; 106:980–987
38. Landolt AM, Haller D, Lomax N, et al. Octreotide may act as a radioprotective agent in acromegaly. J Clin Endocrinol Metab 2000;85: 1287–1289
39. Landolt AM, Lomax N. Gamma knife radiosurgery for prolactinomas. J Neurosurg 2000;93(Suppl 3):14–18
40. Mauermann WJ, Sheehan JP, Chernavvsky DR, Laws ER, Steiner L, Vance ML. Gamma Knife surgery for adrenocorticotropic hormone-producing pituitary adenomas after bilateral adrenalectomy. J Neurosurg 2007;106:988–993
41. Pollock BE, Jacob JT, Brown PD, Nippoldt TB. Radiosurgery of growth hormone-producing pituitary adenomas: factors associated with biochemical remission. J Neurosurg 2007;106:833–838
42. Pollock BE, Nippoldt TB, Stafford SL, Foote RL, Abboud CF. Results of stereotactic radiosurgery in patients with hormone-producing pituitary adenomas: factors associated with endocrine normalization. J Neurosurg 2002;97:525–530
43. Pollock BE, Young WF Jr. Stereotactic radiosurgery for patients with ACTH-producing pituitary adenomas after prior adrenalectomy. Int J Radiat Oncol Biol Phys 2002;54:839–841
44. Pouratian N, Sheehan J, Jagannathan J, Laws ER Jr, Steiner L, Vance ML. Gamma knife radiosurgery for medically and surgically refractory prolactinomas. Neurosurgery 2006;59:255–266, discussion 255–266
45. Kong DS, Lee JI, Lim H, et al. The efficacy of fractionated radiotherapy and stereotactic radiosurgery for pituitary adenomas: long-term results of 125 consecutive patients treated in a single institution. Cancer 2007;110:854–860
46. Landolt AM, Haller D, Lomax N, et al. Stereotactic radiosurgery for recurrent surgically treated acromegaly: comparison with fractionated radiotherapy. J Neurosurg 1998;88:1002–1008
47. Pollock BE, Brown PD, Nippoldt TB, Young WF Jr. Pituitary tumor type affects the chance of biochemical remission after radiosurgery of hormone-secreting pituitary adenomas. Neurosurgery 2008;62:1271–1276, discussion 1276–1278
48. Leber KA, Berglöff J, Pendl G. Dose-response tolerance of the visual pathways and cranial nerves of the cavernous sinus to stereotactic radiosurgery. J Neurosurg 1998;88:43–50
49. Stafford SL, Pollock BE, Leavitt JA, et al. A study on the radiation tolerance of the optic nerves and chiasm after stereotactic radiosurgery. Int J Radiat Oncol Biol Phys 2003;55:1177–1181
50. Vladyka V, Liscák R, Novotný J Jr, Marek J, Jezková J. Radiation tolerance of functioning pituitary tissue in gamma knife surgery for pituitary adenomas. Neurosurgery 2003;52:309–316, discussion 316–317
51. Leenstra JL, Tanaka S, Kline RW, et al. Factors associated with endocrine deficits after stereotactic radiosurgery of pituitary adenomas. Neurosurgery 2010;67:27–32, discussion 32–33

26 Atypical Adenoma, Pituitary Carcinoma, and the Role of Chemotherapy in the Management of Refractory Pituitary Adenoma

Tannaz Moin, William H. Yong, and Anthony Heaney

Pituitary Tumor Classification

Pituitary adenomas are the most common intracranial tumors, and although they may cause significant morbidity due to hormonal hypersecretion or local mass effect, the overwhelming majority are typical adenomas confined to the sella. Pituitary carcinomas are very rare and are diagnosed when cerebrospinal or systemic metastasis is demonstrated. Pituitary carcinomas exhibit increased mitoses, K_i-67 labeling index (LI) >3%, and prominent nuclear staining for p53. Atypical adenomas are tumors that display a more aggressive phenotype characterized by early recurrence, local invasion of surrounding structures, or progression despite surgical resection, medical therapy, and radiotherapy.[1] Like pituitary carcinomas, they are characterized by increased mitoses, K_i-67 LI >3%, and nuclear staining for p53. Atypical adenomas are believed to represent a biologically intermediate stage in tumor progression along the continuum from benign adenomas to carcinomas.[2]

However, the term *atypical adenoma* should not be confused with the term *invasive adenoma* as applied in the literature. Invasive pituitary adenomas, which infiltrate and destroy the dura, bone, blood vessels, and nerve sheaths, are relatively commonly encountered, with a variable incidence of 5 to 20%.[3,4] If pituitary tumors exhibiting microscopic dural invasion are also included, up to 69% of microadenomas and 94% of macroadenomas can be termed invasive.[5]

The 2004 edition of the World Health Organization (WHO) text *Histological Typing of Endocrine Tumors* incorporated advances in immunohistochemistry as a primary feature of distinction among these pituitary tumor types (**Table 26.1**). However, histopathologic evaluation of these tumors is not always able to clearly distinguish pituitary carcinomas from atypical pituitary tumors and typical adenomas.

Information about presentation, management, and treatment of atypical pituitary tumors and carcinomas is sparse and derived largely from isolated case reports and is thus somewhat limited. This chapter provides a general overview of the presenting features of each tumor type and discusses treatment options and outcomes for pituitary carcinomas based on this albeit scant and occasionally anecdotal literature.

Pituitary Carcinomas

Epidemiology and Presenting Symptoms

Pituitary carcinoma is defined by the presence of a pituitary tumor that is either noncontiguous with the primary sellar tumor or has spread to sites distant from the primary. They are very uncommon and represent fewer than 0.2% of pituitary tumors. Up until 2008, there were only 124 reports of pituitary carcinoma in the literature describing a total of 154 patients.[6–8] Due to the often silent nature of pituitary metastatic lesions, some cases may be missed, a contention supported by the diagnosis of pituitary carcinoma only after autopsy in up to 75% of cases reported prior to 1994.[9] Occasionally, cancers of the breast, lung, kidney, and colon can metastasize to the sella or pituitary gland and are difficult to distinguish from primary disease.[10,11] However, metastatic pituitary lesions typically cause partial or panhypopituitarism, particularly diabetes insipidus, which is rarely seen in primary pituitary carcinomas.[10]

No gender or ethnic predilection has been reported for pituitary carcinomas, and patients typically present in the third to fifth decades of life.[8,12] Patients usually present with nonendocrine complaints due to local mass effect from the primary lesion, such as visual disturbances, with diplopia reported in 47% of cases and headaches in 27% of patients.[8] As would be expected, the endocrine findings differ significantly depending on the type of tumor. Although nonfunctioning pituitary tumors are the most commonly encountered pituitary tumors, for unclear reasons the two most commonly occurring pituitary carcinomas are prolactin (PRL)-secreting

Table 26.1 Pituitary Tumor Classification

	Typical	Atypical	Carcinoma
WHO Criteria	K_i-67 <3%	K_i-67 ≥3%* Increased mitoses Extensive p53 staining	K_i-67 >3% Increased mitoses Extensive p53 staining Metastasis
Size	Micro/macroadenoma	Micro/macroadenoma	Macroadenoma
Invasiveness	±	+	+

Abbreviations: WHO, World Health Organization.
*, may not be present.

and corticotroph-secreting carcinomas.[8,12–14] Growth hormone (GH)- and gonadotropin-secreting carcinomas occur much less frequently, and, although reported, thyrotropin-secreting carcinomas are exceedingly rare.

Prolactin-Secreting Carcinoma

There are no particular factors that help differentiate PRL-secreting adenomas that will follow a benign course from those that will progress to carcinoma.[15] Like their benign counterparts, PRL-secreting carcinomas present with PRL-mediated symptoms of amenorrhea, galactorrhea, or impotence, and PRL levels are largely similar to those in patients with typical macroadenomas.[12] However, with disease progression, patients usually demonstrate persistently increasing PRL levels despite appropriate therapy, which is uncharacteristic of typical adenomas that usually respond extremely well to D2-agonist therapy in 85% of cases.[16] In one series serum PRL levels ranged between 6 and 21,560 ng/mL.[8]

Corticotroph Carcinoma

Most adrenocorticotropic hormone (ACTH)-secreting pituitary carcinomas present with distant metastases and typical features of ACTH and cortisol excess, including moon facies, central obesity, abdominal striae, hypertension, diabetes, osteoporosis, altered menses, and delayed wound healing.[8,13,17] Cases have also been reported in the setting of Nelson's syndrome, whereby the ACTH-secreting pituitary tumor grows rapidly following adrenalectomy in patients with Cushing's disease, leading to markedly elevated ACTH levels, often in excess of 100,000 pg/mL.[8,18] In other cases of ACTH-secreting pituitary carcinomas clinical signs of Cushing's syndrome are absent, characteristic of so-called silent corticotroph tumors, which even when nonmetastatic and confined to the sella often run an indolent course.[19,20]

Growth Hormone–Secreting Carcinoma

As of 2001, there were only 10 reported cases of GH-secreting carcinomas presenting with clinical manifestations of acromegaly and elevated levels of GH and insulin-like growth factor-1/somatomedin C (IGF-1/SmC).[21,22] Unlike other pituitary carcinomas, GH-secreting carcinomas present at a relatively younger age, with an age range of 24 to 56.[12]

Gonadotroph Carcinoma

Gonadotroph carcinomas are rare, with only a few published reports, in which clinical symptoms included sexual impotence in males and oligomenorrhea in females.[23–26] Variable levels of serum of luteinizing hormone, follicle-stimulating hormone, and α-subunit have been reported.[23] Interestingly, one reported case presented with partial hypopituitarism, which as noted previously is an uncommon feature of pituitary carcinomas.[23]

Thyrotropin-Secreting Carcinoma

The first case of thyrotropin (thyroid-stimulating hormone [TSH])-secreting carcinoma was reported in 1993.[27] On histology, the primary lesion stained positively for PRL, TSH, and α-subunit. Serum TSH levels were elevated and ranged from 16 to 31 mU/mL (normal 0.4–4.6 mU/L) and α-subunit levels were very high, ranging from 125 to 150 ng/mL (normal <5 ng/mL). A possible case of a PRL- and TSH-co-secreting carcinoma was reported in 2007, although immunostaining of a resected brain metastasis was positive for PRL only.[14] As of 2007, no other cases have been reported in the English-language literature, making this the rarest subtype of pituitary carcinoma.

Evaluation and Management

In the setting of atypical or suspected pituitary carcinoma, the extent of central nervous system (CNS) disease is best defined by magnetic resonance imaging (MRI).[28] Pituitary carcinomas usually present in the setting of a known macroadenoma, exhibit significant suprasellar extension, and invade into either or both cavernous sinuses.[8] Unless the index of suspicion is high, cervical or more distant spine imaging is not routinely performed, and evaluation is best guided by clinical symptoms (e.g., neck pain) or if there is discordance between the volume of tumor discernible and the biochemical markers. It is important to note that neuroimaging cannot distinguish a carcinoma from an adenoma, unless cerebrospinal metastasis is evident.[29] Furthermore, systemic metastasis are not infrequently found incidentally during computed tomography (CT)/MRI scans for seemingly unrelated symptoms.

Pituitary carcinomas can metastasize either locally within the CNS via invasion into the subarachnoid space, leading to tumor seeding, or systemically via lymphatic and hematogenous spread.[30,31] The extent of involvement can vary from a single lesion to widespread dissemination.[13] Previously reported sites of metastasis have included the cerebral cortex, cerebellum, spinal cord, leptomeninges, eyes, heart, lung, cervical lymph nodes, pancreas, liver, kidney, pelvic lymph nodes, ovary, myometrium, and bone.[32–35] There are also reports of metastatic pituitary carcinoma cells isolated from both cerebrospinal fluid (CSF) and pleural effusions.[27,36]

Pituitary carcinomas tend to disseminate systemically rather than via craniospinal spread, with a reported frequency of 47% for systemic metastases, 40% for craniospinal metastases, and 13% exhibiting both.[8] Systemic metastasis appear to be more common in PRL-secreting carcinomas (71% in one series) with ACTH-secreting carcinomas exhibiting the second highest rates (57% in the same series), with a predilection for the liver.[8] In contrast, GH-secreting carcinomas more commonly present with cerebrospinal metastasis, although it must be acknowledged that the number of patients included is low.[12]

Tumorigenesis

The mechanisms involved in the transformation of a typical pituitary tumor to an atypical tumor and particularly to pituitary carcinoma are poorly understood. Previously, concern was voiced that changes induced following radiation therapy or manipulation during surgical procedures played a role in the progression of these tumors. However, given the large numbers of pituitary adenomas that are routinely resected or irradiated in comparison with the small number of pituitary carcinomas reported, this relationship is unsubstantiated. Pituitary carcinomas are now thought to transform via progressive genetic mutations that arise in pituitary adenomas.[1,12,26]

The time interval, or latency period, between the initial diagnosis of a pituitary adenoma and the occurrence of metastatic carcinoma varies considerably, ranging from 4 months to 18 years (mean 6.6 years).[8] Some studies have identified variable latency periods for different tumor subtypes, with patients with ACTH-secreting adenomas having latency periods twice as long as those with PRL-secreting adenomas (9.5 versus 4.7 years).[8]

Role of Molecular Markers in Pituitary Tumors

Cell Atypia and Mitoses

Given the typically low proliferation rates in pituitary adenomas, most generally accepted morphologic and histologic criteria of tumor aggressiveness, such as the number of mitoses, the degree of nuclear pleomorphism or atypia, and necrosis, are of limited use in distinguishing pituitary carcinomas from typical or atypical pituitary tumors.[37–39] For example, the presence of mitoses, which is considered a reliable marker of growth in many tumor tissues, may be scarce in aggressive pituitary tumors, and many of these changes are observed in both pituitary adenomas and carcinomas, which makes them of limited predictive value.[7,36]

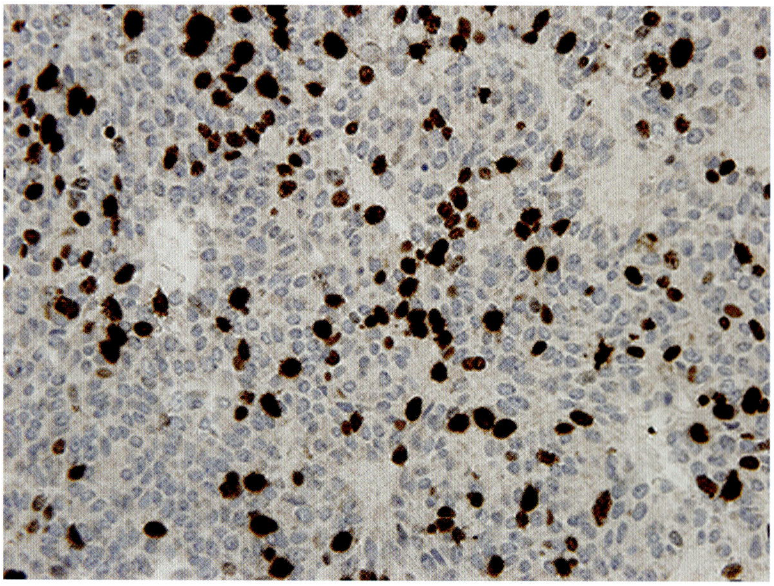

Fig. 26.1 Immunostaining for the proliferative marker K_i-67 in an atypical pituitary adenoma highlights approximately 25% of nuclei, a significantly higher index than the 1 to 2% immunopositivity of the usual adenoma. Original magnification (400×).

K_i-67

K_i-67 is a well-validated marker of cell proliferation, and it is expressed in cells during the G1, G2/M, and S-phase. It can be readily detected immunohistochemically using the MIB-1 monoclonal antibody to determine the K_i-67 LI, defined as the percentage of immunopositive nuclei (**Fig. 26.1**). Some studies have proposed a threshold K_i-67 LI of 3% to distinguish invasive from noninvasive adenomas, which reportedly has a 97% specificity and 73% sensitivity and positive and negative predictive values of 96% and 80%, respectively.[3] In one study, mean K_i-67 LI was 11.91 ± 3.41% in seven cases of pituitary carcinoma, compared with 1.37 ± 0.15% in noninvasive adenomas.[3] However, other studies have not demonstrated such a clear correlation between K_i-67 and invasion, so the role of K_i-67 in differentiating typical from atypical pituitary tumors or likelihood of recurrence remains unclear.[40] Nonetheless, K_i-67 LI is now a component of the WHO classification of pituitary adenomas, and the authors routinely analyze this marker in pituitary adenomas and believe it complements the other more standard methods to distinguish typical from atypical pituitary adenomas, and enables improved patient follow-up by "flagging" potentially recurrent pituitary tumors. Some experts have even proposed that large pituitary tumors exhibiting K_i-67 LI of greater than 10% should routinely be classified as atypical independent of other WHO criteria and followed more closely.[41]

Proliferating Cell Nuclear Antigen

The proliferating cell nuclear antigen (PCNA) is an accessory protein to DNA polymerase required for cell division and has also been employed as a proliferative marker in pituitary tumors. For example, significantly higher values have been noted in metastatic tumors with median of 72% (range 8–98%) compared with adenomas with median of 53% (range 0–93%).[42] However, PCNA is technically more difficult to quantitate, so results are less reliable than those for K_i-67 LI and therefore it has not gained widespread use.

Molecular Pathogenesis: Oncogenes and Tumor Suppressor Genes

p53 Protein

The p53 protein (also known as protein 53 or tumor protein 53) is a widely studied tumor suppressor gene that is commonly mutated in many human cancers and encodes a nuclear phosphoprotein essential for cell proliferation. p53 mutations commonly occur in breast and lung cancers but have not been reported in pituitary carcinomas. However, several studies have documented abundant immunohistochemical p53 expression in pituitary carcinomas and have found that nuclear p53 immunoreactivity correlates with pituitary tumor invasiveness.[43] In one study that included seven pituitary carcinomas, all carcinomas exhibited p53 immunopositivity compared with five of the 70 cases of pituitary adenomas (7.1%).[44] Despite considerable intra- and intertumoral variability, which is a limitation, p53 expression, like K_i-67, is included in the 2004 WHO criteria because correlation with tumor invasiveness can be of diagnostic and therapeutic utility.[44,45]

Other Markers

p27 is a cyclin-dependent kinase inhibitor that regulates cell division by preventing cyclin activation. Increased methylation of CpG islands on the p27 promoter results in lower p27 expression and has been reported in pituitary carcinomas (median 22.8%) compared with invasive adenomas (median 41.7%).[41] Additionally, point mutations in oncogenic *H-ras* have been identified in pituitary tumor metastasis, although few studies exist.[45]

Treatment

Pituitary carcinomas are generally associated with a poor prognosis, and most patients die within 1 year despite administration of maximal multimodal therapies.[46] Overall, patients with systemic metastases seem to have a worse prognosis compared with patients with CNS metastases.[8,12,14] In one series, median survival of patients with systemic disease was 1 year, whereas those with CSF spread lived an average of 2.6 years.[47] Standard treatment options include surgery, which may allow for temporary relief of mass-related symptoms. Radiotherapy is typically used when surgical options have been exhausted or to treat residual tumor after subtotal tumor resection. Medical therapy such as dopamine agonists can be used for PRL-secreting carcinomas, although pituitary carcinomas are typically partially or totally resistant to D2-agonist therapy. Somatostatin analogues have also been employed for GH-secreting carcinomas, although there is little evidence indicating real tumor effect in most cases.

Over the past few years, limited data have emerged on the role of chemotherapy in pituitary carcinomas from small studies and case reports. Given the rarity of cases, no randomized studies have been conducted, and protocols and inclusion or exclusion criteria have varied widely. Although pituitary carcinomas have a high proliferation index, they seem to retain certain aspects of well-differentiated tumors, or in some way are importantly different from other cancers because they do not respond to the standard chemotherapy regimens that are used in adenocarcinomas or sarcomas.[48] Although many single-agent and combination chemotherapy regimens have been tried over many years, the most commonly reported cytotoxic drugs utilized in pituitary carcinomas include chloroethylcyclohexylnitrosourea and 5-fluorouracil (CCNU + 5-FU), and more recently temozolomide (TMZ).

Other cytotoxic drugs employed in pituitary carcinomas include cisplatin, carboplatin, etoposide, Adriamycin, α-interferon, dacarbazine, cyclophosphamide, procarbazine, vincristine, mitotane, and methotrexate. The reported response rates to chemotherapy have been conflicting.[13] For instance, although transient responses in disease progression, such as declining hormone levels, reduced tumor size, diminishment/loss of metastasis, and even pain relief have been reported, these responses are short-lived (**Table 26.2** and **26.3**).

Table 26.2 Reported Cases of Pituitary Carcinomas Treated with Chemotherapy

Case	Tumor	Disease Burden	Treatment	Chemotherapy	Response/ Outcome	Reference
1	ACTH	Liver, lung, mediastinum, ilea, hip, sacral-lumbar spine	Surgery, RDT, BC, cyproheptadine	Cyclophosphamide, Adriamycin, 5-FU × 4 cycles	Alive at 39 mo	Kaiser, 1983[59]
2	GH	Occipital lobe, pons, cerebellopontine angles, spinal cord	3 surgeries, RDT, BC	Cisplatin, vinblastine, bleomycin × 1 cycle	Died <1 mo after chemo	Hashimoto, 1986[36]
3	GH	Right frontal lobe	4 surgeries, RDT	Methotrexate, 5-FU	Alive with no recurrence at 24 mo	Asai, 1988[60]
4	ACTH	Liver, lung, olfactory bulb	3 surguries, RDT	Mitotane, carmofur	Died within 4 mo	Nawata, 1990[61]
5	PRL	Frontal lobe, right ventricle, cerebellopontine angle, vertebral artery	4 surgeries, RDT, BC	CCNU, procarbazine, etoposide × 9 cycles	Initial response but progression, ↑ PRL 500,000, died 12 mo after chemo	Petterson, 1992[62]
6	PRL	Liver, lungs, hilar nodes	9 surgeries, RDT, BC, quinagolide, I^{125} implantation, octreotide	Etoposide, cisplatin, tamoxifen CCNU, 5-FU, folinic acid × 2 cycles	Progression and death within 1 mo	Walker, 1993[15]
7	PRL	Thoracic-lumbar vertebrae, femur	Surgery, RDT, BC, pergolide	CCNU, 5-FU, folinic acid × 1 cycle	Progression with death within a few weeks	Walker, 1993[15]
8	TSH	Lung, liver, bone, base of brain	3 surgeries, RDT, BC, Sandostatin LAR, octreotide	5-FU, Adriamycin, cyclophosphamide × 2 cycles	Initial response?, but progression and death within 2 mo of chemo	Mixson, 1993[27]
9	FSH, LH	Thoracic, lumbar spine, frontal lobe	2 surgeries, RDT	Cisplatin, etoposide × 6 cycles	Initially stable then progression and death 15 mo after chemo	Beauchesne,1995[25]
10	PRL	Ovaries, myometrium, pelvic LN, oral submucosa	2 surgeries, BC, RDT	Cisplatin, etoposide × 2 cycles, CCNU, procarbazine, vincristine × 2 cycles, tamoxifen	Initial progression but then ↓ PRL levels, alive 10 mo after chemo	Gollard, 1995[63]
11	PRL	Oral, ovaries, myometrium, LN	Surgery, RDT	Cisplatinum, procarbazine, CCNU, vincristine	Alive at 1.25 yr	Pernicone, 1997[8]
12	PRL	Spinal subarachnoid	Surgery, RDT, DA	Cisplatinum, procarbazine, CCNU, vincristine	Died within 1.8 yr	Pernicone, 1997[8]

Table 26.2 (*Continued*) Reported Cases of Pituitary Carcinomas Treated with Chemotherapy

Case	Tumor	Disease Burden	Treatment	Chemotherapy	Response/ Outcome	Reference
13	Null cell	Femur, liver	Surgery	Cisplatinum, procarbazine, CCNU, vincristine	Died within 4 yr	Pernicone, 1997[8]
14	PRL	Ethmoid sinus, LN, orbit, jaw, skull, thoracic spine	BC, surgery, cabergoline, octreotide	Carboplatin and etoposide × 3 cycles	Died 3 mo after chemo	Hurel, 1997[64]
15	PRL	Liver, lungs	Surgery, RDT	CCNU + 5-FU × 2 cycles	↓ PRL 550,000 to 90,000 but progression and death 3 mo after chemo	Kaltsas, 1998[46]
16	PRL	Thoracic, lumbar spine	RDT	CCNU + 5-FU × 1 cycle	Died 6 mo after chemo	Kaltsas, 199[46]
17	PRL	Frontal lobe, parietal lobe, orbit	Surgery, RDT	CCNU + 5-FU × 6 cycles; carboplatin × 8 cycles; 5-FU, α-IFN × 8 cycles; carboplatin, α -INF × 8 cycles	Died 11 yr after chemo	Kaltsas, 1998[46]
18	ACTH	Thoracic spine, liver	Surgery, RDT	CCNU + 5-FU × 6 cycles, carboplatin × 6 cycles, DTIC × 2 cycles	Died 3 yr after chemo	Kaltsas, 1998[46]
19	FSH, LH	Sella, cavernous sinus, temporoparietal lobe	2 surgeries, RDT, octreotide	Cyclophosphamide, Adriamycin, DTIC × 7 cycles	Died 4 mo after chemo	McCutcheon, 2000[23]
20	FSH, LH	Ribs, spine	BC, RDT, surgery	Cyclophosphamide, vincristine, dacarbazine × 7 cycles	Slight ↓ tumor, but new metastasis in ribs, alive at publication	Roncaroli, 2003[24]
21	PRL	Cerebellopontine angle, cervical spine	Cabergoline, RDT, 2 surgeries	TMZ	↓ PRL, size of tumor, alive 24 mo after chemo	Lim, 2006[50]
22	LH	Cervical, thoracic spine, ribs	3 surgeries, RDT, radiosurgery	TMZ × 12 cycles pegylated IFN × 1 mo	↓ tumor size and pain, asymptomatic 16 mo after chemo	Fadul, 2006[48]
23	PRL	Cervical, thoracic spine	BC, surgery, proton beam radiation, spine radiation, octreotide, I^{131} MIBG	Carboplatin, paclitaxel, etoposide × 2 cycles, TMZ × 10 cycles	↓ PRL 694 to 50, asymptomatic 15 mo after chemo	Fadul, 2006[48]
24	Null cell, pediatric	Leptomeninges, frontal lobe, sellar, posterior fossa, subarachnoid, cervicothoracic spine	Surgery	TMZ × 1 cycle	Died 2 mo after chemo	Guzel, 2008[65]

(*Continued on page 278*)

Table 26.2 (*Continued*) Reported Cases of Pituitary Carcinomas Treated with Chemotherapy

Case	Tumor	Disease Burden	Treatment	Chemotherapy	Response/ Outcome	Reference
25	PRL	LN	Carbergoline, surgery, Sandostatin, RDT	TMZ × 23 cycles	↓ PRL 738 to 78, ↓ tumor 62%, mets disappeared, alive 34 mo after chemo	Hagen, 2009[52]
26	ACTH/ Nelson's	Skull, occiput, ear, cervical spine	2 surgeries, RDT, GKRT	TMZ × 6 cycles	↓ ACTH 2472 to 389, ↓ tumor, alive 6 mo after chemo	Moyes, 2009[66]
27	PRL	LN	4 surgeries, RDT, DA	TMZ	Died	Raverot, 2010[67]
28	Null cell	Spinal metastasis	2 surgeries, RDT	TMZ × 7 cycles	Progressive disease, died	Bush, 2010[55]

Abbreviations: ACTH, adrenocorticotropic hormone; BC, bromocriptine; CCNU, chloroethylcyclohexylnitrosourea; chemo, chemotherapy; DA, dopamine agonist; DTIC, dacarbazine; FSH, follicle-stimulating hormone; 5-FU, 5-fluorouracil; GH, growth hormone; GKRT, GammaKnife stereotactic radiosurgery; LAR, long-acting release; LH, luteinizing hormone; LN, lymph node; mets, metastasis; MIBG, metaiodobenzylguanidine; PRL, prolactin; RDT, radiation therapy; TMZ, temozolomide; TSH, thyroid-stimulating hormone.
Partially adapted from Kaltsas GA, Grossman AB Malignant pituitary tumors. Pituitary 1998;1:69–81; and McCutcheon IE, Pieper DR, Fuller G, Benjamin RS, Friend KE, Gagel RF. Pituitary carcinoma containing gonadotropins: treatment by radical excision and chemotherapy: case report. Neurosurgery 2000;46:1233–1240.

CCNU + 5-FU

CCNU (also known as lomustine or CeeNU) is an alkylating agent that inhibits DNA and RNA synthesis by blocking the methylation of deoxyuridylic acid. CCNU has been used for many years to treat breast, colon, rectum, and pancreas cancer. The CCNU + 5-FU combination regimen has been used in a small series that included four cases of pituitary carcinoma, three of which had initial surgery followed by external-beam radiotherapy and one case with radiotherapy alone.[46] Patients received a median of two cycles (range 1–6), and the regimen was generally well tolerated. Unfortunately, overall response rate was disappointing, as three of the patients developed disease progression during treatment. Survival ranged from 3 to 65 months, indicating that some patients may have had slowing of disease progression, but given that the natural history is typically 12 months, all four patients eventually died.

Temozolomide (TMZ)

Temozolomide is an alkylating agent that is nonenzymatically converted to the active metabolite MTIC [(methyltriazene-1-yl)-imidazole-4-carboxamide]. The cytotoxic effects of MTIC are manifested through alkylation of DNA at the O^6,N^7 guanine positions, depleting the DNA repair enzyme O^6-methylguanine-DNA methyltransferase (MGMT). TMZ was originally approved for use in refractory glioblastoma multiforme, where it has transformed the outcome for these patients, although long-term survival is poor. The first demonstrated use of TMZ in pituitary carcinoma to have significant efficacy was reported in a patient with a PRL-secreting carcinoma that had progressed despite multiple surgeries, prospective radiation therapy, and high-dose medical therapy in 2006.[49,50] Previous studies in gliomas had suggested a correlation between TMZ response and methylation status of MGMT, and this association has also been examined in pituitary carcinomas.[51–54] However, a recent study describing seven patients treated with TMZ reported disease progression in a patient whose tumor exhibited low MGMT expression and therefore would have been predicted to respond to TMZ, so the relationship between MGMT and TMZ is unclear in pituitary carcinomas.[55]

Based on the limited data available in the literature, TMZ appears to be effective in all pituitary tumor subtypes regardless of hormonal status, although most cases treated to date are representative of the epidemiology of these tumors, with PRL- and ACTH-secreting tumors being most commonly treated. Although promising, studies are now needed to better determine the value of TMZ in treatment of pituitary carcinomas. Most studies have reported short-term treatment periods, although a few long-term responses have also been reported.[47]

Whereas initially TMZ was employed in the treatment of pituitary carcinoma, increasingly it is also being used to treat recurrent pituitary adenomas.[56] This raises several questions. First, cytotoxic agents such as TMZ are generally employed in disease states, such as glioma, where patient

Table 26.3 Reported Cases of Pituitary Adenomas Treated with Chemotherapy

Case	Tumor	Disease Burden	Treatment	Chemotherapy	Response/Outcome	Reference
1	ACTH	Invasive	2 surgeries, RDT, BC, sodium valproate	Procarbazine, etoposide, CCNU × 12 wk	Control of disease	Vaughan, 1985[68]
2	GH	Invasive	3 surgeries, RDT, BC	Doxorubicin, CCNU × 4 cycles	Remission	Kasperlik-Zaluska, 1987[69]
3	PRL	Invasive	2 surgeries, RDT	CCNU + 5-FU × 2 cycles	↓ PRL 21078 to 4746, died 6 mo after chemo from unrelated cause	Kaltsas, 1998[12]
4	GH	Invasive	2 surgeries, RDT	CCNU + 5-FU × 2 cycles	Alive 5 yr after chemo	Kaltsas, 1998[12]
5	ACTH	Invasive	2 surgeries, RDT	CCNU + 5-FU × 4 cycles, carboplatin/5-FU × 6 cycles	Alive 4 yr after chemo	Kaltsas, 1998[12]
6	PRL	Invasive	5 surgeries, RDT, DA	TMZ × 7 cycles	↓ PRL 1838 to 30, ↓ tumor	Kovacs, 2007[70] Syro, 2006[71]
7	PRL	Invasive	BC, surgery, RDT, cabergoline, GKRT, octreotide, octreotide LAR	TMZ × 26 cycles	↓ PRL 7000 to 260, ↓ tumor	Neff, 2007[56]
8	Null cell	Invasive	–	TMZ	No response	Kovacs, 2008[72]
9	ACTH	Invasive	Surgery	TMZ	↓ tumor, alive 16 months after chemo	Mohammed, 2009[73]
10	ACTH	Invasive→ carcinoma	2 surgeries, RDT	TMZ × 12 cycles	↓ tumor, ↓ ACTH 136 to 21, 4 mo after TMZ presented with ↑ tumor and mets S1	Mohammed, 2009[73]
11	Null cell	Invasive	RDT	TMZ	↓ tumor, alive 10 mo after chemo	Mohammed, 2009[73]
12	PRL	Invasive	BC, cabergoline,	TMZ × 12 cycles	↓ PRL 650 to 18, ↓ tumor 80%, alive 12 mo after chemo	Hagen, 2009[52]
13	Null cell	Invasive	6 surgeries, RDT, Sandostatin LAR, cabergoline	TMZ × 15 cycles	↓ tumor 55%, alive at publication	Hagen, 2009[52]
14	LH	Invasive	3 surgeries	TMZ × 5 cycles	↓ tumor, died 6 mo after chemo	Syro 2009[74]
15	Null cell	Invasive	Surgery	TMZ × 10 cycles	↓ tumor 20%	Bush, 2010[55]
16	ACTH	Invasive	3 surgeries, GKRT	TMZ × 11 cycles	↓ ACTH 221 to 18, ↓ tumor 80%	Bush, 2010[55]
17	FSH, LH	Invasive	3 surgeries, RDT	TMZ × 12 cycles	Stable tumor size	Bush, 2010[55]
18	Null cell	Invasive	2 surgeries	TMZ × 10 cycles	Stable tumor size	Bush, 2010[55]
19	PRL	Invasive	2 surgeries, GKRT	TMZ × 11 cycles	↓ PRL 5702 to 121, ↓ tumor 80%	Bush, 2010[55]
20	Null cell	Invasive	3 surgeries, RDT, GKRT	TMZ × 2 cycles temodar/ thalidomine	Died but cause unrelated to pituitary tumor	Bush, 2010[55]

Abbreviations: ACTH, adrenocorticotropic hormone; BC, bromocriptine; CCNU, chloroethylcyclohexylnitrosourea; chemo, chemotherapy; DA, dopamine agonist; DTIC, dacarbazine; FSH, follicle-stimulating hormone; GH, growth hormone; GKRT, GammaKnife stereotactic radiosurgery; LAR, long-acting release; LH, luteinizing hormone; LN, lymph node; mets, metastasis; PRL, prolactin; RDT, radiation therapy; TMZ, temozolomide; TSH, thyroid-stimulating hormone; –, not available.

prognosis is limited and measured in months rather than years. In patients with recurrent pituitary tumors or even TMZ-responsive pituitary cancers, the question arises as to how long TMZ treatment should be continued. This is a concern, as alkylating agents such as TMZ are associated with an increased risk of secondary malignancy, particularly hematologic disorders such as leukemia and lymphoma. Although this risk is small, it may become relevant in pituitary tumor patients who will potentially be treated for many years.

A further related issue is what the dosing regimen of TMZ should be in responsive patients who have exhibited stable disease for a period of time. In the authors' limited experience, stopping TMZ in a patient with pituitary carcinoma resulted in tumor recurrence after 18 months, which implies that some therapy may be needed long-term. It is unclear at this juncture whether intermittent dosing or low-dose continuous therapy would offer stabilization of disease in some or all of these patients and if such a schedule would ameliorate the risk of secondary malignancy. Although the rarity of pituitary carcinoma is clear, and large-scale randomized trials will likely not be possible, it is important that the long-term effects of TMZ therapy be better understood before the drug is more broadly used in recurrent or invasive pituitary tumors, which are not by definition pituitary cancers or atypical by histopathologic evaluation.

Recently some data have also emerged about the use of mammalian target of rapamycin (mTOR) inhibitors, rapamycin and its orally bioavailable analogue everolimus. Rapamycin is produced by the bacterium *Streptomyces hygroscopicus* and was initially developed as an antifungal agent but was later found to have immunosuppressive and antineoplastic properties.[57] In 2009, rapamycin and everolimus were first shown to decrease the number of viable cells and inhibit proliferation of rat pituitary cells and human pituitary cells derived from GH-secreting adenomas.[52] In a more recent in vitro study containing 40 nonfunctioning pituitary adenomas, everolimus significantly reduced cell viability (by approximately 40%, $p < .05$ versus control) and promoted apoptosis (+30%, $p < .05$ versus control).[58] Although more data are needed, mTOR inhibitors may be a promising and novel form of antiproliferative therapy.

Overall, there remain many unanswered questions regarding the long-term management of pituitary carcinomas. Because randomized control studies are technically challenging unless global clinical trials are conducted, treatment options at present must be based on available case reports. Most studies have shown that chemotherapy, although not capable in most situations of offering full or partial disease regression, can lead to disease stabilization (i.e., nonprogression), which in this setting is an acceptable outcome. Other options that have offered enhanced efficacy in other cancers, including the use of combination conventional chemotherapy with kinase-based agents, are as yet unexplored in pituitary carcinomas but may offer additional improved therapeutic options for these rare but rapidly fatal cancers.

References

1. Mamelak AN, Carmichael JD, Park P, Bannykh S, Fan X, Bonert HV. Atypical pituitary adenoma with malignant features. Pituitary 2008 [Epub ahead of print]
2. Amar AP, Hinton DR, Krieger MD, Weiss MH. Invasive pituitary adenomas: significance of proliferation parameters. Pituitary 1999;2: 117–122
3. Thapar K, Kovacs K, Scheithauer BW, et al. Proliferative activity and invasiveness among pituitary adenomas and carcinomas: an analysis using the MIB-1 antibody. Neurosurgery 1996;38:99–106, discussion 106–107
4. Scheithauer BW, Kovacs KT, Laws ER Jr, Randall RV. Pathology of invasive pituitary tumors with special reference to functional classification. J Neurosurg 1986;65:733–744
5. Kontogeorgos G. Predictive markers of pituitary adenoma behavior. Neuroendocrinology 2006;83:179–188
6. Roncaroli F, Scheithauer BW, Horvath E, et al. Silent subtype 3 carcinoma of the pituitary: a case report. Neuropathol Appl Neurobiol 2010;36:90–94
7. Kontogeorgos G. Classification and pathology of pituitary tumors. Endocrine 2005;28:27–35
8. Pernicone PJ, Scheithauer BW, Sebo TJ, et al. Pituitary carcinoma: a clinicopathologic study of 15 cases. Cancer 1997;79:804–812
9. Cusimano MD, Ohori P, Martinez AJ, Jungreis C, Wright DC. Pituitary carcinoma. Skull Base Surg 1994;4:46–51
10. Nudleman KL, Choi B, Kusske JA. Primary pituitary carcinoma: a clinical pathological study. Neurosurgery 1985;16:90–95
11. Komninos J, Vlassopoulou V, Protopapa D, et al. Tumors metastatic to the pituitary gland: case report and literature review. J Clin Endocrinol Metab 2004;89:574–580
12. Heaney AP, Melmed S. Pituitary tumors: molecular targets and new medical therapies. Nature Rev Can 2004;4:285–294
13. Scheithauer BW, Fereidooni F, Horvath E, et al. Pituitary carcinoma: an ultrastructural study of eleven cases. Ultrastruct Pathol 2001;25:227–242
14. Brown RL, Muzzafar T, Wollman R, Weiss RE. A pituitary carcinoma secreting TSH and prolactin: a non-secreting adenoma gone awry. Eur J Endocrinol 2006;154:639–643
15. Walker JD, Grossman A, Anderson JV, et al. Malignant prolactinoma with extracranial metastases: a report of three cases. Clin Endocrinol (Oxf) 1993;38:411–419
16. Webster J, Piscitelli G, Polli A, Ferrari CI, Ismail I, Scanlon MF; Cabergoline Comparative Study Group. A comparison of cabergoline and bromocriptine in the treatment of hyperprolactinemic amenorrhea. N Engl J Med 1994;331:904–909
17. Sheldon WH, Golden A, Bondy PK. Cushing's syndrome produced by a poultry basophil carcinoma with hepatic metastases. Am J Med 1954;17:134–142
18. Petrini L, Gasperi M, Pilosu R, Marcello A, Martino E. Long-term treatment of Nelson's syndrome by octreotide: a case report. J Endocrinol Invest 1994;17:135–139
19. Roncaroli F, Scheithauer BW, Young WF, et al. Silent corticotroph carcinoma of the adenohypophysis: a report of five cases. Am J Surg Pathol 2003;27:477–486

20. Al-Sarraj A, King P, Lantos HP. Atypical pituitary adenomas (silinet corticotroph pituitary adenoma). Neuropathol Appl Neurobiol 2002;28: 157–158
21. le Roux CW, Mulla A, Meeran K. Pituitary carcinoma as a cause of acromegaly. N Engl J Med 2001;345:1645–1646
22. Mountcastle RB, Roof BS, Mayfield RK, et al. Pituitary adenocarcinoma in an acromegalic patient: response to bromocriptine and pituitary testing: a review of the literature on 36 cases of pituitary carcinoma. Am J Med Sci 1989;298:109–118
23. McCutcheon IE, Pieper DR, Fuller GN, Benjamin RS, Friend KE, Gagel RF. Pituitary carcinoma containing gonadotropins: treatment by radical excision and cytotoxic chemotherapy: case report. Neurosurgery 2000;46:1233–1239, discussion 1239–1240
24. Roncaroli F, Nosé V, Scheithauer BW, et al. Gonadotropic pituitary carcinoma: HER-2/neu expression and gene amplification. Report of two cases. J Neurosurg 2003;99:402–408
25. Beauchesne P, Trouillas J, Barral F, Brunon J. Gonadotropic pituitary carcinoma: case report. Neurosurgery 1995;37:810–815, discussion 815–816
26. Spertini F, Deruaz JP, Perentes E, Pelet B, Gomez F. Luteinizing hormone (LH) and prolactin-releasing pituitary tumor: possible malignant transformation of the LH cell line. J Clin Endocrinol Metab 1986;62:849–854
27. Mixson AJ, Friedman TC, Katz DA, et al. Thyrotropin-secreting pituitary carcinoma. J Clin Endocrinol Metab 1993;76:529–533
28. Ragel BT, Couldwell WT. Pituitary carcinoma: a review of the literature. Neurosurg Focus 2004;16:E7
29. Lopes MB, Scheithauer BW, Schiff D. Pituitary carcinoma: diagnosis and treatment. Endocrine 2005;28:115–121
30. Saeger W, Lubke D. Pituitary carcinomas. Endocr Pathol 1996;7: 21–35
31. Garrão AF, Sobrinho LG, Pedro-Oliveira, et al. ACTH-producing carcinoma of the pituitary with haematogenic metastases. Eur J Endocrinol 1997;137:176–180
32. Frost AR, Tenner S, Tenner M, Rollhauser C, Tabbara SO. ACTH-producing pituitary carcinoma presenting as the cauda equina syndrome. Arch Pathol Lab Med 1995;119:93–96
33. Ayuk J, Natarajan G, Geh JI, Mitchell RD, Gittoes NJ. Pituitary carcinoma with a single metastasis causing cervical spinal cord compression. Case report. J Neurosurg Spine 2005;2:349–353
34. Cartwright DM, Miller TR, Nasr AJ. Fine-needle aspiration biopsy of pituitary carcinoma with cervical lymph node metastases: a report of two cases and review of the literature. Diagn Cytopathol 1994;11:68–73
35. Moberg A. A case of pituitary chromophobe adenoma with metastases in the heart. Acta Pathol Microbiol Scand 1959;45:243–249
36. Hashimoto N, Handa H, Nishi S. Intracranial and intraspinal dissemination from a growth hormone-secreting pituitary tumor. Case report. J Neurosurg 1986;64:140–144
37. Thapar K, Kovacs K, Muller PJ. Clinical-pathological correlations of pituitary tumours. Baillieres Clin Endocrinol Metab 1995;9:243–270
38. Challa VR, Marshall RB, Hopkins MB III, Kelly DL Jr, Civantos F. Pathobiologic study of pituitary tumors: report of 62 cases with a review of the recent literature. Hum Pathol 1985;16:873–884
39. Saeger W, Lüdecke DK, Buchfelder M, Fahlbusch R, Quabbe HJ, Petersenn S. Pathohistological classification of pituitary tumors: 10 years of experience with the German Pituitary Tumor Registry. Eur J Endocrinol 2007;156:203–216
40. Salehi F, Agur A, Scheithauer BW, Kovacs K, Lloyd RV, Cusimano M. Ki-67 in pituitary neoplasms: a review—part I. Neurosurgery 2009;65:429–437, discussion 437
41. Kovacs K. The 2004 WHO classification of pituitary tumors: comments. Acta Neuropathol 2006;111:62–63
42. Scheithauer BW, Gaffey TA, Lloyd RV, et al. Pathobiology of pituitary adenomas and carcinomas. Neurosurgery 2006;59:341–353, discussion 341–353
43. Tanizaki Y, Jin L, Scheithauer BW, Kovacs K, Roncaroli F, Lloyd RV. P53 gene mutations in pituitary carcinomas. Endocr Pathol 2007; 18:217–222
44. Thapar K, Scheithauer BW, Kovacs K, Pernicone PJ, Laws ER Jr. p53 expression in pituitary adenomas and carcinomas: correlation with invasiveness and tumor growth fractions. Neurosurgery 1996;38:765–770, discussion 770–771
45. Pei L, Melmed S, Scheithauer B, Kovacs K, Prager D. H-ras mutations in human pituitary carcinoma metastases. J Clin Endocrinol Metab 1994;78:842–846
46. Kaltsas GA, Mukherjee JJ, Plowman PN, Monson JP, Grossman AB, Besser GM. The role of cytotoxic chemotherapy in the management of aggressive and malignant pituitary tumors. J Clin Endocrinol Metab 1998;83:4233–4238
47. Scheithauer BW, Kurtkaya-Yapicier O, Kovacs KT, Young WF Jr, Lloyd RV. Pituitary carcinoma: a clinicopathological review. Neurosurgery 2005;56:1066–1074, discussion 1066–1074
48. Fadul CE, Kominsky AL, Meyer LP, et al. Long-term response of pituitary carcinoma to temozolomide. Report of two cases. J Neurosurg 2006;105:621–626
49. Zhu Y, Shahinian H, Bonert V, Lim S, Heaney A. Temodar: Novel Treatment for Pituitary Carcinoma. Endocrine Society Annual Meeting 2004;OR:43–45
50. Lim S, Shahinian H, Maya MM, Yong W, Heaney AP. Temozolomide: a novel treatment for pituitary carcinoma. Lancet Oncol 2006;7:518–520
51. McCormack AI, McDonald KL, Gill AJ, et al. Low O6-methylguanine-DNA methyltransferase (MGMT) expression and response to temozolomide in aggressive pituitary tumours. Clin Endocrinol (Oxf) 2009;71:226–233
52. Hagen C, Schroeder HD, Hansen S, Hagen C, Andersen M. Temozolomide treatment of a pituitary carcinoma and two pituitary macroadenomas resistant to conventional therapy. Eur J Endocrinol 2009;161:631–637
53. Kovacs K, Horvath E, Syro LV, et al. Temozolomide therapy in a man with an aggressive prolactin-secreting pituitary neoplasm: Morphological findings. Hum Pathol 2007;38:185–189
54. Kovacs K, Scheithauer BW, Lombardero M, et al. MGMT immunoexpression predicts responsiveness of pituitary tumors to temozolomide therapy. Acta Neuropathol 2008;115:261–262
55. Bush ZM, Longtine JA, Cunningham T, et al. Temozolomide treatment for aggressive pituitary tumors: correlation of clinical outcome with O(6)-methylguanine methyltransferase (MGMT) promoter methylation and expression. J Clin Endocrinol Metab 2010;95:E280–E290
56. Neff LM, Weil M, Cole A, et al. Temozolomide in the treatment of an invasive prolactinoma resistant to dopamine agonists. Pituitary 2007;10:81–86
57. Gorshtein A, Rubinfeld H, Kendler E, et al. Mammalian target of rapamycin inhibitors rapamycin and RAD001 (everolimus) induce antiproliferative effects in GH-secreting pituitary tumor cells in vitro. Endocr Relat Cancer 2009;16:1017–1027

58. Zatelli MC, Minoia M, Filieri C, et al. Effect of everolimus on cell viability in nonfunctioning pituitary adenomas. J Clin Endocrinol Metab 2010;95:968–976
59. Kaiser FE, Orth DN, Mukai K, Oppenheimer JH. A pituitary parasellar tumor with extracranial metastases and high, partially suppressible levels of adrenocorticotropin and related peptides. J Clin Endocrinol Metab 1983;57:649–653
60. Asai A, Matsutani M, Funada N, Takakura K. Malignant growth hormone-secreting pituitary adenoma with hematogenous dural metastasis: case report. Neurosurgery 1988;22(6 Pt 1):1091–1094
61. Nawata H, Higuchi K, Ikuyama S, et al. Corticotropin-releasing hormone- and adrenocorticotropin-producing pituitary carcinoma with metastases to the liver and lung in a patient with Cushing's disease. J Clin Endocrinol Metab 1990;71:1068–1073
62. Petterson T, MacFarlane IA, MacKenzie JM, Shaw MDM. Prolactin secreting pituitary carcinoma. J Neurol Neurosurg Psychiatry 1992;55:1205–1206
63. Gollard R, Kosty M, Cheney C, Copeland B, Bordin G. Prolactin-secreting pituitary carcinoma with implants in the cheek pouch and metastases to the ovaries. A case report and literature review. Cancer 1995;76:1814–1820
64. Hurel SJ, Harris PE, McNicol AM, Foster S, Kelly WF, Baylis PH. Metastatic prolactinoma: effect of octreotide, cabergoline, carboplatin and etoposide; immunocytochemical analysis of proto-oncogene expression. J Clin Endocrinol Metab 1997;82:2962–2965
65. Guzel A, Tatli M, Senturk S, Guzel E, Cayli SR, Sav A. Pituitary carcinoma presenting with multiple metastases: case report. J Child Neurol 2008;23:1467–1471
66. Moyes VJ, Alusi G, Sabin HI, et al. Treatment of Nelson's syndrome with temozolomide. Eur J Endocrinol 2009;160:115–119
67. Raverot G, Wierinckx A, Dantony E, et al; HYPOPRONOS. Prognostic factors in prolactin pituitary tumors: clinical, histological, and molecular data from a series of 94 patients with a long postoperative follow-up. J Clin Endocrinol Metab 2010;95:1708–1716
68. Vaughan NJ, Laroche CM, Goodman I, Davies MJ, Jenkins JS. Pituitary Cushing's disease arising from a previously non-functional corticotrophic chromophobe adenoma. Clin Endocrinol (Oxf) 1985;22:147–153
69. Kasperlik-Zaluska AA, Wislawski J, Kaniewska J, Zborzil J, Frankiewicz E, Zgliczyński S. Cytostatics for acromegaly. Marked improvement in a patient with an invasive pituitary tumour. Acta Endocrinol (Copenh) 1987;116:347–349
70. Kovacs K, Horvath E, Syro LV, et al. Temozolomide therapy in a man with an aggressive prolactin-secreting pituitary neoplasm: Morphological findings. Hum Pathol 2007;38:185–189
71. Syro LV, Uribe H, Penagos LC, et al. Antitumour effects of temozolomide in a man with a large, invasive prolactin-producing pituitary neoplasm. Clin Endocrinol (Oxf) 2006;65:552–553
72. Kovacs K, Scheithauer BW, Lombardero M, et al. MGMT immunoexpression predicts responsiveness of pituitary tumors to temozolomide therapy. Acta Neuropathol 2008;115:261–262
73. Mohammed S, Kovacs K, Mason W, Smyth H, Cusimano MD. Use of temozolomide in aggressive pituitary tumors: case report. Neurosurgery 2009;64:E773–E774, discussion E774
74. Syro LV, Scheithauer BW, Ortiz LD, et al. Effect of temozolomide in a patient with recurring oncocytic gonadotrophic pituitary adenoma. Hormones (Athens) 2009;8:303–306

27 The Utility of Intraoperative MRI in Pituitary Surgery

Rudolf Fahlbusch and Vincenzo Paternó

Summarizing the past one and half decades of intraoperative magnetic resonance imaging (IMRI), its utility has been documented mainly in the treatment of pituitary adenomas, although benefit has also been shown in other parasellar tumors such as craniopharyngiomas. For adenomas, 30 to 40% of totally resectable tumors achieve total removal, which could not be obtained at the primary procedure without IMRI.

In addition to other advanced technologies that have been introduced into the operating room in recent years for transsphenoidal surgery such as neuronavigation[1–5] and endoscopy,[6–8] IMRI[5,9–14] is used as an immediate intraoperative quality control, evaluating the extent of tumor removal during the surgical procedure, which allows us to extend resections in those cases where tumor remnants are documented.[9–14]

In one third of macroadenomas, both low-field and especially high-field 1.5-tesla (T) IMRI scanners are able to document adenoma remnants as small as 3 to 4 mm for high-field scanners; these remnants were hidden to the surgeon's eye in folds of the descending diaphragm sella.

The development of IMRI imaging started in the mid-1990s. The application was pioneered by Black et al,[6] who operated in continuously running magnetic field using the so-called double-doughnut system, whereas the 0.2-T open MRI installations in Erlangen and Heidelberg represented the concept of transporting the patient into the magnet while performing surgery outside the strong magnetic field. The evolution from low-field to high-field MR scanners led to a renaissance of the idea of intraoperative imaging in transsphenoidal surgery for resection control and high-quality intraoperative images. High-field MRI has a clear advantage in image resolution compared with the intraoperative low- and mid-field MR system (0.12–0.5T).[16,17]

Not only patients with large tumors but also those with smaller adenomas, especially those extending against and into the cavernous sinus, can profit from IMRI control.

Not only hormonally inactive but also larger hormonally active tumors, in acromegaly and Cushing's disease, profit from IMRI, by an increased rate of complete tumor removal as well as a higher role of endocrine normalization and "near normalization."[18] In nonfunctioning tumors, there are no hormonal markers available that would enable an early prognosis of outcome.

Because in the great majority of cases the excellent IMRI resolution of images (mainly obtained by 1.5 T) permits comprehensive evaluation of the relevant anatomy, the conventional postoperative MRI scan performed 2 to 3 months after surgery (without artifact) can be avoided.

Operating Room Setup

Today several different industrial companies offer low-field (0.15 T, Medtronic, Minneapolis, MN; 0.2 T, Siemens AG Medical Solutions, Hannover, Germany), mid-field (0.3 T, Hitachi; 0.5 T, General Electric, Hannover, Germany), high-field (1.5 T, General Electric, Philips [Andover, MA], Siemens), and ultra-high-field (3 T, General Electric, Philips, Siemens) scanners. The senior author started with a 0.2-T system (Magnetom Open, Siemens) in 1996, followed by a 1.5-T system (Sonata, Siemens) in 2002 in Erlangen.

We now present our current system, the "INI Brain Suite," an operating theater with a 1.5-T Magnetom Espree scanner (Siemens), which was installed in 2006/2007 at the International Neuroscience Institute (INI) in Hannover, Germany. This is a high-field MRI scanner with a superconductive 1.5-T magnet with a length of 160 cm and an inner bore diameter of 70 cm equipped with a gradient system having a field strength of up to 40 mT/m (effective 69 mT/m) and an effective slew rate of up to 200 T/m/s effective. This was the first "open" 1.5-T MRI used for therapeutic purposes.

A rotatable surgical table (Trumpf, Saalfeld, Germany) is adapted to the scanner to allow for a special surgical MRI tabletop. This surgical table can be locked into various positions. The principal surgical position is at 160 degrees, with the patient's head at the 5-gauss (G) line (distance of 4 m to the center of the scanner). As soon as the rotating mechanism has been locked, the height of the table, the angle of tilt, and the lateral tilt can be modified. The table movements are controlled remotely. Only the rotation about the table axis to turn the table into the axis of the scanner is performed manually, for safety reasons.

MRI-compatible ventilation (Aestiva 5/MRI, General Electric) and MRI-compatible monitoring are available for control of anesthesia and for wireless 2.4-GHz data transfer from the radiofrequency-shielded cabin. The perfusions and infusion pumps are shielded for MRI compatibility.

Our endoscopic equipment includes a 0- and 30-degree, 4-mm rigid endoscope Hopkins II (Karl Storz, Tuttlingen, Germany), a full high-definition (HD) camera IMAGE1 H3-Z, and a wide-view HD screen. The use of the endoscope in our "BrainSuite" operating room, with 1.5-T MRI, performing surgery at the 5-G line, is similar to its use in a normal routinely operating theater without IMRI.

In the majority of cases, microscopic tumor removal is performed with the ceiling-mounted Pentero C Multivision microscope (Zeiss, Oberkochen, Germany). The holding device is placed in the middle line within the 5-G line; the microscope itself can have a flexible position in connection with the preferred position of the operating field (as far as we know, we were the first to test this MRI-compatible ceiling-mounted Zeiss Pentero system).

Navigation is indicated in tumors with either encased arteries or loss of anatomical landmarks as occurs in reoperations. We use the BrainLab integrated VectorVision Sky Navigation System (BrianLab, Heimstetten, Germany) with a ceiling-mounted infrared camera and touch-screen display. The patient is placed in a special ceramic head-holding system (**Fig. 27.1A**), and the registration is done automatically through an integrated special coil system. A fiberoptic connection ensures MR-compatible integration into the radiofrequency room. The camera used to monitor the position of the microscope and other instruments is also ceiling-mounted, as well as the touch screen, which is used to operate the navigation system. Two 50-inch flat-screen monitors mounted on the left wall of the BrainSuite are available for viewing the images from the microscope and the MR console, as well as various software applications.

The microscope and endoscope video is recorded using Medimage software (Vepro, Pfungstadt, Germany) in parallel in the MR control room. The instrument table and the various rotating stools (Trumpf, Ditzingen, Germany) are fully MR compatible.

The procedures for emergency magnet quenching and for monitoring of oxygen levels in the operating room are the same as those in standard clinical MRI installations.

Transsphenoidal Surgery and Intraoperative MRI

In our current series of pituitary adenomas, 95% of tumors are approached via the direct endonasal transsphenoidal approach. Head fixation is not required, and imaging is performed using a standard U-shaped large flexible coil that is adapted and draped to the head (**Fig. 27.1B**).

The surgeon, using Cushing's positioning for transsphenoidal surgery, is standing behind the patient's head (**Fig. 27.1C**). A schematic outline of the operating room was published previously.[11,19]

The whole transsphenoidal procedure is identical to that performed in regular operating rooms. The sublabial and unilateral paraseptal approaches to the sphenoidal sinus are used less frequently. We generally prefer the direct endonasal transsphenoidal approach with endoscope assistance. The entrance into the sphenoid sinus is guided by endoscopic visualization, as well as identification of the sellar floor and the carotid arteries. Furthermore, the endoscope is very helpful during resection of tumor remnants in the

A

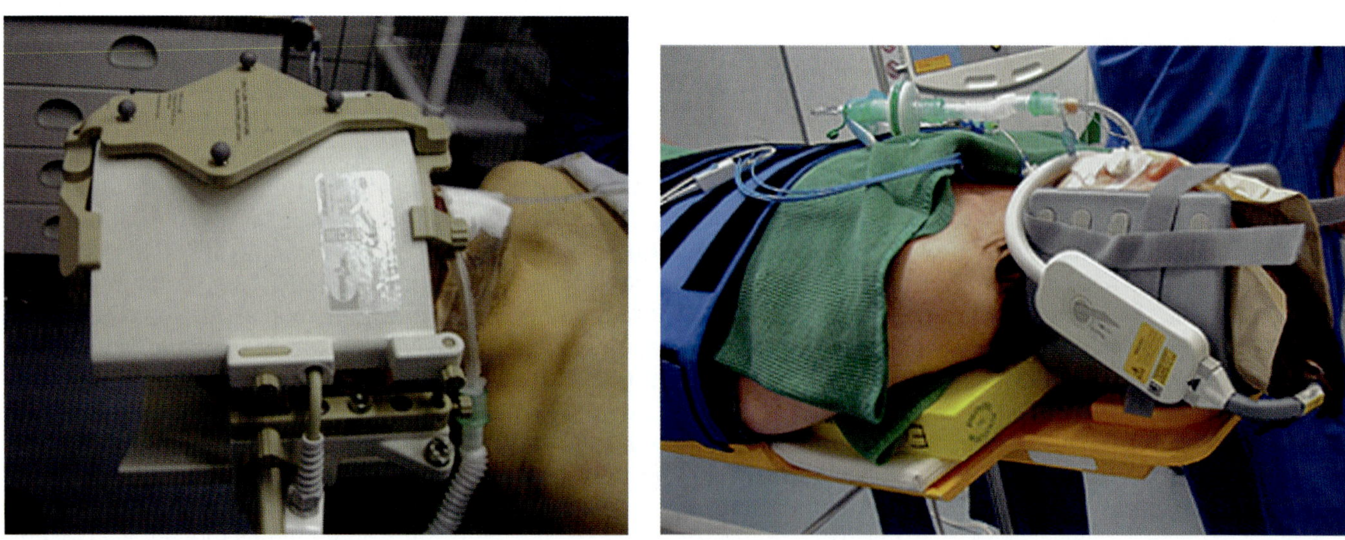

B

Fig. 27.1 **(A)** A rigid navigated magnetic resonance (MR) coil is used to hold the head in a fixed position during the surgical procedure. **(B)** A flexible MR coil is placed around the head, so that the head can be moved during surgery without restrictions; a coil-preamplifier is attached to the flexible coil by a tape.

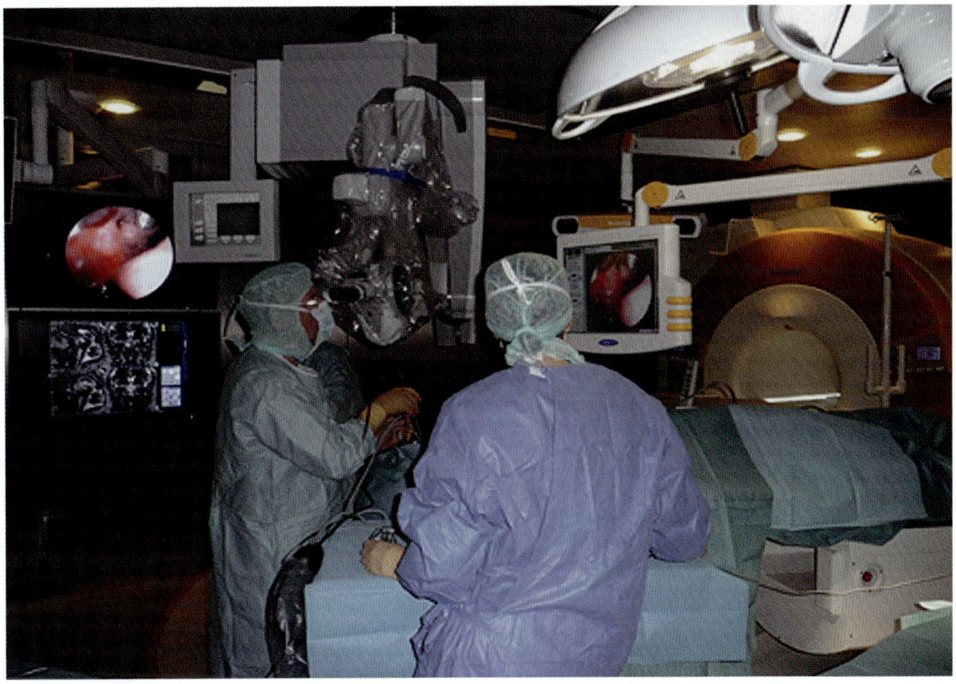
C

Fig. 27.1 (*Continued*) **(C)** The intraoperative scenario in our MR operating room for microneurosurgical procedures. The head is placed at the 5-G red line; the surgeon is standing behind the head (Cushing's position). The microscope and its associated monitor are secured to the ceiling of the operating room, on the left side of the surgeon and the instrument tables, with the endoscope and the nurses stationed on the right side of the surgeon. The anesthesiologist's workstation is located in the right corner of the operating room, opposite the end of the MRI table. The circuit for the endotracheal tube is connected to an MRI-compatible anesthesia machine. Many standard surgical instruments can be used between the 5- and 20-G magnetic field lines. Two 50-inch plasma monitors are located on the left wall of the operating room. A movable MRI-compatible navigation monitor and infrared navigation arm are located close to the left middle part of right wall. An extra 21-inch LCD monitor is attached to the ceiling on the left side of the operating room.

cavernous sinus and in folds of the descending diaphragm, supplementing microsurgical tumor removal.

Less frequently, we have performed a purely endoscopic resection of an adenoma, although purely endoscopic surgery is frequently used during the removal of other parasellar tumors such as chordomas centered in the clivus.

Porcelain-coated drills are used, especially to avoid metal artifacts during imaging, to open the sphenoid sinus and to remove the sellar floor. Transsphenoidal surgery is routinely accompanied by endonasal endoscopic inspection using 0- and 30-degree, 4-mm rigid endoscopes to visualize the surgical site, which is projected on a ceiling-mounted monitor or through the eyepiece of the microscope. Selective adenomectomy is achieved in all patients. In general, regular operating microinstruments are used during the transsphenoidal surgery at the 5-G line. In contrast to earlier years when we used an MRI-compatible nasal speculum for intraoperative imaging, the direct endoscopic-assisted endonasal approach permits us to examine the sella without the speculum, by installing a simple piece of cotton as a placeholder in the nasal cavity. If necessary, especially in cases with defects of the diaphragm sella and cerebrospinal fluid (CSF) leaks, the sellar floor was covered at the end of surgery with fascia or subcutaneous fat tissue, which was obtained during the same surgical session from the right thigh positioned within the 5-G perimeter. For safety reasons, we used fully MRI-compatible instruments to obtain the fascia. In the case of intraoperative CSF leakage, temporary lumbar drainage is utilized. In direct endonasal surgery, no nasal packing is necessary.

The timing of intraoperative imaging is decided by the neurosurgeon; intraoperative imaging is performed either when the neurosurgeon has the impression that a complete tumor removal was done or, in the case of incomplete tumor removal, when he thinks no further removal at this stage of surgery is possible using the transsphenoidal approach. Just before intraoperative imaging, the opened sellar floor is covered with a flat piece of bone wax for better delineation of the sella outlines in the intraoperative images, minimizing artifacts caused by blood from the sphenoid sinus or the nasal cavity. Then the surgical site is covered with a sterile drape, and the MRI table is rotated 160 degrees into the scanner. The time between the decision for intraoperative MRI and the actual start of imaging is approximately 2 minutes.

After the patient is moved into the center of the scanner, certain circuits are switched off, including the fluorescent lamps and the operating microscope. The imaging starts with a localizer sequence (field of view [FOV], 280 mm; repeat time [TR], 20 milliseconds; echo time [TE], 50 milliseconds; scan time, 9 seconds). A T2-weighted, half-Fourier, single-shot turbo spin echo sequence (slice thickness, 5 mm; FOV, 230 mm; TR, 1000 milliseconds; TE, 89 milliseconds; scan time, 25 second at five acquisitions) is performed in coronal and sagittal orientation to give a quick overview of the operative site. Afterward, T1-weighted coronal and sagittal spin echo sequences are acquired (slice thickness, 3 mm; FOV, 270 mm; TR, 450 milliseconds; TE, 12 milliseconds; scan time, 4 minutes 57 seconds at four acquisitions). In addition, high-resolution T2-weighted turbo spin echo sequences with an in-plane resolution of 0.6 × 0.4 mm are obtained (slice thickness, 3 mm; FOV, 230 mm; TR, 4000 milliseconds; TE, 97 milliseconds; scan time, 6 minutes 6 seconds at three acquisitions).

If the intraoperative imaging depicts some remaining tumor (which was not detected by endoscopic inspection before) that appears to be accessible for further resection, surgery is continued. After further resection, a repeated intraoperative MRI scan is performed before closure. The identical imaging protocol is applied for preoperative, as well as postoperative, imaging in the first week after surgery and after 3 months.

Scanning at the identical pre- and intraoperative image slice position enables comparing pre- and intraoperative images in a side-by-side display. In this way fibrin glue, applied for hemostasis, can be identified and differentiated from tumor remnants. Furthermore, the use of porcelain-coated drills prevents extensive drilling artifacts, which would otherwise obscure the image and interfere with interpretation. Because T2-weighted imaging proved to be superior in identification of tumor remnants, and additional T1-weighted imaging did not provide any further information, T1-weighted imaging was omitted from the intraoperative imaging protocol in most patients.

The criterion for selecting patients was pituitary macroadenoma with or without suprasellar extension. All patients had preoperative high-field, contrast-enhanced MRI scans focused on the sellar region to determine extension of tumor growth and invasion of adjacent structures.

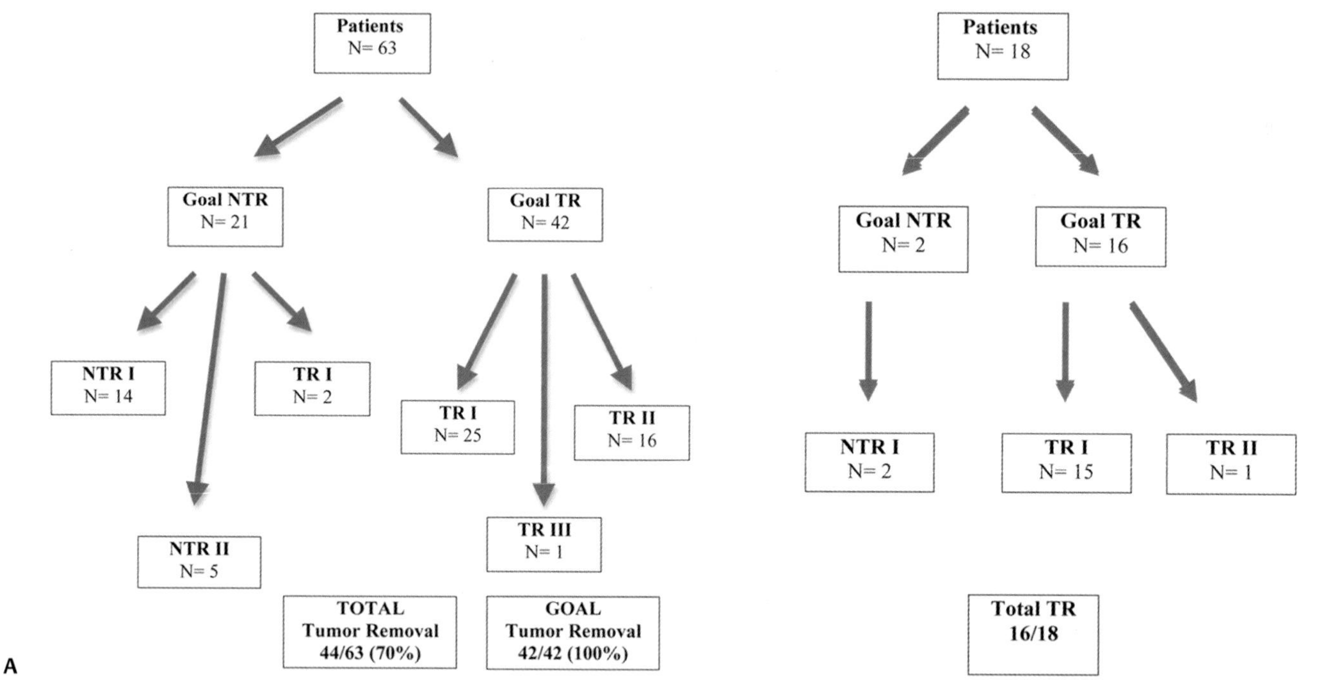

Fig. 27.2 **(A)** Overview of the result of the 63 patients undergoing surgical removal of pituitary adenomas through trans-cranial (2 cases) and trans-sphenoidal approaches (61 cases) using intra-operative high field MRI. In a group of 63 patients, we planned preoperatively to achieve a total tumor resection (Goal TR) in 42 cases and a non total tumor resection (Goal NTR) in 21 patients. After the first intraoperative MRI control, we achieved our goal respectively in 25 cases and 14 cases; we were also able to improve our goal, obtaining total tumor removal in 2 patients, which were preoperatively schedule in the Goal NTR group. After the second intraoperative MRI control, we achieved our goal respectively in 16 cases and we needed a third intraoperative MRI control to achieve the last total tumor resection. In 5 cases, we needed a second intraoperative MRI control to complete the partial tumor resection achieving the NTR. In our series we achieved a total tumour resection, in about 70% of our patients (44/63). We achieved a total tumor resection, in 100% of our Goal TR group (42/42), also profiting from iop MRI in about 40% (17/42), of those patients in which the total tumor resection was possible to achieve after the first control. **(B)** Overview of the result of 18 patients undergoing surgical removal of craniopharingioma through trans-cranial (14 cases) and trans-sphenoidal (4 cases) approaches using intra-operative high-field MRI. In a group of 18 patients, we planned preoperatively to achieve a total tumour resection in 16 cases and a non total tumour resection in 2 patients. After the first intra-operative MRI control, we achieved our goal respectively in 15 cases and in 2 cases: we needed a second intra-operative MRI control to achieve the last ultimate tumour resection. In our series we achieved a total tumour resection in almost 90% of our patients.

Table 27.1 Intraoperative MRI in 398 Pituitary Adenomas and Craniopharyngiomas (Personal Experience of the Senior Author)

Period	1996–2001 ER	2002–2005 ER	March 2007–February 2010 INI
IMRI	0.2 T Magnetom	1.5 T Sonata	1.5 T Espree
Pituitary adenoma	61	203	63
Craniopharyngioma	26	27	18

Abbreviations: ER, Erlangen University; INI, International Neuroscience Institute; MRI, magnetic resonance imaging.

In tumors with parasellar extension, we differentiated between (1) displacement of the cavernous sinus, (2) focal invasion with protrusion through the middle wall of the cavernous sinus, and (3) general invasiveness. Tumor parts located in the lateral part of the cavernous sinus, lateral from the carotid artery, were regarded as not totally resectable (NTR).

Patients with nonsecreting residual tumor remnants were followed closely with postoperative MRI; if tumor growth was detected, patients were scheduled for stereotactic radiosurgery. In patients with secreting tumors, further medical therapy or stereotactic radiosurgery was recommended.

Current Results

The senior author started using IMRI in 1996 in Erlangen, Germany, and has used it in nearly 400 patients with pituitary tumors (**Table 27.1**).

Between February 2007 and February 2010, a consecutive series of 81 patients (35 female and 46 male; ages 3 to 84 years) who harbored 63 pituitary macroadenomas and 18 craniopharyngiomas underwent mainly transsphenoidal surgery at the International Neuroscience Institute, Hannover, Germany.

To evaluate the extent of adenoma removal, high-field MRI was performed during sella exploration once in 58 cases, twice in 22 cases, and three times in one case (**Fig. 27.2**). All patients underwent a comprehensive preoperative and postoperative endocrinologic and ophthalmologic evaluation. Endocrinologic findings were documented as partial pituitary functions (hypogonadism, hypothyroidism, hypocortisolism, and diabetes insipidus).

Before surgery, all patients gave their informed consent for intraoperative MRI.

Tumor visualization with the high-field 1.5-T IMRI Espree scanner in the operating room with the patient under anesthesia was very good and provided even better congruency with the preoperative high-field MRI (1.5 T) (**Figs. 27.3** and **27.4**).

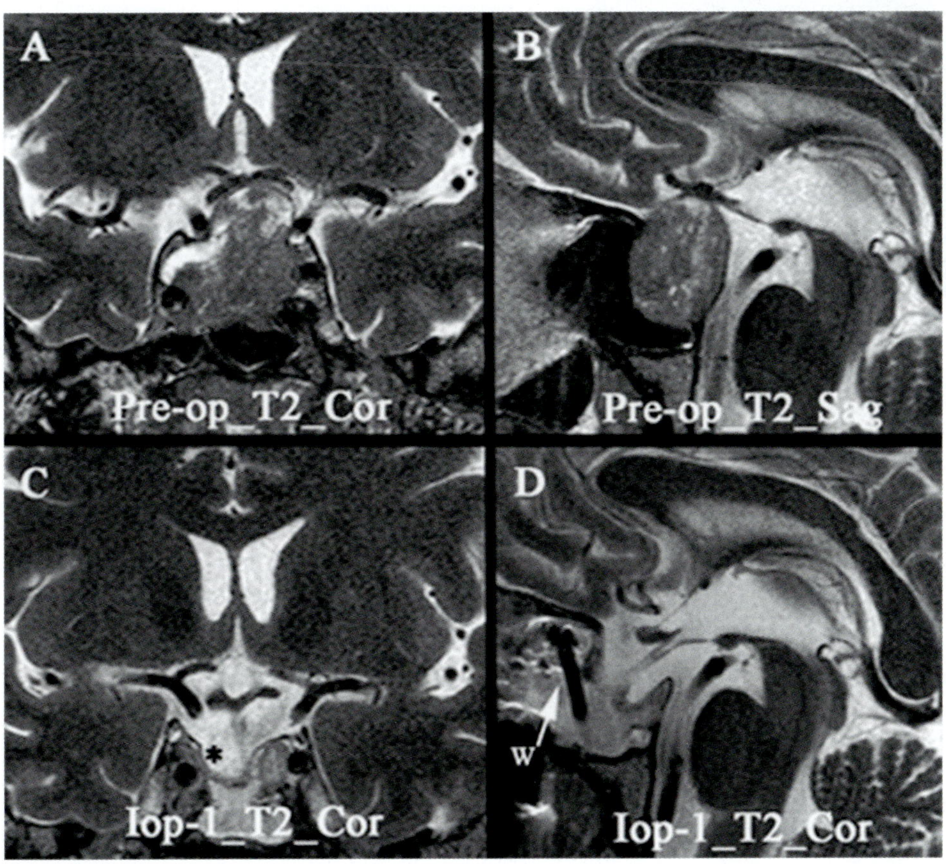

Fig. 27.3 Patient K.S., a 56-year-old woman. **(A,B)** Preoperative: Intra- and suprasellar hormonally inactive pituitary adenoma. **(C,D)** Intraoperative 1: Complete tumor removal, with descent of the infundibulum and diaphragma sellae to the middle of the sella and preserved pituitary gland below the diaphragma and in the posterior sella part. *, decompressed middle wall of the cavernous sinus; W, wax.

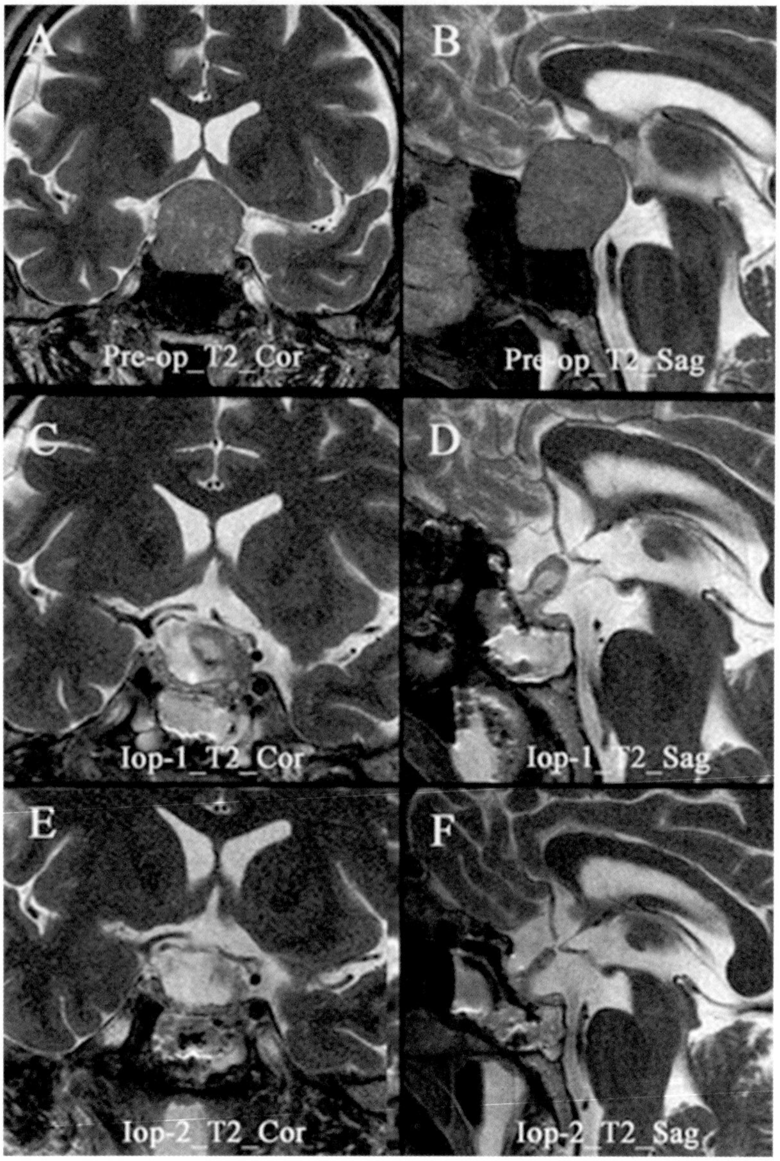

Fig. 27.4 Patient N.A., a 46-year-old man. **(A,B)** Preoperative: Intra- and suprasellar hormonally inactive pituitary adenoma; initial chiasma syndrome and secondary hypoadrenalism. **(C,D)** Intraoperative 1: Intraoperative asymmetric incomplete descent of the diaphragma sellae with attachment to the pituitary stalk. Small tumor remnant is seen in the fold of the diaphragma anterior to the pituitary stalk. **(E,F)** Intraoperative 2: Complete selective adenomectomy, with preservation of the pituitary gland in the middle lateral left position. Normalization of adrenal function.

Preoperatively we distinguished between totally and NTR tumors. NTR was defined as invasion of the lateral part of the cavernous sinus, asymmetrical suprasellar extension, and generally invasive pituitary adenomas.

In eight of 65 patients (12%) in whom tumors had encased the carotid arteries, or the sphenoid sinus was only poorly pneumatized, we used the integrated navigation system for the surgical transsphenoidal approach and intraoperative guidance for tumor removal; for the transcranial approach, we used navigation in 16 of 16 patients.

A total of 39 of 81 patients (48%) had uni- or bilateral cavernous sinus invasion on preoperative MRI. Therefore, intended complete resection was considered to be possible only in 58 of 81 patients (72%). According to tumor residuals, detected by IMRI, further surgery was required in a total of 23 of these 81 patients (28%) (**Fig. 27.5**). An additional tumor resection was possible in 18 of 58 patients (31%) with intended complete tumor resection. In two of 23 patients (9%) in whom incomplete tumor resection was initially planned, total resectability was achieved based on the intraoperative finding; no extensive invasion but rather displacement of the cavernous sinus was found.

In 23 of 81 patients (28%), IMRI control showed accessible residual tumors requiring further resection; 18 of them

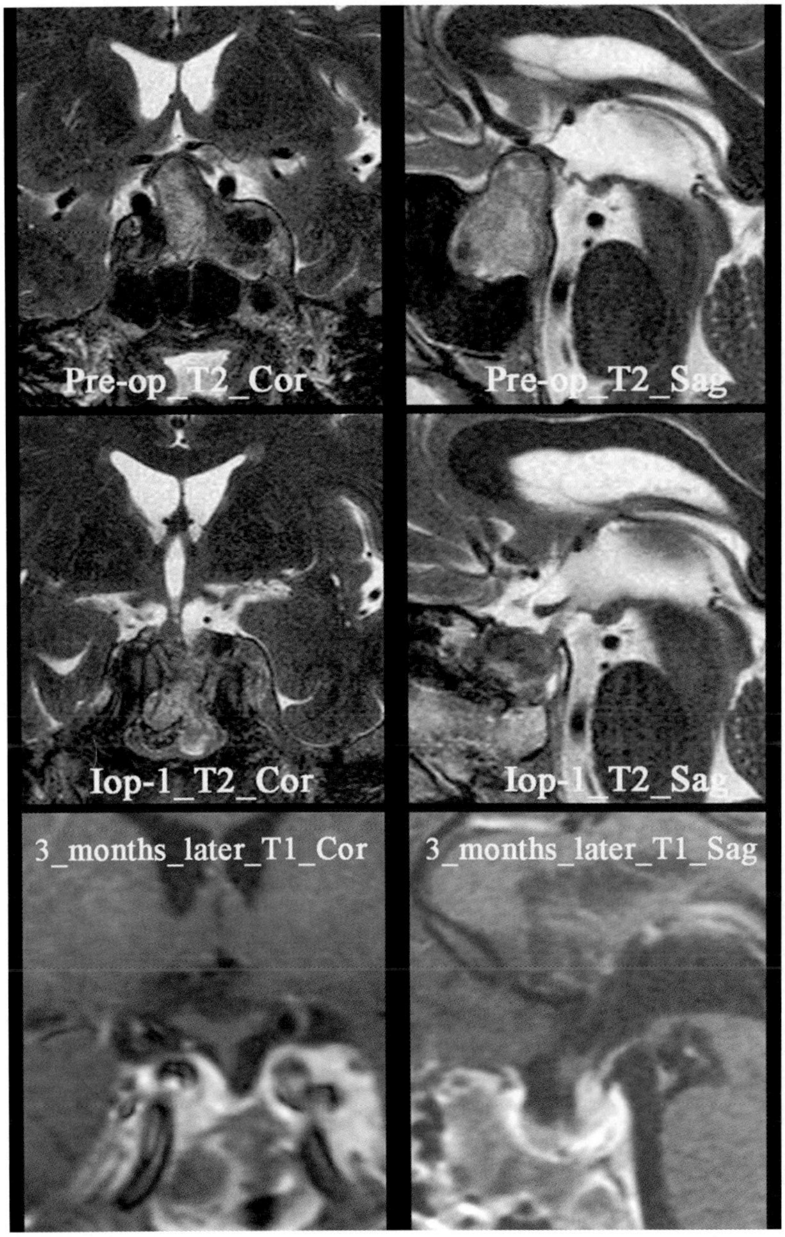

A,B

C,D

E,F

Fig. 27.5 Patient L.A., a 53-year-old man. **(A,B)** Preoperative: Intrasellar and irregular suprasellar and invasive left cavernous sinus prolactin-producing pituitary adenoma. Nonresponder after dopaminergic therapy over a period of 4 months. Secondary hypogonadism. **(C,D)** Intraoperative 1: Complete resection of intra- and suprasellar tumors part. Normalization of chiasma syndrome. Descent and preservation of the pituitary gland located in the right and middle sella part. Nonresectable firm tumor part in the cavernous sinus, mainly lateral to the carotid artery. **(E,F)** Postoperative: Control after 3 months. Preservation of pituitary function and a decrease in but not normalization of the prolactin levels. Gamma-knife therapy.

achieved a complete resection, and the other five achieved a partial tumor resection. This group benefits the most from the use of IMRI.

After tumor resection, the final IMRI scan demonstrated adequate decompression of the optic pathway in all patients.

Implementation of IMRI led to an increased operative time of either 20 or 40 minutes, depending on whether one or two MRI scans were acquired. Sensitivity of the IMRI was of 100% for those tumors located in the suprasellar, intrasellar, and lateral parasellar regions.

In seven patients (9%), the intraoperative interpretation of IMRI was equivocal; thus, it was difficult to distinguish between very small tumor remnants and perioperative changes and artifacts produced by blood and fibrin glue.

For craniopharyngiomas, we found high-field IMRI helpful in achieving complete tumor resection for both intra- and suprasellar tumors and also for laterally located solid tumors that were misdiagnosed as middle cavernous sinus wall (**Fig. 27.6**).[20] In frontolateral craniotomoies, we rarely overlooked tumor remnants of supra- and retrosellar-

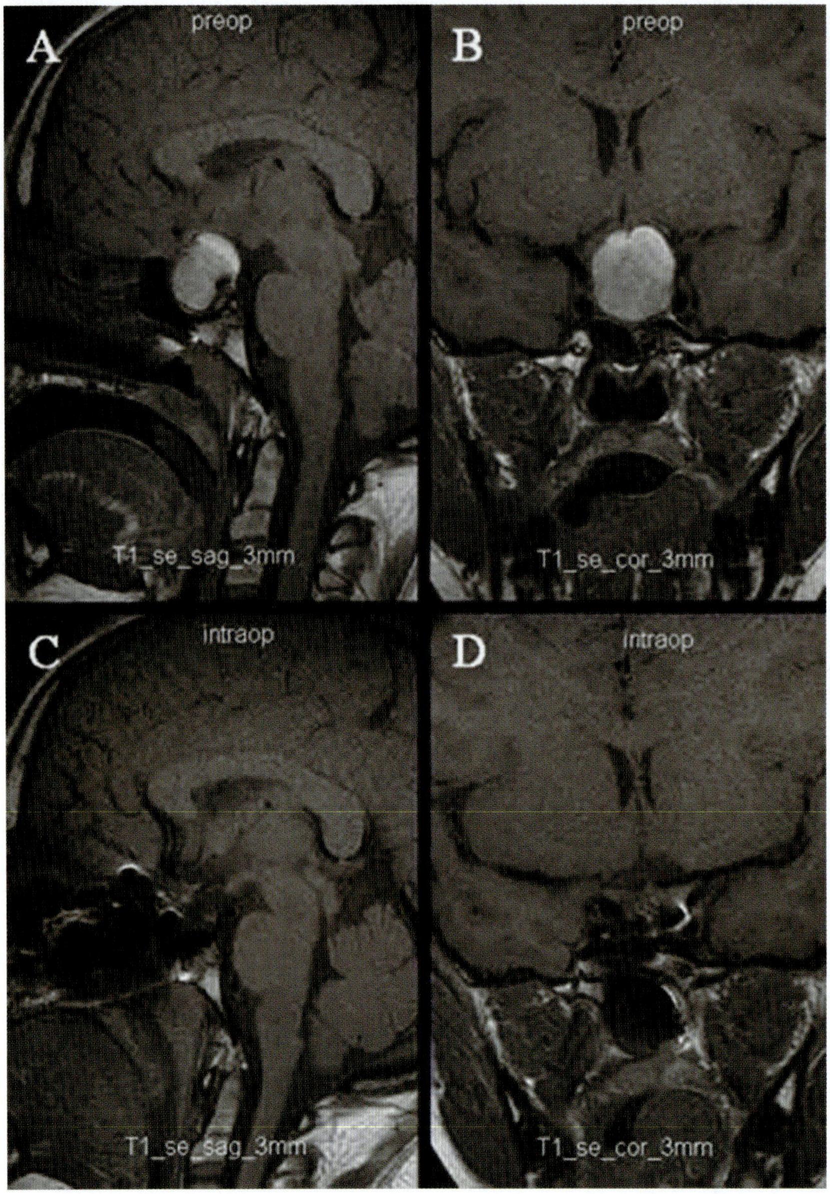

Fig. 27.6 Patient T.A.M., a 15-year-old girl. **(A,B)** Preoperative: Intra- and suprasellar, mixed solid and cystic craniopharyngioma. Dorsal calcified plate, loss of visual acuity, and temporal hemianopsia of the left eye. Panhypopituitarism. Direct transnasal transsphenoidal microscopic, endoscopic assisted approach. **(C,D)** Intraoperative 1: Complete tumor removal. Descending of the optic chiasma, normalization of the chiasma syndrome, no improvement of the pituitary function.

located craniopharyngiomas; however, IMRI helped us identify and preserve the pituitary stalk (**Fig. 27.7**).

Comparison of high-field MRI performed intraoperatively and 3 months later demonstrated very high predictive value for intraoperative examination (preoperative = intraoperative = 3 months postoperative MRI). This comparison also applies to our current experience, which is that the 3-month postoperative MRI scans are no longer necessary in most patients with complete resected pituitary adenomas (**Fig. 27.8**).

In our experience intraoperative high-field MRI in transsphenoidal surgery is a safe and reliable technique. We have not observed any infections in this series and no adverse events related to intraoperative high-field MRI; there were no accidents caused by the ferromagnetic instruments.

Discussion

Utility of IMRI in pituitary surgery has been proven by an increasing number of surgeons who find that imaging guidance and control are necessary in challenging cases.[8,21]

For more than 10 years, neurosurgeons around the world have been acquiring experience with IMRI in operating rooms, starting with low-field MRI. We estimate that currently there are a total of 150 intraoperative MRI installations, of which

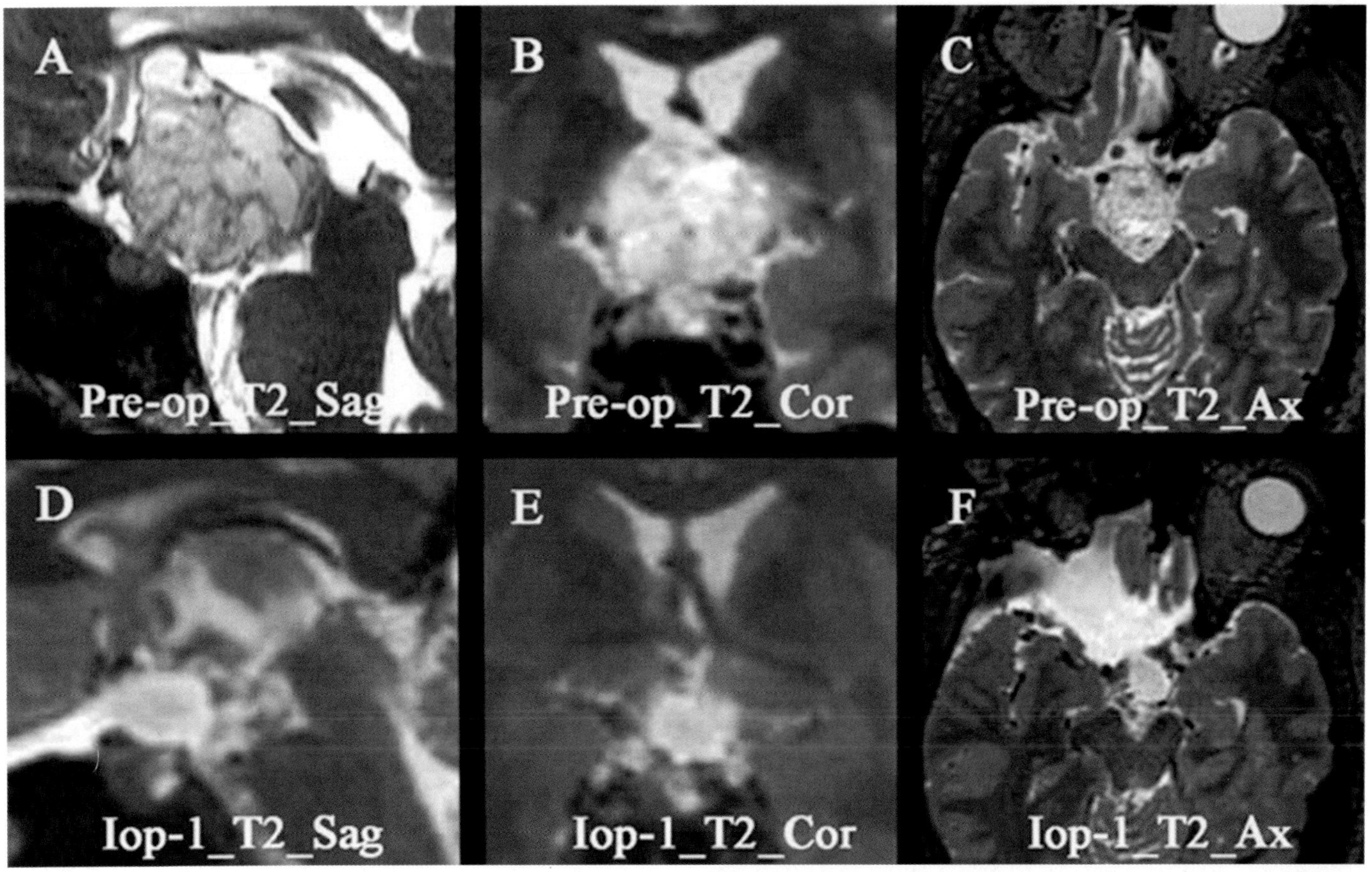

Fig. 27.7 Patient C.C., a 38-year-old man. **(A–C)** Preoperative: Mainly solid supra- and retrosellar craniopharyngioma. Navigated frontolateral craniotomy with translamina terminalis and right parachiasmatic approach. **(D–F)** Intraoperative: Complete tumor removal, with preservation of the pituitary stalk and retrosellar displacement. Pre- and postoperative incomplete pituitary insufficiency. No postoperative deterioration.

approximately 60% appear to be low-field and 40% high-field scanners.

High-field (1.5 T) and ultra-high-field (3 T) IMRI scanners are already becoming available from several manufacturers for clinical applications. Compared with low-field (0.15 and 0.2 T) and middle-field (0.4 T),[16] conventional high-field MRI units offer the advantage of a higher signal-to-noise ratio, which allows higher spatial resolution, and thus the images provide details approaching those of a histologic specimen.[17,22]

The lateral tumor's extension into the parasellar space, which occurs in 30 to 45% of pituitary adenomas, is the most common limiting factor in the resection of these tumors, especially in case of cavernous sinus invasion. The invasive parasellar growth of sella lesions through the medial border of the cavernous sinus is important for surgical planning, but visualization of the fine structure of the medial cavernous sinus border is often unsatisfactory with standard MRI. Therefore, prediction of cavernous sinus invasion based on MRI may rely on indirect signs such as encasement of the intracavernous internal carotid artery (ICA), replacement of the medial cavernous sinus compartment by tumor tissue, or tumor growth beyond a tangential line joining the intracavernous and supraclinoid segments of the ICA. Large sella tumors may flatten the normal pituitary gland so that it could be difficult to recognize it on preoperative conventional MRI. The preoperative knowledge of its position in relation to the lesion may be crucial for preserving its integrity and function.

Due to its higher resolution, 3-T MRI may enable the delineation of parasellar anatomy in such detail that the medial cavernous sinus border may be visible, which is particularly important for surgery for laterally invasive sellar lesions, and also provides optimal imaging during intraoperative navigation.[22] However, there are no data available that convincingly demonstrate that the 3-T IMRI is superior to the 1.5-T IMRI in imaging of pituitary lesions. This question could be

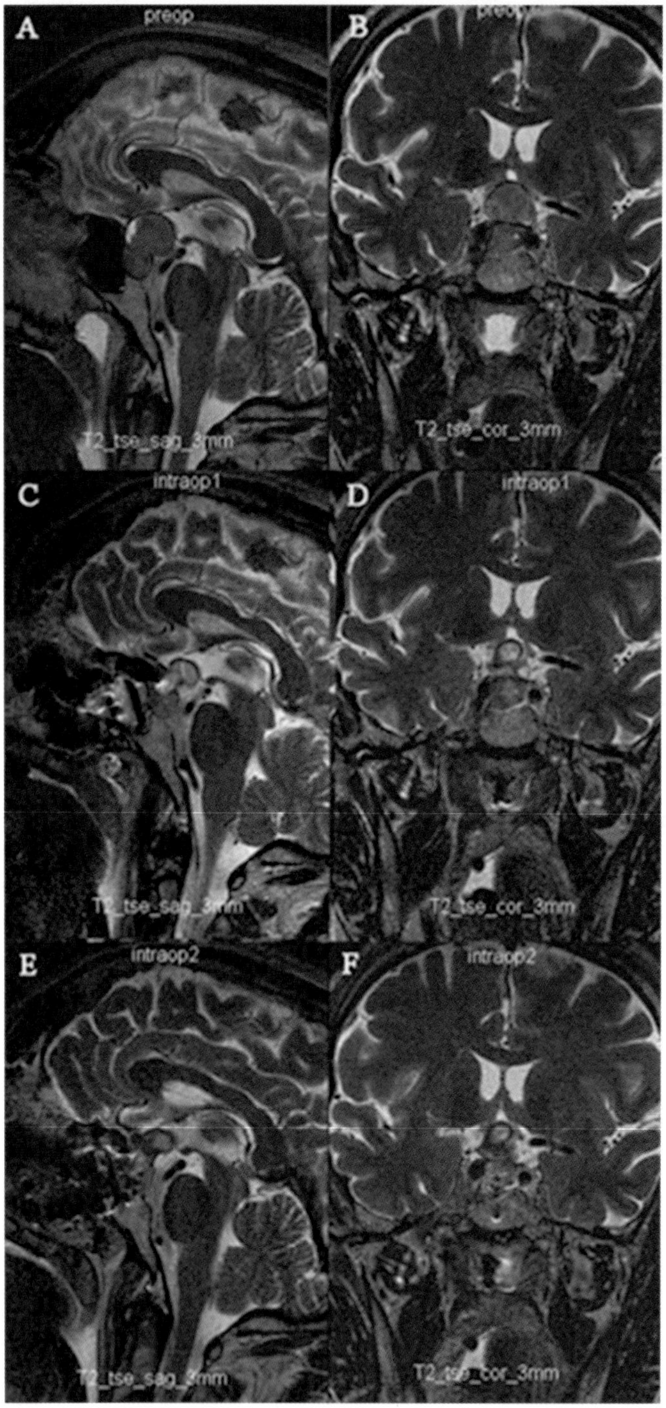

Fig. 27.8 Patient K.R., a 60-year-old man. **(A,B)** Preoperative: Intra- and mainly suprasellar, mixed solid and cystic, prolactin-producing pituitary adenoma, with old blood component. Almost amaurotic on the right side and progressive visual deficit on the left side. Direct transnasal transsphenoidal microscopic, endoscopic-assisted approach. **(C,D)** Intraoperative 1: Intraoperative asymmetric incomplete descent of diaphragm sella. Optimal optic chiasma decompression. Two small right dorsolateral tumor remnants. **(E,F)** Intraoperative 2: Complete tumor removal, with preservation of pituitary gland, left laterally dislocated.

answered by the introduction of useful head coils and solving the current problem of geometric distortion.

The intraoperative assessment of the completeness of tumor resection is often very difficult. Intraoperative surgical assessment based on direct visualization as well as the surgeon's eyes and experience is the standard. In the relatively small size of the operative field, the extensive recesses of the sella are often invisible, even with modern endoscopic techniques and even for expert neurosurgeons.

The application of all this technology increases the operating times only by a minimal amount. Except for the interruption of surgery for scanning, IMRI offers the opportunity for improved cure rates. The learning curve of the operating team is such that more frequent use of IMRI clearly improves scanning time and reduces unnecessary delays. Techniques for positioning and optimizing image quality are refined with increased experience.

The ability of IMRI to assess the extent of resection of pituitary macroadenomas depends also on its ability to provide technically adequate images for interpretation during an operation, which makes it easy to differentiate residual tumor from the adjacent anatomical structures (e.g., optic chiasm, infundibulum, and normal gland) and from artifacts caused by surgery. We prefer T2-weighted images for obtaining rapid information about large remnants, and then we continue with surgery without having to perform multiple sequences such as T1.

Application of a piece of bone wax at the position of the removed sellar floor followed by saline irrigation, which remains in the cavity during imaging, prevents problems with image interpretation such as blood mimicking tumor remnants.

Other practices to define the tumor cavity by implantation of Gelfoam are discussed elsewhere.[23,24]

Intraoperative high-field MRI scanning increases the rate of complete removal of macroadenomas, so that we improved our previous rate[25] from 60 to 100% in the resectable tumors in which complete tumor removal seemed to be possible via the transsphenoidal approach. In our actual series, we achieved in 70% of our patients (44 of 63) a total tumor resection. Also, we achieved a total tumor resection successfully in 100% of our goal TR group (42/42). In addition, in 40% (17/42) of patients the total tumor resection was achieved after the first IMRI scan.

In the literature, improvement rates for total resections are described in 30 to 40% of cases[16,19,26]; higher resection rates are reported in series using high-field IMRI in contrast to lower resection rates in series using low-field IMRI.[9,16]

From our point of view and personal experience, early postoperative MRI outside the operating room directly after finishing surgery or 1 hour later can be helpful in rare selected cases, when fortunately, and in general surprisingly, no early artifacts are visible, but it is not an alternative to intraoperative imaging. Normally, too many artifacts (blood, plastic material, etc.) impair sufficient image interpretation.[27] Only images performed 2 to 3 months after surgery provide definitively reliable information about the extent of resection. The main disadvantage, however, is the missed opportunity for continuing tumor resection afforded by IMRI. Comparing the result of intraoperative imaging and scanning after 3 months, the rate of false-positives was very low at 6%, and there were no false-negative findings.

As important as IMRI is for experienced neurosurgeons during pituitary surgery, it is even more important for neurosurgeons with less experience in this field.

The utility of IMRI is also based on many ergonomic and financial considerations. The cost-benefit ratio also includes construction costs and the costs of shielding of the operating room, the available investment budget to purchase the IMRI system, and the requirements to use the scanner either strictly for intraoperative scans or also for diagnostic purposes.[28] A shared-resource magnetic resonance operating suite that facilitates performance of both neurosurgical and diagnostic procedures in a single unit greatly improves the cost-benefit ratio.[4] Only a few 1.5-T and even fewer 3-T MRI systems (in Istanbul, Praga, Calgary, Brussels) are currently used in patients with pituitary tumors, and such a huge investment is only reasonable if the installation is used intensively. After installation of such a system, the additional costs for a single surgical procedure are lower.

Conclusion

The utility of intraoperative MRI scanning in pituitary tumors has been documented by a significant increase in the rate of totally resectable adenomas. Intraoperative imaging results in immediate intraoperative quality control, and immediately after surgery the surgical results are apparent. During the postoperative phase, there is no psychological stress for the patient and no waiting time, which is normally 3 months, to obtain an artifact-free MRI. In cases of residual tumor, immediate planning for further management is possible so that the surgical procedure can be continued or plans can be made for surveillance, transcranial resection, or treatment with antiproliferance substance or radiotherapy.

Whatever future developments and improvements may occur in IMRI for pituitary surgery, there are sufficient tools available today to improve traditional surgical results significantly.

References

1. Dina TS, Feaster SH, Laws ER Jr, Davis DO. MR of the pituitary gland postsurgery: serial MR studies following transsphenoidal resection. AJNR Am J Neuroradiol 1993;14:763–769
2. Elias WJ, Chadduck JB, Alden TD, Laws ER Jr. Frameless stereotaxy for transsphenoidal surgery. Neurosurgery 1999;45:271–275, discussion 275–277
3. Gerlach R, du Mesnil de Rochemont R, Gasser T, et al. Feasibility of Polestar N20, an ultra-low-field intraoperative magnetic resonance imaging system in resection control of pituitary macroadenomas: lessons learned from the first 40 cases. Neurosurgery 2008;63:272–284, discussion 284–285
4. McPherson CM, Bohinski RJ, Dagnew E, Warnick RE, Tew JM. Tumor resection in a shared-resource magnetic resonance operating room: experience at the University of Cincinnati. Acta Neurochir Suppl (Wien) 2003;85:39–44
5. Schulder M, Sernas TJ, Carmel PW. Cranial surgery and navigation with a compact intraoperative MRI system. Acta Neurochir Suppl (Wien) 2003;85:79–86
6. Black PM, Moriarty T, Alexander E III, et al. Development and implementation of intraoperative magnetic resonance imaging and its

neurosurgical applications. Neurosurgery 1997;41:831–842, discussion 842–845

7. Fahlbusch R, Ganslandt O, Buchfelder M, Schott W, Nimsky C. Intraoperative magnetic resonance imaging during transsphenoidal surgery. J Neurosurg 2001;95:381–390
8. Schwartz TH, Stieg PE, Anand VK. Endoscopic transsphenoidal pituitary surgery with intraoperative magnetic resonance imaging. Neurosurgery 2006;58(1, Suppl):ONS44–ONS51, discussion ONS44–ONS51
9. Arita K, Kurisu K, Tominaga A, et al. Trans-sellar color Doppler ultrasonography during transsphenoidal surgery. Neurosurgery 1998;42: 81–85, discussion 86
10. Cappabianca P, Cavallo LM, Colao A, de Divitiis E. Surgical complications associated with the endoscopic endonasal transsphenoidal approach for pituitary adenomas. J Neurosurg 2002;97:293–298
11. Doppman JL, Ram Z, Shawker TH, Oldfield EH. Intraoperative US of the pituitary gland. Work in progress. Radiology 1994;192:111–115
12. Hardy J, Wigser SM. Trans-sphenoidal surgery of pituitary fossa tumors with televised radiofluoroscopic control. J Neurosurg 1965; 23:612–619
13. Lasio G, Ferroli P, Felisati G, Broggi G. Image-guided endoscopic transnasal removal of recurrent pituitary adenomas. Neurosurgery 2002;51:132–136, discussion 136–137
14. Martin CH, Schwartz R, Jolesz F, Black PM. Transsphenoidal resection of pituitary adenomas in an intraoperative MRI unit. Pituitary 1999;2:155–162
15. Anand VK, Schwartz TH, Hiltzik DH, Kacker A. Endoscopic transsphenoidal pituitary surgery with real-time intraoperative magnetic resonance imaging. Am J Rhinol 2006;20:401–405
16. Jho HD, Alfieri A. Endoscopic endonasal pituitary surgery: evolution of surgical technique and equipment in 150 operations. Minim Invasive Neurosurg 2001;44:1–12
17. Nimsky C, Ganslandt O, Fahlbusch R. Comparing 0.2 tesla with 1.5 tesla intraoperative magnetic resonance imaging analysis of setup, workflow, and efficiency. Acad Radiol 2005;12:1065–1079
18. Dort JC, Sutherland GR. Intraoperative magnetic resonance imaging for skull base surgery. Laryngoscope 2001;111:1570–1575
19. Jane JA Jr, Thapar K, Alden TD, Laws ER Jr. Fluoroscopic frameless stereotaxy for transsphenoidal surgery. Neurosurgery 2001; 48:1302–1307, discussion 1307–1308
20. Nimsky C, Ganslandt O, Hofmann B, Fahlbusch R. Limited benefit of intraoperative low-field magnetic resonance imaging in craniopharyngioma surgery. Neurosurgery 2003;53:72–80, discussion 80–81
21. Pergolizzi RS Jr, Nabavi A, Schwartz RB, et al. Intra-operative MR guidance during trans-sphenoidal pituitary resection: preliminary results. J Magn Reson Imaging 2001;13:136–141
22. Nimsky C, Ganslandt O, Von Keller B, Romstöck J, Fahlbusch R. Intraoperative high-field-strength MR imaging: implementation and experience in 200 patients. Radiology 2004;233:67–78
23. Bohinski RJ, Warnick RE, Gaskill-Shipley MF, et al. Intraoperative magnetic resonance imaging to determine the extent of resection of pituitary macroadenomas during transsphenoidal microsurgery. Neurosurgery 2001;49:1133–1143, discussion 1143–1144
24. Fahlbusch R, Keller B, Ganslandt O, Kreutzer J, Nimsky C. Transsphenoidal surgery in acromegaly investigated by intraoperative high-field magnetic resonance imaging. Eur J Endocrinol 2005;153:239–248
25. Nimsky C, von Keller B, Ganslandt O, Fahlbusch R. Intraoperative high-field magnetic resonance imaging in transsphenoidal surgery of hormonally inactive pituitary macroadenomas. Neurosurgery 2006;59:105–114, discussion 105–114
26. Knosp E, Steiner E, Kitz K, Matula C. Pituitary adenomas with invasion of the cavernous sinus space: a magnetic resonance imaging classification compared with surgical findings. Neurosurgery 1993;33:610–617, discussion 617–618
27. Kiliç T, Ekinci G, Seker A, Elmaci I, Erzen C, Pamir MN. Determining optimal MRI follow-up after transsphenoidal surgery for pituitary adenoma: scan at 24 hours postsurgery provides reliable information. Acta Neurochir (Wien) 2001;143:1103–1126
28. Wolfsberger S, Ba-Ssalamah A, Pinker K, et al. Application of three-tesla magnetic resonance imaging for diagnosis and surgery of sellar lesions. J Neurosurg 2004;100:278–286

28 Limited Utility of Intraoperative MRI in Endoscopic Pituitary Surgery

Ilya Laufer, Vijay K. Anand, and Theodore H. Schwartz

Pituitary neoplasms represent 15 to 20% of all intracranial tumors. The overwhelming majority of pituitary tumors are low-grade adenomas. As with most low-grade neoplasms, total resection may be curative and therefore represents the goal of pituitary surgery.[1] Additional goals of pituitary surgery are decompression of the optic apparatus and preservation or restoration of normal pituitary function.[2] Unfortunately, large operative series show recurrence rates of 5 to 20% in various types of pituitary adenomas and gross total resection rates of 30 to 90%, signifying that complete cure may not always be possible.[1] This may be attributed to the tumor's invasion of the cavernous sinus, or envelopment of the carotid artery or the visual apparatus, leading to the surgeon's intentionally leaving residual tumor or to the surgeon's inability to visualize tumor remnants during the operation and leaving unintentional residual tumor. Attempts to evacuate tumor that is adherent to vital structures may lead to devastating complications and generally should be avoided, although sharp dissection in these situations may be feasible. On the other hand, incomplete visualization of the tumor may lead to postoperative residual tumor that could have been safely removed during the initial operation. Residual tumor requires treatment with radiation therapy, repeat operation, or pharmacotherapy, all of which could have been avoided had the residual tumor been appreciated during the first operation. These factors serve as a great impetus to continually improve the surgeon's ability to visualize pituitary tumors and the surrounding structures.

Neurosurgeons employ numerous adjuncts to safely maximize the extent of tumor evacuation. Intraoperative ultrasound and echo probes permit the localization of the carotid arteries[3] as well as localization of residual tumor.[4,5] Intraoperative magnetic resonance imaging (IMRI), which continues to proliferate as high-power imaging units become more available and affordable, provides the surgeon with the ability to evaluate the extent of resection radiographically while the patient is still under anesthesia. A "second look" can be performed during the first operation to remove any residual tumor.[6–11] Likewise, evolving hematomas, although rare in occurrence, can be visualized and treated before the patient leaves the operating room. Finally, endoscopy has increased the size of the operative field, permitting surgeons to see around corners by bringing the light source and the scope lens directly into the operative field and using angled scopes to see structures that are not in the direct line of sight.[12–17] Both IMRI and endoscopy have similar functions, which increases the ability of the surgeon to remove the entire tumor safely. This chapter discusses the issues that will be involved in definitively determining whether one technology achieves this goal more effectively than the other or whether they provide complementary information.

■ Intraoperative MRI

MRI technology, in combination with stereotaxis, was introduced into the operating room to maximize the safety and efficacy of surgery. In skull base surgery, it allows precise localization of vital structures such as the carotid artery and cranial nerves. Exact determination of their location in three-dimensional space in reference to the lesion boundaries and the resection cavity maximizes the surgeon's ability to avoid and preserve those structures. Furthermore, MRI allows visualization of certain portions of the lesion that extend beyond normal lines of sight, such as the suprasellar cistern or the superior lateral aspect of the sella. Although conventional stereotaxis based on preoperative imaging also allows similar functions, any intraoperative shift of the anatomy renders these images useless. IMRI permits the surgeon to update the images and thus update the basis of stereotactic space. In addition, the appearance and consistency of certain portions of the lesion may not be readily discerned from normal tissue with the naked eye or magnification and may become apparent only with MRI after administration of intravenous contrast. Thus, intraoperative imaging may significantly enhance the safety of the operation as well as allow maximal resection of the lesion.[18]

The first intraoperative MR unit was introduced at the Brigham and Women's Hospital (Boston, MA) and was described by Black et al.[19] Since then, numerous IMRI suites have been introduced with a wide range of magnet strengths. Many of the high-power magnet suites rely on the principle of bringing the operating room to the MR suite. The patients may be positioned in the MRI donut, with the operation taking place within the confines of the imager. Alternatively, various permutations of moving imagers and operating room tables have been implemented to remove the patient from the imaging core and to allow comfortable positioning of the surgeon and staff. Although special nonferromagnetic instruments are required to operate in the proximity of the MRI donut, standard instruments may be used outside of the "fringe field," generally several feet away from the magnet.

Alternatively, several MR imagers were designed with the principle of bringing the imaging technology into the operating room, while attempting to alter as little of the standard operating room setup as possible. Such magnets generally have low magnetic field strength and may be stored under the operating table. Standard operating instruments may be used.

Low-Field-Strength IMRI

Low-field-strength imagers require minimal alteration of the operating room setup and workflow. The PoleStar N20 (Medtronic Navigation, Louisville, CO) uses a 0.15-tesla (T) magnet and has two vertical magnet poles (**Fig. 28.1**). The imager is mobile and may be stored in a recessed steel cage when not in use, allowing the operating room to be used for any procedure under standard protocols without MRI precautions. During IMRI-aided operations, the device is positioned under the patient's head and elevated to the operating field when imaging is desired. The imager allows a 15- × 20-cm field of view and does not impose restrictions on the positioning of the patient, enabling a full-lateral head position if required. Standard ferromagnetic instruments may be used when the imager is lowered but must be removed from the operating field during image acquisition. The mean additional time that was attributed to implementation of this imager has been reported as 1.1 hour, with a range of 0.5 to 2 hours.[10]

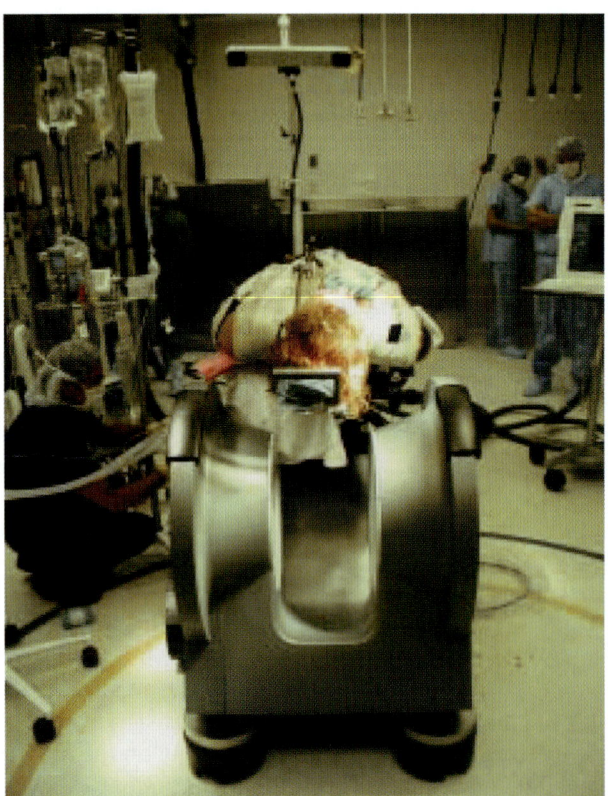

Fig. 28.1 An 0.15-Tesla imager installed at the University of Medicine and Dentistry of New Jersey Medical School.

A larger, nonmobile 0.2-T imager has been implemented at the University of Toronto. This imager also employs two vertical magnet poles. However, because the magnet is not mobile, the operating room table is moved into the imaging field when required and the operation is performed outside of the magnet to allow convenient access for two surgeons. Nonferromagnetic instruments are used inside the magnet, and regular instruments are used when the patient's head is 60 to 90 cm outside of the field. A specially designed nonferromagnetic nasal speculum and endoscopes are used in transsphenoidal surgery.[6]

An alternative 0.2-T imager (Open Viva, Siemens Medical Solutions, Hannover, Germany) uses two horizontally positioned magnets mounted on a C-arm (**Fig. 28.2**). The operating table has tilting and rotating capabilities allowing for placing the patient in Trendelenburg and reverse Trendelenburg positions and tilting the operating field to obtain optimal visualization. Standard operating instruments may be used when outside of the magnet field. However, when endoscopy was used, MR-compatible scope, light-source, camera, and LCD display were required. An average imaging time of 35 minutes was reported.[8]

The surgical team in the Oulu University Hospital in Finland has been using a 0.23-T, horizontally open imager. The magnet has fast shutdown and power-up capabilities (6 minutes). Thus, the operation is performed with the magnet turned off. When imaging is desired, non–MRI-compatible instruments, including electrocautery, endoscopes, operating microscope, and ferromagnetic instruments, are moved outside of the 5-mT line or into an adjacent room, and the magnet is turned on. Each imaging session requires approximately 30 to 40 minutes.[20]

Finally, a 0.3-T imaging unit (AIRIS II, Hitachi Medical Corp., Tokyo, Japan) has been actively employed at the University of Cincinnati Medical Center. The imager is similar to open-MRI systems that use two horizontal magnets. This imager is housed in a room that is adjacent to the standard operating room. The operation may take place in the standard operating room, and the patient is transported to the scanner through a sterile corridor, or the operation may be performed in the MRI room with the patient's head positioned either within the imaging isocenter or outside of it. Each intraoperative scanning session added approximately 20 minutes to the operative time. Such setup allows the use

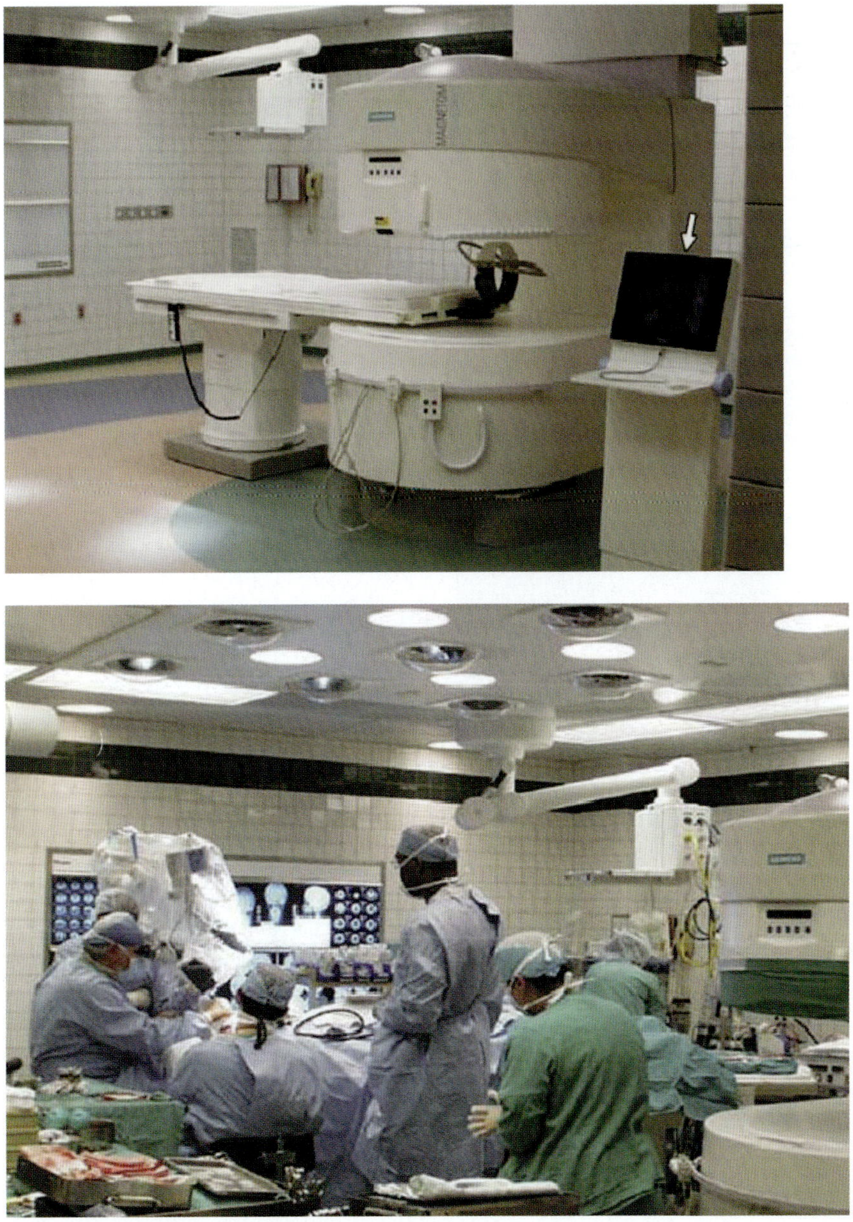

A

B

Fig. 28.2 **(A)** A 0.2-Tesla open intraoperative imager installed at the University Hospitals of Cleveland/Case Western Reserve University. **(B)** When the operating table is outside of the scanner, standard operating room instruments may be used.

of the MR imager for nonoperative imaging, although a 1-hour sterile cleansing procedure must be performed prior to operative imaging.[21]

Mid-Field-Strength IMRI

Several centers employ a 0.5-T "double-donut" imaging system (Signa SP, General Electric Medical Systems, Milwaukee, WI) that was first used at the Brigham and Women's Hospital (**Fig. 28.3**). The system uses two vertically oriented circular magnets with a vertical gap between them. The vertical gap between the two donuts allows access to the operative field for two surgeons. Because the patient's head is positioned in the magnet isocenter at all times, all of the operating instruments and the microscope must be MR-compatible. This machine allows real-time imaging while operating without moving the patient or the imager.[11,19]

High-Field Strength IMRI

A mobile 1.5-T imager was developed in Calgary, Canada (Innovative Magnetic Resonance Imaging Systems, Inc., Winnipeg, Manitoba, Canada). The ceiling-mounted magnet may be moved into the surgical field when imaging is desired (**Fig. 28.4**). This allows the use of standard operating equipment during the operations, as long as the ferromagnetic equipment is moved into the fringe zone during imaging. This imager avoids the movement of the patient

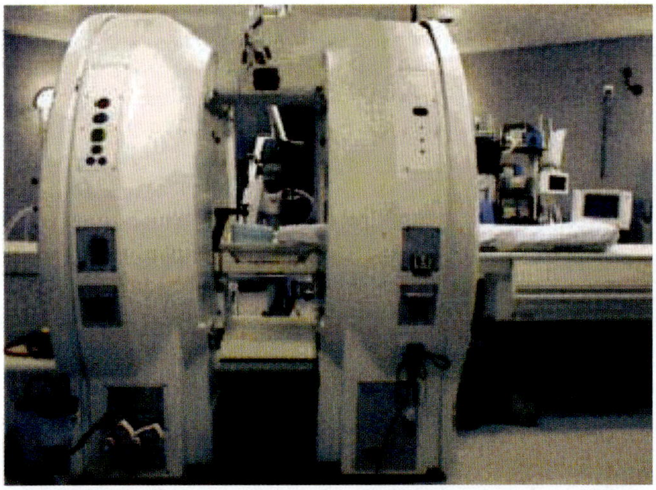

A

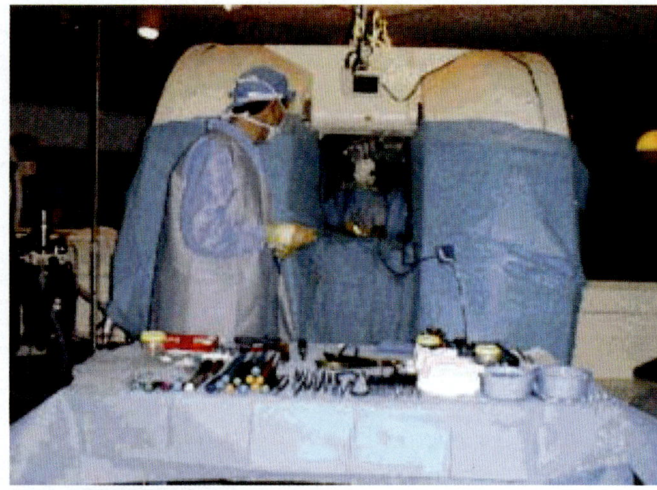

B

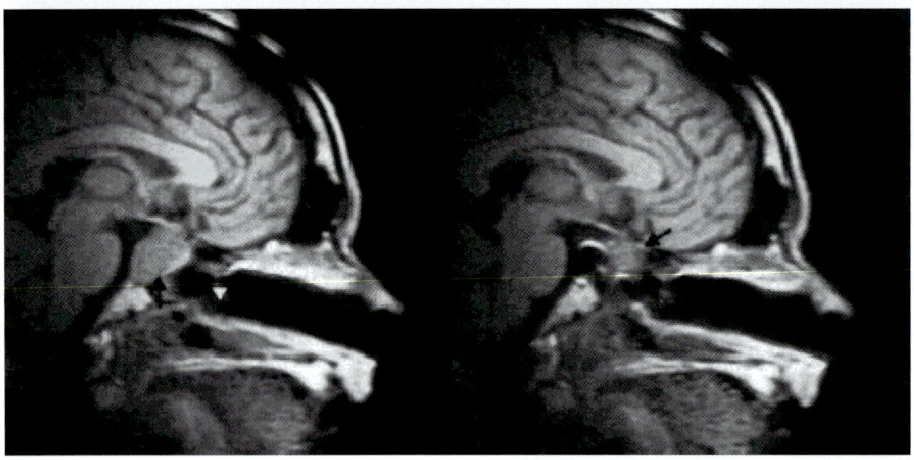

C

Fig. 28.3 **(A)** A 0.5-Tesla imager installed at Brigham and Women's Hospital (Boston, MA). **(B)** The open design of the imager allows the surgeon to have access to the patient while imaging is in progress. **(C)** Intraoperative images of a sella tumor pre-resection and after partial resection with residual tumor identified.

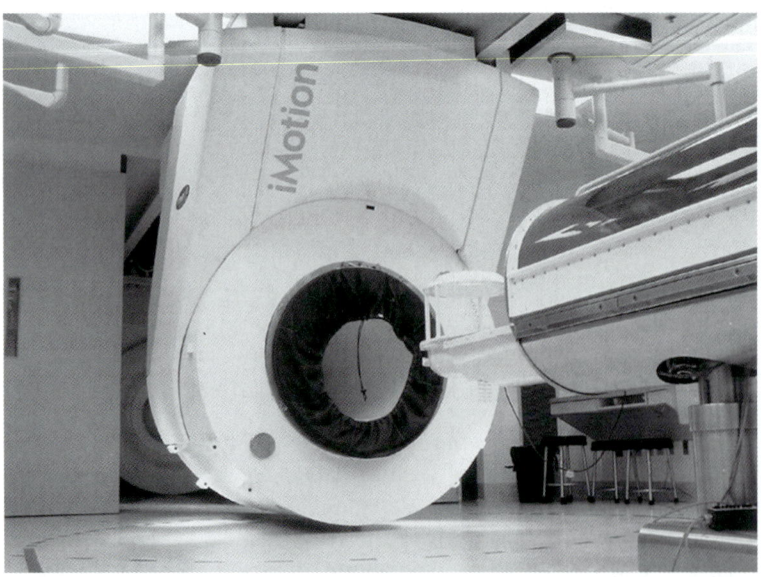

A

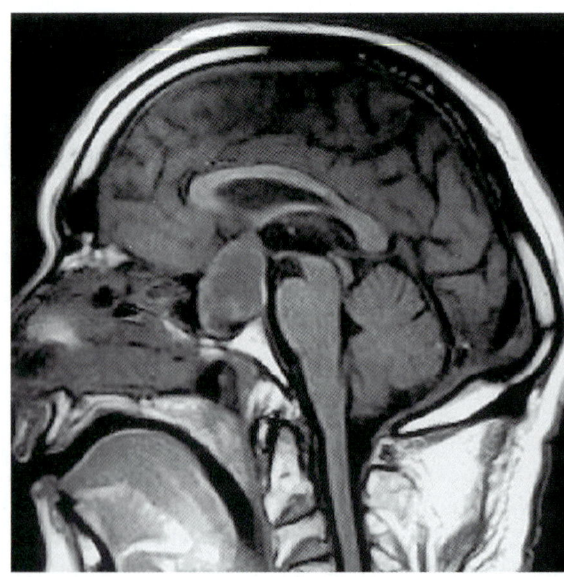

B

Fig. 28.4 **(A)** A 1.5-Tesla imager installed at the University of Calgary. The imager slides along a ceiling-mounted rail system, bringing the system to the operating field when required. **(B)** Image obtained prior to the start of resection shows a large pituitary tumor with suprasellar extension.

during the operation, potentially improving the safety of the procedure.[7] Positioning of the imager, acquisition of a set of T1-weighted images, and reexposure of the surgical field require approximately 25 minutes.

A different 1.5-T imager (Magnetom Sonata Maestro Class, Siemens Medical Solutions) has been developed in Erlangen, Germany (**Fig. 28.5**). The imager resembles standard stationary MR imagers and uses a rotating surgical table that can be rotated into and out of the imager. The operation is performed with the patient's head at the 0.5-mT line using standard operating equipment. The table height, as well as the longitudinal and lateral angles, may be modified.[9] This imaging system has permitted integration of functional imaging[22] and spectroscopy[23] into the intraoperative imaging sequences.

A similar 1.5-T imaging system (Intera I/T, Philips Medical Solutions, Best, Netherlands) has been employed at the University of Minnesota Medical Center. However, the authors prefer to perform the entire operation within the magnetic field using nonferromagnetic instrumentation, thus minimizing patient movement. It was estimated that tumor resection with intraoperative imaging took one-third longer than standard resection.[24] The same group is currently exploring applications of a 3-T magnet (Intera, Philips Medical Systems) in the operating room.[25]

The use of IMRI requires several substantial modifications to the operating room environment. The operating room must have radiofrequency shielding, and standard MR precautions must be taken by all staff. All electronic equipment plugged into wall outlets must be shut down, and in some circumstances plugs must even be removed from sockets. In some suites, a single switch can be created that will shut down all electronic equipment. Battery-operated devices are often acceptable and produce little electromagnetic noise. An alternative to shielding the entire operating room is the use of local radiofrequency shields that can be placed over the patient during imaging.[7] MR-compatible ventilators and anesthesia-delivery machines must be employed. Care must be taken to prevent contact of any cables with the patient's skin to avoid burns. Furthermore, all transducers must be kept outside of the scanner to avoid artifacts. A process of "troubleshooting" is often required to find sources of noise that may escape even the most careful of room designs. Although initial scans may need to be repeated several times until all sources of noise are eliminated, eventually the process can be done more rapidly.

Pituitary Surgery Outcomes

Operative Series Without IMRI

Operative gross total resection rates and postoperative recurrences vary with the type of pituitary adenoma. In addition, the size, grade, and stage of the tumor have been shown to correlate with residual and recurrence rates. A large series of 4050 patients with various adenoma subtypes that spanned 23 years of practice had total resection rates that ranged from 74 to 92% and increased with the surgeon's experience and technologic advances. The resection rate increased from 47% in patients with grade IV adenomas to 97% in grade I adenomas. In this series, 3286 patients with long-term MRI follow-up showed that 196 patients had residual tumor, of which 16 progressed with time. An additional 18 patients had tumor recurrence with a mean follow-up of 7.2 years.[2]

An operative series of 429 prolactinomas, with mean follow-up of 38 months, showed overall radiographic tumor control in 85% of patients and hormonal recovery in 52% of patients. In patients with invasive adenomas, only 39% underwent gross total resection, whereas 86% of patients with noninvasive adenomas had gross total resection.[26]

Several groups have reported on their experience with surgical treatment of growth hormone–secreting adenomas. A series of 139 patients with a median follow-up of 5.6 years showed an overall 68% endocrinologic remission rate, with 91% remission in microadenomas and 60% remission in macroadenomas. Furthermore, seven patients (7.4%) with initial surgical remission had evidence of endocrinologic recurrence.[27] A series of 254 patients showed postoperative remission in 76% of patients, with nine of these patients having disease recurrence. Follow-up of 41 patients from the postoperative persistent-disease group revealed that only 11 had persistent disease after pharmacologic and radiation therapy.[28] Finally, a series of 125 patients with acromegaly with 5.4 years of postsurgical follow-up showed 71% remission after surgery and radiation therapy. Gross total tumor evacuation was documented in 100% of microadenomas and in 82% of macroadenomas. An overall recurrence rate was noted in 5.4% of patients, all occurring in patients with macroadenomas.[29]

An operative series of 122 patients with Cushing's disease resulted in endocrinologic remission in 67% of patients with macroadenomas and in 91% of patients with microadenomas; 16% of patients with postoperative remission were noted to suffer a recurrence.[30] A larger series of 426 patients showed a similar recurrence rate of 15% in patients who had postoperative remission of Cushing's disease. Eighty-nine percent of patients who, by the surgeon's impression, had complete tumor resection achieved long-term disease control.[31]

Finally, a large series of nonfunctioning pituitary adenomas showed residual tumor in 36% of cases. Fourteen percent of these patients underwent repeat surgery to obtain adequate decompression of neural structures. Median follow-up of 53 months revealed recurrence in 83 of 436 patients (19%).

Operative Series with IMRI

Because MRI is a relatively new addition to the operating room, case series that specifically examine the role of IMRI

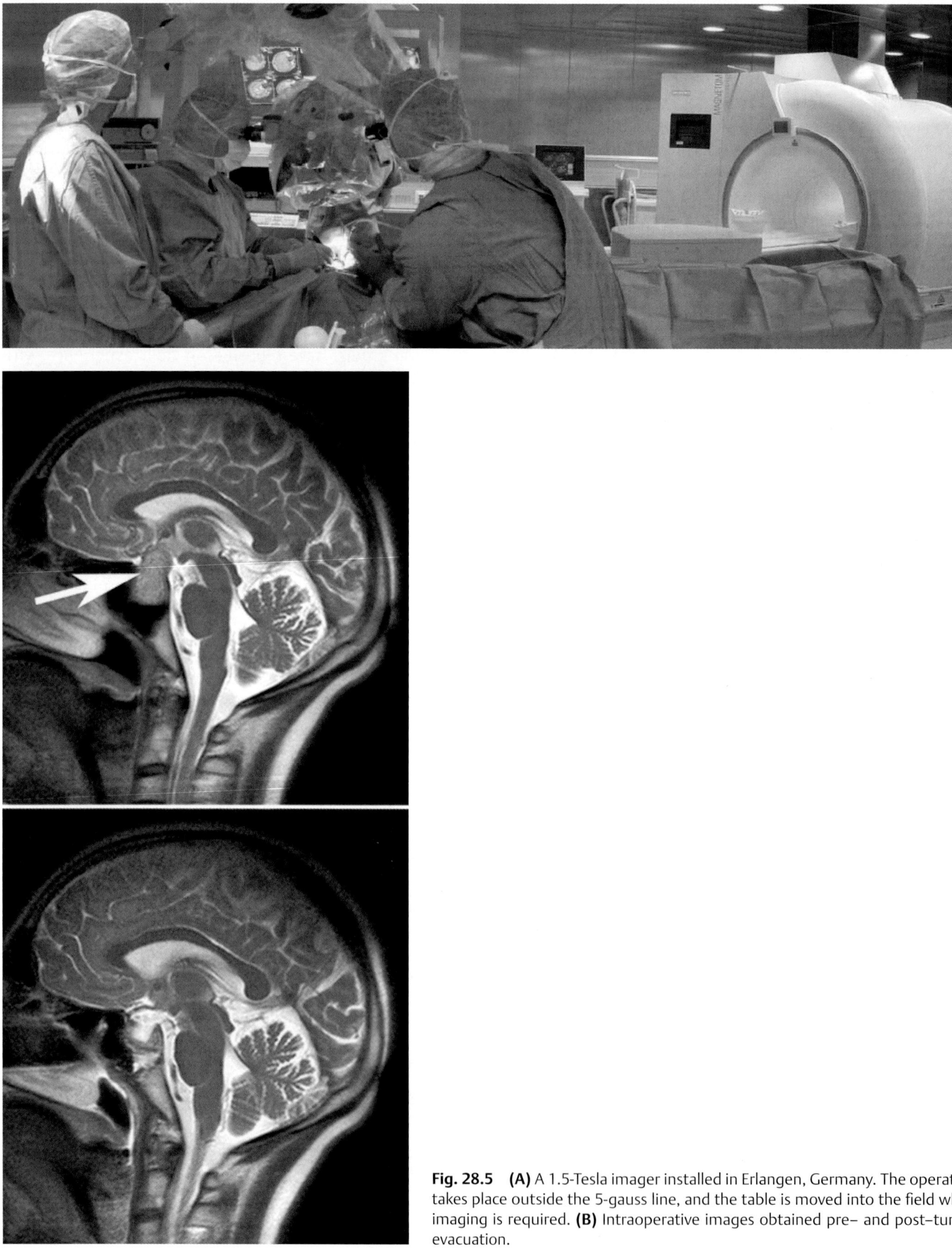

A

B

Fig. 28.5 **(A)** A 1.5-Tesla imager installed in Erlangen, Germany. The operation takes place outside the 5-gauss line, and the table is moved into the field when imaging is required. **(B)** Intraoperative images obtained pre– and post–tumor evacuation.

in resection of pituitary tumors generally include significantly fewer patients than the operative series mentioned in the previous section and much shorter follow-up times. Pergolizzi et al[32] published their experience with 17 patients who underwent transnasal pituitary resection with the assistance of the 0.5-T Signa SP system. Eight patients underwent primary resection, whereas the remaining nine were undergoing resection of recurrent or residual tumor. Preoperatively, sagittal and coronal T1-weighted spin echo images were obtained to guide the approach. Subsequently, additional T1-weighted sagittal sequences were obtained to determine the extent of tumor evacuation. Contrast-enhanced imaging was performed toward the end of the resection to precisely localize residual tumor. Upon resection completion, a T1 sagittal and a gradient echo sequence were performed to evaluate the extent of resection and to make certain that an evolving hematoma was not visualized. Final imaging showed residual tumor that was not visualized by the surgeon in seven cases (41%), leading to complete evacuation of the tumor remnants in all patients. The postresection gradient echo sequence diagnosed an expanding hematoma after the fat graft was put in place. The hematoma was evacuated, and complete hemostasis was achieved prior to completion of the operation.[33] An intraoperative injury to the intracavernous carotid artery that occurred during resection of tumor adherent to the cavernous wall was rapidly localized with MRI, and as hemostasis was obtained, distal flow was visualized and preserved. The patient accrual and follow-up period in this study span 3 years, and no recurrence was noted during this period.[32]

Dort and Sutherland[34] reported their experience with skull base surgery using the 1.5-T mobile ceiling-mounted intraoperative imager. Thirty-one patients were included in the series, with 15 patients having pituitary adenomas with suprasellar extension. Interdissection images revealed unexpected residual tumor in nine (60%) patients, and in eight of them the surgeons were able to complete the resection, resulting in 93% of patients having a gross total resection.

Thirty patients with macroadenomas underwent tumor resection with the aid of the 0.3-T AIRIS II imager. The authors occasionally used MRI to guide the approach. After resection, a localizing T1-weighted sagittal sequence was obtained, followed by pre- and postcontrast coronal sequences. In one patient with a recurrent tumor, brisk bleeding was encountered during tumor evacuation, and MRI showed a large hemorrhage with intraventricular extension. The operation was converted to a craniotomy and an A1 injury was identified. In the remaining 29 patients, the authors found the expected and desired extent of resection in only 10 patients (34%), with the remaining patients undergoing additional exploration and tumor evacuation.[35]

Operative Series Combining Endoscopy and IMRI

The Erlangen group has reported the largest operative series of IMRI-assisted pituitary adenoma resections. Tumor resection was performed using an operating microscope with endoscopic assistance. The group initially reported its experience with a 0.2-T imager in 44 patients[36] and subsequently, after advancing to a 1.5-T Magnetom Sonata imager, has reported on its experience resecting 106 hormonally inactive macroadenomas[37] and 23 growth hormone–secreting adenomas.[38] After obtaining localizer sequences, the authors obtained T1-weighted sagittal and coronal spin echo sequences followed by high-resolution T2-weighted turbo spin echo sequences. Each imaging session caused an approximately 15-minute-long interruption in the operation. Irrigation of the sellar floor with saline and application of bone wax to mimic the sellar floor decreased imaging artifact from pooled blood and air. Porcelain-coated drills also decreased imaging artifact. In the nonfunctioning macroadenoma group, initial postresection imaging showed total resection in 49 patients. Among the remaining 57 patients, 37 underwent additional evacuation of the imaged remnants. In the overall group, total resection was intended in 85 patients and intraoperative imaging increased the proportion of successful total resection from 58% to 82%. Among the 23 acromegalic patients, complete resection was intended in 18 patients. In eight of these patients, additional tumor evacuation increased the endocrinologic remission rate from 33% to 44%.

In our institution, pituitary surgery is performed using purely endoscopic technique. A combination of aggressive endoscopic resection and intraoperative imaging with PoleStar N10 0.12-T imager was performed in 15 patients. In three patients, IMRI revealed tumor remnants that were subsequently visualized with a 45-degree endoscope and resected, leading to completion of tumor evacuation. In an additional four patients, IMRI showed signal that was suspicious for unintended residual tumor, which upon further inspection turned out to be arachnoid folds and pooled blood. In three patients residual tumor was intentionally left in the cavernous sinus, and in the remaining five patients total resection was confirmed with initial intraoperative imaging. These results were confirmed with follow-up 1.5-T imaging at 3 months after the operation.[39] The relatively high rate of unnecessary reexploration (27%) led us to question routine intraoperative scanning with our low-field imager. As our experience and confidence increased with the use of angled endoscopes and increasing employment of extended transsphenoidal approaches, such as the transtuberculum and transplanum approaches, which allowed direct visualization in the suprasellar space, our center has abandoned low-field IMRI in favor of direct visualization using endoscope-assisted surgery. It is our impression that the combination of extended approaches with angled endoscopes will obviate the need for IMRI in most cases, and the few cases in which it might be helpful do not justify its use in all cases, given the extra time and expense it entails.

Endoscopic surgery has become an indispensable part of modern pituitary surgery. Multiple large operative series have shown that a purely endoscopic technique produces excellent tumor control results, comparable to microsurgical technique. Importantly, patient satisfaction and recovery times may be better after endoscopic surgery compared with traditional microscopic techniques.[12–17,40,41] Although the results with high-power magnets seem promising in endoscope-assisted pituitary surgery, low-power magnets may not be as useful. With popularization of endoscope-assisted and purely endoscopic surgery, the role for low-Tesla MR imagers in pituitary surgery may decrease and the role for high-Tesla magnets needs further investigation. Careful examination of preoperative MR images and thorough endoscopic exploration of all suspicious areas should result in adequate tumor resection in most cases. This should also avoid the unnecessary reexploration that occasionally results from the blood and arachnoid artifact with low-power magnets. However, high-power magnets may be beneficial in pituitary surgery if they have adequate resolution to differentiate tumor remnants from postsurgical artifact.

In macroadenomas where complete evacuation is not the goal, intraoperative imaging may be useful to determine whether the extent of decompression of the normal pituitary gland or the optic apparatus is sufficient. If the goal is to decompress the optic apparatus and to deliver postoperative radiation therapy to the residual tumor, intraoperative imaging with a high-power magnet may be useful in determining whether an adequate distance between remaining tumor and the optic chiasm was achieved.[42]

Currently, most of the intraoperative imaging systems incorporate frameless stereotaxy. Thus, all of the required preoperative and postoperative imaging may be performed using the intraoperative scanner at the time of surgery. Prior to the start of the operation, the initial navigation sequences may be acquired. Subsequently, needle biopsy, cyst aspiration, catheter positioning, tumor resection, or even deep brain stimulator insertion may be performed.[23,43] The extent of tumor resection or stimulator or catheter placement can then be evaluated intraoperatively and appropriate adjustments made prior to completion of the operation. Finally, the degree of final tumor resection may be assessed in the operating room, obviating the need for postoperative scanning. If required, postoperative adjuvant treatment can be discussed and planned immediately after the operation, rather than at the time of delayed postoperative imaging.

Financial Considerations

A few authors have addressed the financial justification of IMRI. Hall et al[44] reported a 55% decrease in the duration of hospital stay in patients who underwent first-time surgery for resection of brain tumors and a 31% decrease in patients with repeat resections. They also reported a 14% decrease in total hospital costs for patients with first-time resections. Schulder et al[10] also reported a decreased hospital stay in patients who underwent IMRI-assisted tumor resection, which, however, did not translate into a reduction in total hospitalization costs. The estimated cost of installation of a high-strength MR imager has been estimated at around $5 to $6 million[37] and remains to be validated through a decreased number of reoperations and recurrences, a decreased number of postsurgical adjuvant treatments, and a shorter and less complicated hospital stay. Ultimately, superior clinical outcomes and extended survival may be sufficient justification for this costly technology.

The role of intraoperative MRI in surgery of the sella remains to be defined. Intraoperative imaging may result in more complete resection of pituitary lesions, particularly in lesions with suprasellar extension. However, it is unclear how the use of IMRI influences the surgeon's decision to stop tumor evacuation and whether in such instances surgeons are more likely to be less aggressive with the resection, knowing that they will continue the operation after the imagining is completed. High-power MRI may be useful in select cases where the tumor is hidden from view by anatomical structures or where the degree of decompression of vital structures must be assessed. Endoscopy and IMRI are rapidly becoming part of the armamentarium of neurosurgeons. The large microsurgical series with extensive follow-up times and information about outcomes specifically related to tumor grades and hormonal activity are difficult to compare with the currently available publications describing the experience with endoscopy and IMRI. The endoscopic and intraoperative imaging series are limited by smaller numbers, paucity of grade and hormonal activity information, and much shorter follow-up times. However, both technologies show great promise and have already become incorporated into many academic centers. Long-term outcome studies are in progress to validate and assess the efficacy and relative contributions of each technique.

References

1. Kreutzer J, Fahlbusch R. Diagnosis and treatment of pituitary tumors. Curr Opin Neurol 2004;17:693–703
2. Shou XF, Li SQ, Wang YF, Zhao Y, Jia PF, Zhou LF. Treatment of pituitary adenomas with a transsphenoidal approach. Neurosurgery 2005;56:249–256, discussion 249–256
3. Dusick JR, Esposito F, Malkasian D, Kelly DF. Avoidance of carotid artery injuries in transsphenoidal surgery with the Doppler probe and micro-hook blades. Neurosurgery 2007;60(4, Suppl 2):322–328, discussion 328–329
4. Ram Z, Bruck B, Hadani M. Ultrasound in pituitary tumor surgery. Pituitary 1999;2:133–138
5. Suzuki R, Asai J, Nagashima G, et al. Transcranial echo-guided transsphenoidal surgical approach for the removal of large macroadenomas. J Neurosurg 2004;100:68–72

6. Bernstein M, Al-Anazi AR, Kucharczyk W, Manninen P, Bronskill M, Henkelman M. Brain tumor surgery with the Toronto open magnetic resonance imaging system: preliminary results for 36 patients and analysis of advantages, disadvantages, and future prospects. Neurosurgery 2000;46:900–907, discussion 907–909
7. Kaibara T, Saunders JK, Sutherland GR. Advances in mobile intraoperative magnetic resonance imaging. Neurosurgery 2000;47:131–137, discussion 137–138
8. Lewin JS, Nour SG, Meyers ML, et al. Intraoperative MRI with a rotating, tiltable surgical table: a time use study and clinical results in 122 patients. AJR Am J Roentgenol 2007;189:1096–1103
9. Nimsky C, Ganslandt O, Von Keller B, Romstöck J, Fahlbusch R. Intraoperative high-field-strength MR imaging: implementation and experience in 200 patients. Radiology 2004;233:67–78
10. Schulder M, Salas S, Brimacombe M, et al. Cranial surgery with an expanded compact intraoperative magnetic resonance imager. Technical note. J Neurosurg 2006;104:611–617
11. Seifert V, Zimmermann M, Trantakis C, et al. Open MRI-guided neurosurgery. Acta Neurochir (Wien) 1999;141:455–464
12. Cappabianca P, Cavallo LM, Colao A, et al. Endoscopic endonasal transsphenoidal approach: outcome analysis of 100 consecutive procedures. Minim Invasive Neurosurg 2002;45:193–200
13. Cappabianca P, Cavallo LM, de Divitiis O, Solari D, Esposito F, Colao A: Endoscopic pituitary surgery. Pituitary 2008;11(4):385–390
14. Jarrahy R, Berci G, Shahinian HK. Assessment of the efficacy of endoscopy in pituitary adenoma resection. Arch Otolaryngol Head Neck Surg 2000;126:1487–1490
15. Jho HD, Alfieri A. Endoscopic endonasal pituitary surgery: evolution of surgical technique and equipment in 150 operations. Minim Invasive Neurosurg 2001;44:1–12
16. Jho HD, Carrau RL. Endoscopic endonasal transsphenoidal surgery: experience with 50 patients. J Neurosurg 1997;87:44–51
17. Nasseri SS, Kasperbauer JL, Strome SE, McCaffrey TV, Atkinson JL, Meyer FB. Endoscopic transnasal pituitary surgery: report on 180 cases. Am J Rhinol 2001;15:281–287
18. Schwartz TH. Intraoperative magnetic resonance imaging in the surgical treatment of epilepsy. In: Broderick PA, Rahni DN, Kolodny EH, eds. Bioimaging in Neurodegeneration. Totowa, NJ: Humana Press; 2005:177–192
19. Black PM, Moriarty T, Alexander E III, et al. Development and implementation of intraoperative magnetic resonance imaging and its neurosurgical applications. Neurosurgery 1997;41:831–842, discussion 842–845
20. Yrjänä SK, Tuominen J, Koivukangas J. Intraoperative magnetic resonance imaging in neurosurgery. Acta Radiol 2007;48:540–549
21. Bohinski RJ, Kokkino AK, Warnick RE, et al. Glioma resection in a shared-resource magnetic resonance operating room after optimal image-guided frameless stereotactic resection. Neurosurgery 2001;48:731–742, discussion 742–744
22. Gasser T, Ganslandt O, Sandalcioglu E, Stolke D, Fahlbusch R, Nimsky C. Intraoperative functional MRI: implementation and preliminary experience. Neuroimage 2005;26:685–693
23. Hall WA, Truwit CL. Intraoperative MR-guided neurosurgery. J Magn Reson Imaging 2008;27:368–375
24. Martin AJ, Hall WA, Liu H, et al. Brain tumor resection: intraoperative monitoring with high-field-strength MR imaging-initial results. Radiology 2000;215:221–228
25. Hall WA, Galicich W, Bergman T, Truwit CL. 3-Tesla intraoperative MR imaging for neurosurgery. J Neurooncol 2006;77:297–303
26. Ozgen T, Oruckaptan HH, Ozcan OE, Acikgoz B. Prolactin secreting pituitary adenomas: analysis of 429 surgically treated patients, effect of adjuvant treatment modalities and review of the literature. Acta Neurochir (Wien) 1999;141:1287–1294
27. Ahmed S, Elsheikh M, Stratton IM, Page RC, Adams CB, Wass JA. Outcome of transsphenoidal surgery for acromegaly and its relationship to surgical experience. Clin Endocrinol (Oxf) 1999;50:561–567
28. Abosch A, Tyrrell JB, Lamborn KR, Hannegan LT, Applebury CB, Wilson CB. Transsphenoidal microsurgery for growth hormone-secreting pituitary adenomas: initial outcome and long-term results. J Clin Endocrinol Metab 1998;83:3411–3418
29. Freda PU, Wardlaw SL, Post KD. Long-term endocrinological follow-up evaluation in 115 patients who underwent transsphenoidal surgery for acromegaly. J Neurosurg 1998;89:353–358
30. Blevins LS Jr, Christy JH, Khajavi M, Tindall GT. Outcomes of therapy for Cushing's disease due to adrenocorticotropin-secreting pituitary macroadenomas. J Clin Endocrinol Metab 1998;83:63–67
31. Hofmann BM, Hlavac M, Martinez R, Buchfelder M, Müller OA, Fahlbusch R. Long-term results after microsurgery for Cushing disease: experience with 426 primary operations over 35 years. J Neurosurg 2008;108:9–18
32. Pergolizzi RS Jr, Nabavi A, Schwartz RB, et al. Intra-operative MR guidance during trans-sphenoidal pituitary resection: preliminary results. J Magn Reson Imaging 2001;13:136–141
33. Martin CH, Schwartz R, Jolesz F, Black PM. Transsphenoidal resection of pituitary adenomas in an intraoperative MRI unit. Pituitary 1999;2:155–162
34. Dort JC, Sutherland GR. Intraoperative magnetic resonance imaging for skull base surgery. Laryngoscope 2001;111:1570–1575
35. Bohinski RJ, Warnick RE, Gaskill-Shipley MF, et al. Intraoperative magnetic resonance imaging to determine the extent of resection of pituitary macroadenomas during transsphenoidal microsurgery. Neurosurgery 2001;49:1133–1143, discussion 1143–1144
36. Fahlbusch R, Ganslandt O, Buchfelder M, Schott W, Nimsky C. Intraoperative magnetic resonance imaging during transsphenoidal surgery. J Neurosurg 2001;95:381–390
37. Nimsky C, von Keller B, Ganslandt O, Fahlbusch R. Intraoperative high-field magnetic resonance imaging in transsphenoidal surgery of hormonally inactive pituitary macroadenomas. Neurosurgery 2006;59:105–114, discussion 105–114
38. Fahlbusch R, Keller B, Ganslandt O, Kreutzer J, Nimsky C. Transsphenoidal surgery in acromegaly investigated by intraoperative high-field magnetic resonance imaging. Eur J Endocrinol 2005;153:239–248
39. Schwartz TH, Stieg PE, Anand VK. Endoscopic transsphenoidal pituitary surgery with intraoperative magnetic resonance imaging. Neurosurgery 2006;58(1, Suppl)ONS44–ONS51, discussion ONS44–ONS51
40. Jain AK, Gupta AK, Pathak A, Bhansali A, Bapuraj JR. Excision of pituitary adenomas: randomized comparison of surgical modalities. Br J Neurosurg 2007;21:328–331
41. Kawamata T, Iseki H, Ishizaki R, Hori T. Minimally invasive endoscope-assisted endonasal trans-sphenoidal microsurgery for pituitary

tumors: experience with 215 cases comparing with sublabial transsphenoidal approach. Neurol Res 2002;24:259–265

42. Jones J, Ruge J. Intraoperative magnetic resonance imaging in pituitary macroadenoma surgery: an assessment of visual outcome. Neurosurg Focus 2007;23:E12
43. Martin AJ, Larson PS, Ostrem JL, et al. Placement of deep brain stimulator electrodes using real-time high-field interventional magnetic resonance imaging. Magn Reson Med 2005;54:1107–1114
44. Hall WA, Kowalik K, Liu H, Truwit CL, Kucharezyk J. Costs and benefits of intraoperative MR-guided brain tumor resection. Acta Neurochir Suppl (Wien) 2003;85:137–142

29 The Role of Stereotactic Navigation in Endoscopic Pituitary Surgery

Abtin Tabaee, Vijay K. Anand, and Theodore H. Schwartz

Advances in instrumentation including specialized dissectors, powered drills and microdebriders, straight and angled rigid endoscopes, and high-definition monitors have provided a solution to the various challenges of endoscopic pituitary surgery, including its cavitary nature, dissection of bony and soft tissue structures, proximity of the target site to critical neurovascular structures, and limited vectors of motion. Inherent to endoscopic surgery is the ability to maintain robust visualization throughout the procedure. The absolute need for anatomical orientation remains an ongoing focus of development in endoscopic pituitary surgery.

Although modern endoscopes and monitors provide a magnified panoramic view of the operative field, several limitations continue to exist, the largest of which is the inability to see through bone or tissue to predict what anatomy lies just beyond the penetration of visible light. The two-dimensional view of current systems lacks the depth perception afforded by microscopic surgery. Additionally, the cavitary nature of endoscopic surgery implies that only limited perspectives are available, especially early in the course of the procedure. Anatomical structures are dissected in an anterior to posterior trajectory, in comparison to open access surgery, where circumferential anatomical exposure is possible. Finally, the separation of target sites by bony boundaries requires transgression of a given structure before successful arrival at the target is confirmed. Examples of these boundaries include the anterior face of the sphenoid sinus and the floor of the sella. Surgical experience, preoperative imaging studies, and the stability of anatomical landmarks are more than adequate to maintain orientation in the majority of patients. However, the potential for anatomical disorientation and inadvertent injury to surrounding neurovascular structures exists. Certain situations are identified as potentially higher risk, including anatomical variants, revision surgery, and complex pathology. The need for increased anatomical information is the theoretical basis for stereotactic navigation in endoscopic pituitary surgery. The triplanar radiographic correlate of the surgical field allows for an improved understanding of the relationship of a given structure to its surrounding anatomy. The radiographic information provided by neuronavigation complements the endoscopic view and has the potential to result in improved outcomes. This chapter reviews the history, technology, indications, clinical use, limitations, recent advances, and future directions of stereotactic navigation in endoscopic pituitary surgery.

History

The historical landmarks in stereotactic neuronavigation have been based on adaptation of diagnostic radiology to the operating room. The earliest neuronavigational device was described in 1908 and utilized a rigid frame for fixing the head and a system of levers and pulleys to predict the location of intracranial structures based on external landmarks of the skull.[1] The application of plain radiography to stereotaxy was described by Spiegel and Wycis in the 1940s, and although conceptually similar to modern neuronavigation, this device lacked sufficient accuracy for practical use.[2] The era of modern image guidance began in the 1970s with the incorporation of computed tomography (CT). The CT-based system described by Bergstrom and Greitz[3] in 1976 utilized a fixed metal ring worn by the patient during both the scan and the procedure. Although this allowed for improved accuracy, it also blocked complete surgical access. The practical refinements over the ensuing decade, including semirigid articulating arms, frameless systems, and incorporation of magnetic resonance imaging (MRI)-based data sets, increased the utility of neuronavigation.[4–7] Reductions in the cost and improvements in the flexibility of these devices resulted in their widespread adoption for neurosurgical procedures during the 1980s and 1990s, including for microscopic transsphenoidal surgery.[8] The popularity of image-guided surgery significantly broadened with its application to endoscopic sinus surgery (ESS) in the 1990s. Similar to transcranial surgery, ESS involves surgical dissection within stable bony confines, namely the paranasal sinuses and skull base. This allows for maintenance of accuracy throughout the procedure. The use of image guidance in ESS has been described for a variety of indications including revision procedures, anatomical variations, cerebrospinal fluid leak closure, endoscopic tumor resection, endoscopic orbital surgery, and endoscopic skull base surgery.[9–14] The inability of traditional image guidance to reflect intraoperative changes has led to interest in incorporation of "real-time" imaging modalities into the operating room. Multiple modalities used for intraoperative imaging have been reported over the past 50 years including x-ray fluoroscopy,[15] gas cisternography,[16] ultrasound,[17,18] Doppler ultrasound,[19] CT scan,[20] and MRI.[21–23] These technologies have the potential to provide critical information, including the necessary extent of resection and the presence of residual tumor. However, as explored in this chapter, the role of these technologies in endoscopic pituitary surgery is currently evolving.

Technology and Practical Use

The field of neuronavigation is, in large part, driven by a continual stream of technologic advancements. Although the specific solutions offered by the different commercially available systems vary, the basic tenets of image guidance are similar. The hardware component houses the computer workstation, a monitor for image display, and an interactive component that communicates between the surgical team and the computer (**Fig. 29.1**). The last varies among the systems, with examples including keyboard, mouse, and touch-screen models. The tracking device interfaces between the patient and computer and enables navigation to be performed during the surgery. Three different models of surgical tracking have been described. The earliest systems were mechanical and relied on the use of rigid and semirigid arms. The cumbersome nature and limited degrees of motion associated with these systems eventually resulted in their obsolescence. Modern systems are based on either line-of-sight or electromagnetic technology. Line-of-sight technology utilizes light-emitting diodes and infrared communication between the computer workstation and the tracking device, whereas electromagnetic technology achieves this with radiofrequency emission. The practical limitation of the infrared systems is the need to maintain an unobstructed spatial path between the tracking device and the cameras on the computer workstation. In contrast,

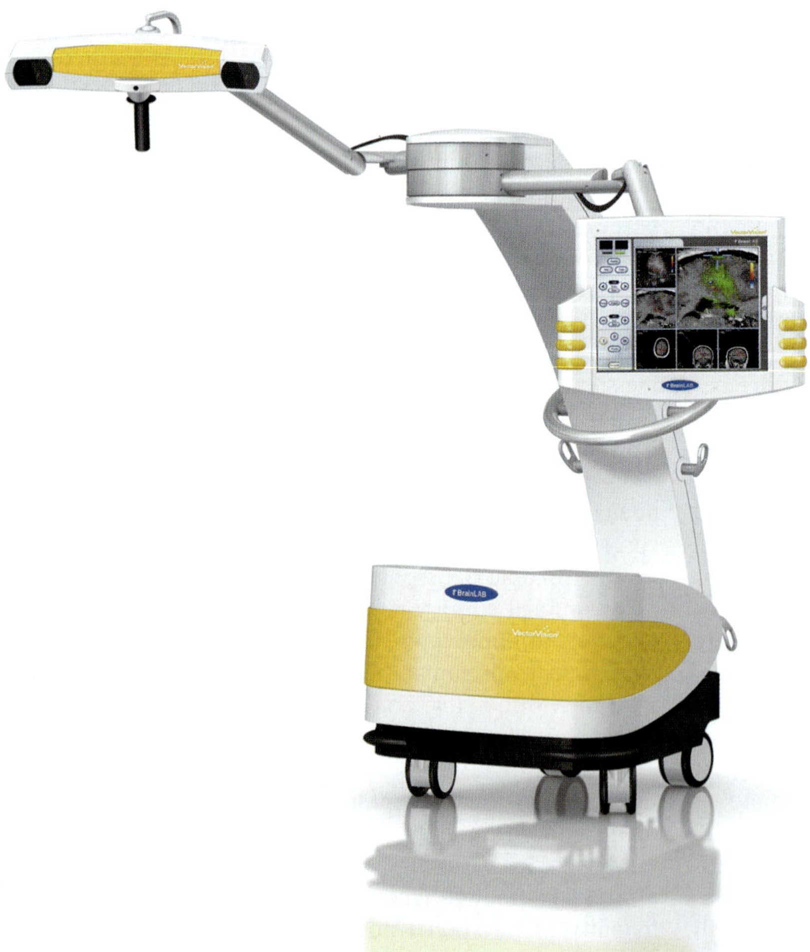

Fig. 29.1 The computer workstation, visualization screen, and infrared tracking sensors. The direct line of sight required for this type of system contrasts with the radiofrequency emission used in electromagnetic based systems. (BrainLab VectorVision[2], image courtesy of BrainLab AG.)

electromagnetic systems require a direct communication between the tracking device and the computer, typically in the form of cables. An additional distinction of electromagnetic systems is the potential for interference with ferromagnetic instrumentation.

Similar to operating systems for personal computers, those used in image guidance are continually upgraded with newer generations. Specialty-specific parameters (e.g., for neurosurgery, otolaryngology, and spine surgery) are incorporated in the workstation. Newer generations of operating systems include more refined parameters for the registration, manipulation, and display of radiographic data. The software component is the patient's radiographic data set. Reformatting and manipulation of these images allow for the creation of triplanar views, three-dimensional (3D) models, and different window settings (e.g., soft tissue, bone). The choice of the imaging modality that is used for tracking is at the discretion of the surgeon.

The individual steps of performing image-guided surgery require coordination by the entire surgical team. The decision to perform image-guided surgery is at the discretion of the surgeon and is further explored in the surgical indications section below. The patient undergoes the appropriate imaging study. Specific protocols for these scans are utilized typically with 1-mm-thick slices around the area of the surgical field. Inclusion of fiducial markers or headsets varies depending on the system. Coordination with the imaging center is required for the correct performance of the study, as the formatting of these scans differs from traditional diagnostic studies. The images are transferred to the computer workstation and reviewed by the surgical team preoperatively to confirm that the indicated study was performed with the correct formatting and that the anatomical area of interest is well displayed. Successful transfer of images is additionally confirmed with reproduction of a 3D model of the patient's face. Distortion of this model indicates an error either with the protocol used for the scan or the transfer of the raw data onto the computer workstation. Surgical planning including visualization of 3D reconstructions and determining the surgical trajectory can be performed at this point.

Once the patient is brought into the operating room and anesthetized, registration and calibration are performed. Registration is defined as the 3D correlation of radiographic images with the surgical anatomy. This critical step allows for accurate navigation during the procedure. The method of registration varies based on the image guidance system and may incorporate adhesive fiducial markers, disposable head set, rigid fixation in a neurosurgical pins with attachment of the reference array to the head frame, specialized rigid pin with reference array placed directly into the skull, and elastic headband. Calibration refers to the preparation of neuronavigational instruments for intraoperative tracking. The instruments available for neuronavigation were initially limited to suctions and straight probes. However, modern systems allow for tracking with the complete array of standard surgical instrumentation including dissection and powered instrumentation (e.g., microdebriders, drills). During the course of the procedure, neuronavigational tracking is performed at the discretion of the surgical team; potential applications are discussed below. The possibility of degradation in accuracy exists, especially with longer procedures, and re-registration is indicated if this occurs. Some of the currently available systems additionally perform automatic re-registration at fixed time intervals throughout the surgery.

Following the surgery, neuronavigation is billed under the Current Procedural Terminology (CPT) code 61795, Stereotactic Computer-Assisted Volumetric (Navigational) Procedure, Intracranial, Extracranial, or Spinal. It is classified as an "add-on" code and must be linked with the primary procedure codes. Additionally, adequate documentation of its use must be detailed in the operative report, including the indications for its use, downloading and verification of images, intraoperative registration, calibration, and intraoperative tracking.

Clinical Indications

The indications for neuronavigation in endoscopic pituitary surgery are based on the need for additional anatomical information during potentially complex dissections. In the majority of patients, surgical experience and preoperative radiographic studies are adequate. Image guidance in this setting provides little additional information and may serve a confirmatory role only (**Fig. 29.2**). This is especially true in patients undergoing primary surgery for tumors confined to the sella and without significant anatomical variants. Although the surgical team may elect to utilize image guidance in selected cases, there are benefits to routine inclusion even if a minimal role is anticipated. Familiarity with the equipment including management of technical problems is enhanced by its regular use. This greatly increases the comfort level and ability to correctly interpret the conveyed information during critical moments. Additionally, the potential for unanticipated situations where image guidance aids in anatomical orientation exists even in routine cases.

The role of image guidance in endoscopic pituitary surgery potentially encompasses all aspects of the surgery including presurgical planning, surgical approach, tumor resection, and skull base reconstruction. Toggling through the electronic radiographic display preoperatively allows the surgical team to understand the triplanar anatomical relationships in a more dynamic sense than would be possible with hardcopy images. This is further enhanced with data manipulation including changing of the window settings and creation of 3D reconstructions. The trajectory and anticipated area of required exposure can be planned.

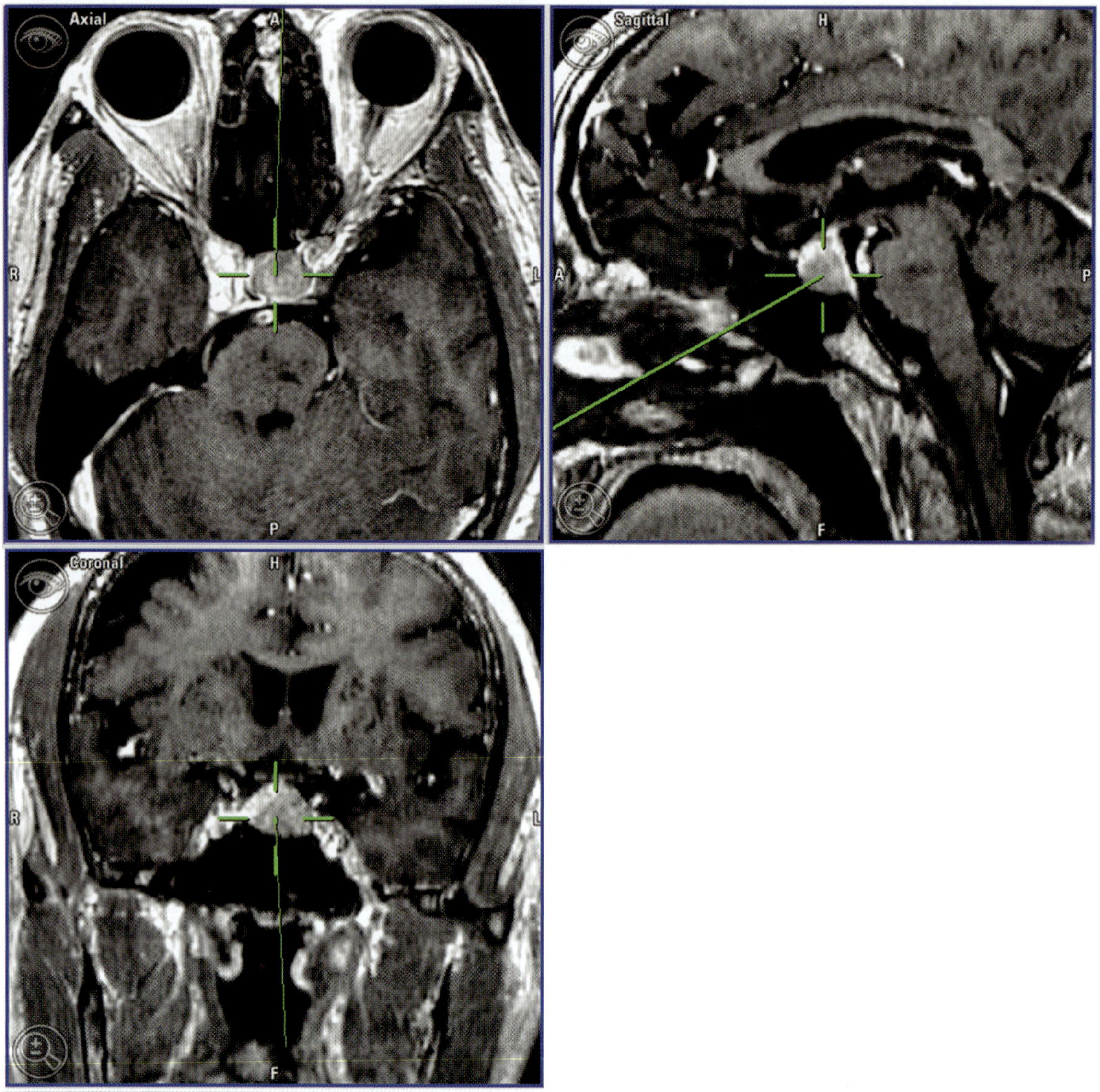

A B C

Fig. 29.2 **(A)** Axial, **(B)** sagittal, and **(C)** coronal magnetic resonance imaging (MRI) scans in a patient undergoing image-guided surgery for pituitary macroadenoma. Image guidance may have only a confirmatory role in patients with pneumatized sphenoid sinuses, no significant anatomical variations, and adenomas confined to the sella.

The endoscopic approach to the sella is facilitated by image guidance including confirmation of the anterior face of the sphenoid sinus, sellar floor, sphenoidal portion of the internal carotid arteries, and optic nerves. The expected location and anatomical boundaries of the tumor may be defined with image guidance, which thereby assists in determining the extent of necessary sellar opening. Specific situations where image guidance has greater utility include revision surgery,[24] anatomical variants, and extended procedures.[25] The anatomical disorientation that can occur in revision surgery may result from adhesion formation, removal or displacement of normal surgical landmarks, and the presence of reconstruction material. Anatomical variants associated with increased surgical complexity during the surgical approach include poor pneumatization of the sphenoid sinus including the conchal variant, the presence of multiple intersinus septa, dehiscence of the internal carotid artery or optic nerves, medial location of the cavernous portions of the internal carotid arteries, presence of aberrant posterior ethmoid cells within the sphenoid sinus (Onodi cell), surgery in pediatric patients, and comorbid sinonasal disease including inflammatory chronic sinusitis. Finally, the bony opening required in lesions with extrasellar extension can be defined by image guidance. For example, in patients with "giant" macroadenomas, an adequate exposure encompassing the sella, tuberculum sellae, and planum sphenoidale

(**Fig. 29.3**) may be delineated with image guidance prior to visualization of the tumor itself.

Neuronavigation may be used for exploration of the tumor cavity following opening of the sellar floor including confirmation of the cavernous portion of the internal carotid arteries. However, the accuracy of image guidance based on preoperative images alone quickly degrades in this setting secondary to soft tissue shifts, tumor resection, and loss of cerebrospinal fluid. Finally, the bony margins of the sellar defect can be defined for planning of the surgical reconstruction at the conclusion of the procedure. The millimetric grid function allows for measurement of the skull base defect and assists in preparation of the reconstructive graft materials.

Limitations and Recent Advances

The limitations associated with neuronavigation include those related to accuracy, anatomical disorientation, radiographic information, cost, and outcomes literature. Accuracy in image guidance refers to the difference between the true position of a point in space compared with its predicted radiographic position. The various methods of measuring accuracy differ based on the points of reference. Target registration error refers to the difference between an anatomical point and its radiographic position. Fiducial localization error is a similar calculation but is based on the position of a fiducial marker, rather than an anatomical point. Fiducial registration error is the difference between the position

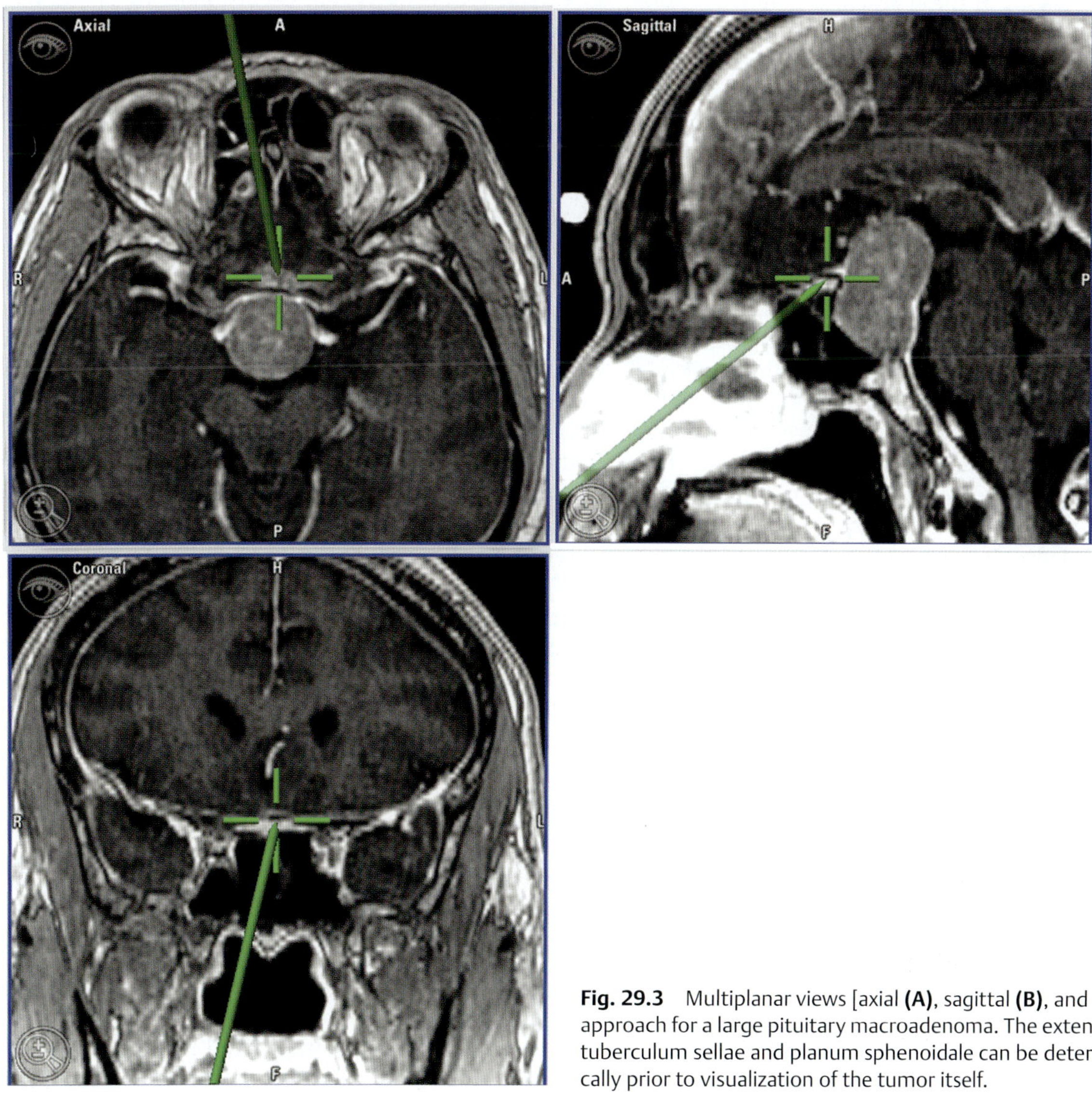

A B C

Fig. 29.3 Multiplanar views [axial **(A)**, sagittal **(B)**, and coronal **(C)**] of the approach for a large pituitary macroadenoma. The extent of removal of the tuberculum sellae and planum sphenoidale can be determined stereotactically prior to visualization of the tumor itself.

of a fiducial point and its predicted radiographic location following registration, which in turn is calculated by image-guidance software in terms of a root-mean-square value. Modern generations of image-guidance systems have improved the fidelity and reproducibility related to accuracy by incorporating improved imaging data sets, increased fiducial points, improved three-dimensionality of fiducial points, and automation of the registration process.[26] Although multiple studies have confirmed a reproducible accuracy of image guidance systems to within 2 mm,[27–30] this is balanced against the anatomical precision necessary for skull base surgery where millimetric distances may be critical.

The potential for anatomically misleading information is inherent to all image-guidance systems, especially those based on preoperative imaging studies. Several factors including limitations in accuracy, structural shifting, and registration error may result in a disparity between intraoperative findings and the information conveyed by the image-guidance system. In these situations, surgical judgment and experience remain paramount. Additionally, image guidance will not compensate for deficiencies in technique and anatomical knowledge. Despite its useful role in endoscopic surgery, image guidance, therefore, remains only an adjunct to surgery.

The costs associated with image guidance are based both on fixed capital expenses and those incurred with use. The cost of the image-guidance systems varies depending on the model and ranges from approximately $100,000 to $200,000 for the most commonly used systems to greater than $1,000,000 for intraoperative MRI. The per-case costs of stereotactic surgery include those related to the additional imaging studies, the single-use items that are used during the procedure, and the increase in procedure time. The last may be as little as 15 minutes for routine procedures or over an hour for intraoperative MRI.[24] However, a meaningful cost-benefit analysis would require data regarding the impact of image guidance on surgical outcomes including tumor control and perioperative complications. Unfortunately, impracticalities with study design including ethical issues with randomization, large numbers of patients required to achieve adequate statistical power, duration, and costs of the study preclude the performance of an appropriately designed study to address these questions.

Image guidance in endoscopic pituitary surgery is most commonly based on either preoperative CT or MRI studies. The robust definition of bony anatomy by CT imaging is countered by its relatively poor soft tissue resolution. This contrasts with MRI, where the reverse is true. If a single-study modality is used for neuronavigation, the choice of CT versus MRI is based on the intraoperative needs. CT scan may be more useful in patients with complex sinonasal anatomy including revision surgery or conchal-type sphenoid sinus pneumatization. This contrasts in patients with complex intracranial anatomy including large macroadenomas or medial location of the cavernous portion of the internal carotid arteries. Combining the two modalities with "fusion" technology optimizes the strengths of both studies. To perform image fusion, the patient initially undergoes CT and MRI studies with the correct protocol. The images are then fused on the computer workstation manually, semiautomatically, or fully automatically depending on the system and user preference. In endoscopic skull base surgery, the CT images are used for the sinonasal anatomy and the MRI images are used for the intracranial anatomy. Other imaging modalities may be incorporated including vascular (MR angiography) and functional studies (positron emission tomography). The need for two different scans limits the use of fusion technology to select cases.

Regardless of the imaging modality of choice, any neuronavigation based on preoperative scans is limited by its failure to reflect intraoperative changes. Significant degradation of accuracy is expected throughout the procedure from soft tissue shifts that occur following opening of the sellar floor, resection of the tumor, and decompression of cerebrospinal fluid cisterns. The intracranial aspects of the surgery, in particular, are poorly represented by preoperative imaging. These include the extent of residual tumor and the relationship of the tumor to the cavernous sinus laterally and the anterior cerebral circulation superiorly. This has led to renewed interest in intraoperative image acquisition for neuronavigation.

Intraoperative fluoroscopy has a well-established role in transsphenoidal surgery. Acquisition of intraoperative video fluoroscopic data in the sagittal plane is obtained through an intraoperative C-arm. The boundaries of the sella can be defined and the trajectory of the approach to the sella can be confirmed.[31] The low-cost and high-quality triplanar radiographic images represent advantages of modern fluoroscopic equipment. However, the attendant radiation exposure[32,33] and the lack of soft tissue resolution have spurred interest in other intraoperative imaging modalities.

Transcranial ultrasonography has been preliminarily described for resection of large macroadenomas. This technique involves placement of the ultrasound probe through a frontal bur hole craniotomy. Dynamic visualization of the tumor and intracranial vascular structures is possible. However, the need for a separate craniotomy and limited image resolution may limit this technology from widespread adoption.[34] This has led to interest in intraoperative transsphenoidal sonography. Ultrasonographic visualization of sellar anatomy with the use of a modified pediatric transesophageal echocardiography probe has been described.[35] This approach has the potential to allow for dynamic visualization of the intracranial anatomy in a minimally invasive way. Although a learning curve related to the interpretation of these images by the surgical team is expected, the relative speed of image acquisition and the ability to visualize dynamic blood flow represent advantages compared with other intraoperative imaging modalities. To date, the most practical use of sonographic technology in endoscopic pituitary surgery utilizes a bayoneted micro-Doppler. Gross localization of the cavernous internal carotid arteries is based on the relative strength of the pulsation sound. Although no visual anatomical data are afforded, an estimation of proximity both prior to the initial sellar opening and within the tumor cavity itself may avoid catastrophic injury. Additional benefits include relative ease of use and low cost.[36]

Intraoperative CT scan for pituitary and skull base lesions has been previously described and has the potential for acquiring real-time radiographic information regarding the presence of residual tumor and the relationship of the tumor to critical neurovascular structures.[37] The inclusion of radiographic contrast is possible and would better delineate these structures. Although the image resolution of intraoperative CT improves on that of fluoroscopy, millimetric soft tissue detail is not possible. The adaptation of MRI to the operating room represents the most recent advance in image guidance. The ability to acquire high-resolution intraoperative imaging allows for determination of critical issues including extent of resection and location of radiographically visible disease.[22,23] This topic is further explored in a separate chapter in this book.

Future Directions

The future development of endoscopic pituitary surgery is based on several forces including cumulative clinical experience, reporting of outcomes literature, and continued technologic advancements. The last is particularly true of image guidance, which has continuously evolved during its short history. Several practical measures have been already achieved and will continue to be refined. These include automatic and semiautomatic registration, touch screens, voice activation, and sophisticated software manipulation of the radiographic studies. The increasing popularity and demand for use of image guidance in a variety of procedures has resulted in the manufacturing of different models designed to fit the complexity of procedures. These factors may result in a more favorable cost structure. Image guidance will likely continue to adapt to the variability in surgical volume and hospital resources in different institutions. The integration of image guidance to the physical infrastructure of the operating room allows for a more streamlined approach and is most applicable to tertiary-care medical centers. In contrast, portable units that may be easily transported allow for image-guided surgery in smaller, low-volume institutions. The ultimate solution for both cost and portability may involve formatting of image guidance for use on personal computers.

Although robotic surgery has been more fully developed in other disciplines, several applications are potentially possible with image-guided endoscopic pituitary surgery. The most simplistic model utilizes a robotic system as an endoscope holder. This frees a surgical hand while providing a stable field of view. Dynamic movement of the endoscope is achieved with robotic control.[38] Several models exist for inclusion of robotic technology for actual performance of the surgery including automatic, semiautomatic, and fully controlled. The potential benefits of robotic technology include reproducible accuracy and lack of surgical fatigue.[39] Adaptation of robotic technology to surgery of the sella is augmented by the localization information conveyed by both endoscopy and image guidance. However, several practical limitations exist with current robotic systems, including size, cost, lack of appropriate instrumentation, and undetermined clinical need.

Virtual endoscopy, although currently in its early stages, has the potential to revolutionize endoscopic surgery. Computerized images of routine studies including CT and MRI can be manipulated to create virtual 3D reconstructions including both traditional anatomical models and endoscopic views. The latter has the potential to allow for a robust virtual representation of surgical anatomy including the paranasal sinuses, internal carotid arteries, and sella.[40] The virtual endoscopic views may be reviewed for surgical planning, as is done with traditional image studies. Three-dimensional virtual reality representations of critical structures may potentially be superimposed on the endoscopic view during the course of surgery. For example, the outline of the pituitary tumor and internal carotid arteries may be projected onto the endoscopic view of the sphenoid sinus prior to the skull base openings.[41] In the future, this technology may be merged with surgery simulators and allow for virtual endoscopic surgery. The potential ramifications of this for facilitating teaching and improving surgical outcomes may be profound.

References

1. Horsley V, Clarke RH. The structure and functions of the cerebellum examined by a new method. Brain 1908;31:45–124
2. Spiegel EA, Wycis HT, Marks M, Lee AJ. Stereotaxic apparatus for operations on the human brain. Science 1947;106:349–350
3. Bergström M, Greitz T. Stereotaxic computed tomography. AJR Am J Roentgenol 1976;127:167–170
4. Roberts DW, Strohbehn JW, Hatch JF, Murray W, Kettenberger H. A frameless stereotaxic integration of computerized tomographic imaging and the operating microscope. J Neurosurg 1986;65:545–549
5. Watanabe E, Mayanagi Y, Kosugi Y, Manaka S, Takakura K. Open surgery assisted by the neuronavigator, a stereotactic, articulated, sensitive arm. Neurosurgery 1991;28:792–799, discussion 799–800
6. Leggett WB, Greenberg MM, Gannon WE, et al. The Viewing Wand: a new system for three dimensional computed tomography-correlated intraoperative localization. Curr Surg 1991;48:674–678

7. Guthrie BL, Adler JR Jr. Computer-assisted preoperative planning, interactive surgery, and frameless stereotaxy. Clin Neurosurg 1992;38:112–131
8. Elias WJ, Chadduck JB, Alden TD, Laws ER Jr. Frameless stereotaxy for transsphenoidal surgery. Neurosurgery 1999;45:271–275, discussion 275–277
9. Anon JB, Lipman SP, Oppenheim D, Halt RA. Computer-assisted endoscopic sinus surgery. Laryngoscope 1994;104:901–905
10. Senior BA, Lanza DC, Kennedy DW, Weinstein GS. Computer-assisted resection of benign sinonasal tumors with skull base and orbital extension. Arch Otolaryngol Head Neck Surg 1997;123:706–711
11. Tabaee A, Kassenoff TL, Kacker A, Anand VK. The efficacy of computer assisted surgery in the endoscopic management of cerebrospinal fluid rhinorrhea. Otolaryngol Head Neck Surg 2005;133:936–943
12. Dubin MR, Tabaee A, Scruggs JT, Kazim M, Close LG. Image-guided endoscopic orbital decompression for Graves' orbitopathy. Ann Otol Rhinol Laryngol 2008;117:177–185
13. Kacker A, Tabaee A, Anand V. Computer-assisted surgical navigation in revision endoscopic sinus surgery. Otolaryngol Clin North Am 2005;38:473–482, vi
14. Tabaee A, Kacker A, Kassenoff TL, Anand V. Outcome of computer-assisted sinus surgery: a 5-year study. Am J Rhinol 2003;17:291–297
15. Hardy J, Wigser SM. Trans-sphenoidal surgery of pituitary fossa tumors with televised radiofluoroscopic control. J Neurosurg 1965;23:612–619
16. Nesbakken R, Reinlie S, Eldevik OP. Intraoperative gas cisternography and gas dissection in the operative treatment of pituitary tumors. A methodological description. Eur Surg Res 1984;16(Suppl 2): 73–79
17. Atkinson JL, Kasperbauer JL, James EM, Lane JI, Nippoldt TB. Transcranial-transdural real-time ultrasonography during transsphenoidal resection of a large pituitary tumor. Case report. J Neurosurg 2000;93:129–131
18. Ram Z, Shawker TH, Bradford MH, Doppman JL, Oldfield EH. Intraoperative ultrasound-directed resection of pituitary tumors. J Neurosurg 1995;83:225–230
19. Arita K, Kurisu K, Tominaga A, et al. Trans-sellar color Doppler ultrasonography during transsphenoidal surgery. Neurosurgery 1998;42:81–85, discussion 86
20. Batra PS, Kanowitz SJ, Citardi MJ. Clinical utility of intraoperative volume computed tomography scanner for endoscopic sinonasal and skull base procedures. Am J Rhinol 2008;22:511–515
21. Black PM, Moriarty T, Alexander E III, et al. Development and implementation of intraoperative magnetic resonance imaging and its neurosurgical applications. Neurosurgery 1997;41:831–842, discussion 842–845
22. Fahlbusch R, Ganslandt O, Buchfelder M, Schott W, Nimsky C. Intraoperative magnetic resonance imaging during transsphenoidal surgery. J Neurosurg 2001;95:381–390
23. Schwartz TH, Stieg PE, Anand VK. Endoscopic transsphenoidal pituitary surgery with intraoperative magnetic resonance imaging. Neurosurgery 2006;58(1, Suppl):ONS44–ONS51, discussion ONS44–ONS51
24. Lasio G, Ferroli P, Felisati G, Broggi G. Image-guided endoscopic transnasal removal of recurrent pituitary adenomas. Neurosurgery 2002;51:132–136, discussion 136–137
25. Jagannathan J, Prevedello DM, Ayer VS, Dumont AS, Jane JA Jr, Laws ER. Computer-assisted frameless stereotaxy in transsphenoidal surgery at a single institution: review of 176 cases. Neurosurg Focus 2006;20:E9
26. Citardi MJ, Batra PS. Image-guided sinus surgery: current concepts and technology. Otolaryngol Clin North Am 2005;38:439–452, vi
27. Metson R, Gliklich RE, Cosenza M. A comparison of image guidance systems for sinus surgery. Laryngoscope 1998;108(8 Pt 1):1164–1170
28. Germano IM, Villalobos H, Silvers A, Post KD. Clinical use of the optical digitizer for intracranial neuronavigation. Neurosurgery 1999;45:261–269, discussion 269–270
29. Kaus M, Steinmeier R, Sporer T, Ganslandt O, Fahlbusch R. Technical accuracy of a neuronavigation system measured with a high-precision mechanical micromanipulator. Neurosurgery 1997;41: 1431–1436, discussion 1436–1437
30. Gong J, Mohr G, Vézina JL. Endoscopic pituitary surgery with and without image guidance: an experimental comparison. Surg Neurol 2007;67:572–578, discussion 578
31. Jane JA Jr, Thapar K, Alden TD, Laws ER Jr. Fluoroscopic frameless stereotaxy for transsphenoidal surgery. Neurosurgery 2001;48:1302–1307, discussion 1307–1308
32. Ulmer S, Schulz E, Moeller B, et al. Radiation dose of the lens in transsphenoidal pituitary surgery: pros and cons of a conventional setup using fluoroscopic guidance and CT-based neuronavigation. AJNR Am J Neuroradiol 2007;28:1559–1564
33. Manarey CR, Anand VK. Radiation dosimetry of the FluoroCAT scan for real-time endoscopic sinus surgery. Otolaryngol Head Neck Surg 2006;135:409–412
34. Suzuki R, Asai J, Nagashima G, et al. Transcranial echo-guided transsphenoidal surgical approach for the removal of large macroadenomas. J Neurosurg 2004;100:68–72
35. Arita K, Kurisu K, Tominaga A, et al. Trans-sellar color Doppler ultrasonography during transsphenoidal surgery. Neurosurgery 1998;42:81–85, discussion 86
36. Dusick JR, Esposito F, Malkasian D, Kelly DF. Avoidance of carotid artery injuries in transsphenoidal surgery with the Doppler probe and micro-hook blades. Neurosurgery 2007;60(4, Suppl 2):322–328, discussion 328–329
37. Okudera H, Takemae T, Kobayashi S. Intraoperative computed tomographic scanning during transsphenoidal surgery: technical note. Neurosurgery 1993;32:1041–1043
38. Nathan CO, Chakradeo V, Malhotra K, D'Agostino H, Patwardhan R. The voice-controlled robotic assist scope holder AESOP for the endoscopic approach to the sella. Skull Base 2006;16:123–131
39. Bumm K, Wurm J, Rachinger J, et al. An automated robotic approach with redundant navigation for minimal invasive extended transsphenoidal skull base surgery. Minim Invasive Neurosurg 2005;48: 159–164
40. Wolfsberger S, Neubauer A, Bühler K, et al. Advanced virtual endoscopy for endoscopic transsphenoidal pituitary surgery. Neurosurgery 2006;59:1001–1009, discussion 1009–1010
41. Kawamata T, Iseki H, Shibasaki T, Hori T. Endoscopic augmented reality navigation system for endonasal transsphenoidal surgery to treat pituitary tumors: technical note. Neurosurgery 2002;50:1393–1397

30 Anesthesia Considerations

Patricia Fogarty Mack

Patients with pituitary disease can pose many unique challenges to the anesthesiologist. The endocrine diseases that often accompany pituitary masses may cause changes in the patient's airway, cardiovascular system, and various metabolic pathways. Such changes require specific preoperative evaluation and consideration throughout the perioperative period.

Many patients presenting with pituitary tumors suffer from functional adenomas. Although there are many subtypes of functional adenoma, the two that have the most impact on anesthetic management are those that secrete growth hormone, leading to acromegaly, and adrenocorticotropic hormone (ACTH), leading to Cushing's disease.

Airway Management

Airway management is a primary concern of the anesthesiologist, and both acromegaly and Cushing's disease may affect the ability to secure the airway.[1–3] In two large reviews, the incidence of difficult intubation for acromegalics was 10%[4] and 9.1%.[5] In contrast, the incidence of difficult intubation in patients with Cushing's disease, prolactinoma, or nonsecretory pituitary tumors was no different from that in the general population (1 to 4%).[5]

Acromegaly manifests with enlargement of the facial bones, especially the mandible,[2] as well as hypertrophy of the laryngeal and pharyngeal soft tissue.[6,7] Hypertrophy of the periepiglottic folds and calcinosis of the larynx may be seen, as may recurrent laryngeal nerve paresis.[8] These anatomical changes may serve to make intubation technically difficult.

Four grades of airway involvement in acromegaly have been described: grade 1, no involvement; grade 2, soft tissue hypertrophy of the nasopharynx without glottic involvement; grade 3, glottic stenosis or vocal cord paresis; and grade 4, both soft tissue hypertrophy and glottic stenosis.[9] The difficulties with intubation and ventilation were so commonly encountered in patients with grades 3 and 4 that in the past routine tracheostomy was recommended.[10] The advent of awake fiberoptic bronchoscopic intubation as well as the increased use of alternative intubating devices has rendered the preoperative tracheostomy a rare occurrence.

Even in those patients whose anatomy does not appear to be difficult, such as patients with Mallampati class I or II airways, there may be a 20% incidence of difficult intubation.[11] In Nemergut and Zuo's[5] review, fully 50% of the Mallampati class I and II patients went on to be difficult intubations.[5]

Additionally, acromegalic patients also commonly suffer from obstructive sleep apnea. This occurs in 25% of female and 70% of male acromegalic patients and may manifest as snoring or daytime somnolence.[12] This incidence of sleep apnea must be considered in planning the induction of anesthesia, as it may compromise the ease of mask ventilation. It is also important in the postoperative period, as those patients with obstructive sleep apnea are known to have an increased incidence of postoperative ventilatory compromise.[13]

Of patients with Cushing's disease, 33% also suffer from obstructive sleep apnea, with 18% of patients having severe sleep apnea.[14] Many patients with Cushing's disease become morbidly obese and may suffer from gastroesophageal reflux and delayed gastric emptying. This leads many anesthesiologists to consider rapid sequence or awake intubation in this population as well.

Airway concerns actually may be increased postoperatively due to the presence of nasal packing, rendering postoperative mask ventilation less effective if necessary. Blind placement of any type of nasal airway, nasogastric tube, or nasal endotracheal tube is absolutely contraindicated in the immediate postoperative period.[15] Thus, judicious titration of postoperative pain medication is essential to avoid the need for mask ventilation or any manipulation of the airway.

Over time, there may be regression of hypertrophied tissues in the acromegalic patient, and impaired vocal cord function may improve within 10 days of surgery.[16,17] In the patient with Cushing's disease, weight loss after surgery may lead to improvement in airway and ventilatory function.

Other pituitary tumors, for example prolactinoma or nonsecretory tumors, pose no additional risk of difficult intubation or ventilation.

Cardiovascular Concerns

The leading cause of death in untreated acromegaly is cardiac dysfunction.[18] In acromegaly several cardiac manifestations of disease may occur, including endothelial dysfunction, left ventricular (LV) dysfunction, and dysrhythmia.[19] Small-vessel coronary artery disease has been described in the acromegalic population,[20] and endothelial-dependent vasodilation is impaired.[21] Thus, any anginal symptoms should be considered as evidence for ischemia even in a patient with no independent risk factors.

Acromegalic cardiomyopathy is defined as cardiomyopathy secondary to chronic growth hormone excess in the absence of other causes. Incidence of acromegalic cardiomyopathy is 3 to 4 cases/million/year. Cardiomegaly with concentric hypertrophy and an increase in LV mass with normal LV dimensions are consistent findings. The heart may weigh up to 1300 g, whereas normal is less than 250 g.[20] The severity of the hypertrophy is related to the duration of disease, and if LV dilatation occurs, the prognosis worsens. Left untreated, acromegalic cardiomyopathy progresses through three stages. In the early stage there is increased contractility and decreased systemic vascular resistance, leading to an increased cardiac output.[22,23] There may be significant LV diastolic dysfunction in spite of the normal LV mass.[22] In the intermediate stage, biventricular hypertrophy develops and diastolic dysfunction becomes evident.[24] Although there is preserved systolic function at rest, the patient will have impaired exercise tolerance. The late stage of acromegalic cardiomyopathy is marked by dilatation of the ventricles, depressed systolic function, and congestive heart failure.[3,22,23]

If treatment occurs in the early or intermediate stage, ventricular hypertrophy may resolve, although diastolic dysfunction may persist, which is consistent with the histologic finding of interstitial fibrosis. At the time of diagnosis, 10% of patients have signs of high-output heart failure with diminished ejection fraction, and 3% have significant systolic dysfunction.[25]

As far as cardiac rhythm is concerned, the frequency and severity of ventricular dysrhythmia are significantly greater in acromegalics than in controls and appear to be correlated with LV mass.[26] In addition, it has been variously reported that 18 to 60% of acromegalic patients suffer from hypertension.[18,27–30] In addition to a direct effect from growth hormone, contributing factors are an increase in sympathetic tone, cardiac hyperkinesis, an increase in plasma volume, a reduction in atrial natriuretic peptide secretion, and hyperinsulinemia.[31–36] Even in those patients with normal blood pressure, half have LV hypertrophy.[37] Not surprisingly, many have diastolic dysfunction, with preserved systolic function.

In contrast to the acromegalic patient, the cardiovascular manifestations of Cushing's disease are predominantly the consequence of the Cushing patient's predisposition to significant hypertension. Up to 80% of Cushing's patients have hypertension, with 50% having diastolic pressures >100 mm Hg if untreated.[38] This propensity for hypertension is the direct result of excessive levels of corticosteroids.[39,40] Hydrocortisone increases hepatic production of angiotensinogen, activating the renin-angiotensin system and increasing plasma volume.[40] Furthermore, glucocorticoids lead to an increase in angiotensin II receptors on vascular smooth muscle cells.[41] This in turn leads to an augmented response to both endogenous and perhaps exogenous catecholamines. Finally, glucocorticoid inhibition of vascular smooth muscle phospholipase A_2 reduces the production of vasodilatory prostaglandins.[42]

Left ventricular hypertrophy, the expected consequence of hypertension, is far more severe in patients with Cushing's disease than in those with essential hypertension, suggesting a direct effect of elevated cortisol levels. In addition, the incidence of asymmetric LV hypertrophy, with greater hypertrophy of the intraventricular septum, is also higher.[43] Diastolic dysfunction occurs in at least 40% of Cushing's disease patients.[44] Electrocardiogram (ECG) changes include LV strain pattern. Most ECG and echocardiographic abnormalities return to normal within 1 year after resection of ACTH-secreting adenoma.[45]

In view of these potentially severe cardiac abnormalities, it may be prudent to obtain a resting ECG and echocardiogram in all patients with acromegaly and Cushing's disease regardless of the patient's age.

Other Preoperative Concerns

Other functional pituitary adenomas include thyrotropic adenoma, prolactinoma, and gonadotroph adenoma. Thyrotropic adenomas represent only 2.8% of all pituitary tumors and may cause hyperthyroidism.[46] The signs and symptoms of hyperthyroidism are usually present and a goiter may even be observed. As patients are often treated for another cause of hyperthyroidism, the pituitary tumor can be large at the time of presentation, with 60% being locally invasive. Signs and symptoms of hyperthyroidism should be controlled medically prior to presentation for surgery.

There are no specific airway or cardiovascular concerns for patients with prolactinoma or gonadotroph adenoma. These patients often present with nonspecific symptoms. Women with prolactinoma usually present with amenorrhea, galactorrhea, and infertility.[3] Many tumors (90%) respond to bromocriptine (dopamine agonist) therapy and thus do not require surgery. In men, however, prolactinomas present with erectile dysfunction, premature ejaculation, and loss of libido. These nonspecific symptoms may lead to a delayed diagnosis, and the patient may develop symptoms of macroadenoma.[47]

Once a tumor becomes a macroadenoma, the patient may present with symptoms of a sellar mass. These symptoms include headache, visual loss (bitemporal hemianopsia) from compression of the optic chiasm, and hypopituitarism from compression of the anterior pituitary.[47] In extreme cases, especially if the tumor obstructs the third ventricle, the patient may present with symptoms of increased intracranial pressure (ICP). If symptoms of intracranial hypertension are present, care must be taken to avoid further increases in the ICP secondary to anesthesia management.

Hematologic and Metabolic Concerns

Although most patients presenting with pituitary tumors have an extensive hematologic, metabolic, and endocrinologic evaluation as part of their tumor workup, several studies are of particular importance to the anesthesiologist and should be obtained as close to the time of surgery as practical. These include baseline hemoglobin, as these cases can occasionally entail significant hemorrhage. Coagulation studies are not indicated unless the patient has a history consistent with an increased risk of bleeding. Serum electrolytes should be obtained to rule out hyponatremia, which may result from diabetes insipidus (DI) caused by posterior pituitary dysfunction. Serum glucose and perhaps hemoglobin A_{1c} are useful in patients with Cushing's disease. Fully 60% of patients with Cushing's disease have glucose intolerance and 33% have diabetes mellitus.[48] Furthermore, blood glucose may be increased in acromegaly secondary to insulin resistance.[49] The "tightness" of perioperative glucose control is controversial; however, there is clear evidence that hyperglycemia is undesirable during periods of neuronal ischemia.[50–52] A thyroid panel, to ensure euthyroid state, and a pregnancy test, especially in amenorrheic women, should also be obtained. Finally, an active type and screen are recommended.[3,53]

If panhypopituitarism is present, the patient should be given thyroid replacement and hydrocortisone. These medications should be continued on the morning of surgery.[3,53] All patients should be given corticosteroid replacement with the exception of those with Cushing's disease. In Cushing's patients hydrocortisone is withheld and serum cortisol levels are obtained every 6 hours after resection. A decrease in serum cortisol serves as biochemical confirmation of successful surgical resection.[54]

Intraoperative Management

The anesthesia management of the patient is impacted by the surgical approach. For tumors with significant extrasellar extension, a craniotomy may be required, and anesthesia management for craniotomy is extensively discussed elsewhere. This section focuses on the anesthesia management of the pituitary tumor via the transnasal approach. Although traditionally performed with the assistance of an operating microscope, commonly this procedure is now performed with endoscope-guided surgical exposure and localization using a frameless stereotactic system.

Monitoring

Traditionally, placement of an arterial line was not considered necessary for transsphenoidal resection of pituitary tumor. An arterial line was reserved for patients who had significant cardiovascular disease or cardiovascular sequelae of acromegaly. Although usually not necessary prior to induction of anesthesia, an arterial line may be useful in quickly noting and responding to hemodynamic changes associated with intranasal injection or application of vasoactive substances, as well as with the rare, but potentially catastrophic, occurrence of massive hemorrhage if the carotid or another artery is perforated during the operation. Finally, an arterial line provides access for blood samples, which may be useful in the management of diabetes mellitus and DI. Of note, radial artery catheterization may have increased risk in acromegalic patients, especially those with symptoms of carpal tunnel syndrome. Fifty percent of patients have been found to have diminished ulnar blood flow.[55] Thus an Allen's test is recommended in acromegalic patients.

A monitor of central venous pressure is rarely indicated and is reserved for those with significant compromise in cardiac function.

Adequate intravenous access is important because of the rare occurrence of abrupt hemorrhage. Similarly, all patients should have crossmatched blood available.

It should be noted that most navigation systems employed for proper localization of the tumor use infrared light, which may interfere with the pulse oximeter waveform. If one covers the pulse oximeter probe with foil (one can use a wrapper from an alcohol swab) to isolate it from the navigation system, the waveform will return to normal.[56]

Airway Management

As discussed above, both the acromegaly and Cushing's disease patients may present challenges with ventilation by mask as well as intubation. As such, it is important for the anesthesiologist to consider an awake intubation, especially in the acromegalic. If the anesthesiologist does not think an awake intubation is indicated, it would be prudent to have an alternative airway device available should direct laryngoscopy prove difficult. Such devices include but are not limited to the gum elastic bougie,[5] intubating laryngeal mask airway (LMA),[57] the GlideScope (Verathon, Bothell, WA), the Airtraq (Prodol Meditec, San Jose, CA), the Bullard laryngoscope (Gyrus Acmis, Norwalk, OH), and the fiberoptic bronchoscope. The use of these devices should be determined by the level of comfort of the anesthesiologist. Obviously, the endonasal surgical approach precludes the use of nasal intubation.

In our experience an oral RAE tube (a preformed tube named after its inventors, Drs. Ring, Adair, and Elwyn) is helpful, although not essential, in reducing the amount of pressure placed on the tube by the surgeon and the assistant surgeon. One possible problem with the use of the oral RAE tube is that the depth of the tube (centimeters) at the lip is determined by the diameter of the tube. Although the large tongue of the acromegalic may require the preformed bend in the tube to be at a greater depth, the presence of laryngeal or subglottic stenosis may preclude the diameter of tube that is necessary. For example, in a 7.0-mm-diameter endotracheal tube the bend is at 20 cm from the tip. It would take an 8.5-mm-diameter endotracheal tube if one wanted to place the tip of the tube at 22 cm from the lip. An additional disadvantage of the RAE tube is that the preformed bend may make navigating a fiberoptic bronchoscope more difficult. In our practice the tube is generally secured down the left side of the chin, as the anesthesiologist is positioned on the left side of the patient during the operation.

Maintenance of Anesthesia: Planning for Emergence

The emergence from anesthesia after transsphenoidal pituitary surgery must be carefully planned from the start of the procedure. Of the several anesthesia techniques commonly employed for pituitary surgery, all have the goal of having a pain-free patient with a patent airway. In addition, the patient should be alert enough to avoid any airway obstruction and to perform a postoperative neurologic exam promptly postextubation. Several anesthesia plans may facilitate this goal. One suitable plan for anesthesia maintenance is a remifentanil infusion combined with either volatile agent (sevoflurane/isoflurane/desflurane) or propofol infusion. Remifentanil is ideally suited for this patient population due to the varied levels of surgical stimuli throughout the procedure as well as the potential lack of surgical pain in the immediate postoperative period due to residual intraoperative local anesthesia effect. Because remifentanil is an esterase metabolized narcotic, it will be entirely eliminated shortly after cessation of the infusion, no matter how long the infusion is administered. This may reduce the risk of airway obstruction in patients who may already have sleep apnea and are now unable to breathe through their nasal passage secondary to packing and postsurgical edema. A clinical comparison of remifentanil versus isoflurane anesthesia documented a faster time to awakening in the remifentanil group as well as a decreased requirement of labetalol in the perioperative period.[58] Another study comparing a remifentanil–propofol combination versus a remifentanil–sevoflurane combination found a faster emergence in the sevoflurane group.[59] Many different anesthesia regimens may be employed to achieve the goal of an awake patient who is capable of maintaining an adequate airway.

Neuromuscular Blockade

Many anesthesiologists do not use muscle relaxants when the patient's head is fixated in a rigid pin fixation device.[58] It is our practice, however, to maintain paralysis via administration of muscle relaxants. Not all surgeons utilize a Mayfield or similar head fixation device. During entry into the sella, during tumor resection, and while hemostasis is established, the endoscope may be fixed to rigid arm, which is secured to the operating table. Thus, the surgeon would not be able to remove the endoscope rapidly in case of patient movement or coughing. Paralysis may be accomplished using either infusion or bolus dosing of neuromuscular relaxants while monitoring the neuromuscular junction. Upon removal of the endoscope from the nasal cavity, neuromuscular blockade may be allowed to wear off, with reversal of neuromuscular blockade administered at the conclusion of surgery.

■ Intraoperative Emergencies

Hemodynamic Instability and Myocardial Ischemia

Hemodynamic variability is common during transsphenoidal surgery because of cardiovascular responses modulated by stimulation of the trigeminal nerve[60] as well as the infiltration or topical application of vasoactive agents to diminish bleeding. Increased cortisol levels predispose the Cushing's patient to hypertension via activation of the angiotensin system. Such patients may be expected to have an augmented response to the application of topical vasoconstrictors.[61] In patients with acromegalic cardiomyopathy, the increase in afterload induced by oxymetazoline (Afrin), phenylephrine, or cocaine may lead to acute decompensation.

Cocaine solution 4 to 10% has long been used for both vasoconstriction and analgesia in endoscopic sinus surgery. There are several case reports, even in young adults, of myocardial ischemia and infarction, perhaps secondary to coronary artery spasm, in the setting of intraoperative use of topical cocaine.[62–65] Cocaine has also been suggested as a cause for postoperative delirium[66] and acute glaucoma.[67]

Phenylephrine, oxymetazoline, as well as the combination of lidocaine or bupivacaine with epinephrine have also been used to provide hemostasis and analgesia. Complications such as visual loss[68,69] and profound hypertension[61,70] have been attributed to the intranasal injection of local anesthesia in combination with epinephrine. Hypertension and tachycardia are secondary to a marked increase of up to 400% in plasma catecholamines within minutes of intranasal epinephrine infiltration.[71,72]

A review of 100 patients at the Mayo Clinic noted an average increase in systolic and diastolic blood pressures of 60 and 23 mm Hg, respectively, following intranasal injection of local anesthesia with epinephrine.[73] No relationship was found between the dose of epinephrine and the severity of hypertension, nor was there any episode of cardiac dysrhythmia, persistent myocardial ischemia, or myocardial infarction noted in this cohort.[74]

In contrast to the intuitive expectation of hypertension following epinephrine injection, significant hypotension has also been noted. Hemodynamic instability following infiltration with a local anesthetic containing epinephrine may be marked by a profound hypotension for 1 to 2 minutes.[75] Studies in both craniotomy and sinus surgery patients suggest that when patients develop hypotension following epinephrine injection it is self-limited and often followed by hypertension.[76,77] Further, it has been suggested that light general anesthesia is more effective than fluid bolus in ameliorating this hypertension.[78]

Multiple studies have been performed in the otorhinolaryngology patient population to determine the safety and efficacy of various combinations of drugs for vasoconstriction and analgesia.[78–82] Institutional and surgeon preferences often determine the selection of vasoconstricting agents.

It is critical to monitor for myocardial ischemia during the time when local anesthesia and vasoconstrictive agents are injected into or applied to the endonasal mucosa. If ST segment monitoring and alarms are available, the baseline levels of the PR segment and ST segment should be obtained and alarms activated. If extreme tachycardia, severe hypertension, or myocardial ischemia is detected, cocaine-soaked pledgets should be removed from the nasal cavity and injection of other vasoconstricting agents suspended.

Treatment of α-agonist–induced hypertension must also be judicious. Cardiogenic shock and pulmonary edema leading to cardiac arrest and even death have been reported in both children and adults receiving β-blockade to treat α-agonist–induced hypertension.[83,84] Because hypertension secondary to α-agonist–induced vasoconstriction preferentially shifts blood from the peripheral to the pulmonary circulation, left ventricular end-diastolic volume and pressure increase. Maintenance of contractility is important in this setting to prevent severe pulmonary edema. Theoretically, the negative inotropic consequences of calcium channel blockers or a significant increase in volatile anesthetic agent may have the same untoward effects as β-blockade.[84]

Thus, treatment of profound hypertension secondary to cocaine, phenylephrine, oxymetazoline, and even epinephrine may be more appropriately treated with α-antagonists such as sodium nitroprusside and phentolamine. Sublingual or intravenous infusion of nitroglycerin may be administered if myocardial ischemia occurs.

Arterial Injury

A rare but serious complication of transsphenoidal resection of pituitary and intracranial masses is injury to the internal carotid artery or to another artery, such as the ophthalmic artery.[85–87] The anesthesiologist for these cases must always anticipate that such injury is a possibility. Thus the anesthesiologist must ensure adequate venous access for rapid blood transfusion as well as the availability of sufficient crossmatched blood. If such an injury should occur, prompt volume and blood resuscitation is essential. If the injury to the artery cannot be repaired, the surgeon may decide to pack the bleeding vessel and transport the patient to the interventional radiology suite for embolization of the injured vessel.

Blood pressure management may be complicated by the need to assist the surgeon in the controlling the hemorrhage by avoiding hypertension, counterbalanced by the need to provide adequate cerebral perfusion pressure. An arterial line would be helpful in guiding volume resuscitation, blood transfusion, and blood pressure management in the setting of arterial injury.

Postoperative Management

Emergence from Anesthesia

In general, patients are extubated at the conclusion of transsphenoidal surgery. As discussed previously, the anesthesia is planned from the outset to maximize patient responsiveness as well as the patient's ability to maintain the airway. The criteria for extubation include a hemodynamically stable patient, appropriate respiratory rate and tidal volume during spontaneous ventilation, adequate reversal of neuromuscular blockade, adequate air movement (leak) around the endotracheal tube when the cuff is deflated, and the ability of the patient to follow commands. Other extubation criteria may be required in addition. Upon extubation, it is prudent to ensure the ability of the patient, who may have preexisting sleep apnea, to maintain adequate ventilation. Obviously, postoperative placement of a nasal airway is contraindicated. In addition, continuous positive airway pressure or bilevel positive airway pressure via a face mask would not be possible in the immediate postoperative period due to the risk of disrupting the surgical closure and possible pneumocephalus. If the patient has preexisting sleep apnea, it may be prudent for the patient to remain in a monitored setting overnight to ensure adequate ventilation.

With the technique described above, the patient generally does not require significant narcotic supplementation in the immediate postoperative period. As the local anesthesia wears off, however, patients require pain medication, which must be titrated judiciously, especially in the patient with sleep apnea. Use of postoperative morphine in the postanesthesia care unit (PACU) has been found to average between 5.2 and 6.7 mg in transsphenoidal surgery patients.[88] Bilateral infraorbital nerve blocks have been reported to decrease postoperative narcotic use.[89,90]

Postoperative Nausea and Vomiting Prophylaxis

Single-agent antiemetic prophylaxis was not found to reduce the incidence of postoperative emesis (7.5%) in a retrospective cohort of transsphenoidal surgery patients.[88] The need for rescue medication in the PACU for either nausea or emesis was reduced significantly, however. This population did not involve patients undergoing an endoscopic endonasal approach and also included cases of craniopharyngioma. In our institution we believe it is important to employ prophylaxis against postoperative nausea and vomiting in these patients. Even if a throat pack is used to prevent intraoperative bleeding from draining into the stomach, postoperative oozing may continue and even a small amount of blood swallowed by the patient may lead to nausea and vomiting. In a vicious circle, the straining from vomiting may lead to further venous oozing. It is our practice to aggressively administer prophylaxis against nausea and vomiting in a multimodal fashion with pharmaceuticals of different mechanisms of action. We also apply gentle careful orogastric suctioning immediately upon conclusion of the surgery. Obviously, nasogastric suction is contraindicated.

Diabetes Insipidus

Diabetes insipidus (DI) is a common complication of transsphenoidal pituitary surgery, with 31% of patients experiencing at least transient DI.[91] Review of a cohort of patients who have undergone minimally invasive endoscopic pituitary resection revealed a 13.6% rate of postoperative transient DI and a 2.7% rate of permanent DI.[92] In most cases the onset occurs 24 to 48 hours after surgery and resolves within 7 days.[92] The postoperative management of DI is discussed in detail in Chapter 34. Infrequently, however, DI presents intraoperatively with a voluminous increase in urine output. DI is characterized as an inability to concentrate the urine in the face of dehydration. Thus it is necessary to ensure that the increase in urine output is not secondary to overhydration or hyperglycemia. Laboratory findings consistent with DI would be a low urine specific gravity, a urine osmolality lower than plasma osmolality, and a serum sodium >145 mEq/L. Only in rare instances would it be necessary to give vasopressin intraoperatively.

References

1. Seidman PA, Kofke WA, Policare R, Young M. Anaesthetic complications of acromegaly. Br J Anaesth 2000;84:179–182
2. Melmed S. Acromegaly. N Engl J Med 1990;322:966–977
3. Nemergut EC, Dumont AS, Barry UT, Laws ER. Perioperative management of patients undergoing transsphenoidal pituitary surgery. Anesth Analg 2005;101:1170–1181
4. Schmitt H, Buchfelder M, Radespiel-Tröger M, Fahlbusch R. Difficult intubation in acromegalic patients: incidence and predictability. Anesthesiology 2000;93:110–114
5. Nemergut EC, Zuo Z. Airway management in patients with pituitary disease: a review of 746 patients. J Neurosurg Anesthesiol 2006;18:73–77
6. Kitahata LM. Airway difficulties associated with anaesthesia in acromegaly. Three case reports. Br J Anaesth 1971;43:1187–1190
7. Williams RG, Richards SH, Mills RG, Eccles R. Voice changes in acromegaly. Laryngoscope 1994;104:484–487
8. Edge WG, Whitwam JG. Chondro-calcinosis and difficult intubation in acromegaly. Anaesthesia 1981;36:677–680
9. Southwick JP, Katz J. Unusual airway difficulty in the acromegalic patient—indications for tracheostomy. Anesthesiology 1979;51:72–73
10. Ovassapian A, Doka JC, Romsa DE. Acromegaly—use of fiberoptic laryngoscopy to avoid tracheostomy. Anesthesiology 1981;54:429–430
11. Hakala P, Randell T, Valli H. Laryngoscopy and fibreoptic intubation in acromegalic patients. Br J Anaesth 1998;80:345–347
12. Fatti LM, Scacchi M, Pincelli AI, Lavezzi E, Cavagnini F. Prevalence and pathogenesis of sleep apnea and lung disease in acromegaly. Pituitary 2001;4:259–262
13. Piper JG, Dirks BA, Traynelis VC, VanGilder JC. Perioperative management and surgical outcome of the acromegalic patient with sleep apnea. Neurosurgery 1995;36:70–74, discussion 74–75
14. Shipley JE, Schteingart DE, Tandon R, Starkman MN. Sleep architecture and sleep apnea in patients with Cushing's disease. Sleep 1992;15:514–518
15. Paul M, Dueck M, Kampe S, Petzke F, Ladra A. Intracranial placement of a nasotracheal tube after transnasal trans-sphenoidal surgery. Br J Anaesth 2003;91:601–604
16. Pelttari L, Polo O, Rauhala E, et al. Nocturnal breathing abnormalities in acromegaly after adenomectomy. Clin Endocrinol (Oxf) 1995;43:175–182
17. Wilson CB. Role of surgery in the management of pituitary tumors. Neurosurg Clin N Am 1990;1:139–159
18. Rajasoorya C, Holdaway IM, Wrightson P, Scott DJ, Ibbertson HK. Determinants of clinical outcome and survival in acromegaly. Clin Endocrinol (Oxf) 1994;41:95–102
19. Clayton RN. Cardiovascular function in acromegaly. Endocr Rev 2003;24:272–277
20. Lie JT. Pathology of the heart in acromegaly: anatomic findings in 27 autopsied patients. Am Heart J 1980;100:41–52
21. Maison P, Démolis P, Young J, Schaison G, Giudicelli JF, Chanson P. Vascular reactivity in acromegalic patients: preliminary evidence for regional endothelial dysfunction and increased sympathetic vasoconstriction. Clin Endocrinol (Oxf) 2000;53:445–451
22. Herrmann BL, Bruch C, Saller B, et al. Acromegaly: evidence for a direct relation between disease activity and cardiac dysfunction in patients without ventricular hypertrophy. Clin Endocrinol (Oxf) 2002;56:595–602
23. Rossi L, Thiene G, Caragaro L, Giordano R, Lauro S. Dysrhythmias and sudden death in acromegalic heart disease. A clinicopathologic study. Chest 1977;72:495–498
24. Fazio S, Cittadini A, Sabatini D, et al. Evidence for biventricular involvement in acromegaly: a Doppler echocardiographic study. Eur Heart J 1993;14:26–33
25. Schwarz ER, Jammula P, Gupta R, Rosanio S. A case and review of acromegaly-induced cardiomyopathy and the relationship between growth hormone and heart failure: cause or cure or neither or both? J Cardiovasc Pharmacol Ther 2006;11:232–244
26. Kahaly G, Olshausen KV, Mohr-Kahaly S, et al. Arrhythmia profile in acromegaly. Eur Heart J 1992;13:51–56
27. Colao A, Ferone D, Marzullo P, Lombardi G. Systemic complications of acromegaly: epidemiology, pathogenesis, and management. Endocr Rev 2004;25:102–152
28. Colao A, Baldelli R, Marzullo P, et al. Systemic hypertension and impaired glucose tolerance are independently correlated to the

severity of the acromegalic cardiomyopathy. J Clin Endocrinol Metab 2000;85:193–199
29. McGuffin WL Jr, Sherman BM, Roth F, et al. Acromegaly and cardiovascular disorders. A prospective study. Ann Intern Med 1974;81:11–18
30. Bondanelli M, Ambrosio MR, degli Uberti EC. Pathogenesis and prevalence of hypertension in acromegaly. Pituitary 2001;4:239–249
31. Thuesen L, Christensen SE, Weeke J, Orskov H, Henningsen P. A hyperkinetic heart in uncomplicated active acromegaly. Explanation of hypertension in acromegalic patients? Acta Med Scand 1988;223:337–343
32. Ho KY, Kelly JJ. Role of growth hormone in fluid homeostasis. Horm Res 1991;36(Suppl 1):44–48
33. Møller J, Møller N, Frandsen E, Wolthers T, Jørgensen JO, Christiansen JS. Blockade of the renin-angiotensin-aldosterone system prevents growth hormone-induced fluid retention in humans. Am J Physiol 1997;272(5 Pt 1):E803–E808
34. Ikeda T, Terasawa H, Ishimura M, et al. Correlation between blood pressure and plasma insulin in acromegaly. J Intern Med 1993;234:61–63
35. Bondanelli M, Ambrosio MR, Franceschetti P, Margutti A, Trasforini G, Degli Uberti EC. Diurnal rhythm of plasma catecholamines in acromegaly. J Clin Endocrinol Metab 1999;84:2458–2467
36. Wickman A, Friberg P, Adams MA, et al. Induction of growth hormone receptor and insulin-like growth factor-I mRNA in aorta and caval vein during hemodynamic challenge. Hypertension 1997;29(1 Pt 1):123–130
37. López-Velasco R, Escobar-Morreale HF, Vega B, et al. Cardiac involvement in acromegaly: specific myocardiopathy or consequence of systemic hypertension? J Clin Endocrinol Metab 1997;82:1047–1053
38. Ross EJ, Marshall-Jones P, Friedman M. Cushing's syndrome: diagnostic criteria. QJM 1966;35:149–192
39. Pirpiris M, Yeung S, Dewar E, Jennings GL, Whitworth JA. Hydrocortisone-induced hypertension in men. The role of cardiac output. Am J Hypertens 1993;6:287–294
40. Mantero F, Boscaro M. Glucocorticoid-dependent hypertension. J Steroid Biochem Mol Biol 1992;43:409–413
41. Sato A, Suzuki H, Murakami M, Nakazato Y, Iwaita Y, Saruta T. Glucocorticoid increases angiotensin II type 1 receptor and its gene expression. Hypertension 1994;23:25–30
42. Sato A, Suzuki H, Iwaita Y, Nakazato Y, Kato H, Saruta T. Potentiation of inositol trisphosphate production by dexamethasone. Hypertension 1992;19:109–115
43. Sugihara N, Shimizu M, Shimizu K, et al. Disproportionate hypertrophy of the interventricular septum and its regression in Cushing's syndrome. Report of three cases. Intern Med 1992;31:407–413
44. Muiesan ML, Lupia M, Salvetti M, et al. Left ventricular structural and functional characteristics in Cushing's syndrome. J Am Coll Cardiol 2003;41:2275–2279
45. Sugihara N, Shimizu M, Kita Y, et al. Cardiac characteristics and postoperative courses in Cushing's syndrome. Am J Cardiol 1992;69:1475–1480
46. Mindermann T, Wilson CB. Thyrotropin-producing pituitary adenomas. J Neurosurg 1993;79:521–527
47. Melmed S, Braunstein GD, Chang RJ, Becker DP. Pituitary tumors secreting growth hormone and prolactin. Ann Intern Med 1986;105:238–253
48. Smith M, Hirsch NP. Pituitary disease and anaesthesia. Br J Anaesth 2000;85:3–14
49. Seidman PA, Kofke WA, Policare R, Young M. Anaesthetic complications of acromegaly. Br J Anaesth 2000;84:179–182
50. Baird TA, Parsons MW, Phanh T, et al. Persistent poststroke hyperglycemia is independently associated with infarct expansion and worse clinical outcome. Stroke 2003;34:2208–2214
51. Lindsberg PJ, Roine RO. Hyperglycemia in acute stroke. Stroke 2004;35:363–364
52. Sieber FE. The neurologic implications of diabetic hyperglycemia during surgical procedures at increased risk for brain ischemia. J Clin Anesth 1997;9:334–340
53. Vance ML. Perioperative management of patients undergoing pituitary surgery. Endocrinol Metab Clin North Am 2003;32:355–365
54. Jane JA Jr, Thapar K, Kaptain GJ, Maartens N, Laws ER Jr. Pituitary surgery: transsphenoidal approach. Neurosurgery 2002;51:435–442, discussion 442–444
55. Campkin TV. Radial artery cannulation. Potential hazard in patients with acromegaly. Anaesthesia 1980;35:1008–1009
56. Mathes AM, Kreuer S, Schneider SO, Ziegeler S, Grundmann U. The performance of six pulse oximeters in the environment of neuronavigation. Anesth Analg 2008;107:541–544
57. Law-Koune JD, Liu N, Szekely B, Fischler M. Using the intubating laryngeal mask airway for ventilation and endotracheal intubation in anesthetized and unparalyzed acromegalic patients. J Neurosurg Anesthesiol 2004;16:11–13
58. Gemma M, Tommasino C, Cozzi S, et al. Remifentanil provides hemodynamic stability and faster awakening time in transsphenoidal surgery. Anesth Analg 2002;94:163–168
59. Cafiero T, Cavallo LM, Frangiosa A, et al. Clinical comparison of remifentanil-sevoflurane vs. remifentanil-propofol for endoscopic endonasal transphenoidal surgery. Eur J Anaesthesiol 2007;24:441–446
60. Abou-Madi MN, Trop D, Barnes J. Aetiology and control of cardiovascular reactions during trans-sphenoidal resection of pituitary microadenomas. Can Anaesth Soc J 1980;27:491–495
61. Keegan MT, Atkinson JLD, Kasperbauer JL, Lanier WL. Exaggerated hemodynamic responses to nasal injection and awakening from anesthesia in a Cushingoid patient having transsphenoidal hypophysectomy. J Neurosurg Anesthesiol 2000;12:225–229
62. Kara CO, Kaftan A, Atalay H, Pinar HS, Oğmen G. Cardiovascular safety of cocaine anaesthesia in the presence of adrenaline during septal surgery. J Otolaryngol 2001;30:145–148
63. Makaryus JN, Makaryus AN, Johnson M. Acute myocardial infarction following the use of intranasal anesthetic cocaine. South Med J 2006;99:759–761
64. Ross GS, Bell J. Myocardial infarction associated with inappropriate use of topical cocaine as treatment for epistaxis. Am J Emerg Med 1992;10:219–222
65. Laffey JG, Neligan P, Ormonde G. Prolonged perioperative myocardial ischemia in a young male: due to topical intranasal cocaine? J Clin Anesth 1999;11:419–424
66. Audu PB, Curtis N, Armstead V. An unusual case of emergence delirium. J Clin Anesth 2004;16:545–547
67. Hari CK, Roblin DG, Clayton MI, Nair RG. Acute angle closure glaucoma precipitated by intranasal application of cocaine. J Laryngol Otol 1999;113:250–251
68. Savino PJ, Burde RM, Mills RP. Visual loss following intranasal anesthetic injection. J Clin Neuroophthalmol 1990;10:140–144
69. Maaranen TH, Mäntyjärvi MI. Central retinal artery occlusion after a local anesthetic with adrenaline on nasal mucosa. J Neuroophthalmol 2000;20:234–235
70. Chelliah YR, Manninen PH. Hazards of epinephrine in transsphenoidal pituitary surgery. J Neurosurg Anesthesiol 2002;14:43–46

71. Taylor S, Achola K, Smith G. Plasma catecholamine concentrations. The effects of infiltration with local analgesics and vasoconstrictors during nasal operations. Anaesthesia 1984;39:520–523
72. John G, Low JM, Tan PE, van Hasselt CA. Plasma catecholamine levels during functional endoscopic sinus surgery. Clin Otolaryngol Allied Sci 1995;20:213–215
73. Pasternak JJ, Atkinson JL, Kasperbauer JL, Lanier WL. Hemodynamic responses to epinephrine-containing local anesthetic injection and to emergence from general anesthesia in transsphenoidal hypophysectomy patients. J Neurosurg Anesthesiol 2004;16:189–195
74. Yang JJ, Li WY, Jil Q, et al. Local anesthesia for functional endoscopic sinus surgery employing small volumes of epinephrine-containing solutions of lidocaine produces profound hypotension. Acta Anaesthesiol Scand 2005;49:1471–1476
75. Yang JJ, Zheng J, Liu HJ, Liu YX, Shen JC, Zhou ZQ. Epinephrine infiltration on nasal field causes significant hemodynamic changes: hypotension episode monitored by impedance-cardiography under general anesthesia. J Pharm Pharm Sci 2006;9:190–197
76. Yang JJ, Cheng HL, Shang RJ, et al. Hemodynamic changes due to infiltration of the scalp with epinephrine-containing lidocaine solution: a hypotensive episode before craniotomy. J Neurosurg Anesthesiol 2007;19:31–37
77. Li WY, Zhou ZQ, Ji JF, Li ZQ, Yang JJ, Shang RJ. Relatively light general anesthesia is more effective than fluid expansion in reducing the severity of epinephrine-induced hypotension during functional endoscopic sinus surgery. Chin Med J (Engl) 2007;120:1299–1302
78. Katz RI, Hovagim AR, Finkelstein HS, Grinberg Y, Boccio RV, Poppers PJ. A comparison of cocaine, lidocaine with epinephrine, and oxymetazoline for prevention of epistaxis on nasotracheal intubation. J Clin Anesth 1990;2:16–20
79. Dunlevy TM, O'Malley TP, Postma GN. Optimal concentration of epinephrine for vasoconstriction in neck surgery. Laryngoscope 1996;106:1412–1414
80. Moore MA, Weiskopf RB, Eger EI II, Wilson C, Lu G. Arrhythmogenic doses of epinephrine are similar during desflurane or isoflurane anesthesia in humans. Anesthesiology 1993;79:943–947
81. Drivas EI, Hajiioannou JK, Lachanas VA, Bizaki AJ, Kyrmizakis DE, Bizakis JG. Cocaine versus tetracaine in septoplasty: a prospective, randomized, controlled trial. J Laryngol Otol 2007;121:130–133
82. Benjamin E, Wong DKK, Choa D. "Moffett's" solution: a review of the evidence and scientific basis for the topical preparation of the nose. Clin Otolaryngol Allied Sci 2004;29:582–587
83. Schwalm J-D, Hamstra J, Mulji A, Velianou JL. Cardiogenic shock following nasal septoplasty: a case report and review of the literature. Can J Anaesth 2008;55:376–379
84. Groudine SB, Hollinger I, Jones J, DeBouno BA; The Phenylephrine Advisory Committee. New York State guidelines on the topical use of phenylephrine in the operating room. Anesthesiology 2000;92: 859–864
85. Pepper JP, Wadhwa AK, Tsai F, Shibuya T, Wong BJ. Cavernous carotid injury during functional endoscopic sinus surgery: case presentations and guidelines for optimal management. Am J Rhinol 2007;21:105–109
86. Weidenbecher M, Huk WJ, Iro H. Internal carotid artery injury during functional endoscopic sinus surgery and its management. Eur Arch Otorhinolaryngol 2005;262:640–645
87. Gadhinglajkar SV, Sreedhar R, Bhattacharya RN. Carotid artery injury during transsphenoidal resection of pituitary tumor: anesthesia perspective. J Neurosurg Anesthesiol 2003;15:323–326
88. Flynn BC, Nemergut EC. Postoperative nausea and vomiting and pain after transsphenoidal surgery: a review of 877 patients. Anesth Analg 2006;103:162–167
89. McAdam D, Muro K, Suresh S. The use of infraorbital nerve block for postoperative pain control after transsphenoidal hypophysectomy. Reg Anesth Pain Med 2005;30:572–573
90. Higashizawa T, Koga Y. Effect of infraorbital nerve block under general anesthesia on consumption of isoflurane and postoperative pain in endoscopic endonasal maxillary sinus surgery. J Anesth 2001;15:136–138
91. Hensen J, Henig A, Fahlbusch R, Meyer M, Boehnert M, Buchfelder M. Prevalence, predictors and patterns of postoperative polyuria and hyponatraemia in the immediate course after transsphenoidal surgery for pituitary adenomas. Clin Endocrinol (Oxf) 1999;50: 431–439
92. Sigounas DG, Sharpless JL, Cheng DM, Johnson TG, Senior BA, Ewend MG. Predictors and incidence of central diabetes insipidus after endoscopic pituitary surgery. Neurosurgery 2008;62:71–78, discussion 78–79

31 Managing Postoperative Sinusitis

Ameet Singh, Madeleine R. Schaberg, Gurston G. Nyquist, and Vijay K. Anand

Postoperative care of the nasal and paranasal sinuses after endoscopic pituitary and skull base surgery is based on many of the well-established principles in endoscopic sinus surgery for inflammatory disease. The chief goals include maximizing wound healing, restoring mucociliary clearance, maintaining ostia patency, preventing scar formation, and avoiding rhinosinusitis.[1] Although all of the above-mentioned goals are important, none is more critical than the preservation and rapid healing of the skull base. This is important to prevent serious complications such as cerebrospinal fluid (CSF) leaks, tension pneumocephalus, and meningitis.[2,3]

The otolaryngologist plays a crucial role in promoting wound healing of the skull base reconstruction during the postoperative period. Excessive crusting and rhinosinusitis secondary to impaired mucociliary clearance, synechia formation, and obstruction of sinus ostia may occur without adequate surveillance and intervention. Medical management includes saline irrigation, topical or oral antibiotics, nasal steroid sprays, decongestants, and mucolytics. In addition, postoperative nasal endoscopy with debridement is imperative for enhancing sinonasal healing and preventing sinonasal complications. Proper medical and surgical management of the sinonasal cavity provides the best opportunity for rapid and safe healing after endoscopic skull base surgery.

Sinonasal Management

Postoperative management of the sinonasal cavity is individualized based on the operative intervention and the patient's wound-healing capabilities. The surgical approach, extent of surgery, presence of an intraoperative CSF leak, complexity of skull base reconstruction, and the patient's comorbidities help to guide the postoperative management strategy. For example, extended transplanum, transtuberculum approaches to resect sellar-suprasellar pituitary macroadenomas require a greater amount of postoperative sinonasal care than resection of smaller intrasellar pituitary microadenomas. More extensive surgical dissection through the sinonasal cavity often requires a longer amount of time for wound healing and establishment of mucociliary clearance. Most approaches for pituitary adenomas require limited dissection, and therefore no more than 4 to 6 weeks is required for complete wound healing. Patient comorbidities such as diabetes, chronic renal failure, and chronic steroid use may prolong healing of the sinonasal cavity and skull base. Skull base reconstruction with biomaterials may prolong postoperative healing compared with the use of a vascularized pedicled flap (**Fig. 31.1**). A meticulous mucosa-preserving surgical approach usually results in

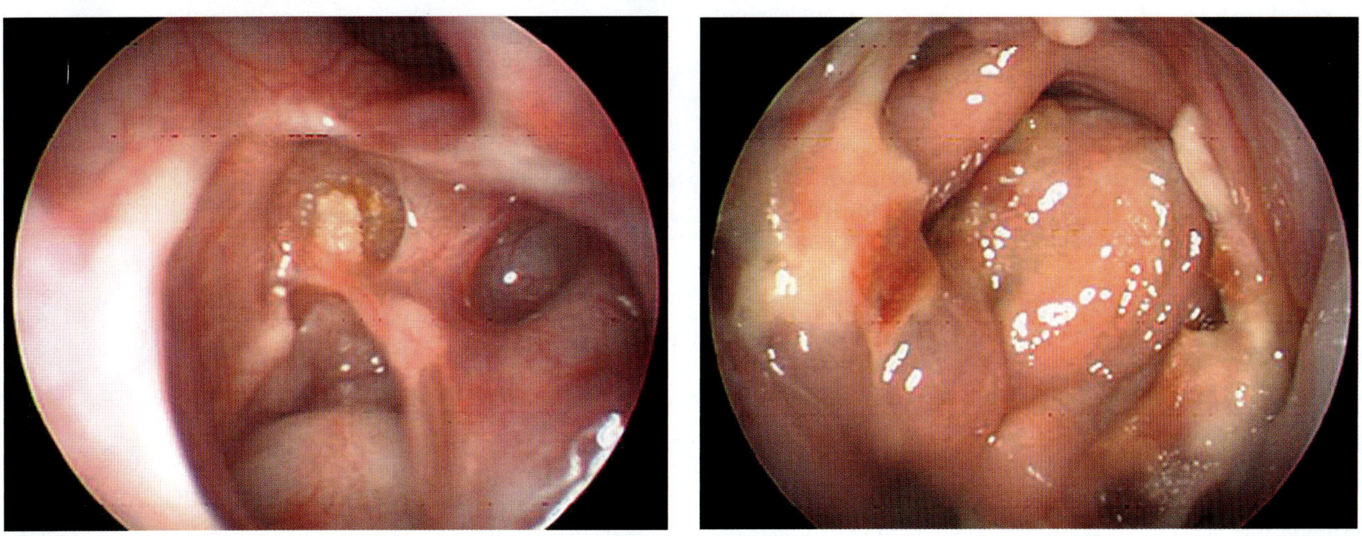

A B

Fig. 31.1 **(A)** Incomplete mucosalization of the skull base at 6 weeks after skull base reconstruction with a biomaterial implant. **(B)** Healing of the skull base at 2 weeks after skull base reconstruction with a vascularized nasoseptal flap for an extended approach to a pituitary adenoma.

decreased crusting, scarring, and obstruction of natural sinus ostia. Finally, rare intraoperative or postoperative complications such as bleeding, rhinosinusitis, and CSF leaks may also alter the postoperative management of the sinonasal cavity.

Perioperative Management

The vast majority of patients after endoscopic pituitary and skull base surgery are admitted to the intensive care unit in the immediate postoperative period for observation. These patients often require frequent neurologic examinations, occasional lumbar drainage management, and monitoring for diabetes insipidus, CSF leaks, and pneumocephalus. Telfa nasal packs are placed anteriorly in the nasal cavities to wick blood in the immediate postoperative period. These packs are removed 24 to 48 hours after the surgical procedure, preferably prior to obtaining the postoperative magnetic resonance imaging (MRI). The head of the bed is kept elevated, usually no more than 30 degrees from the supine position. Ice packs are placed around the nose and face for comfort as needed. A face tent provides mist humidification to the sinonasal cavity and decreases patient discomfort. Nasal cannulae are strictly avoided during the postoperative period. Delivery of oxygen through a nasal cannula has the potential of causing a tension pneumocephalus, a serious and potentially devastating complication of endonasal, intracranial approaches (**Fig. 31.2**). Nasal sprays and irrigation should be avoided during the first postoperative week because they may cause bleeding or displace materials used for skull base reconstruction.

All patients are given perioperative antibiotics for 24 to 48 hours after surgery. A series of 90 patients undergoing endoscopic skull base surgery who received a single dose of perioperative antibiotics yielded no cases of intracranial infections or meningitis.[4] These results are encouraging because skull base reconstruction entails transport of the grafts (fat, fascia lata, Medpor [Porex, Newnan, GA]) though the nasal cavity, considered to be a contaminated field. The potential ramifications of infection in these patients include meningitis, intracranial abscesses, and vascular compromise.

Patients are advised to avoid nose blowing, sneezing with their mouth open, sipping through straws, and heavy lifting or other strenuous activity, to adhere to a bowel regimen of stool softeners, and to avoid any maneuvers that may increase their intracranial pressure. Patients are also instructed to avoid hot showers to prevent vasodilation of intranasal vessels and subsequent bleeding. Patients are usually discharged with a prescription for an antibiotic and pain control along with a follow-up appointment with the otolaryngologist in 1 week.

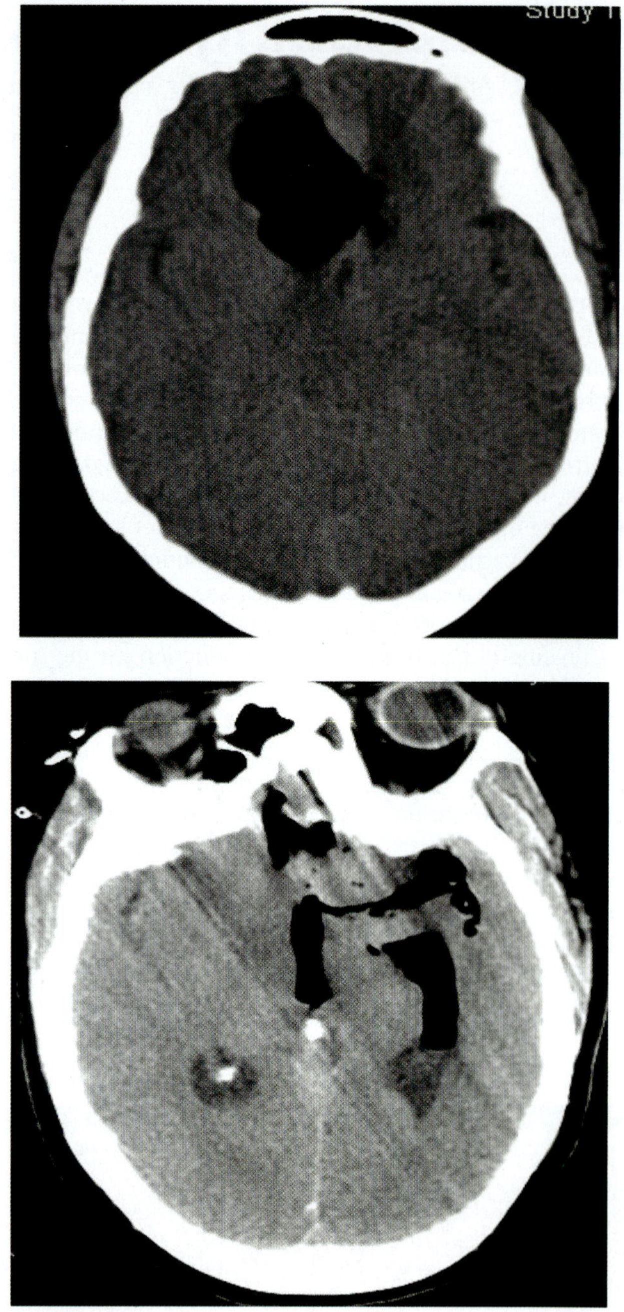

A

B

Fig. 31.2 Delivery of oxygen with nasal cannula after endoscopic skull base surgery resulted in **(A)** tension pneumocephalus at the base of the frontal lobe, which may enter into **(B)** the subarachnoid space and intraventricularly.

Postoperative Management

Postoperative sinonasal care begins with the otolaryngologist, approximately 1 week after discharge from the hospital. Gentle postoperative endoscopic debridement of the sinonasal cavity is performed. This includes removing crusting, old blood, mucoid secretions, and breakdown products from hemostatic agents and tissue. The sphenoid sinus cavity is carefully inspected for a CSF leak, and secretions are gently suctioned, without instrumenting the skull base. Any crusting along the reconstruction site is left in place until subsequent visits when the scabs are no longer adherent to the skull base. Scabs are never aggressively debrided from the skull base in the early postoperative visits as this may precipitate bleeding or a CSF leak.

Vestibular sores or abrasions to the nasal ala and vestibule are extremely rare. However, if present, they should be treated with local wound care and topical antibiotic ointment. Patients are also placed on a gentamicin nasal spray (80 mg in 1000 mL of saline) three times a day for 4 weeks to decrease mucosal edema and bacterial colony count, as well as to improve nasal mucociliary function and nasal hygiene.[5] Systemic absorption of intraoperative gentamicin nasal irrigation has been studied and appears to be below systemic therapeutic levels.[6] Patients are typically seen in the office 3 and 6 weeks after discharge from the hospital. Follow-up visits consist of postoperative sinonasal debridements, lysis of synechia, and examination of the skull base. A cranial nerve exam is performed in addition to evaluate for meningeal signs or symptoms as well as the presence of CSF rhinorrhea. Extended skull base approaches require more frequent and lengthier postoperative follow-up visits to remove crusting and ensure good mucosal healing.

Management of Sinonasal Complications

Bleeding

Postoperative bleeding rarely requires intervention if meticulous hemostasis is maintained intraoperatively. In our series of pituitary and anterior skull base cases, there was a 2% incidence of postoperative epistaxis. Minor postoperative bleeding is expected and usually does not require any treatment other than mist humidification and frequent changing of the nasal drip pad. In rare cases, a moderate amount of bleeding may be controlled with placement of a hemostatic matrix or intranasal packing. Endoscopic visualization of the origin is recommended for expedient hemostatic control and to avoid jeopardizing the skull base reconstruction. In some circumstances, if the patient is cooperative, local anesthesia and electrocautery can be applied under endoscopic guidance to control the bleeding. If the bleeding is brisk, located deeper in the nasal cavity, and difficult to identify despite endoscopic visualization, controlling the hemorrhage in the operating room is preferable. This is particularly important in the immediate postoperative period, given the risk of displacing the skull base reconstruction materials if a nasal pack is placed without adequate visualization. Moreover, although rare, depending on the extent of intracranial dissection especially within the cavernous sinus, unidentified bleeding deep in the nasal cavity may represent an intracranial source.

In endoscopic pituitary surgery, particular attention must be directed to the posterior nasal and posterior septal branches off the sphenopalatine artery. For extended transethmoidal, transcribriform, or transorbital procedures, attention should be directed to branches of the anterior and posterior ethmoidal arteries. Suspected bleeding from the ethmoidal arteries necessitates immediate evaluation of the eye to rule out a retrobulbar hematoma. In the extremely rare event of a sentinel bleed suggestive of bleeding from the carotid artery, immediate intranasal packing and insertion of a Foley balloon should be initiated to tamponade the bleed. A hemodynamically stable patient should be taken emergently for angiography. An unstable patient should be emergently taken to the operating room for carotid ligation.

Crusting

Crusting almost always occurs after endoscopic pituitary surgery. However, it is usually limited to the nasal cavity along the free mucosal edges of the posterior septum and sphenoid rostrum. Crusting may be more extensive in extended skull base procedures for larger pituitary adenomas, given the greater amount of sinonasal dissection and mucosal damage (**Fig. 31.3**). Postoperative debridement after endoscopic skull base surgery is important to improve mucosal healing, encourage mucociliary function, decrease synechia formation, prevent sinonasal obstruction, avoid acute or chronic rhinosinusitis, and improve patient comfort. The

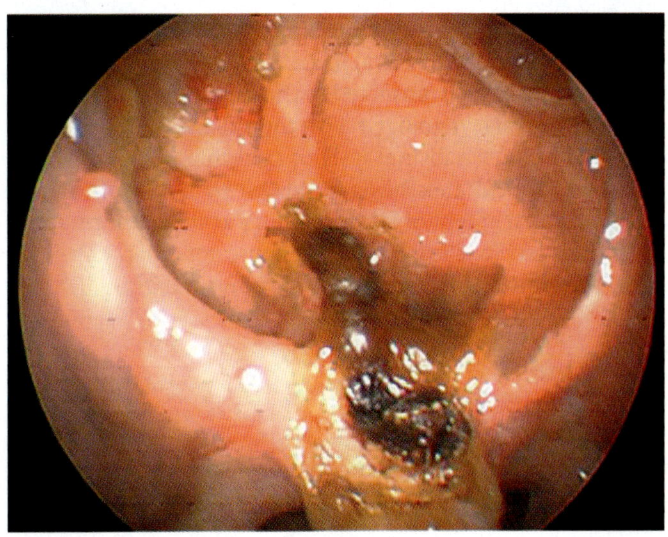

Fig. 31.3 Crusting noted in the postoperative period after an extended endoscopic approach to pituitary adenoma.

disadvantages include bleeding, mucosal avulsion, and minor discomfort.

Multiple studies evaluating the advantages and disadvantages of postoperative debridement in endoscopic sinus surgery have been conducted. A randomized, blinded clinical trial evaluating postoperative debridement in patients undergoing endoscopic sinus surgery was published in 2006.[7] Sixty patients were divided into two groups; one group used saline nasal irrigation during the postoperative period (control group), and the other used saline irrigation and underwent weekly postoperative debridements. At 12 weeks postoperatively, the debridement group experienced a slightly longer duration of pain (2.7 days versus 2.3 days), but less nasal obstruction and fewer synechiae over time.[8] Patients experience similar benefits and disadvantages with postoperative debridement after endoscopic pituitary surgery. Overaggressive debridement especially at the skull base should be absolutely avoided.

Patients are encouraged to maintain good nasal hygiene with the use of nasal sprays, irrigation, moisturization of the nose, and mist humidification. Initial experience suggests that these remedies should be used a week after surgery, approximately, after the initial postoperative visit with the otolaryngologist.

Synechia

Postoperative synechia may occur in the sinonasal cavity after endoscopic pituitary and skull base surgery, despite meticulous surgical and postoperative care. Synechia may be found between the posterior nasal septum and middle turbinate/lateral nasal wall after the transnasal, transsphenoidal approach to the sella. Lateral approaches to the sphenoid sinus or transpterygoid approaches to the pterygopalatine or infratemporal fossa may result in synechia between the middle turbinate and lateral nasal wall. Soft, immature synechia may be easily transected in the early postoperative period by the otolaryngologist with topical anesthesia. Mature synechia require a formal lysis of synechia, which involves topical and local anesthesia, followed by resection of scar tissue and placement of Silastic splints to avoid reformation. Lysis of synechia is important to ensure good nasal air flow, prevent sinonasal obstruction, and rhinosinusitis.

Rhinosinusitis

Acute Rhinosinusitis

Acute rhinosinusitis is rare and unusual after endoscopic pituitary or skull base surgery. In our series the incidence of postoperative rhinosinusitis (based on American Academy of Otolaryngology–Head and Neck Surgery guidelines) was less than 2% for endoscopic pituitary surgery. More common was crusting, accompanied with mucoid or purulent secretions without significant mucosal inflammation. Typically, postoperative debridement of the sinonasal cavity in addition to topical nasal therapy is sufficient to improve nasal hygiene. Occasionally, inflammation of the nose and sinuses accompanied by purulent secretions may occur, resulting in acute rhinosinusitis. In general, acute rhinosinusitis is defined as symptomatic inflammation of the nose and paranasal sinuses, or more specifically 10 days or more of purulent nasal drainage accompanied by nasal obstruction, facial pain and pressure, or both.[9]

Medical management with antibiotics is well supported in the literature to eradicate bacteria from the sinuses, hasten recovery, and improve quality of life.[9] Adjunctive treatments, which include decongestants, corticosteroids, saline irrigation, and mucolytics, may provide symptomatic relief to patients. Nasal steroid sprays have been shown to reduce mean symptom scores in nonsevere acute rhinosinusitis.[10] However, topical therapy, including nasal sprays and irrigation, must be used cautiously in the immediate postoperative period to avoid disturbing the skull base reconstruction, specifically hastening the dissolution of dural and tissue sealants. Adequate assessment of pain and appropriate treatment with analgesics must also be initiated.

Evidence for deferring antibiotics in patients with acute bacterial rhinosinusitis with mild symptoms (temperature <100°F) exists in the literature. This strategy is based primarily on comparing antibiotics versus placebo for acute rhinosinusitis, showing spontaneous improvement in 62 to 69% of patients after 7 to 14 days, spontaneous cure in 19 to 39%, and improvement in 13 to 19% when antibiotics are used.[9] Although this may apply in patients with acute bacterial rhinosinusitis, it is probably an unwise strategy after endoscopic pituitary and skull base surgery. Because meningitis is a possibility in the setting of acute bacterial rhinosinusitis, it must be treated aggressively in patients after endoscopic pituitary surgery.

Although amoxicillin is the first-line therapy for acute bacterial rhinosinusitis, it may not be the appropriate choice in patients after endoscopic pituitary and skull base surgery. This is particularly true because these patients have usually received antibiotics while in the hospital, thereby increasing the risk of antibiotic-resistant bacteria. In addition, amoxicillin is ineffective against β-lactamase–producing *Moraxella catarrhalis* and *Haemophilus influenzae* (approximately 80% and 30% of isolates, respectively).[9] High-dose amoxicillin-clavulanate (4 g per day amoxicillin equivalent), a respiratory fluoroquinolone (levofloxacin, moxifloxacin), macrolides, or a third-generation cephalosporin (ceftriaxone) may be a better choice for antibiotic therapy in these patients.

Endoscopic culture-directed treatment of acute bacterial rhinosinusitis has improved treatment strategies.[11] This technique may be particularly important for patients with acute bacterial rhinosinusitis after endoscopic pituitary or skull base surgery. Studies in patients with acute bacterial rhinosinusitis after endoscopic sinus surgery have shown that most postoperative infections were present as de novo infections by bacteria other than colonizing bacteria.[12] Given this information, the best treatment for acute bacterial rhinosinusitis may be with endoscopic culture-directed antibiotics.

Topical therapy, including nasal sprays and irrigation as well as postoperative surgical debridements, needs to be performed cautiously given the potential for intracranial spread of infection. This is certainly not the case after the skull base is well healed but is a more significant consideration during the acute postoperative period. Nasal sprays and irrigation may displace the multilayer reconstruction but are more likely to hasten the breakdown of dural and tissue sealants. Postoperative debridements must also proceed with significant caution given the risk of disturbing the multilayered skull base reconstruction. A small piece of crust in the posterior nasal cavity could be tightly tethered to one of the layers of the multilayered skull base reconstruction. Any attempt to remove this crust could disturb the skull base reconstruction, resulting in a potential CSF leak or one-way valve causing pneumocephalus. Care should be exercised during endoscopic debridement to avoid a traumatic CSF leak.

Meningitis is a rare but possible complication in the setting of acute bacterial rhinosinusitis. The recent literature points to a rate of less than 3% for intracranial complications such as meningitis, CSF leaks, and pneumocephalus in the perioperative period after endoscopic endonasal skull base surgery including extended approaches.[2]

Chronic Rhinosinusitis

Chronic rhinosinusitis in patients after endoscopic pituitary and skull base surgery is usually limited to the sphenoid sinus, in which case it is known as sphenoiditis, and the symptoms manifested are more frequently retro-orbital headache, visual changes, meningitis, and nasal obstruction.[13] The symptoms of sphenoid sinusitis tend to be insidious, and a high index of suspicion must be maintained for diagnosis. The pathophysiology of sphenoid sinusitis in the postsurgical patient is varied. It can be due to mechanical obstruction of the sphenoid ostia, synechiae, decreased mucociliary clearance, or mucocele formation.

The incidence of postoperative sinusitis following transsphenoidal pituitary surgery was first addressed by the Johns Hopkins group in the early 1980s. In their large series of more than 100 cases, the incidence of postoperative sinusitis following the sublabial transseptal approach was 15%.[14] All patients in this cohort were successfully managed medically. In a 2005 review of 200 cases of both endoscopic and sublabial transseptal transsphenoidal pituitary surgery, Batra et al[15] reported an incidence of 7.5%. Of the 10 patients with sphenoid sinusitis, half were managed medically, with the other half requiring surgery (one report of a sphenoid sinus mucocele. Senior et al[16] looked at a large cohort of more than 170 patients who underwent a purely endoscopic transsphenoidal approach and found the incidence of postsurgical sphenoid sinusitis to be 5.7%. In his group of patients, all but one were treated effectively with oral and topical antibiotics. The one patient whose condition did not resolve required surgery for bilateral sphenoid mucoceles. Interestingly, Lu et al[17] recently published their results with a series of more than 300 patients who underwent purely endonasal endoscopic transsphenoidal surgery. They had a 6.2% rate of sphenoid sinusitis, 65% of which resolved with medical management; the remaining required surgery (one mucocele was reported).

An incidence of between 6% and 15% is thus supported by the otolaryngologic literature.[13–16] In the most recent series, however, in which the trend has been away from the sublabial transseptal approach and toward the purely endoscopic approach, the incidence has decreased to the 6 to 8% range.[15–17] The neurosurgical literature reports a slightly decreased incidence, ranging from 1 to 4%.[18,19] It is unclear if the reasons for the decreased incidence is secondary to inadequate follow-up.

Determining the exact incidence remains difficult due to the small number of cases as well as the varied surgical approaches and closure materials used. This is further complicated by the fact that many of these patients receive postoperative radiation, and this may play a role in sphenoid sinusitis unrelated to the surgery itself. Of utmost importance are awareness and continued postoperative follow-up in these patients.

Role of Imaging in Diagnosis

Computed Tomography

Imaging is an important diagnostic tool in the evaluation of patients after endoscopic pituitary surgery. Sphenoid abnormalities remain visible on computed tomography (CT) in the early postoperative period due to postsurgical inflammation, debris, blood, and mucus retention.[20] These immediate postoperative inflammatory changes, however, resolve on CT scan by 3 months.[21] Batra et al[15] reported that in 90% of patients with postoperative sinusitis, CT was critical in their diagnosis, with findings ranging from mucosal thickening to opacification. Of note is that in this series the CT scans were performed after the patient had been having symptoms for an average of 3 years. Performing CTs in the immediate postoperative period is nonillustrative due to the expected inflammatory changes. Therefore, endoscopic findings are more valuable in diagnosing sinusitis during this period. Imaging with CT remains crucial in detecting mucoceles.

Magnetic Resonance Imaging

Magnetic resonance imaging (MRI) enables improved soft tissue differentiation based on density. MRI can assist in the diagnosis of a patient with symptoms clinically suggestive of sphenoid sinusitis. Inflamed mucosa appears as a low signal on T1 and high signal on T2 due to its high water content, whereas fibrosis has a low signal content on T1 and T2. In a study by Stickney et al,[22] in which MRIs were performed at varying intervals after transsphenoidal surgery, abnormalities continued long after 3 months. Early scans, performed 1 to 12 weeks after surgery, showed large effusions in all patients and 100% were characterized as abnormal with high T1 signal. Intermediate scans, performed 6 to 18 months after surgery, were abnormal in 71% of patients and showed continued thickened mucosa but with low T1 signal. Late scans, performed 2 to 3 years after surgery, were abnormal in 78% of patients and were similar to the scans performed at 6 to 18 months with thickened mucosa and low T1 signal. Thus the MRI characteristics last far longer than 3 months after surgery and are consistent with fibrotic rather than inflamed mucosa.

Treatment for Postoperative Sinusitis: When Is Surgery Necessary?

Uncomplicated Sphenoiditis

The cornerstone of treatment for uncomplicated sphenoid sinusitis is medical therapy, as previously discussed. Broad-spectrum antibiotics are instituted along with steroid nasal sprays and decongestants for 14 days with resolution of symptoms expected within 3 months.

Complicated Sphenoiditis

Complicated sphenoid sinusitis, referring to any sphenoiditis that is refractory to over 3 months of medical therapy, requires surgical management. This term also applies to any condition that has resulted in neurologic or ophthalmologic complications secondary to an ascending infection or a sphenoid sinus mucocele. If the ostia have significant stenosis or scarring, surgery may also be indicated depending on the nature of the obstruction. Surgical intervention entails enlarging the sphenoidotomy and removal of debris to improve drainage and restore mucociliary flow.

Role of Intravenous Antibiotics

Intravenous antibiotics have been used in the treatment of select patients with persistent chronic sinusitis.[23] Their use on an outpatient long-term basis, typically a 6-week course of treatment, has reasonable effectiveness with a low incidence of complications.[24] In the setting of sinusitis following skull base surgery, it is indicated in the most rare cases of refractory sinusitis or in the treatment of clinically significant methicillin-resistant *Staphylococcus aureus* sinusitis.

Skull Base Reconstruction

A variety of materials and techniques have been used in endoscopic skull base reconstruction after endoscopic pituitary surgery. Materials include autografts, allografts, and homografts. Techniques include single-layer, multilayer, onlay, inlay, gasket-seal, and pedicled vascularized grafts, among others.[3,25] Failure of skull base reconstruction may result in CSF leaks, meningitis, or pneumocephalus. Postoperative management after endoscopic pituitary surgery emphasizes the rapid healing of the skull base. Topical nasal therapy must be used with caution while concurrently keeping the cavity moist to promote skull base healing. Postoperative debridement near the skull base reconstruction must proceed with caution because removing a crust may displace the graft and result in a CSF leak or pneumocephalus. Rigid grafts such as Medpor prothesis and titanium plates that partially extrude after endoscopic pituitary surgery should be left alone and removed only if and when they fall into the sphenoid sinus (**Fig. 31.4**) or become a source of infection. Early experience appears to suggest that mucosa-preserving dissection and use of autogenous grafts or vascularized pedicled flaps are preferable for rapid healing of the skull base after endoscopic pituitary surgery.

Conclusion

Postoperative management after endoscopic pituitary surgery closely approximates the care received by patients after endoscopic sinus surgery. Preservation and rapid healing of

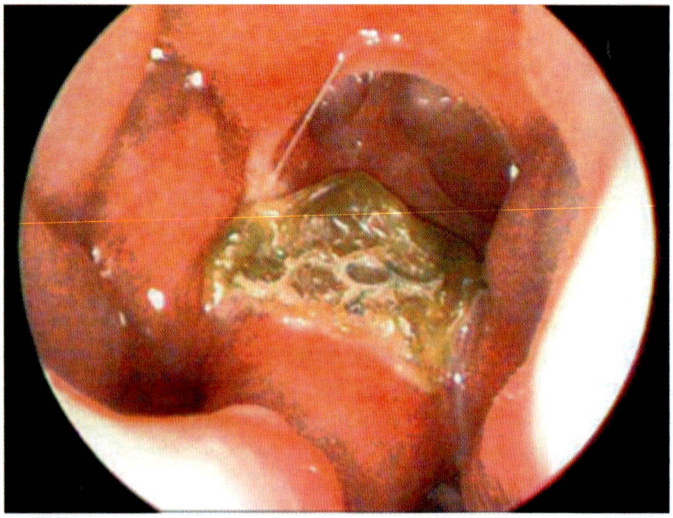

Fig. 31.4 Extrusion of a titanium plate into the sphenoid sinus after endoscopic pituitary surgery.

the skull base accounts for the major difference in the postoperative management of the two groups. Postoperative topical therapy and debridement must proceed with caution in light of the skull base reconstruction. The surgical approach, extent of surgery, complexity of skull base reconstruction, patient comorbidities, and complications guide the postoperative management strategy for these patients.

References

1. Kuhn FA, Citardi MJ. Advances in postoperative care following functional endoscopic sinus surgery. Otolaryngol Clin North Am 1997;30:479–490
2. Harvey RJ, Smith JE, Wise SK, Patel SJ, Frankel BM, Schlosser RJ. Intracranial complications before and after endoscopic skull base reconstruction. Am J Rhinol 2008;22:516–521
3. Tabaee A, Anand VK, Brown SM, Lin JW, Schwartz TH. Algorithm for reconstruction after endoscopic pituitary and skull base surgery. Laryngoscope 2007;117:1133–1137
4. Brown SM, Anand VK, Tabaee A, Schwartz TH. Role of perioperative antibiotics in endoscopic skull base surgery. Laryngoscope 2007;117:1528–1532
5. Kida Y. Gentamicin and CFTR. N Engl J Med 2003;349:2570
6. Wong KK, Marglani O, Westerberg BD, Javer AR. Systemic absorption of topical gentamicin sinus irrigation. J Otolaryngol Head Neck Surg 2008;37:395–398
7. Bugten V, Nordgård S, Steinsvåg S. The effects of debridement after endoscopic sinus surgery. Laryngoscope 2006;116:2037–2043
8. Thaler ER. Postoperative care after endoscopic sinus surgery. Arch Otolaryngol Head Neck Surg 2002;128:1204–1206
9. Rosenfeld RM, Andes D, Bhattacharyya N, et al. Clinical practice guideline: adult sinusitis. Otolaryngol Head Neck Surg 2007;137(3, Suppl):S1–S31
10. Meltzer EO, Bachert C, Staudinger H. Treating acute rhinosinusitis: comparing efficacy and safety of mometasone furoate nasal spray, amoxicillin, and placebo. J Allergy Clin Immunol 2005;116:1289–1295
11. Cincik H, Ferguson BJ. The impact of endoscopic cultures on care in rhinosinusitis. Laryngoscope 2006;116:1562–1568
12. Bhattacharyya N, Gopal HV, Lee KH. Bacterial infection after endoscopic sinus surgery: a controlled prospective study. Laryngoscope 2004;114:765–767
13. Sethi DS. Isolated sphenoid lesions: diagnosis and management. Otolaryngol Head Neck Surg 1999;120:730–736
14. Kennedy DW, Cohn ES, Papel ID, Holliday MJ. Transsphenoidal approach to the sella: the Johns Hopkins experience. Laryngoscope 1984;94:1066–1074
15. Batra PS, Citardi MJ, Lanza DC. Isolated sphenoid sinusitis after transsphenoidal hypophysectomy. Am J Rhinol 2005;19:185–189
16. Senior BA, Ebert CS, Bednarski KK, et al. Minimally invasive pituitary surgery. Laryngoscope 2008;118:1842–1855
17. Lu YJ, Chang CN, Pai PC, Wei KC, Chuang CC. Isolated sphenoid sinusitis or mucocele: a potential complication of endonasal transsphenoidal surgery. J Neurooncol 2009;91:63–67
18. Cappabianca P, Cavallo LM, Colao A, de Divitiis E. Surgical complications associated with the endoscopic endonasal transsphenoidal approach for pituitary adenomas. J Neurosurg 2002;97:293–298
19. Jho HD. Endoscopic transsphenoidal surgery. J Neurooncol 2001;54:187–195
20. Dolinskas CA, Simeone FA. Transsphenoidal hypophysectomy: postsurgical CT findings. AJR Am J Roentgenol 1985;144:487–492
21. Tazawa S. [CT after transsphenoidal surgery]. Nippon Igaku Hoshasen Gakkai Zasshi 1991;51:234–244
22. Stickney KO, Weymuller EA Jr, Mayberg M. MRI evaluation of the sphenoid sinus after transsphenoidal approach to the pituitary. Laryngoscope 1994;104(1 Pt 1):1–4
23. Anand V, Levine H, Friedman M, et al. Intravenous antibiotics for refractory rhinosinusitis in nonsurgical patients: preliminary findings of a prospective study. Am J Rhinol 2003;17:363–368
24. Lin JW, Kacker A, Anand VK, Levine H. Catheter- and antibiotic-related complications of ambulatory intravenous antibiotic therapy for chronic refractory rhinosinusitis. Am J Rhinol 2005;19:365–369
25. Leng LZ, Brown S, Anand VK, Schwartz TH. "Gasket-seal" watertight closure in minimal-access endoscopic cranial base surgery. Neurosurgery 2008;62(5, Suppl 2):E342–E343, discussion E343

32 Managing Carotid Injury During Transsphenoidal Surgery

Jared Knopman, Athos Patsalides, Y. Pierre Gobin, and Howard A. Riina

The transsphenoidal approach is a routine, widely accepted, and safe operative procedure; however, serious vascular injuries may occur during both the approach and the resection of pathology. Rates of complication are related to surgical volume, with incidences directly correlated with the surgeon's experience. Carotid injury is a rare but potentially life-threatening complication of the transsphenoidal approach. Although an uncommon occurrence, approximately 12% of pituitary surgeons have experienced this complication at some point in their practice.[1] A detailed preoperative knowledge of the sphenoid and sellar anatomy as well as the use of intraoperative neuronavigation help to prevent pitfalls during the transsphenoidal approach, yet arterial injuries can still occur, particularly in the management of complex lesions. The ability to quickly and effectively treat vascular injuries is imperative in attaining a satisfactory outcome. This requires the support of multiple medical subspecialties as well as access to available endovascular technologies. This chapter reviews the vascular anatomy of the sellar and suprasellar region and discusses the types of vascular injuries most commonly seen with the transsphenoidal approach and their immediate intraoperative and postoperative endovascular management.

Vascular Anatomy of the Pituitary Region

The cavernous segment of the carotid artery originates lateral to the posterior clinoid process, where it enters the sinus and traverses it in a forward and horizontal direction for approximately 2 cm. It then turns upward medial to the anterior clinoid process as it exits the roof of the cavernous sinus and the dural ring. It is the most medial structure within the cavernous sinus. In approximately 14% of reviewed cases, the shortest distance between the bilateral carotid arteries was within the sellar component of the cavernous-carotid artery.[2] In 4% of cases, the shortest distance was within the sphenoid component of the cavernous-carotid segment.[2]

The relationship between the sella and the cavernous segment of the carotid artery, specifically the distance separating the medial edge of the carotid artery and the lateral surface of the pituitary gland, is a crucial factor to consider during transsphenoidal surgery. In a review of cadaveric cases, the distance between the lateral aspect of the pituitary and the artery varied from 1 to 7 mm (average, 2.3 mm).[2] However, a separation between the gland and the artery is not always present, and in one fourth of reviewed cases the cavernous segment of the carotid artery protruded through the medial wall of the cavernous sinus to directly abut and indent the pituitary gland.[3,4] This results in not only herniation of the gland in a contralateral position but also conforming of the pituitary to the wall of the artery, with protrusion both above and below the vessel. The same phenomenon applies to a sellar tumor, in which the artery may become invaginated by the expanding mass, even if the tumor is small and does not invade the cavernous sinus.

Multiple arterial branches arise from the cavernous segment of the internal carotid artery. The meningohypophyseal trunk, the most proximal branch, arises lateral to the dorsum sellae just as the artery turns anterior from the foramen lacerum. The meningohypophyseal trunk gives rise to three arteries: the tentorial artery; the inferior hypophyseal artery, which supplies the pituitary capsule and anastomoses with the contralateral vessel; and the dorsal meningeal artery. The inferolateral trunk arises from the lateral side of the horizontal segment of the cavernous-carotid artery in 84% of cases but may infrequently branch from the meningohypophyseal trunk as well.[3,5]

Given the ability to extend the transsphenoidal approach across the planum sphenoidale and into the suprasellar compartments, the suprasellar relationship and morphology of the anterior circulation to a large sellar tumor are of crucial importance during preoperative planning. Numerous arteries, including the internal carotid and basilar artery, as well as the circle of Willis and its branches, may be deformed from mass effect by the expanding tumor. In 82% of cadaveric cases, the shortest distance between the bilateral internal carotid arteries was noted in the supraclinoid segment.[4] The internal carotid artery exits the cavernous sinus along the medial aspect of the anterior clinoid process as it reaches the anterior incisural space. It then proceeds posteriorly, superiorly, and laterally to its bifurcation below the anterior perforated substance. As it courses lateral to the optic nerve, creating the opticocarotid space in between, it feeds multiple small arterial branches to the optic nerve, chiasm, tract, and floor of the third ventricle. The superior hypophyseal artery, which courses medially below the floor of the third ventricle to anastomose with the contralateral vessel around the infundibulum, is a branch from the ophthalmic segment of the internal carotid artery. The next intradural branch of the internal carotid artery is the ophthalmic artery, which enters the optic canal below the optic nerve. This is followed by the posterior communicating artery, which branches from the posterior wall of the internal carotid artery and travels posteromedially below the optic tracts and floor of the third ventricle. Finally, the anterior choroidal artery originates immediately above the posterior communicating artery, also from the posterior wall of the internal carotid artery, but takes a posterolateral course below the optic tracts. The internal carotid artery ends in a bifurcation with the anterior cerebral artery coursing medially above the optic nerve and chiasm to the interhemispheric fissure, where it joins its contralateral vessel via the anterior communicating artery. The anterior cerebral artery is of particular importance when performing extended suprasellar approaches for tumors as they will likely be displaced or encased by the lesion.

Vascular Injuries to the Carotid Artery

Vascular injury during transsphenoidal surgery can occur during both the surgical approach as well as the resection of tumor. The most effective management of vascular injury is prevention through detailed preoperative and intraoperative technique. It is critical for the operative surgeon to remain in the midline during the approach and have an intimate knowledge of the relationship between the vasculature and the surrounding bony structures. Entry into the sphenoid sinus may be complicated by a carotid artery that bulges into the space or is actually exposed to the sinus without any bony protection, a phenomenon seen in 4% of specimens.[4] Preoperative magnetic resonance imaging and computed tomography angiography (CTA) are noninvasive methods to accurately assess the relationship among vascular, bony, and soft tissue structures. Vascular abnormalities on these studies can then be followed by digital subtraction angiography (DSA) for further elucidation. In addition, these imaging modalities can be coupled to intraoperative neuronavigation to ensure that a midline approach is adhered to beyond the vomer, an especially important tool in abnormal sphenoid sinus anatomy such as cases of honeycomb configuration, nonpneumatized sphenoid bone, and oblique sphenoid septum. Other predisposing surgical difficulties include cavernous sinus invasion by the tumor, previous transsphenoidal surgery, radiation therapy, and bromocriptine therapy. Patients with acromegaly may also be at higher risk for injury secondary to distortion of nasal and sinus anatomy as well as a tendency to have tortuous ectatic arteries that may protrude into the sella.[6] In addition, previous inflammatory conditions in the vicinity of the sella such as cerebrospinal fluid rhinorrhea or meningitis may weaken the carotid wall, predisposing it to iatrogenic injury.

Surgical Control of Intraoperative Hemorrhage

Despite proper preoperative planning and meticulous intraoperative technique, injuries to the vascular structures of the anterior circulation will inevitably occur, especially if one performs many surgeries for complex sellar pathology. The early recognition of such an injury as well as the coordinated and effective steps taken from that point are critical in limiting the morbidity and mortality associated with these events.

The first step is to control the hemorrhage to prevent excessive blood loss. Upon encountering the torrential arterial bleeding from inadvertent laceration or perforation, the natural first step is aspiration of blood with the appropriate-size sucker and application of a cottonoid with pressure to the site of injury. Concomitantly, the anesthesiologist should resuscitate the patient with intravenous fluids, pressors, and blood products as needed. In addition, direct manual compression on the cervical carotid artery ipsilateral to the side of injury can help to diminish the proximal pressure on the arteriotomy, potentially facilitating hemostasis. With endoscopic surgery, the endoscopic view may become obscured by blood. The use of two suctions, one in each nostril, and constant irrigation of the lens will facilitate visualization. If the endoscope is on a scope-holder, it is important to have an extra set of hands to control the scope so that it can be removed and cleaned or moved above the rising pool of blood or down toward the arteriotomy as needed.

Fukushima and Maroon[7] describe a surgical technique for intrasellar control and hemostasis of an injured carotid artery. After temporary control with the aforementioned method, they slowly replace the cottonoid with a piece of shredded Teflon, millimeter by millimeter, until an artificial wall is made over the laceration. This can be layered by taking another piece of Teflon, which has been dipped in semisolid methylmethacrylate, and applying it over the first piece. Pressure is maintained for approximately 1½ to 3 minutes while polymerization occurs. The edge of the impregnated Teflon can then be inserted under the bony ridge of the sellar floor to buttress the entire system, with the option of adding a small titanium miniplate under the bony edge for even further reinforcement. This technique retains the advantage of controlling the hemorrhage specifically at the site of injury within the sella and offering a permanent compressive construct that does not need to be removed, thereby introducing risk of rebleeding. Direct cautery of the arteriotomy can be attempted if it is small. Even in situations of successful control of hemorrhage, postoperative vascular imaging, in particular angiography, is essential to rule out vascular anomalies that may have developed regardless of the type of vascular control attained.

In situations where quick and effective immediate control of the hemorrhage cannot be obtained through direct surgical means, a Fogarty balloon catheter can be inserted through the nares into the sphenoid sinus, and inflated to tamponade the exsanguination until definitive angiographic intervention can be undertaken. In addition, this may lower the risk of "overpacking" with hemostatic material, which can be associated with carotid occlusion, carotid stenosis, and basilar artery compression.

If an extended transsphenoidal approach has been performed with a large opening into the intracranial cavity, it is sometimes prudent to obtain a computed tomography (CT) scan of the head with the patient intubated prior to proceeding to angiography, to rule out an extensive intracranial hemorrhage that may need to be addressed via a craniotomy.

Endovascular Evaluation and Treatment of Vascular Injuries

The patient can be brought intubated from the operating room directly to the angiography suite. The most commonly encountered internal carotid artery injuries after transsphenoidal surgery include thrombosis/emboli, stenosis, pseudoaneurysm formation, and cavernous-carotid fistula (CCF) (**Fig. 32.1**). Even if the immediate postoperative angiogram is normal in appearance, repeat angiography should be undertaken after nasal packing is removed and before the patient is discharged to rule out delayed formation of a vascular anomaly such as a pseudoaneurysm.

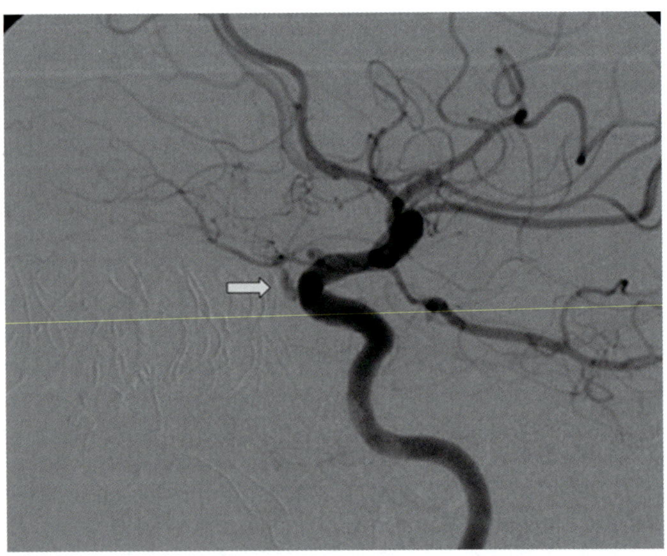

Fig. 32.1 Lateral view of a right internal carotid artery angiogram demonstrating extravasation of contrast from an iatrogenic injury to the cavernous segment of the right internal carotid artery after transsphenoidal surgery. The arrow points to the pseudoaneurysm of the cavernous carotid artery.

Carotid Occlusion, Stenosis, and Pseudoaneurysm Formation

Carotid occlusions and stenoses are most commonly the result of overpacking during initial attempts at hemostasis. However, the variable degree and reversibility of visualized occlusion and stenosis in certain cases lend evidence to the fact that temporary host reactions such as local vasospasm, hematoma formation, and dissection also play a role in certain cases of occlusion and stenosis. The danger of recanalization of these anomalies lies in the risk of subsequent distal cerebral emboli, pseudoaneurysm formation, and recurrent hemorrhagic episodes. Therefore, patients with postoperative carotid stenoses and occlusions should receive definitive endovascular treatment, occasionally with parent-vessel occlusion, to nullify the risk of delayed complications.

Pseudoaneurysms represent a dangerous and unstable vascular anomaly encountered after transsphenoidal surgery. They are most often positioned medially, and their thin walls predispose them to rapid growth and frequent rupture. In some cases, the aneurysmal "wall" may be formed only by a clot with no real arterial tissue. The most common presenting sign is epistaxis, which can be delayed. These lesions may be catheterized and embolized in selective patients; however, the risk for procedure-related rupture as well as the lack of protection afforded from incomplete embolization often mandate parent-vessel occlusion.

Endovascular Carotid Occlusion

The most commonly used and effective treatment for iatrogenic injury to the internal carotid artery after transsphenoidal surgery is endovascular carotid occlusion in the case of larger injuries that cannot be endovascularly reconstructed. The endovascular approach is simple and can be performed immediately after the diagnostic images are obtained. Controlled endovascular embolization is more reliable than direct surgical packing of the internal carotid artery and permits balloon test occlusion to minimize ischemic risks.

The patient is brought to the angiography suite and placed in a supine position on the angiography table. Both groins are prepped and draped in a sterile fashion, and the bilateral common femoral arteries are accessed with a 19-gauge needle. The needles are exchanged for arterial sheaths that are attached to a continuous heparinized saline flush. A guide catheter is advanced through each sheath over a guidewire into each internal carotid artery. Depending on the hemodynamic stability and hemorrhagic state of the patient, weight-based systemic heparin is dosed intravenously. In cases where a balloon test occlusion needs to be performed, a balloon microcatheter is then advanced over a microwire into the high cervical segment of the internal carotid artery ipsilateral to the side of injury. With the balloon inflated until occlusion of the injured vessel, biplane angiography is performed over the cranium after injection of contrast into the contralateral/normal internal carotid artery (**Fig. 32.2**).

In formal balloon test occlusion cases, neurophysiologic testing is performed on the patient at sequential time intervals and with controlled drops in mean arterial pressure to ensure adequate collateral circulation through the anterior communicating artery and the circle of Willis to the contralateral circulation. This can be performed in awake patients who have elective DSA after being stabilized in the immediate setting. However, these elective physiologic tests are more difficult to apply in the setting of life-threatening hemorrhage, where the patient is likely still intubated and under general anesthesia from the operation, and too unstable for systematic drops in blood pressure. Therefore, cerebral blood flow based on imaging during angiography is used to estimate the patient's tolerance to subsequent carotid occlusion. In patients for whom balloon test occlusion fails, either through neurophysiologic testing or cerebral blood flow imaging, surgical bypass remains a subsequent option, provided they are hemodynamically stable and the epistaxis/hemorrhage is well controlled. In addition, angiography performed through the vertebral artery can demonstrate collateral supply to the anterior circulation via retrograde flow through a patent posterior communicating artery.

When vessel occlusion is required, endovascular embolization can be performed safely and quickly with the use of detachable platinum coils. A microcatheter is navigated over a microwire into the internal carotid artery. Embolization of the vessel must occur both above and below the injury, thereby "trapping" the perforation. Distal coils are deployed just before the branch point of the ophthalmic artery. Placement adjacent to a branch vessel ensures that blood flow is not static in the vicinity of the coil mass, decreasing the chance for thrombus formation, propagation, and emboli. The microcatheter is then retracted to the petrous/cavernous segment proximal to the site of arterial injury, and the next set of coils are deployed until total occlusion is achieved (**Fig. 32.3**).

Cavernous-Carotid Fistulas

Iatrogenic CCFs rarely close spontaneously and often require invasive therapeutic intervention. Indications and timing for treatment are based on the severity of the symptoms, which can include decreasing visual acuity, external ophthalmoplegia, proptosis, hemorrhage, cortical venous drainage, intolerable bruit/headache, and ischemia related to vascular steal phenomenon. The pattern of venous drainage in the CCF typically dictates the symptom or sign seen in the patient. Venous drainage can extend anteriorly into the ophthalmic veins, inferiorly into the pterygoid venous plexus, posteriorly into the petrosal sinuses, superiorly into the cortical veins via the sphenoparietal sinus, and across the circular sinus into the contralateral cavernous sinus. Often, a mixed venous drainage pattern is seen.

As opposed to the previously mentioned arterial injuries, CCF treatment can often be performed without sacrificing the parent vessel. This represents an evolution from previous

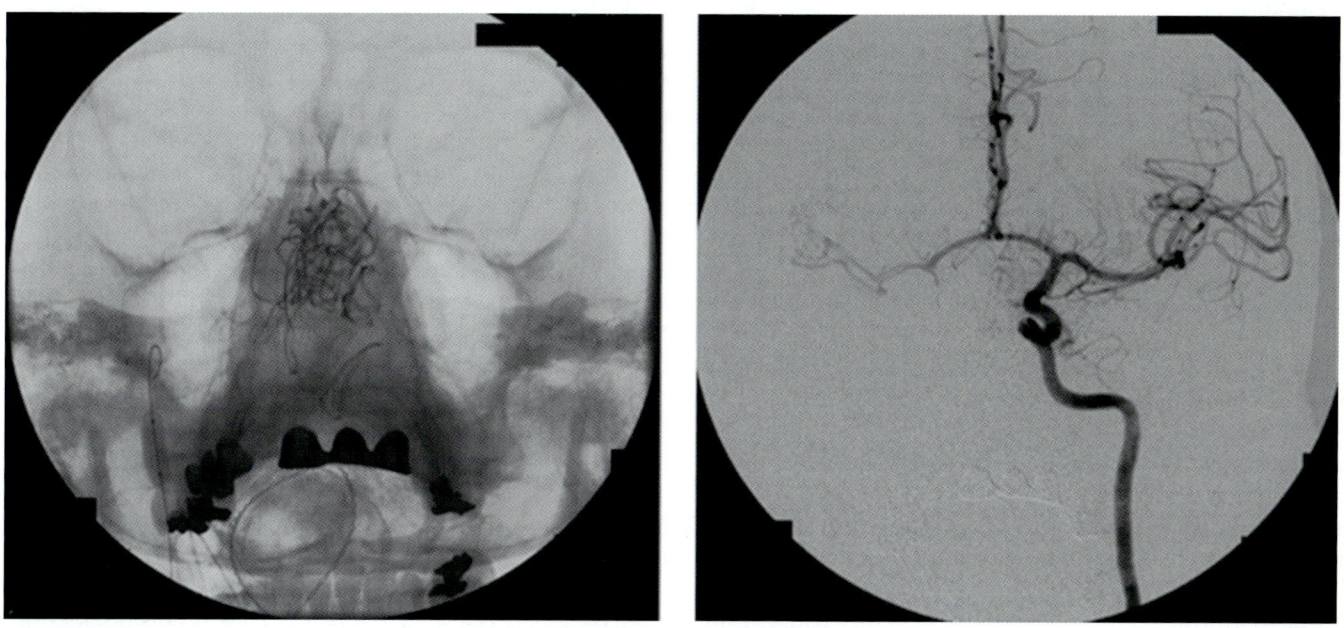

A B

Fig. 32.2 Unsubtracted **(A)** and subtracted **(B)** anteroposterior views of the left internal carotid artery angiogram with balloon inflated to occlusion within the right internal carotid artery, demonstrating brisk contralateral cross-filling through a patent anterior communicating artery to the right anterior and middle cerebral artery distributions. Note the packing within the sphenoid from the operating room.

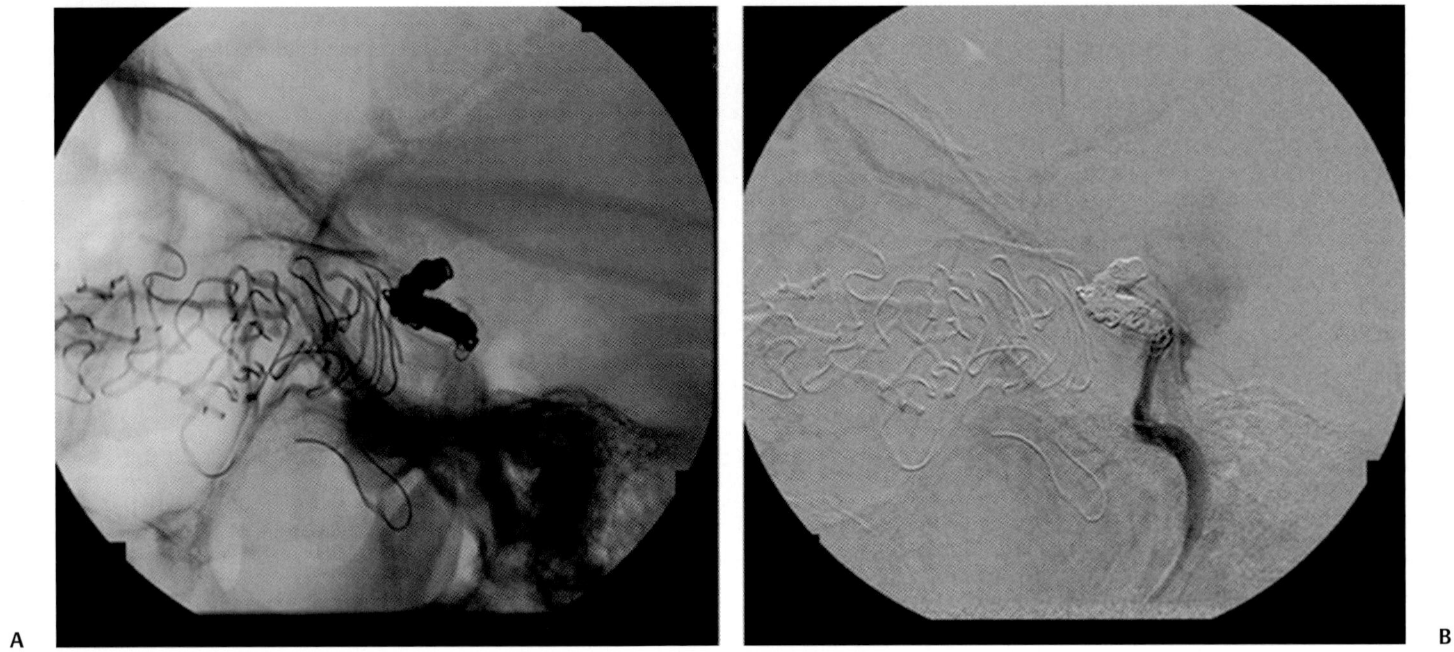

Fig. 32.3 **(A)** Unsubtracted and subtracted **(B)** lateral views of right internal carotid artery angiogram after parent-vessel coil embolization spanning from the ophthalmic segment to the petrous segment of the right internal carotid artery. Note no anterograde flow of contrast beyond the coil mass or continued extravasation. Also note the artifact produced by the cottonoids packed into the sphenoid in the operating room.

modalities of treatment, including carotid occlusion, which runs the risk of recurrence by not obliterating the fistula. This is largely secondary to advances in both imaging and device technology.

Endovascular therapy can be performed transarterially or transvenously. Specific manual maneuvers can be employed to visualize the morphology of a high-flow fistula. These include ipsilateral compression of the internal carotid artery to slow the flow during same side or contralateral injection (Allcock maneuver). The use of detachable platinum coils or liquid embolic material such as acrylic (*N*-butyl cyanoacrylate, TruFill; Codman, Boston, MA) or Onyx (ev3 Endovascular Inc., Irvine, CA) ensures precise embolization at the level of the fistulous connection. Often, the flow into a traumatic CCF is rapid and requires the initial placement of detachable coils within the fistula to slow flow to a rate that liquid embolic material can be used without anterograde migration into the venous drainage system. However, care must be taken not to decrease the pressure gradient between the carotid artery and the fistula to such a degree that forward flow embolic material will reflux into the carotid artery and embolize into the distal intracranial circulation.

In favorable venous anatomy, transvenous embolization can be performed at the cavernous fistulous connection, most commonly via the ipsilateral jugular vein and inferior petrosal sinus. Both detachable coils and liquid embolic agents have been used successfully. During transvenous approaches, it is typical to inject contrast through an arterial catheter in the ipsilateral internal carotid artery to localize the site of fistulous connection and confirm adequate closure.

A principal risk involved with the transvenous approach includes perforation of the relatively thin-walled venous structures during catheterization. Although many "arterialized" venous structures build up thicker layers in longstanding CCFs, the acute formation of a traumatic CCF after transsphenoidal surgery does not lend itself to such a morphologic change. Perforation of a vein, combined with the high flow of arterialized blood into that vein, can result in rapid and severe subarachnoid hemorrhage. Alternatively, venous thrombosis may occur during catheterization. If the cavernous fistula remains open but venous outflow is compromised, the patient may experience worsening ocular symptoms via increased drainage through the superior ophthalmic vein or intracranial hemorrhage from shunting into cortical venous structures.

In situations where the CCF cannot be precisely catheterized due to tortuosity of vasculature, or the site of fistulous connection cannot be clearly identified, endovascular closure of the parent internal carotid artery still remains a feasible option. Often, a formal balloon test occlusion does not need to be performed, as anterograde flow through the ipsilateral internal carotid artery is already diverted fully into the fistula without any distal intracranial runoff.

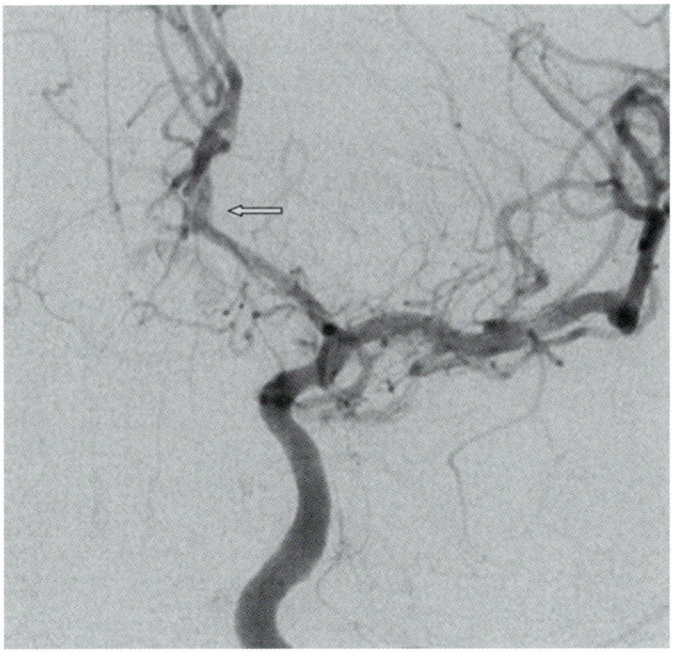

Fig. 32.4 The anteroposterior view of the left internal carotid artery angiogram demonstrating extravasation (*arrow*) of contrast from an iatrogenic injury to the proximal left anterior cerebral artery after transsphenoidal surgery. Note the superior displacement of the left anterior cerebral artery secondary to underlying hematoma formation.

Although total obliteration of a traumatic CCF may not occur during initial treatment, thereby increasing the risk for recurrence, the goal for initial management of this lesion is to alleviate clinical symptoms and stabilize the patient. Follow-up angiography and ophthalmologic examination can be performed on an elective basis from that point forward.

Management of Other Arterial Injuries

Although injury to the cavernous segment of the carotid artery accounts for the vast majority of vascular complications encountered with the transsphenoidal procedure, other arteries may be injured during the both the surgical approach and resection of a lesion. Injuries to the vasculature of the external carotid artery, most notably the sphenopalatine artery, are less frequently recognized but important causes of epistaxis that can be easily treated. The complication usually occurs during opening of the sphenoid ostium with a punch rongeur, as the artery is hidden in the inferior lateral corner of the sphenoidal sinus. Once avulsed, it can be difficult to coagulate because it has a tendency to retract toward the maxilla.[8] This may result in delayed epistaxis that can be life-threatening. Therefore, any patient who presents with epistaxis after transsphenoidal surgery must obtain bilateral external carotid artery angiograms with visualization of the internal maxillary artery to rule out pseudoaneurysm formation from the sphenopalatine artery. Often, the sphenopalatine artery can be safely embolized after knowledge of the surrounding anastomoses so as not to jeopardize flow to collateral branches to the ophthalmic artery or meningeal branches to the carotid artery supplying the trigeminal nerve.

With the application of the transsphenoidal approach to the resection of tumors that spread outside the sellar compartment, injuries to arteries within the intradural compartment may occur. A commonly displaced or encased intradural artery by suprasellar extension of a tumor is the anterior cerebral artery. Iatrogenic perforation or laceration of this artery while dissecting adherent tumor from its wall is particularly devastating, as parent-vessel occlusion will often result in an ipsilateral stroke. Another possibility is avulsion of a small perforator from the anterior cerebral or anterior communicating artery (**Fig. 32.4**). In select cases, when the laceration is small, an angled microcatheter can be advanced over a microwire distal to the site of perforation. The microwire can then be removed and the microcatheter retracted toward the arteriotomy until the tip "pops" into the perforation so it is traversing the subarachnoid space (**Fig. 32.5**). From here, liquid embolic material can be injected to form a plug outside the laceration while preserving distal flow through the anterior cerebral artery (**Fig. 32.6**). In cases of intradural injuries to the arterial circulation, standard subarachnoid hemorrhage vasospasm precautions must be

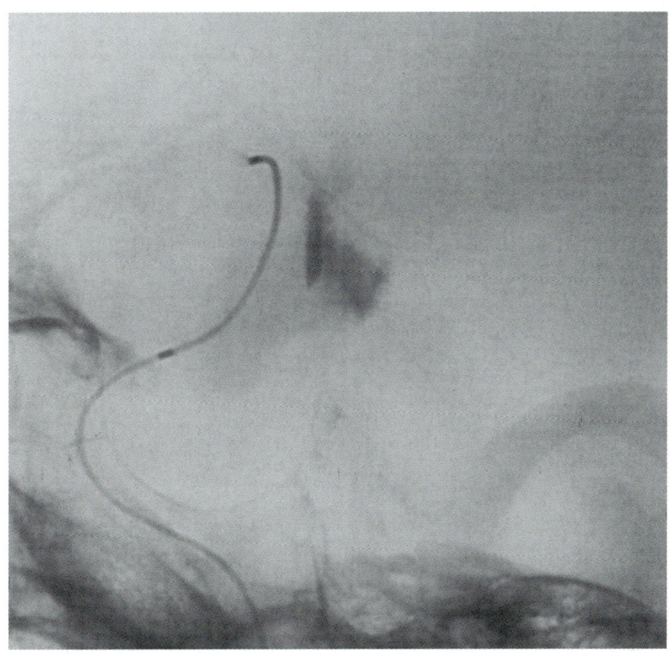

Fig. 32.5 The unsubtracted anteroposterior view of a microcatheter advanced into the left anterior cerebral artery and retracted until it "pops" through the iatrogenic arteriotomy site into the subarachnoid space.

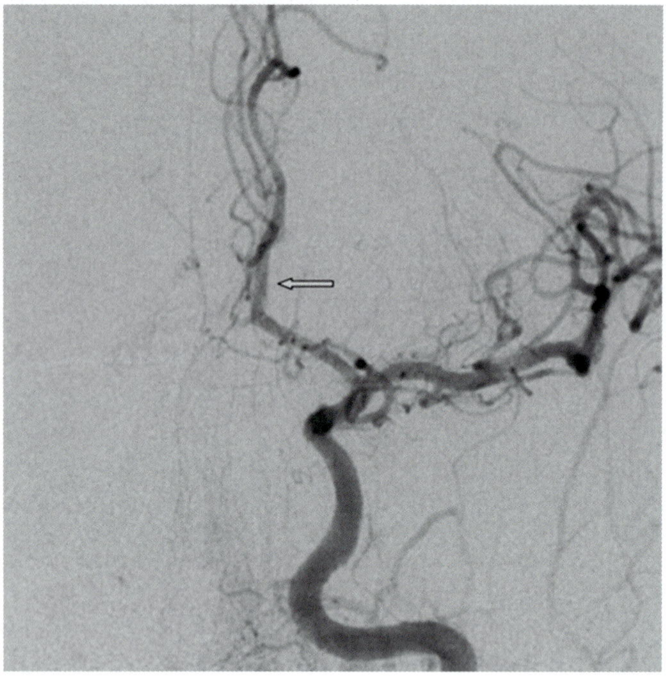

Fig. 32.6 The anteroposterior view of the left internal carotid artery angiogram after *N*-butyl cyanoacrylate glue embolization of the arteriotomy site demonstrating no further extravasation (*arrow*) of contrast and preserved flow into the distal left anterior cerebral artery.

maintained, and the patient should receive intermittent angiographic studies and hyperdynamic volume and pressor therapy in the event of symptomatic vasospasm.

Conclusion

Although the incidence of arterial injury during transsphenoidal surgery is rare, the morbidity and mortality associated with these events are high. A detailed knowledge of the preoperative anatomy of the vagaries of the vasculature and bony landmarks and the intraoperative use of neuronavigation decrease the likelihood of encountering a complication. In the event of an observed injury, immediate surgical stabilization and follow-up angiography are imperative to attaining a satisfactory outcome. With the evolution of endovascular imaging and technology, adequate tools are in place to treat the most commonly encountered arterial injuries, including carotid occlusions, stenoses, pseudoaneurysms, and fistulas. A normal postoperative angiogram mandates repeat follow-up study before discharge, as arterial injuries are often insidious and clinically occult until devastating presentation.

References

1. Ciric I, Ragin A, Baumgartner C, Pierce D. Complications of transsphenoidal surgery: results of a national survey, review of the literature, and personal experience. Neurosurgery 1997;40:225–236, discussion 236–237
2. Rhoton AL. The sellar region. In: Cranial Anatomy and Surgical Approaches. Schaumburg, IL: The Congress of Neurological Surgeons; 2003:363–402
3. Harris FS, Rhoton AL. Anatomy of the cavernous sinus. A microsurgical study. J Neurosurg 1976;45:169–180
4. Renn WH, Rhoton AL Jr. Microsurgical anatomy of the sellar region. J Neurosurg 1975;43:288–298
5. Inoue T, Rhoton AL Jr, Theele D, Barry ME. Surgical approaches to the cavernous sinus: a microsurgical study. Neurosurgery 1990;26: 903–932
6. Hardy J. Traitment chirurgical de l'adenome hypophysaire. In: Neuro-Chirurgie: Acromegalie-Gigantisme. Paris: Masson; 1973:75–99
7. Fukushima T, Maroon JC. Repair of carotid artery perforations during transsphenoidal surgery. Surg Neurol 1998;50:174–177
8. Hardy J, McCutcheon IE. Pituitary macroadenomas. In: Apuzzo MLJ, ed. Brain Surgery: Complication Avoidance and Management. New York: Churchill Livingstone; 1992:276–295

33 Managing Postoperative CSF Leak

Paul A. Gardner, Carl Snyderman, and Juan Fernandez-Miranda

Endoscopic endonasal approaches (EEAs) to the pituitary and parasellar regions have been refined and expanded over the past decade.[1–11] These approaches often create complex and high-flow cerebrospinal fluid (CSF) defects in the dura and skull base. Endoscopic reconstruction of such defects was one of the major challenges of endoscopic endonasal skull base surgery in early case series. Depending on reconstructive technique, tumor type, and surgical approach, rates of postoperative CSF leak vary from 5% to as high as 75%.[12–15] Development of vascularized reconstruction techniques such as the nasal septal mucosal flap[16,17] have lowered these rates to levels similar to those of open approaches.

Sequelae of postoperative CSF leak include meningitis, abscess, and pneumocephalus. Nonclinical sequelae include prolonged hospitalization and increased cost of care. Early repair may help to prevent these sequelae. However, it can be challenging to determine whether or not a patient is actively leaking in the postoperative period. Most postoperative CSF leaks do not become apparent until nasal packing is removed. Rarely, late CSF leaks will occur (weeks to months following surgery) as a consequence of patient activity, excessive debridement, or adjunctive therapy.

The reasons for a postoperative CSF leak are multiple and varied. The most common reasons for failure include high-flow defects, increased intracranial pressure, unsuitable reconstructive material, improper placement of a flap, inadequate recipient bed, and disruption of the repair. There are limited data regarding the optimal treatment strategy for patients with postoperative CSF leak.

Risk Factors for Postoperative CSF Leak

There are several factors that seem to contribute to higher postoperative CSF leak rates. These factors may be related to the disease (Cushing's disease leading to obesity and poor healing) anatomical site (involvement of arachnoid cisterns or ventricles), reconstructive technique, adjuvant therapies, patient comorbidities (obesity, poor nutrition), or the patient's strenuous activities.

Diseases such as Cushing's disease create a disastrous milieu for surgery. Patients are overweight, heal poorly, and are at high risk for perioperative complications such as deep venous thrombosis or cardiac ischemia. As a result, skull base defects require meticulous repair in these settings. We prefer vascularized repair such as a nasoseptal mucosal flap[16,17] even when treating small tumors because of these factors. Fat grafts are also less suitable in these patients because of the poor quality of the fat.

Suprasellar, clival, or parasellar tumors often involve the basal arachnoid cisterns. Resultant wide dissection within these cisterns creates an open space for rapid transit of CSF. This may be one reason that these tumors have a higher risk of a postoperative CSF leak.[14,15] Additionally, increased mixture of blood and CSF intraoperatively contribute to postoperative elevations of CSF pressure. Certainly, tumors such as craniopharyngiomas that extend into the third ventricle create a unique challenge for reconstruction (**Fig. 33.1**). Once again, a vascularized mucosal flap is preferred over avascular reconstructive techniques for separation of a direct communication between the ventricles and paranasal sinuses.

Although small dural defects can be reliably reconstructed using a variety of techniques and materials,[18,19] large or high-flow defects are more demanding. We have observed the greatest success with a combination of an inlay collagen graft and an onlay septal mucosal flap. Alternative vascularized reconstructions may be used when a septal flap is not available. There are many technical factors to consider in performing the reconstruction. These include preparation of the recipient bed, elevation of the flap, placement of the

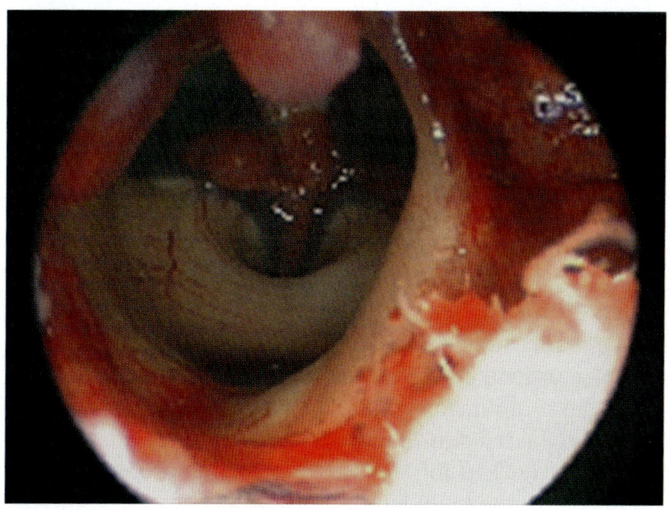

Fig. 33.1 Endoscopic view of the third ventricle following endoscopic endonasal resection of a craniopharyngioma. The resultant direct communication between the ventricular system and sinus cavity presents a unique challenge for reconstruction.

flap, protective coverings (fibrin glue, synthetic glue), and support of the flap (nasal packing, balloon catheter).

Adjuvant treatments such as chemotherapy or radiation can delay or halt postoperative healing. Occasionally, irradiation can lead to necrosis of a well-healed skull base repair. A vascularized repair should be strongly considered when the patient has received prior radiation therapy or the pathology requires postoperative irradiation. A sufficient period of time should pass following preoperative chemotherapy before performing skull base surgery to allow white cell counts to recover. Conversely, postoperative chemotherapy should not be started until healing is complete (minimum of 2 to 3 weeks).

Patient comorbidities should also be considered. Obesity is known to be a risk factor for occult hydrocephalus. It is hypothesized that increased central venous pressure secondary to high intra-abdominal pressure contributes to increased intracranial pressure. In addition, patients of any body habitus can suffer from malnutrition, leading to poor healing. If this is suspected, preoperative prealbumin levels should be checked and, if possible, optimized prior to elective skull base surgery.

Detection of Postoperative CSF Leak

As with any complication, there is no substitute for direct examination of the patient for detection. Reliable patients are able to detect constant, unusual postnasal drainage and may complain of a gagging sensation or frequent cough. It can have an oddly salty or sweet flavor for the patient. This is different from the thick and sometimes vaguely foul-smelling or foul-tasting typical postoperative drainage. Most patients with this history can be tested with direct provocation. This involves having the patient lean forward, with the head lowered, to observe nasal drainage. Unilateral drainage that is clear and watery is usually CSF, but postoperative nasal washes, vasomotor rhinitis, and the CSF/sinus reservoir effect can all provide false positives. Nasal endoscopy may provide clear documentation of a CSF leak, but many leaks are missed due to the absence of drainage with the patient upright and the difficulty of visualizing the operative site. This can often be performed in the clinic or at the bedside.

A reliable adjuvant test is β_2-transferrin (β_2T) testing. β_2T is a protein found almost exclusively in CSF.[20] Suspicious nasal drainage should be collected in an appropriate container (a red-top blood-collection tube at our institution) and checked for the presence of this protein via immunoelectrophoresis. Limitations of the test include the labor cost, delay in results, and limited availability at many hospitals. High sensitivity of the test can lead to false positives if there is retained CSF in the sinuses since the time of surgery. A more rapid test is the measurement of β-trace protein, but this test is not currently available in the United States. Radionuclide studies are not used anymore for detection of CSF leaks because more reliable tests are available. Injection of fluorescein dye into the CSF via a lumbar puncture could also provide objective evidence of a CSF leak but poses additional discomfort to the patient and is rarely necessary. There are other, secondary indicators of postoperative CSF leak. In some patients, especially in the setting of aggressive lumbar drainage, pneumocephalus can occur rather than CSF egress. If there is only a pinhole defect, even tension pneumocephalus can occur, presumably as a result of a ball-valve effect. Any patient with significant or increasing pneumocephalus requires urgent reexploration. Another sequela of CSF leak is meningitis or even abscess. Early onset of infection should raise concern for a persistent CSF fistula and lead to reexploration. However, adjuvant therapies such as lumbar drainage are probably as likely to contribute to meningitis and abscess. Infection can also be a sequela of sinusitis in the absence of a direct communication between the sinonasal tract and CSF space. Unless there is another obvious source, reexploration of the skull base repair should be considered.

Operative Reexploration

Endonasal reexploration is the definitive step for detection and treatment of postoperative CSF leak following endonasal skull base surgery (ESBS). If there is sufficient clinical evidence of a leak, the patient should be taken for reexploration in a timely fashion (<48 hours). In the setting of tension pneumocephalus, this becomes emergent.

Although a wide variety of reconstructive techniques have been used successfully following ESBS, individual success rates will vary and surgeons will have to decide what works best in their hands. As discussed previously, the type of disease, anatomical site, reconstructive technique, adjunctive therapy, and patient comorbidities affect the risk of a CSF leak. The management of a postoperative CSF leak will depend on the primary reconstructive technique as well as other risk factors. There should be a plan for repair prior to reexploration. This plan depends on the technique used for reconstruction. Sometimes the entire repair is redone, but frequently the leak is focal and the repair can be augmented without sacrificing the healing that has already taken place. Generally, if a nonvascularized repair has failed, a vascularized flap should be a part of the reexploration. If a vascularized flap has failed, the solution depends on the reason for failure.

Fluorescein is often used to identify sites of CSF leaks, either by topical application and watching for a washout effect or by intrathecal injection. Although the worldwide experience is extensive and the administration of intrathecal fluorescein is safe (risk of seizures), if proper dosing protocols

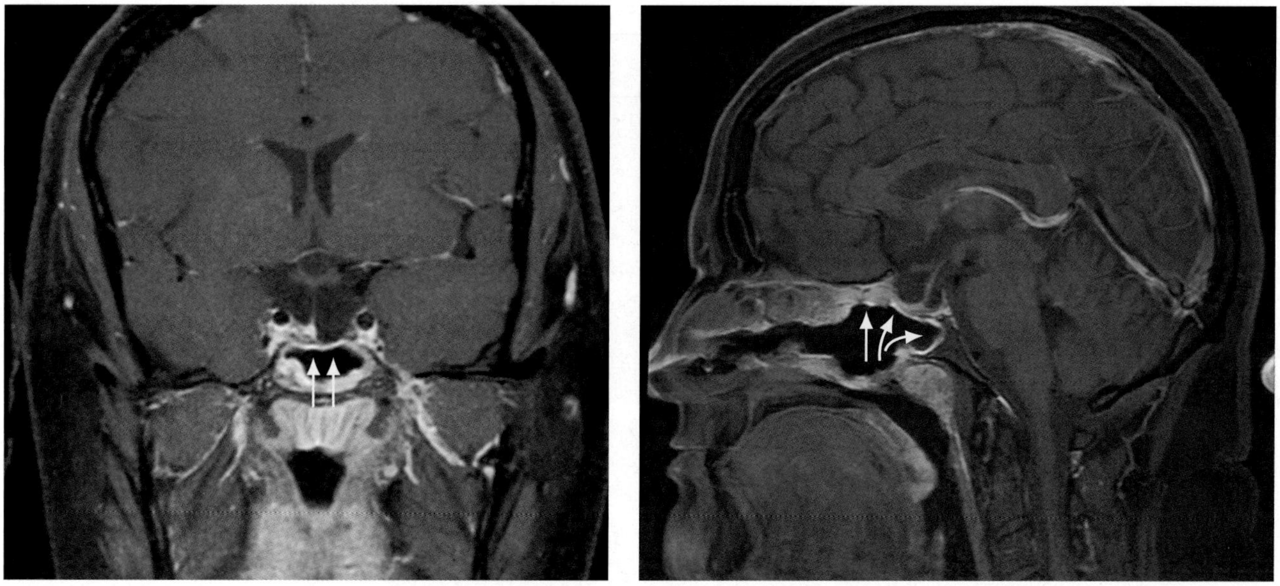

Fig. 33.2 Postoperative magnetic resonance imaging coronal **(A)** and sagittal **(B)** views showing bright enhancement of the nasal septal mucosa flap (*arrows*) used for sellar and anterior skull base reconstruction. The enhancement is indicative of a viable flap.

are followed, we do not use fluorescein at our institution. In virtually all cases, CSF leaks are readily apparent without the need for fluorescein.

Multilayer allograft and free mucosal grafts are quite effective for small leaks, especially following simple pituitary surgery. The addition of a bolster such as Merocel packing or a balloon catheter can prevent graft migration or dislodgment in the early postoperative period. The gasket-seal technique involves wedging a solid synthetic or cartilage graft in place to replace the skull as well as hold the allograft in place.[21] If one of these techniques fails, strong consideration should be given to a vascularized repair as a solution. Alternatively, the entire repair can be augmented or redone with an inlay fascial graft and onlay mucosal or fascial graft. Lumbar drainage should be strongly considered following reexploration.

Vascularized flaps, such as the nasal septal mucosal flap,[16,17] can fail for multiple reasons noted previously: high-flow defects, increased intracranial pressure, unsuitable reconstructive material, improper flap placement, inadequate recipient bed, and disruption of the repair. Flap necrosis is a rare event caused by intraoperative injury to the vascular pedicle. Postoperative magnetic resonance imaging can verify the viability of the flap; enhancement of the mucosa is noted (**Fig. 33.2**). The most common errors relate to flap placement. Care should be taken to confirm that the pedicle of the flap is not twisted and that the mucosal surface of the flap is superficial. Displacement of the flap after placement can occur when the packing is placed (**Fig. 33.3**). If the flap is too small for the defect, it needs to be supplemented with fascial grafts deep to it or onlay fat grafts. Avascular areas of reconstruction that are not covered by the flap are at increased risk for failure. If the flap is too short, tension may pull the edges away from the dural edge. The entirety of the flap pedicle should be in contact with bone; bridging of the pedicle across a sinus cavity will result in contracture and shortening of the flap. The reach of the flap can be augmented by mobilization of the flap pedicle up to the pterygopalatine space or by filling the inferior part of the defect with a fat graft so that the flap can lay flat over it.

Reexploration begins with removal of packing and gentle suctioning of overlying reconstructive materials such as tissue glue and collagen. Careful endoscopic inspection after each layer is debrided should reveal the site of leak. If the leak is not immediately obvious, the entire edge of the graft/flap is sequentially inspected. Valsalva maneuvers to increase intracranial pressure can assist in this process. Rarely, a defect occurs in the center of the flap due to pressure from a bolster or as a result of a septal spur during harvest. Some surgeons use fluorescein routinely to assist in this process.[22] We have not found this to be necessary for detecting postoperative leak. If no leak is identified in the setting of a suspected leak, repeat packing is carefully performed, often with fat to provide a biologic dressing.

Once the site of leak is identified, as previously stated, the repair depends on the type of reconstruction technique used. Typically, the entire repair does not fail; rather, a small leak develops at one of the edges. Small fistulas in an allograft repair can be carefully repacked. However, if a nonvascularized repair has multiple areas or a large area of failed healing, a vascularized rescue should be considered. If the pedicle for the nasal septal flap is still intact, it can be harvested and provides a confident solution in the setting of prior failure. If it is not available, other vascularized options

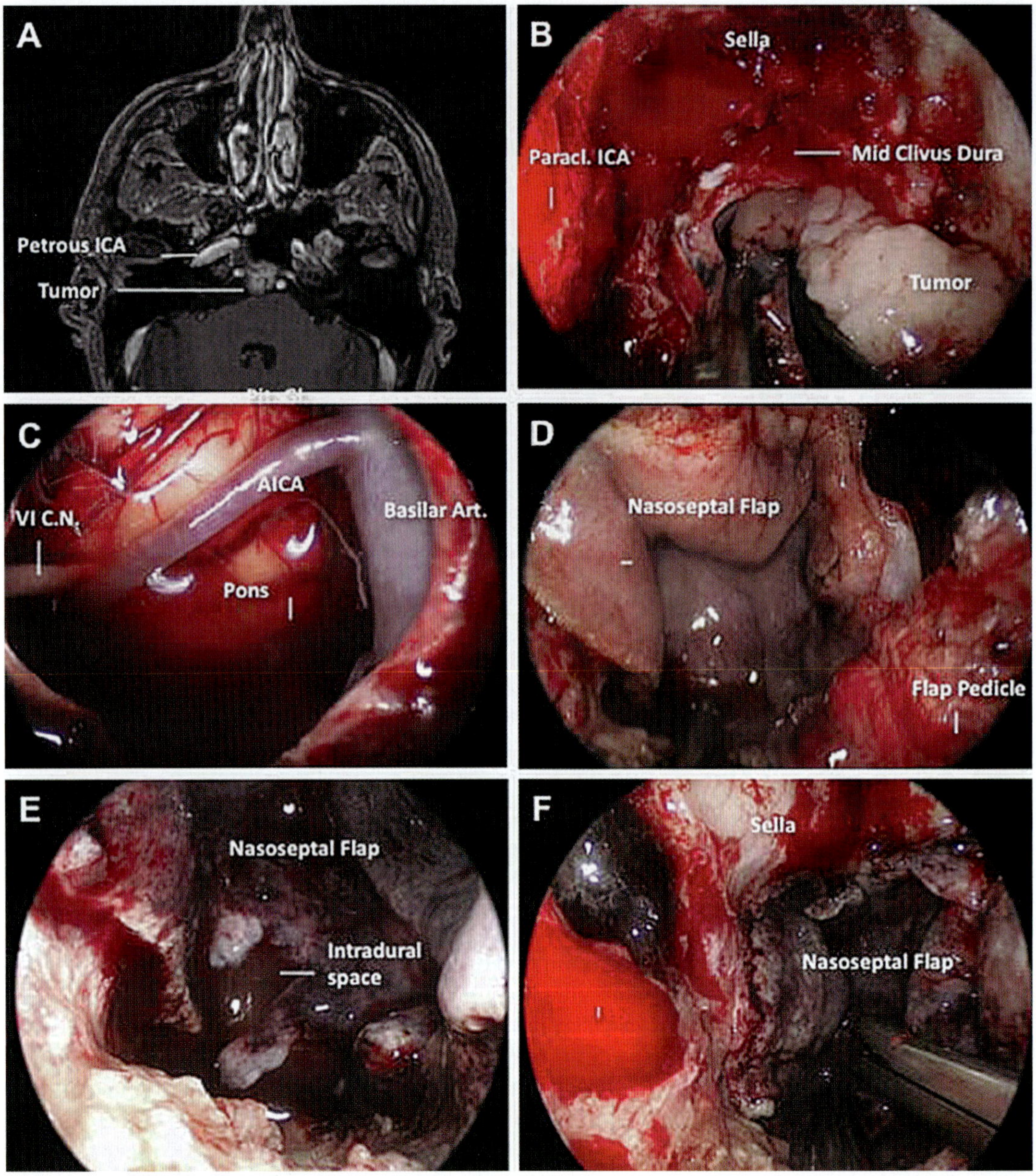

Fig. 33.3 Intraoperative endoscopic view of a displaced nasal septal mucosal flap. **(A)** Preoperative MRI showing a small clival chordoma with dural involvement. **(B)** Intraoperative view during tumor resection. **(C)** Endoscopic view showing the resultant dural defect after tumor and dural resection. **(D)** Endoscopic endonasal view of the nasal septal mucosal flap following initial placement. **(E)** Endoscopic view during reexploration for CSF leak. The inferior edge of the flap clearly does not cover the caudal defect as a result of manipulation during placement of packing or postoperative shift (unusual). **(F)** Endoscopic view showing repositioning of the flap. The patient healed successfully following this reoperation. AICA, anterior inferior cerebellar artery; Art., artery; ICA, internal carotid artery; Paracl., paraclival; VI C.N., cranial nerve VI.

include the middle turbinate flap,[23] inferior turbinate flap,[24] and pericranial flap.[25] If the patient was reconstructed with a vascular flap, the edge of the flap is elevated at the site of the leak and, if it cannot be well positioned, an inlay collagen or AlloDerm (LifeCell, Branchburg, NJ) graft is placed. If the flap cannot be repositioned to cover the defect, fat grafts are placed along the edge and packing is placed. If the flap is malpositioned, it is completely elevated and repositioned.

Role of Lumbar Drainage

Lumbar drainage is commonly used as an adjunct to nonvascularized repairs following extended transsphenoidal surgery as well as initial treatment for a postoperative CSF leak. However, there are no stringent studies that examine the efficacy of lumbar drainage in these settings. Lumbar drainage may allow very small fistulas to heal. However, significant defects that result in postoperative CSF leak are unlikely to respond to lumbar drainage alone, and pneumocephalus can be worsened by CSF diversion. Lumbar drainage also increases the risk of intracranial bacterial infection by reversing the flow of a CSF leak and through contamination of the lumbar catheter. As a result, we prefer to reexplore endonasal skull base defects primarily rather than trialing lumbar drainage. We attribute a low risk of postoperative bacterial intracranial infection following ESBS (1.8%) to multiple factors including early intervention rather than a "wait-and-see" approach.[26]

Conclusion

Postoperative CSF leak rates following endoscopic endonasal skull base surgery have declined dramatically with the introduction of the nasoseptal mucosal flap and other vascularized reconstruction techniques. The management of postoperative CSF leaks requires an understanding of risk factors and reasons for failure of reconstructive techniques. Early detection and reexploration help to minimize the development of infectious complications. Lumbar drainage may be beneficial in the setting of high-flow leaks, but its role has not been well defined by carefully conducted studies.

References

1. Kassam AB, Snyderman CH, Gardner P, Carrau RL, Spiro R. The expanded endonasal approach: a fully endoscopic transnasal approach and resection of the odontoid process: technical case report. Neurosurgery 2005;57(1, Suppl):E213, discussion E213
2. Cavallo LM, Messina A, Cappabianca P, et al. Endoscopic endonasal surgery of the midline skull base: anatomical study and clinical considerations. Neurosurg Focus 2005;19:E2
3. Kassam AB, Snyderman CH, Mintz A, Gardner P, Carrau RL. Expanded endonasal approach: the rostrocaudal axis. Part I. Crista galli to the sella turcica. Neurosurg Focus 2005;19:E3
4. Kassam AB, Snyderman CH, Mintz A, Gardner P, Carrau RL. Expanded endonasal approach: the rostrocaudal axis. Part II. Posterior clinoids to the foramen magnum. Neurosurg Focus 2005;19:E4
5. Kassam AB, Prevedello DM, Thomas A, et al. Endoscopic endonasal pituitary transposition for a transdorsum sellae approach to the interpeduncular cistern. Neurosurgery 2008;62(3, Suppl 1):57–72, discussion 72–74
6. Kassam AB, Gardner PA, Snyderman CH, Carrau RL, Mintz AH, Prevedello DM. Expanded endonasal approach, a fully endoscopic transnasal approach for the resection of midline suprasellar craniopharyngiomas: a new classification based on the infundibulum. J Neurosurg 2008;108:715–728
7. Hofstetter CP, Singh A, Anand VK, Kacker A, Schwartz TH. The endoscopic, endonasal, transmaxillary transpterygoid approach to the pterygopalatine fossa, infratemporal fossa, petrous apex, and the Meckel cave. J Neurosurg 2010;113:967–974
8. Laufer I, Anand VK, Schwartz TH. Endoscopic, endonasal extended transsphenoidal, transplanum transtuberculum approach for resection of suprasellar lesions. J Neurosurg 2007;106:400–406
9. Stammberger H, Anderhuber W, Walch C, Papaefthymiou G. Possibilities and limitations of endoscopic management of nasal and paranasal sinus malignancies. Acta Otorhinolaryngol Belg 1999;53:199–205
10. Cappabianca P, Cavallo LM, Esposito F, De Divitiis O, Messina A, De Divitiis E. Extended endoscopic endonasal approach to the midline skull base: the evolving role of transsphenoidal surgery. Adv Tech Stand Neurosurg 2008;33:151–199
11. de Divitiis E, Cappabianca P, Cavallo LM, Esposito F, de Divitiis O, Messina A. Extended endoscopic transsphenoidal approach for extrasellar craniopharyngiomas. Neurosurgery 2007;61(5, Suppl 2):219–227, discussion 228
12. Stippler M, Gardner PA, Snyderman CH, Carrau RL, Prevedello DM, Kassam AB. Endoscopic endonasal approach for clival chordomas. Neurosurgery 2009;64:268–277, discussion 277–278
13. Greenfield JP, Anand VK, Kacker A, et al. Endoscopic endonasal transethmoidal transcribriform transfovea ethmoidalis approach to the anterior cranial fossa and skull base. Neurosurgery 2010;66:883–892, discussion 892
14. Gardner PA, Kassam AB, Snyderman CH, et al. Outcomes following endoscopic, expanded endonasal resection of suprasellar craniopharyngiomas: a case series. J Neurosurg 2008;109:6–16
15. Gardner PA, Kassam AB, Thomas A, et al. Endoscopic endonasal resection of anterior cranial base meningiomas. Neurosurgery 2008;63:36–52, discussion 52–54
16. Hadad G, Bassagasteguy L, Carrau RL, et al. A novel reconstructive technique after endoscopic expanded endonasal approaches: vascular pedicle nasoseptal flap. Laryngoscope 2006;116:1882–1886
17. Kassam AB, Thomas A, Carrau RL, et al. Endoscopic reconstruction of the cranial base using a pedicled nasoseptal flap. Neurosurgery 2008;63(1, Suppl 1):ONS44–ONS52, discussion ONS52–ONS53
18. Hegazy HM, Carrau RL, Snyderman CH, Kassam A, Zweig J. Transnasal endoscopic repair of cerebrospinal fluid rhinorrhea: a meta-analysis. Laryngoscope 2000;110:1166–1172
19. Zweig JL, Carrau RL, Celin SE, et al. Endoscopic repair of cerebrospinal fluid leaks to the sinonasal tract: predictors of success. Otolaryngol Head Neck Surg 2000;123:195–201
20. Bachmann-Harildstad G. Diagnostic values of beta-2 transferrin and beta-trace protein as markers for cerebrospinal fluid fistula. Rhinology 2008;46:82–85
21. Leng LZ, Brown S, Anand VK, Schwartz TH. "Gasket-seal" watertight closure in minimal-access endoscopic cranial base surgery. Neurosurgery 2008;62(5, Suppl 2):E342–E343, discussion E343
22. Tabaee A, Placantonakis DG, Schwartz TH, Anand VK. Intrathecal fluorescein in endoscopic skull base surgery. Otolaryngol Head Neck Surg 2007;137:316–320
23. Prevedello DM, Barges-Coll J, Fernandez-Miranda JC, et al. Middle turbinate flap for skull base reconstruction: cadaveric feasibility study. Laryngoscope 2009;119:2094–2098
24. Fortes FS, Carrau RL, Snyderman CH, et al. The posterior pedicle inferior turbinate flap: a new vascularized flap for skull base reconstruction. Laryngoscope 2007;117:1329–1332
25. Zanation AM, Snyderman CH, Carrau RL, Kassam AB, Gardner PA, Prevedello DM. Minimally invasive endoscopic pericranial flap: a new method for endonasal skull base reconstruction. Laryngoscope 2009;119:13–18
26. Kono Y, Prevedello DM, Snyderman CH, et al. One thousand endoscopic skull base surgical procedures demystifying the infection potential: incidence and description of postoperative meningitis and brain abscesses. Infect Control Hosp Epidemiol 2011;32:77–83

34 Postoperative and Neurocritical Care Management of Patients after Endonasal Endoscopic Transsphenoidal Pituitary Surgery

Jeffrey P. Greenfield and Theodore H. Schwartz

As the number of transsphenoidal surgeries being performed for an ever-widening array of skull base lesions increases, the recognition and management of the potential postoperative complications these procedures carry with them are of fundamental importance for the neurosurgeons performing the surgeries. Perhaps equally important is the relevance to an ever-widening array of clinicians involved in the postoperative management of these patients. Lesions approached endoscopically through the sphenoid sinus represent a diverse spectrum of disease. Although pituitary tumors remain the lesions most regularly approached endoscopically, experienced surgeons now use the endonasal endoscopic approach to resect meningiomas, chordomas, and craniopharyngiomas and to repair traumatic and spontaneous cerebrospinal fluid (CSF) leaks. In addition, intracranial disease being approached transsphenoidally need not arise from the sella turcica; lesions located anteriorly along the planum sphenoidale, the infundibulum proper, and as inferior as the clivus are now routinely biopsied and resected using these approaches.

This diversity of pathology and location presents serious challenges, as neural structures including the optic nerves and chiasm and pituitary stalk and gland, and their variable blood supplies, are often intimately related to the lesions being resected. Even when these structures remain intact at the conclusion of the procedure, gentle traction, suction, irrigation, or tamponade upon these structures can produce transient effects in the tissue that may affect the patient's postoperative homeostasis. The care of these patients requires vigilance extending beyond assessment of perturbations of the hypothalamic-pituitary axis and visual pathways as postoperative complications that include CSF leak and secondary meningitis or pneumocephaly are significant concerns.

The incidence and complications associated with transsphenoidal surgeries have been studied.[1,2] In a survey-based report,[2] 958 respondent neurosurgeons reported performing transsphenoidal surgery. As one might expect, the incidence of complications was statistically significantly higher among surgeons with less experience performing transsphenoidal surgery. The overall operative mortality rate was 0.9%. The most frequent complications were anterior pituitary insufficiency (19.4%) and diabetes insipidus (DI) (17.8%). The incidence of CSF fistula was 3.9%. Other significant complications, such as carotid artery injuries, hypothalamic injuries, loss of vision, and meningitis, occurred with incidence rates between 1 and 2%.

In this chapter we review the immediate and extended postoperative management of patients undergoing endonasal, endoscopic, transsphenoidal neurosurgical procedures. We focus on the early recognition and appropriate management of fluid balance disorders, endocrine disturbances, CSF fistulas, and other emergent situations one might encounter in the recovery room or intensive care unit postoperatively.

Disorders of Fluid Balance

Understanding the normal metabolism of water and sodium is at the core of managing the patient who has had surgery that transiently or permanently disrupts the hypothalamic-pituitary axis. We explain the pathophysiology of the pathways governing this homeostasis and then examine how perturbations of various aspects of those pathways lead to specific deficits and how best to recognize, diagnose, and definitively treat those deficits.

Pathophysiology of Water and Sodium Metabolism

Total body water content approximates 60% of the body weight of a healthy adult male. Two thirds of total body water is intracellular fluid (ICF) and one third is extracellular fluid (ECF). Of the ECF, 75% is in the interstitial space and the remainder is contained within the vasculature. An average adult with normal kidney function requires 400 to 500 mL of water to excrete a normal 24-hour solute load in maximally concentrated urine. The major intracellular cation is potassium (K^+) at 140 mEq/L. The extracellular concentrations are very tightly regulated at much lower concentrations, 3.5 to 5.0 mEq/L. The major extracellular cation is sodium (Na^+), which has an average serum concentration of 140 mEq/L and an intracellular concentration of 12 mEq/L. Water movement between compartments is controlled by the osmolality of the compartments. The ECF and ICF are both roughly 290 mOsm/kg water. Water movement is secondary to changes in cation concentration, which are regulated by the energy-dependent Na^+/K^+–adenosine triphosphatase (ATPase) responsible for moving Na^+ out of cells in exchange for K^+.

Body fluid osmolality can be precisely determined by this formula: plasma osmolality (mOsm/kg) = $2(Na^+_{plasma})$ + (glucose/18) + (blood urea nitrogen [BUN]/2.8). Na^+ is by far the major determinant of plasma osmolality, and doubling the plasma Na^+ level to get a rough estimate often suffices in emergency situations where quickly raising the plasma osmolality to 300 mOsm/kg to combat intracranial swelling is the major concern. Tight glycemic control must be maintained postoperatively, as hyperglycemia can raise plasma osmolality. Without insulin, glucose remains extracellular, drawing water into the ECF and diluting the serum Na^+ by as much as 1.5 to 2.4 mEq/L for every 100-mg/dL increment in the plasma glucose level above normal.[3]

Thirst mechanisms, antidiuretic hormone (ADH) secretion, and kidney function all regulate a patient's water volume.[4] Receptors in the anterolateral hypothalamus are stimulated by elevations in plasma osmolality and then release ADH from the posterior pituitary. Circulating ADH increases the absorption of water by making the distal nephron permeable to water. The pathways leading to thirst and ADH release are exquisitely sensitive, triggered by as little as a 2% increase in ECF osmolality.

Sodium also regulates total body volume by regulating ECF. When *total* Na^+ in the ECF is low, the ECF volume is low by definition. This is sensed by pressure-dependent receptors in the cardiac atria, resulting in renal sodium retention. Conversely, the carotid sinus and renal juxtaglomerular apparatus respond to high volume secondary to high sodium by increasing natriuresis to adjust volume.

Hyperosmolality and Hypernatremia

After endoscopic endonasal transsphenoidal surgery, the evaluation of a single elevated serum sodium value should focus on the possible presence of DI. Postoperative hypernatremia is due to the loss of body water in excess of body solutes,[5] because of either insufficient water intake or excessive water excretion. The clinical ECF volume status of a patient is crucial to assess. It can be measured by comparing preoperative and current weight, central venous pressure (CVP) if available through a central venous catheter, or strictly measured intakes and outputs. Postoperative laboratory values to assess include plasma electrolytes, glucose, BUN, creatinine, urine electrolytes and osmolality, and urine glucose. As mentioned previously, the marked elevation of plasma glucose, such as occurs in nonketotic hyperglycemic hyperosmolar coma, can result in an elevated plasma osmolality with a normal volume status.

When a postoperative patient is determined to be hyperosmolar by the above criteria, an assessment of the patient's ability to concentrate urine provides useful direction for their care. Disorders of hyperosmolality can be subdivided into those in which renal water conservation mechanisms are intact but are unable to compensate for inadequately replaced losses of hypotonic fluid and those in which renal concentrating defects are a contributing factor to the deficiency of body water. If the urine is appropriately concentrated (>800 mOsm/kg water), the possibility of primary renal cause is eliminated. An inappropriately low urine osmolality (<800 mOsm/kg water) in a hyperosmolar patient indicates that the kidney is unable to concentrate the urine. In the absence of glucosuria or other causes of osmotic diuresis, inadequately concentrated urine in a hyperosmolar patient indicates DI. In the postoperative patient population, this algorithm is often unnecessary to scrutinize due to the knowledge of both normal preoperative fluid homeostasis and intraoperative pituitary stalk manipulation. Nevertheless, if these straightforward values are assessed in all postoperative endoscopic patients, their fluid management will be less complicated and their return to fluid homeostasis, either naturally or pharmacologically, will be expedited.

Diabetes Insipidus and Pathophysiology of Arginine Vasopressin

Hypotonic polyuria due to inadequate arginine vasopressin (AVP) secretion is the definition of DI. Broadly speaking, DI is a syndrome that can be classified as central (acquired or congenital lesion of the hypothalamic-pituitary axis) due to surgery, trauma, infarction, thrombosis, or granulomatous disease, or as nephrogenic (most commonly congenital due to defects in the AVP V^2 receptor or aquaporin-2 water channel). In the postoperative patient, disordered AVP secretion due to manipulation or transection of the pituitary stalk is the etiology unless proven otherwise. L-Arginine vasopressin (AVP, ADH) is synthesized in the bodies of magnocellular neurons in the paired supraoptic nuclei and paraventricular nuclei and is transported in granules down the pituitary stalk to be stored in the posterior pituitary axons terminals. Stores are sufficient for 5 to 10 days of maximum antidiuresis or 1 month of normal antidiuresis. AVP binds to V_2 receptors in the kidney and stimulates the production of cyclic adenosine monophosphate (cAMP), which leads to synthesis of aquaporin-2 water channels in cells of the collecting tubules. AVP secretion maintains plasma osmolality tightly at 280 to 290 mOsm/kg.[6,7]

The presence of DI preoperatively from a pituitary tumor is fairly unusual because AVP synthesis occurs in the hypothalamus. A lesion to the pituitary gland redirects the AVP into the bloodstream closer to its site of synthesis intracranially, rather than in the sella. If DI is present preoperatively, alternative diagnoses should be considered, including craniopharyngioma, meningioma, or disease directly involving the hypothalamus.

A central etiology for DI can be proven in the postoperative hypernatremic patient by evaluating the response to the administration of AVP or the AVP V^2 receptor agonist, desmopressin (deamino-8-D-arginine vasopressin [DDAVP]). An increase in urine osmolality with a concomitant decrease in plasma sodium values after DDAVP administration indicates insufficient endogenous AVP secretion and a central cause for the DI. No response to DDAVP suggests renal resistance to AVP and a nephrogenic cause for the DI. When treating postoperative DI, the premise is to first correct any preexisting water deficits and then to reduce any ongoing urinary water losses. Awake and ambulatory patients with an intact thirst mechanism will have little body water deficit but may still benefit from pharmacologic control of polyuria and polydipsia, especially at night. Hospitalized patients with various degrees of disruption of mental status or thirst mechanisms may have more dangerous hyperosmolality. To establish a patient's water deficit, the following formula is used: water deficit = 0.6 × preoperative weight × $(1-140/[Na^+])$. The osmolality should be corrected over 24 to 48 hours to avoid causing cerebral edema.[7] The fluid can be replaced orally as water or through intravenously administered dextrose 5% in water (D_5W).

Multiple options exist for replacing insufficient AVP in the postoperative patient. Arginine vasopressin (pitressin) is a synthetic form of a naturally occurring human AVP. It has a relatively short half-life and can cause acute increases in blood pressure when administered intravenously. It may have limited usefulness in the immediate management of postoperative DI, but it is not optimal for longer DI management because it requires frequent dosing. A better option is DDAVP. It has a longer half-life and lacks the pressor effects of pitressin.[8,9] It is available as an intranasal form, an oral form, and a parenteral form that can be administered intravenously, intramuscularly, or subcutaneously. The dosage is usually started at 1 to 2 µg subcutaneously or intravenously, urine output should be reduced promptly, and the duration is usually 6 to 12 hours. This patient population also usually receives stress-dose glucocorticoids postoperatively,[10] which sometimes cause acute hyperglycemia and resultant polyuria. This confounding variable should be quickly controlled with appropriate doses of insulin before further treatment is initiated for DI. Postoperative diuresis from excess fluid administration is also a consideration in a polyuric patient. Normal postoperative diuresis is monitored by following serial serum sodium levels. In a patient with stable serum sodium levels, polyuria is managed by gradually weaning the intravenous fluids and continuing to monitor serum sodium levels and urine outputs.

Once DI is definitively diagnosed, antidiuretic management must be initiated. Neurosurgeons performing traditional craniotomies to access sellar or suprasellar lesions may be more reluctant to initiate antidiuresis for fear of worsening cerebral edema caused by retraction during the procedure; by accessing the region through the sphenoid sinus, this fear is allayed. Once therapy has been initiated, the serum sodium level should be measured every 6 hours for the first 24 hours, every 8 hours for the next 24 hours, and every 12 hours thereafter until consecutive measurements indicate the level has stabilized without manipulation of antidiuresis medications. It is preferable to allow a slight return of polyuria when first administering the antidiuresis medication to avoid overtreating transient DI. Overtreatment of transient DI is a major source of preventable postoperative hyponatremia leading to increased length of hospital stay. Urine osmolality and specific gravity are also monitored, often more frequently than serum sodium due to ease of measurement, but every 4 to 6 hours is sufficient.

The well-described "triple-phase" or triphasic pattern of postoperative DI is suggestive of complete stalk transection.[11] In brief, initial DI, which may last hours to days, occurs because of damage to axons and neurons, which release AVP. Once the neurons begin to degenerate, the second phase occurs of uncontrolled AVP release into the bloodstream that causes rapid reversal of fluid homeostasis. This reversal is characterized by sudden hyponatremia on postoperative day 3 or later. The antidiuresis lasts until the supply of endogenous AVP is exhausted and the initial DI reappears in the third phase. To complicate the evaluation further, transient hyponatremia identical to the second phase of the triphasic response can occur in the absence of preceding DI due to damage severe enough to cause uncontrolled release of AVP but not severe enough to impair the secretion initially.[12] In general, DI is not an infrequent postoperative sequela of intranasal endoscopic transsphenoidal surgery, but its acute and measured management should result in a rapid return to fluid homeostasis.

Hypo-osmolality and Hyponatremia

Hypo-osmolality is due to an excess of water relative to solute in the ECF. The evaluation of this clinical entity in a patient who has undergone endonasal endoscopic transsphenoidal surgery is similar to that for hypernatremia: electrolytes, glucose, BUN and creatinine, urine electrolytes, and osmolality. Pseudohyponatremia secondary to elevated plasma lipids or glucose is the only circumstance in which hyponatremia and hypo-osmolality are not synonymous.

In all other cases, once the initial laboratory values are obtained, management of the hyponatremia is based on the ECF volume status of the patient.[13]

Hyponatremia can be present in hypovolemic, euvolemic, or hypervolemic states.[14] Hypovolemic hyponatremia is characterized by deficiencies in both water and sodium; however, proportionally more sodium than water has been lost. Significant ECF fluid losses result in the release of ADH, causing water retention by the kidneys and maintenance or worsening of the hyponatremia.[15] Euvolemic hyponatremia results when total body water is increased and there is no significant change in total body sodium content. Dilutional hyponatremia may result from excessive water intake without sodium retention in the presence of renal failure or, more importantly, nonosmotic ADH secretion as can occur in the postoperative patient.[16] Hyponatremia has been reported in up to 4.5% of all postoperative patients as a result of the combination of non-osmotic ADH release and excessive administration of hypotonic fluids after surgery.[17] Hypervolemic hyponatremia is characterized by an increase in both total body sodium and total body water. This condition is usually associated with heart failure or hepatic cirrhosis and rarely occurs in postoperative neurosurgery patients except in those with preexisting conditions in addition to their neurosurgical lesions.

Syndrome of Inappropriate Antidiuretic Hormone Secretion and Cerebral Salt Wasting

The syndrome of inappropriate antidiuretic hormone secretion (SIADH) is the most common cause of euvolemic hypo-osmolality. SIADH is defined by having true ECF hypo-osmolality and a urine osmolality that is greater than 100 mOsm/Kg H_2O, both occurring at euvolemia. SIADH cannot be diagnosed in a patient who is hypovolemic or edematous. It should be pointed out that AVP secretion might be suppressed in some patients, thereby causing the urine to be dilute even with low plasma osmolality. This situation is sometimes referred to as a "reset osmostat."

The entity referred to as cerebral salt wasting (CSW) often causes considerable confusion in relation to the postoperative neurosurgical patient. CSW in this context is simply the renal loss of sodium after intracranial surgery leading to hyponatremia and a decreased ECF, that is, hypovolemic hyponatremia. SIADH and CSW were treated as a single entity until it became evident that although patients with CSW may have satisfied the initial criteria for SIADH, they were hypovolemic and had normal ADH secretion. In CSW, volume depletion triggers an appropriate ADH release, thereby causing relative water retention and worsening of the salt deficit, compounding the hyponatremia.[18]

Cerebral salt wasting is hypothesized to be due to several mechanisms. One possibility is that modulation of atrial natriuretic peptide or brain natriuretic peptide release from the hypothalamus due to direct injury from surgery causes renal salt wasting and diuresis. Alternatively, a direct neural effect secondary to sympathetic hyperactivity may lead to a cascade of effects including decreased plasma volume and natriuresis due to increased glomerular blood flow and decreased renin release.[19]

The most important factor for differentiating CSW from SIADH is volume status. Patients with CSW lose weight, whereas patients with SIADH gain weight. Patients with CSW have a negative water balance, low CVP, and increased urine sodium; they often have an elevated serum potassium level, a result not seen in SIADH. The first step in the management of CSW is to treat the underlying problem first if it is easily reversible (meningitis, hydrocephalus, pneumocephaly) and then initiate volume replacement with intravenous isotonic saline with the aim of keeping a positive fluid balance. Colloids are useful to increase CVP and draw fluid from the interstitial space. If the hyponatremia does not begin to resolve, oral salt tablets or hypertonic saline may be used to ensure a positive sodium balance. Finally, fludrocortisone, a mineralocorticoid, may be used to enhance sodium reabsorption by directly acting on the tubule, although patients treated with this medication must be monitored for the development of hypokalemia, fluid overload, and hypertension.

Clinical Symptoms of Hyponatremia and Postoperative Management

The osmotic gradient created by plasma hypo-osmolality causes an influx of water from the cerebral vasculature into brain parenchyma, which produces a spectrum of neurologic disorders ranging from mild headache to life-threatening seizures and coma at extremely low levels; patients often do not complain of any symptoms at levels above 125 mEq/L. Perhaps as important as the actual level of plasma osmolality is the time course over which it falls. The rapidity with which the hyponatremia occurs correlates well with the severity of symptoms. Over prolonged periods, the brain can compensate by extruding solutes into the ECF, resulting in patients who are largely asymptomatic despite dangerously low sodium levels in the outpatient setting.

The first step in the management of hyponatremia is the correction of hypovolemia using an isotonic solution of 0.9% NaCl (i.e., normal saline) at the appropriate rate for the patient's depletion. If the patient is not volume depleted but has evidence of primary adrenal insufficiency, has recently used diuretics, or has a markedly decreased urine sodium level, a trial of isotonic saline is also warranted. If SIADH truly is present, all excess NaCl presumably will be excreted and the plasma sodium level will respond to intravenously administered solute. In fact, over a long period of time, this therapy will begin to fail, as water retention will gradually cause the plasma sodium level to drift lower.

Patients who meet all the criteria for SIADH but are still not maximally concentrating their urine (i.e., a low urine osmolality) should simply be observed for a short period of time, as they may be manifesting a very transient SIADH. If there is any concern about adrenal function, glucocorticoid replacement should be initiated or restarted.[19,20] A common oversight is that hypocortisolism can directly cause elevated plasma AVP and has direct renal effects as well, which preclude optimal urinary dilution. It is good practice, therefore, to check adrenal function in postoperative neurosurgical patients for whom the diagnosis of SAIDH is being weighed.[21] The usual mechanism is a rapid adrenocorticotropic hormone (ACTH) stimulation test. Diuresis in response to glucocorticoids is diagnostic for glucocorticoid deficiency-induced hyponatremia. If there is any component of hypervolemia, the patient should be treated by diuresis. If these measures all fail, limited degrees of sodium and free water restriction help to reduce body fluid retention.

The correction of mild hyponatremia has more nuances when compared with life-threatening severe hyponatremia. The risk of the neurologic consequences of hyponatremia must be balanced with the risk of demyelinating the pons as occurs with a too-rapid correction, termed central pontine myelinolysis. Again, the duration over which the symptoms develop is of importance, as the patients at greatest risk from rapid correction are those whose hyponatremia manifested after a very slow decline in the serum sodium level. Alternatively stated, patients who have had rapid postoperative development of hyponatremia require correction more quickly to safe levels, and they are less likely to develop sequelae from this intervention than are those with chronic hyponatremia who are resuscitated overly aggressively. For the intermediate patients who have developed hypo-osmolality over days rather than hours or weeks, the hyponatremia should be corrected very carefully in the range of 0.5 mEq/L/h to 1 to 2 mEq/L/h not to exceed 12 to 18 mEq over the first 24 to 48 hours. Patients with neurologic demise should be more aggressively managed than asymptomatic patients, for whom patience should be rigorously practiced. The plasma sodium levels of these patients will not be raised without infusions of a hypertonic saline of 3% NaCl. A useful rule of thumb for choosing replacement fluid rate is to multiply the patient's weight in kilograms by the desired *rate* of increase to obtain the hourly fluid rate for 3% hypertonic saline. For example, a 50-kg woman will need 25 mL/h of 3% saline to increase serum sodium from 118 to 130 over 24 hours (0.5 mEq/L/h multiplied by 50 kg equals 12 mEq), or 50 mL/h to accomplish an emergent correction from 112 to 124 over 12 hours. The goal should be return to a safe level not necessarily to a normal one. Chronic postsurgical SIADH of the very mild to moderate variety can be treated with fluid restriction or pharmacologically with demeclocycline to decrease urine concentration.

Disturbances of the Hypothalamic-Pituitary-Adrenal Axis

Management of the hypothalamic-pituitary-adrenal (HPA) axis in the postoperative neurosurgical patient varies among neurosurgeons.[22] There is no debate that when a patient manifests any degree of cortisol deficiency preoperatively, stress–dose glucocorticoids must be administered in the preoperative and postoperative settings. At our institution we routinely administer 10 mg of dexamethasone at the time of surgery and two 2-mg oral doses postoperatively before either stopping steroid replacement or resuming preoperative replacement schedules if patients required steroids preoperatively. Other surgeons prefer to administer 50 to 100 mg of hydrocortisone at the time of induction and then several doses postoperatively, followed by a taper to the preoperative regimen. In those patients without laboratory evidence of cortisol deficiency, we administer two postoperative doses of dexamethasone followed by a fasting morning cortisol level on the second postoperative day to assess the integrity of the HPA axis. The assumption is that any manipulation of the pituitary gland can potentiate the transient release of ACTH, even in the absence of gross transection of the pituitary stalk. Withholding postoperative steroids is a legitimate practice as long as serial serum cortisol levels are assessed serially and all clinicians providing the patient's care can quickly identify the symptoms of cortisol deficiency, including, most importantly, hypotension, but also nausea, malaise, hyponatremia, and difficulties with thermoregulation, and can rapidly institute replacement therapy. If there is any question of cortisol deficiency postoperatively, replacement therapy should be instituted. The patient may be weaned if necessary as an outpatient either by the neurosurgeon or, preferably, by an endocrinologist.

In a patient with the preoperative diagnosis of Cushing's disease, the postoperative assessment will establish whether the cortisol level has normalized.[23] Perioperative glucocorticoids are not routinely administered to these patients due to their hypercortisolemic state, but cortisol levels are assessed rigorously at least every 6 hours for the first 24 hours. If any of the signs or symptoms of low cortisol begin to manifest in a postoperative patient with Cushing's disease, in conjunction with a suboptimal cortisol level, then replacement is begun with the assumption that there will be a surgical cure of the hypersecreting tumor. In patients with Cushing's disease, results are often achieved rapidly, as the adenoma creates a chronic suppression of the normal feedback pathways. This prevents the release of corticotropin-releasing factor from the hypothalamus, and as a result there is a very rapid fall of endogenous cortisol secretion once the tumor is excised.

Transsphenoidal surgery for acromegaly creates a similar set of postoperative issues. Growth hormone (GH) levels should be assessed on postoperative days 1 and 2 and should improve significantly when compared with preoperative GH levels. A surgically induced cure generally refers to a random GH level of less than 2.5 μg/L 6 weeks after surgery and normal response to oral glucose tolerance test. With respect to general postoperative management issues in patients with acromegaly, there is a theoretical concern of upper airway obstruction postoperatively in this population due to hypertrophied soft tissue and macroglossia. However, airway management is no different than that for any other postsurgical patient and is managed expectantly with a nasal trumpet if necessary once the anesthesiologist is comfortable that extubation criteria have been satisfied. The pituitary-thyroid axis is also examined postoperatively, and in general preoperative replacement is simply continued in the postoperative period until follow-up testing can be performed at the endocrinologist's discretion. Intraoperative sectioning of the hypophysis dictates postoperative pan replacement of normal pituitary hormones including thyroxine.

Cerebrospinal Fluid Drainage, Fistula Formation, and Meningitis Risk

The transsphenoidal approach to lesions within the sella or parasellar regions poses unique challenges to surgeons with respect to obtaining watertight closures of the CSF space and preventing CSF leaks and meningitis. Synthetic graft, allograft, and autograft, often in combination and in conjunction with dural sealants, are used within the defect with the hope of creating a sterile and leak-proof closure of the operative region when CSF has been encountered intraoperatively.

We rarely use intraoperative lumbar drainage, but we routinely perform a preoperative lumbar puncture to infuse fluorescein into the lumbar cistern for easier visualization of the CSF. Postoperative drainage with a lumbar drain is used only if persistent CSF leak is identified at the conclusion of the surgery. Rarely, in a patient with a difficult body habitus, if we feel there is a high possibility of leak due to the size of defect, concerns with the closure, or a history of recurrent CSF leak, a postoperative drain may be placed while the patient is still under anesthesia to facilitate postoperative management and avoid having to place a drain at the bedside. Despite the creative approaches neurosurgeons have devised to counteract this problem, CSF leak remains a significant hindrance for endoscopic neurosurgeons.

Inspection for CSF leak should be part of the routine evaluation of every patient having surgery through the sphenoid sinus, both in the recovery room and in the days after surgery. Although the discharge of clear fluid from the nose should be easily identifiable as a CSF fistula, the signs are often more subtle. All patients should be asked about the presence of a salty taste in their throats and any sensation of a continuous drip either in their sinuses or at the back of the throat. Leaning the patient's torso and head forward should make a subtle leak more obvious. In addition, the situation can be clarified further by asking the patient to perform a gentle Valsalva maneuver. The patients may also complain of positional headaches from the loss of CSF and experience relief when in a reclined position. If there is enough drainage to collect in a tube, the use of biochemical markers such as β-transferrin, prostaglandin-D synthase, and transthyretin to differentiate CSF from other nasal discharge is warranted. In our experience, CSF fistulas postoperatively are almost always diagnosed without waiting for the laboratory results.

Once a leak has been identified, a nonenhanced computed tomography (CT) scan of the head is necessary to evaluate the possible presence of clinically significant pneumocephaly. This scan is useful both as a baseline and as a way of gauging the immediacy with which intervention in required. Some surgeons prefer immediate reexploration for the benefit of immediate repair and reduced hospital stay, whereas others believe that lumbar drainage is a less invasive approach that allows the majority of leaks to heal. At our institution, we prefer a trial of lumbar drainage before reexploration under general anesthesia. If there is any concern during the initial surgery of a high risk of CSF leak, a lumbar drain is placed at that time. When drains are placed postoperatively, repeat CT scans and frequent neurologic assessments are essential to monitor for pneumocephaly, as continuous CSF drainage from the lumbar cistern can create a pressure gradient that encourages the entrainment of air through the fistula.

Prolonged CSF leak puts patients at risk for developing bacterial meningitis in addition to entraining air intracranially. A large retrospective evaluation of the risk of meningitis with or without lumbar drainage concluded that postoperative external lumbar drainage reduces the risk for meningitis.[24] In this study, all patients with intraoperative CSF leak had postoperative drains placed for 5 days, and the incidence of postoperative meningitis was compared with that in a previously studied series of 228 consecutive patients who underwent transsphenoidal operations without placement of lumbar drains in cases with intraoperative CSF leak. Postoperative meningitis occurred in 0.7% of the operations with drainage compared with 3.1% of the operations without drainage. Similar to the use of CSF drainage, the role of prophylactic antibiotic treatment in transsphenoidal surgery and specifically in patients with CSF rhinorrhea after transsphenoidal surgery remains to be established. We use a prophylactic third-generation cephalosporin during these surgeries as we do for routine craniotomies, typically for 24 hours. The use of broad-spectrum "triple antibiotics" to cover gram-negative and anaerobic organisms is not supported by current evidence-based studies. Patients with lumbar CSF diversion are typically maintained on the cephalosporin for the duration of their drainage.

Other Emergent Postoperative Complications

Injury to the carotid artery is a rare complication but carries with it the potential serious consequences of exsanguination and stroke.[25] If the carotid artery is injured during endonasal, endoscopic transsphenoidal surgery, surgical closure of the defect is highly unlikely. However, with the newer endoscopic bipolar forceps, attempts at primary control have a higher likelihood of success and should be made if possible. If direct control of bleeding cannot be achieved, bleeding must be controlled with pressure through intranasal packing or balloon tamponade with a Fogarty catheter. The hemodynamically stable patient should be brought immediately to the angiography suite for carotid artery evaluation. The sequelae of carotid artery injury may include thrombosis of the vessel and vascular injury to the brain, dissection, or pseudoaneurysm formation, all of which should be treated endovascularly if possible.

All postoperative neurologic deficits must be managed in an equally emergent fashion. New vision loss, a major visual field deficit not present preoperatively, cranial neuropathy, and any unexpected alteration in mental status should be assessed with emergent CT. Overexuberant packing with autologous fat may compress neuronal structures and must be removed if identified on CT. Epistaxis, although of concern for hemorrhage from the operative bed, usually resolves spontaneously; uncontrolled bleeding is usually due to injury of the sphenopalatine artery that may need to be controlled with embolization. Compression of the visual apparatus from hemorrhage or excessive packing/repair needs to be reversed via endoscopic exploration if new postoperative deficit is present. Deficits that are not identified in the recovery room and that develop subacutely may best be evaluated with magnetic resonance imaging to visualize the sella and surrounding structures in detail and in multiple dimensions.

Conclusion

The simplicity and elegance of the transsphenoidal approach to sellar and parasellar pathology must be tempered by vigilance about the abundance of pitfalls that exist when operating in such a constrained space near vital neuroanatomy. Disorders of water balance and anterior pituitary endocrinopathies are by far the most common perioperative events, and their management is the backbone of the perioperative care of patients undergoing endonasal, endoscopic transsphenoidal neurosurgery. Awareness of the basic physiology regulating water balance is crucial both to recognizing potentially dangerous trends and, equally importantly, to not overreacting to normal physiologic homeostasis. Early recognition and constant attention to the details of these patients' disorders usually reveal transient self-limiting events, and an excellent working partnership with the endocrine service makes their management less complicated. Once patients have passed through the acute postoperative period, many of the issues they face can be more smoothly managed on an outpatient basis, including follow-up endocrine testing with an endocrinologist and formal visual field testing with an ophthalmologist. Although the cooperation of physicians from different fields facilitates the long-term care of these patients, it remains the responsibility of the neurosurgeon to understand the pathophysiology and management of the major perioperative complications that can occur in this patient population.

References

1. Black PM, Zervas NT, Candia GL. Incidence and management of complications of transsphenoidal operation for pituitary adenomas. Neurosurgery 1987;20:920–924
2. Ciric I, Ragin A, Baumgartner C, Pierce D. Complications of transsphenoidal surgery: results of a national survey, review of the literature, and personal experience. Neurosurgery 1997;40:225–236, discussion 236–237
3. Katz MA. Hyperglycemia-induced hyponatremia—calculation of expected serum sodium depression. N Engl J Med 1973;289: 843–844
4. Johnson AK, Buggy J. Periventricular preoptic-hypothalamus is vital for thirst and normal water economy. Am J Physiol 1978;234: R122–R129
5. Fujiwara TM, Morgan K, Bichet DG. Molecular biology of diabetes insipidus. Annu Rev Med 1995;46:331–343
6. Robinson AG. Disorders of antidiuretic hormone secretion. Clin Endocrinol Metab 1985;14:55–88
7. Gullans SR, Verbalis JG. Control of brain volume during hyperosmolar and hypoosmolar conditions. Annu Rev Med 1993;44:289–301
8. Seckl JR, Dunger DB, Bevan JS, et al. Vasopressin antagonist in early postoperative diabetes insipidus. Lancet 1990;335:1353–1356
9. Verbalis JG. Management of disorders of water metabolism in patients with pituitary tumors. Pituitary 2002;5:119–132
10. Hout WM, Arafah BM, Salazar R, Selman W. Evaluation of the hypothalamic-pituitary-adrenal axis immediately after pituitary adenomectomy: is perioperative steroid therapy necessary? J Clin Endocrinol Metab 1988;66:1208–1212
11. Dumont AS, Nemergut EC II, Jane JA Jr, Laws ER Jr. Postoperative care following pituitary surgery. J Intensive Care Med 2005;20: 127–140
12. Olson BR, Rubino D, Gumowski J, Oldfield EH. Isolated hyponatremia after transsphenoidal pituitary surgery. J Clin Endocrinol Metab 1995;80:85–91
13. Hensen J, Henig A, Fahlbusch R, Meyer M, Boehnert M, Buchfelder M. Prevalence, predictors and patterns of postoperative polyuria and hyponatraemia in the immediate course after transsphenoidal surgery for pituitary adenomas. Clin Endocrinol (Oxf) 1999;50: 431–439
14. Adrogué HJ, Madias NE. Hyponatremia. N Engl J Med 2000;342: 1581–1589
15. Rabinstein AA, Wijdicks EFM. Hyponatremia in critically ill neurological patients. Neurologist 2003;9:290–300

16. Chung HM, Kluge R, Schrier RW, Anderson RJ. Clinical assessment of extracellular fluid volume in hyponatremia. Am J Med 1987;83:905–908
17. Cusick JF, Hagen TC, Findling JW. Inappropriate secretion of antidiuretic hormone after transsphenoidal surgery for pituitary tumors. N Engl J Med 1984;311:36–38
18. Harrigan MR. Cerebral salt wasting syndrome. Crit Care Clin 2001;17:125–138
19. Carroll PB, McHenry L, Verbalis JG. Isolated adrenocorticotrophic hormone deficiency presenting as chronic hyponatremia. N Y State J Med 1990;90:210–213
20. Fichman MP, Michelakis AM, Horton R. Regulation of aldosterone in the syndrome of inappropriate antidiuretic hormone secretion (SIADH). J Clin Endocrinol Metab 1974;39:136–144
21. Simmons NE, Alden TD, Thorner MO, Laws ER Jr. Serum cortisol response to transsphenoidal surgery for Cushing disease. J Neurosurg 2001;95:1–8
22. Singer PA, Sevilla LJ. Postoperative endocrine management of pituitary tumors. Neurosurg Clin N Am 2003;14:123–138
23. Trainer PJ, Lawrie HS, Verhelst J, et al. Transsphenoidal resection in Cushing's disease: undetectable serum cortisol as the definition of successful treatment. Clin Endocrinol (Oxf) 1993;38:73–78
24. van Aken MO, de Marie S, van der Lely AJ, et al. Risk factors for meningitis after transsphenoidal surgery. Clin Infect Dis 1997;25: 852–856
25. Laws ER Jr. Vascular complications of transsphenoidal surgery. Pituitary 1999;2:163–170

Index

Information in figures and tables is indicated by f and t.

A

B

C

D

E

F

G

H

I

K

L

M

N

O

P

Q

R

S

T

U

V

W

X